T0381477

NCLEX-RN® EXCEL

Ruth A. Wittmann-Price, PhD, RN, CNS, CNE, CHSE, ANEF, FAAN, is the dean of the School of Health Sciences at Francis Marion University, Florence, South Carolina. Dr. Wittman-Price has been an obstetrical/women's health nurse for 38 years. She received her BSN degree from Felician College in Lodi, New Jersey (1981), and her MS as a perinatal clinical nurse specialist (CNS) from Columbia University, New York, New York (1983). Dr. Wittmann-Price completed her PhD in nursing at Widener University, Chester, Pennsylvania (2006), and was awarded the Dean's Award for Excellence. She developed a mid-range nursing theory, Emancipated Decision-Making in Women's Health Care, and has tested her theory in four research studies. International researchers are currently using her theory as the foundation for further studies. Her theory is being used at the University of Limpopo, South Africa, in their campaign, "Finding Solutions for Africa," which helps women and children. Dr. Wittmann-Price was also the appointed research coordinator for Hahnemann University Hospital, Philadelphia, Pennsylvania, and oversaw the evidence-based practice projects for nursing (2007–2010). Hahnemann University Hospital was granted initial Magnet® designation in December of 2009. Dr. Wittmann-Price has taught all levels of nursing students over the past 20 years and has completed an international service-learning trip. She mentors doctor of nursing practice and doctor of philosophy students and is on several committees for both Drexel and Widener Universities. Dr. Wittmann-Price has authored 14 books, two book chapters, and more than 20 articles. She has presented her research regionally, nationally, and internationally. Dr. Wittmann-Price was inducted into the National League for Nursing (NLN) Academy of Nurse Educator Fellows in 2013 and named a fellow of the American Academy of Nursing in October 2015.

Brenda Reap Thompson, MSN, RN, CNE, is an adjunct faculty member at Drexel University, College of Nursing and Health Professions, Philadelphia, Pennsylvania. She received a BSN degree from Gwynedd Mercy University, Gwynedd Valley, Pennsylvania (1982), and an MSN degree (Adult Health and Education) from Villanova University, Villanova, Pennsylvania (1992). In 1990, she was the recipient of the Professional Nurse Traineeship Award at Villanova. Her clinical experience in nursing is in the areas of critical care and emergency health care and she has served as a director of cardiac rehabilitation. She has taught all levels of nursing throughout the past 15 years. Her expertise is in test development and she has had the opportunity to contribute to the development and review of test questions for the National Council Licensure Examination (NCLEX) under the direction of the National Council of State Boards of Nursing. Ms. Thompson was also a clinical safety coordinator in risk management and is an advocate for patient safety and quality improvement. She is a member of the American Society for Professionals in Patient Safety (ASPPS). She is the coeditor and author of *Nursing Concept Care Maps for Safe Patient Care* (2013); she has contributed five book chapters and two refereed abstracts, the latter on the use of standardized patients and the human simulation experience for undergraduate students. She has presented nationally and internationally on test development and construction and the human simulation experience. She is a member of the American Nurses Association, National League for Nursing, and president of the Nu Eta Chapter of Sigma Theta Tau International.

Frances H. Cornelius, PhD, MSN, RN-BC, CNE, is a clinical professor and department chair for advanced role master of science in nursing and complementary and integrative health programs at Drexel University in Philadelphia. She is a board-certified nurse educator and has taught at the college and university level since 1990. She has an extensive clinical background in medical–surgical, psychiatric, oncology, and community health nursing. In addition, Dr. Cornelius has substantial experience in the design, development, and delivery of online, hybrid, and traditional course content as well as the integration of learning technologies into the classroom. Her area of research involves student learning, development of clinical decision-making skills, and clinical competency using handheld mobile devices.

In 2010, Dr. Cornelius was the recipient of the Outstanding Educator in Online Learning Award from Drexel University Online. She is currently a master reviewer for Quality Matters™, a faculty-centered peer-review process that is designed to certify the quality of online and blended courses. She is a National League for Nursing (NLN) Certified Nurse Informaticist and a National Library of Medicine Medical Informatics fellow. Dr. Cornelius is the coeditor of *PDA Connections: Mobile Technology for Health Care Professionals* (2007), an innovative textbook designed to teach health care professionals how to use mobile devices for "point-of-care" access of information. She is the coeditor and author of *Ethical Health Informatics: Challenges and Opportunities* (2016). She is also a coauthor of an innovative series of six National Council Licensure Examination (NCLEX) review books, published by Springer Publishing Company, designed to support development of critical thinking among nursing students using unfolding case studies infused with mobile decision support resources to replicate realistic clinical experiences.

NCLEX-RN® EXCEL

Test Success Through Unfolding Case Study Review

Second Edition

Ruth A. Wittmann-Price, PhD, RN, CNS, CNE, CHSE, ANEF, FAAN

Brenda Reap Thompson, MSN, RN, CNE

Frances H. Cornelius, PhD, MSN, RN-BC, CNE

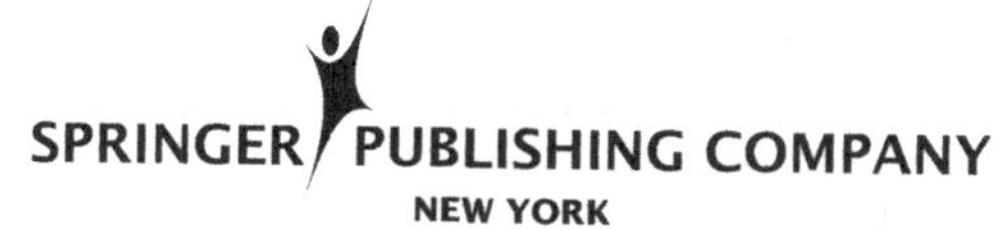

Springer Publishing Company, LLC
11 West 42nd Street
New York, NY 10036
www.springerpub.com

Acquisitions Editor: Elizabeth Nieginski
Composition: Newgen KnowledgeWorks

ISBN: 978-0-8261-2833-1
e-book ISBN: 978-0-8261-2834-8

16 17 18 19/ 5 4 3 2 1

The author and the publisher of this Work have made every effort to use sources believed to be reliable to provide information that is accurate and compatible with the standards generally accepted at the time of publication. Because medical science is continually advancing, our knowledge base continues to expand. Therefore, as new information becomes available, changes in procedures become necessary. We recommend that the reader always consult current research and specific institutional policies before performing any clinical procedure. The author and publisher shall not be liable for any special, consequential, or exemplary damages resulting, in whole or in part, from the readers' use of, or reliance on, the information contained in this book. The publisher has no responsibility for the persistence or accuracy of URLs for external or third-party Internet websites referred to in this publication and does not guarantee that any content on such websites is, or will remain, accurate or appropriate.

Library of Congress Cataloging-in-Publication Data
Names: Wittmann-Price, Ruth A., editor. | Thompson, Brenda Reap., editor. | Cornelius, Frances H., editor. | Preceded by (work): Wittmann-Price, Ruth A. NCLEX-RN excel.
Title: NCLEX-RN excel: test success through unfolding case study review/[edited by] Ruth A. Wittmann-Price, Brenda Reap Thompson, Frances H. Cornelius.
Description: Second edition. | New York, NY: Springer Publishing Company, LLC, [2017] | Preceded by NCLEX-RN excel/ Ruth A. Wittmann-Price, Brenda Reap Thompson. 2010. | Includes bibliographical references and index.
Identifiers: LCCN 2016039691 | ISBN 9780826128331 (paper back) | ISBN 9780826128348 (e-book)
Subjects: | MESH: Nursing Care—methods | Nursing Process | Specialties, Nursing—methods | Examination Questions
Classification: LCC RT51 | NLM WY 18.2 | DDC 610.73—dc23
LC record available at https://lccn.loc.gov/2016039691

Printed in the United States of America by Bradford & Bigelow.

Contents

Contributors

Frances H. Cornelius, PhD, MSN, RN-BC, CNE
Clinical Professor and Department Chair
Advanced Role MSN and Complementary and Integrative Health Programs
Drexel University
Philadelphia, Pennsylvania

Mary Foster Cox, PhD, CPNP-PC
Clinical Assistant Professor
Department of Nursing
University of South Carolina
Columbia, South Carolina

Brian J. Fasolka, PhD, RN, CEN
Assistant Clinical Professor
College of Nursing and Health Professions
Drexel University
Philadelphia, Pennsylvania

Tracy P. George, DNP, APRN-BC, CNE
Assistant Professor
Francis Marion University
Florence, South Carolina

Karen K. Gittings, DNP, RN, CNE
Associate Dean of Health Sciences Chair, Nursing Program
Director of MSN Nurse Educator Track
Associate Professor of Nursing
Francis Marion University
Florence, South Carolina

Maryann Godshall, PhD, CCRN, CPN, CNE
Assistant Clinical Professor
College of Nursing and Health Professions
Drexel University
Philadelphia, Pennsylvania

Mary Gallagher Gordon, PhD, MSN, RN, CNE
Clinical Associate Professor
Assistant Dean, Student and Technology Operations
College of Nursing and Health Professions
Drexel University
Philadelphia, Pennsylvania

Karyn E. Holt, PhD, CNM, NCC
Associate Clinical Professor
Division of Graduate Nursing Advanced Role MSN Department
College of Nursing and Health Professions
Drexel University
Philadelphia, Pennsylvania

Deborah L. Hopla, DNP, APRN-BC
Assistant Professor
Director, MSN/FNP Program
Francis Marion University
Florence, South Carolina

Cheryl Portwood, MSN, RN, NEA-BC, CNE
Assistant Clinical Professor
College of Nursing and Health Professions
Drexel University
Philadelphia, Pennsylvania

Roseann V. Regan, PhD, APRN, BC
Assistant Professor
Gwynedd Mercy University
Gwynedd Valley, Pennsylvania

Nina Russell, DNP, FNP-C, APRN
Nursing Instructor
Francis Marion University
Florence, South Carolina

Brenda Reap Thompson, MSN, RN, CNE
Adjunct Faculty
RN-BSN Degree Completion Program College of Nursing and Health Professions
Drexel University
Philadelphia, Pennsylvania

Roberta Waite, EdD, PMHCNS-BC, FAAN, ANEF
Professor and Assistant Dean
Academic Integration and Evaluation of Community Programs, Doctoral Nursing Department
College of Nursing and Health Professions
Drexel University
Philadelphia, Pennsylvania

Ruth A. Wittmann-Price, PhD, RN, CNS, CNE, CHSE, ANEF, FAAN
Dean
School of Health Sciences
Francis Marion University
Florence, South Carolina

Reviewer

Amanda Myrhen, RN, MSN
Instructor
Francis Marion University
Florence, South Carolina

Foreword

The most important test that any nurse will ever take is the National Council Licensure Examination-RN (NCLEX-RN®), validating safety to practice nursing and opening the door to professional nursing practice opportunities. Therefore, preparation for the NCLEX must begin early in the nursing program and provide a scaffold on which to hang the nursing knowledge and the skill base on which safe practice is built. The authors of this review book understand the scaffolding process and its relationship to NCLEX success. They have watched nursing students struggle with NCLEX preparation and have learned what works and what does not.

Instead of an exhaustive list of questions attached to a snippet of case information, this unique review book presents a group of unfolding case studies that tell stories about real patients, clinical issues, and the role of the nurse in providing high-quality, safe care. Integrated into each unfolding case study are activities to increase comprehension, rapid response terms that highlight important information, and the pharmacological interventions required for the conditions being discussed. This book allows the student to make decisions about the cases as they unfold and encourages the student to "think like a nurse." Practicing the role of the nurse is a novel and beneficial review method of studying for the NCLEX.

There are at least two schools of thought concerning NCLEX preparation. One asserts that passing the NCLEX is the sole responsibility of the student, the program having provided the curriculum and experiences. The second school of thought asserts that the nursing program is a collaborative partner in the student's quest for licensure. Measures focusing on the attainment of licensure must be built into the curriculum from nursing foundations to senior seminar. Every nursing faculty member who teaches undergraduate nursing students needs resource material to use in the course of teaching or to recommend to students as they prepare for the test that will launch their careers.

It is incumbent on every nursing faculty member involved in undergraduate, prelicense nursing education to know and use the resources that will enable the graduate's successful career entry. Given the human and fiscal investment that a student makes while pursuing a nursing career, we need more effective tools to enable success on the licensure examination. Ruth A. Wittmann-Price, Brenda Reap Thompson, and Frances H. Cornelius have developed a creative and engaging approach to NCLEX preparation that has the potential of ensuring success for many more nursing school graduates.

Gloria Ferraro Donnelly, PhD, RN, FAAN
Dean and Professor
College of Nursing and Health Professions
Drexel University
Philadelphia, Pennsylvania

Preface

This book was designed with several purposes in mind. It is foremost a review and remediation workbook for students who are about to take the National Council Licensure Examination-RN (NCLEX-RN®; National Council of State Boards of Nursing, 2016). This book is also a unique case study workbook for instructors to assign to students throughout their course of undergraduate study for the purposes of (a) assisting faculty in delivering content in an innovative format, (b) assisting students in understanding the nature of clinical thinking, and (c) use in simulation environments. The philosophy of this book is to engage students in active learning using unfolding case studies. Carr (2015) states:

> The use of the unfolding case study moves health care provider education from fact-based lecturing to situation-based discussion and decision making as a person's condition or situation changes. Use of the unfolding case facilitates collaborative learning, covers necessary content, and assists students to think beyond the facts and use their clinical imagination. Unfolding case studies require students to begin to grasp the nature of a clinical situation and adjust interventions as the clinical situation unfolds. (p. 283)

In this way, unfolding case studies closely mimic real-life situations in nursing practice and are important situational mental models that are useful in assisting students to problem solve and to actively engage in and use critical-thinking techniques (Kaylor & Strickland, 2015). Unlike other NCLEX-RN preparation books that expect students to answer question after unrelated question, this book builds content into the case scenarios, thereby engaging students in the process of having to consider an evolving, and perhaps increasingly complex, clinical situation before answering each question.

As you, the student, work and twist your mind through the unfolding case studies, you will begin to envision being a practicing registered nurse who is actively problem solving and "thinking like a nurse." Adopting this method of thinking will assist you in developing clinical-thinking skills that are important for NCLEX-RN success in assessment, planning, intervention, and evaluation of patient care. The patient care content areas that are essential to master for NCLEX-RN success—safe and effective care, health promotion, and physiological and psychological integrity—are interwoven throughout the unfolding case studies. You will find this unique format enjoyable; it will help you escape the drudgery of answering multiple-choice question after multiple-choice question, studying flashcards, medical terminology definitions, or simply wasting valuable time applying test-taking tricks.

Let's face it: The NCLEX-RN is a content-driven test. The unfolding case studies presented in this study guide deliver the content intermingled with active learning strategies. Many different evaluative forms are used in this book to help you assess your own learning. The question styles used include all those used on the NCLEX-RN licensing examination, including multiple-choice questions, select all that apply, hot spots, matching, true or false, prioritizing, and calculations. This book also has Rapid Response Tips that help students make easy cognitive connections about content, includes pharmacology principles of each nursing specialty, and has a chapter devoted completely to the review of medication administration principles. The authors have heard and listened to the recommendations of nursing students that continuously ask for a pharmacology review that is applied to clinical situations.

The correct responses to each question related to the case studies are easily accessible at the end of each chapter. The authors suggest that you work through each chapter, then go back and evaluate yourself, paying close attention to the content areas that might require remedial work before taking the NCLEX-RN examination.

The authors are committed to making this the best review book ever to break the endless review cycle of question after question and to support students' ability to walk into the NCLEX-RN examination with confidence. This book was written and compiled by practicing clinicians: nurses who work at the bedside and know how to multitask, prioritize, and lead novice nurses to success. Please provide us with feedback on your experience using this book at cs@springerpub.com. We look forward to hearing from you and to you soon becoming one of our colleagues in nursing.

Ruth A. Wittmann-Price
Brenda Reap Thompson
Frances H. Cornelius

Resources

Carr, K. C. (2015). Using the unfolding case study in midwifery education. *Journal of Midwifery & Women's Health, 60*(3), 283–290. doi:10.1111/jmwh.12293

Kaylor, S. K., & Strickland, H. P. (2015). Unfolding case studies as a formative teaching methodology for novice nursing students. *Journal of Nursing Education, 54*(2), 106–110. doi:10.3928/01484834-20150120-06

National Council of State Boards of Nursing. (2016). Home page. Retrieved from ncsbn.org

CHAPTER 1

Strategies for Studying and Taking Standardized Tests

Ruth A. Wittmann-Price, Brenda Reap Thompson, and Frances H. Cornelius

Always bear in mind that your own resolution to succeed is more important than any one thing.—Abraham Lincoln

Many factors contribute to success in studying and test taking. Once you learn about these, your life becomes much easier because you are "in the know." This chapter briefly, but effectively, reviews key points that are important for all students who are about to embark on a "high-stakes" test.

Motivation

The most important aspect of test taking is studying, and the most important aspect of studying is motivation. Do not worry if you are not always motivated to sit and study. Motivation comes from both internal and external sources and is not always consistent or stable for any one person. External factors that motivate are those that arise from the environment around you. Many different things, people, and issues can be the source of an external motivator, such as grades, parents, and career goals. Internal factors that motivate you to study are those aspects that are part of you and drive you; they are part of your personality makeup. Positive thinking can increase your motivation, as can the task of creating a study schedule and following it seriously so that it becomes part of your routine. The good news is that overall motivation can be improved through the introduction of such strategies. Successful time management, study, and test-taking skills will help you to improve your motivation.

Time Management

Time management is a key strategy that we hear much about these days, probably because everyone's day is so full. You cannot manage time; it just moves forward. But you can manage what you do with your time. Here are some hints that help successful test takers. Use a weekly calendar to schedule study sessions by outlining time frames for all of your other activities: home, school, and appointments. Then find the "unscheduled time" in your calendar. Make these times your study periods, and make them very visible by using color to highlight them either on your paper calendar or in your electronic timekeeper. Make these "study times" priorities. Another strategy is to investigate your learning style to optimize the time you devote to study by applying methods that mesh with your personal learning style (Thompson, 2009). You can use the 3-month calendar template in Table 1.1.

TABLE 1.1 Three-Month Study Calendar

Month ____________________ (Add dates)

Week	Sunday	Monday	Tuesday	Wednesday	Thursday	Friday	Saturday
1							
2							
3							
4							

Month ____________________ (Add dates)

Week	Sunday	Monday	Tuesday	Wednesday	Thursday	Friday	Saturday
1							
2							
3							
4							

Month ____________________ (Add dates)

Week	Sunday	Monday	Tuesday	Wednesday	Thursday	Friday	Saturday
1							
2							
3							
4							

Clearly mark your study times and your NCLEX-RN® test date if you know it.

Learning Styles

Different students learn differently. To maximize your learning potential, it is helpful to determine what type of learner you are. Quite simply, a learning style is an approach to learning; you want to use the style that works best for you. Most learners may have a predominant learning style, but it is possible to have more than one style. The four most common learning styles are defined by the acronym VARK, described by Fleming (2001); VARK stands for:

- Visual (V)
- Auditory (A)
- Read/write (R)
- Kinesthetic (K)

The visual (spatial) learner learns best by what he or she sees, such as pictures, diagrams, flowcharts, timelines, maps, and demonstrations. A good way to learn a topic for a visual learner may be by concept mapping or the use of computer graphics.

If you are an aural/auditory learner, you prefer information that is heard or spoken. You may learn best from lectures, tapes, tutorials, group discussion, speaking, web chats, e-mails, mobile phones, and reading aloud the content you are studying. By reading aloud, you may be able to sort things out and gain understanding (Brancato, 2007; Fleming, 2001).

A read/write learner prefers information offered in the form of written words. This type of learner likes text-based input and output in all of its forms. Students who prefer this method like PowerPoint presentations, the Internet, lists, dictionaries, thesauri, quotations, and anything with written words (Fleming, 2001).

The fourth type of learner is characterized as kinesthetic and uses the body and sense of touch to enhance learning. This type of learner likes to think out issues while working out or exercising. Kinesthetic learners prefer learning content through gaming or acting. This type of learner (Fleming, 2001) appreciates simulation or a real-life experience. Felder and Solomon (1998) refer to these learners as active learners.

It is not hard to find out what type of learning style will work best for you. You can easily use the Internet to search "learning styles," and a variety of self-administered tests are available for self-assessment. Having this insight about yourself is just one more way of becoming a more successful test taker!

Successful Studying

Other studying tips are also helpful for many students. First, eliminate external sources of distraction (TV, radio, phone) while studying. Even though many people feel that they study better with music, there is no evidence to support this notion. Eliminate your internal sources of distraction, such as hunger, thirst, or thoughts about problems that cannot be worked out at that moment. If there is an interpersonal relationship issue bothering you—with a family member, friend, or partner—try to talk it out and clear it up before your scheduled "study time." In addition, do not forget to treat yourself well and take breaks. Take a 10-minute break after each hour of study. During your break, get up and stretch, have a glass of water, or get yourself a snack (Thompson, 2009).

Create a conducive study environment. Get comfortable but not so comfortable that you fall asleep! Use a clean, clear, attractive workspace. Have all the materials that you need assembled so that you won't have to interrupt yourself to look for things like a pen or a stapler.

What to study can pose another dilemma. Many nurse educators suggest that the best way to go is to concentrate on questions of the National Council Licensure Examination-RN (NCLEX-RN®) type. Others propose that you should use material that reviews content. We are suggesting that a combination of the two is best. By completing questions as your only strategy, you may miss important information. Therefore, if you are reviewing information that truly escapes your memory, go back to a reliable source, such as a textbook, and reread that content. Let's face it: Some of the topics learned in the beginning of your professional education may be slightly harder to recall than content learned in the final courses.

Organizing Information

The use of studying frameworks can be helpful in organizing information. One of the best ways to organize information is to think of the answer in terms of the nursing process framework. The nursing process was created as a logical method to solve problems of patient care. *Assessment* is always the first step of the process, because you need to comprehend all aspects of the patient's physical and emotional situation before making a *nursing diagnosis*. Once you have a nursing diagnosis, you can create a nursing *plan*. Then you can confidently carry out that plan by implementing the nursing *interventions*. The only way to know whether those interventions work is to *evaluate* the outcome; then you reassess the situation and the process then starts over again. An example of a question that can be answered by applying the nursing process framework is shown in Exercise 1.1.

EXERCISE 1.1 Multiple-choice:

The physician orders the insertion of a catheter into the patient's abdomen for peritoneal dialysis. In preparing a preoperative teaching plan for this patient, the nurse would initially:

A. Invite the patient's family to join the preoperative teaching session
B. Ask the physician what information was already discussed with the patient
C. Assess the patient's knowledge and understanding about the procedure
D. Have the operative permit signed and then institute the teaching plan

The answer can be found on page 19

Other frameworks may include using mnemonics, and these work well for many students. A familiar one is *ABC* (airway, breathing, and circulation). Exercise 1.2 is a question that lends itself to the mnemonic principle.

EXERCISE 1.2 Multiple-choice:

The nurse is caring for a client who has returned from surgery after a below-the-knee amputation of the right lower extremity. What would the nurse assess first?

A. Temperature

B. Tissue perfusion

C. Pain

D. Orientation

The answer can be found on page 19

Other mnemonics are not so familiar but often helpful, such as VEAL CHOP (see Table 1.2). This mnemonic is further explained in Chapter 4.

Many other methods help learners to understand and remember what they need to know; these include visualization strategies, games, fact sheets, and tables for comparison. For example, Table 1.3 shows a comparison for a patient experiencing midtrimester vaginal bleeding to help a learner remember the primary symptoms.

Establishing Study Groups

Another strategy is to form study groups; these work well for many learners. If you choose to try working with a study group, start with a small one whose members get along well. You can choose a leader who can keep a list of members' contact information and can schedule a time and place that is convenient and comfortable for everyone. Each person

TABLE 1.2 Fetal-Monitoring Basics

V	Variable	C	Cord
E	Early deceleration	H	Head compression
A	Acceleration	O	OK
L	Late deceleration	P	Placental insufficiency

TABLE 1.3 Comparison of Third-Trimester Bleeding

Sign	Placenta Previa	Placental Abruption
Pain	No	Yes
Bleeding	Yes	Not always
Abdomen	Soft	Ridged

should be assigned a role and do some presession preparation. Everyone in the group should take the responsibility of keeping the others on task and using the time together in the most productive manner. This does not mean that the study group cannot take breaks, but breaks should be planned (Thompson, 2009).

Understanding the NCLEX-RN Exam

The NCLEX-RN exam was developed from a specific test plan. Most nursing students know that there are at least 75 questions and possibly as many as 265 (National Council of State Boards of Nursing [NCSBN], 2016). Each NCLEX-RN test also contains 15 test or practice items mixed in with the scored questions. The questions are developed by using Bloom's revised taxonomy (Bloom, Englehart, Furst, Hill, & Drathwohl, 1956) (Table 1.4).

Table 1.5 provides Exercises 1.3 to 1.8, which are examples of NCLEX-RN types of multiple-choice questions at each level of Bloom's taxonomy.

TABLE 1.4 Blooms's Revised Taxonomy

Creating	Generating new ideas, designing, constructing, planning, and producing
Evaluating	Justifying a decision or course of action, checking
Analyzing	Breaking information into parts to explore understandings and relationships
Applying	Implementing, carrying out, using, executing
Understanding	Explaining ideas or concepts, interpreting, summarizing, explaining
Remembering	Recalling information, recognizing, listing, describing

TABLE 1.5 Example Questions Using Bloom's Taxonomy

Level of Bloom's Revised Taxonomy	NCLEX-RN® Type of Multiple-Choice Question
Creating **EXERCISE 1.3**	A group of outpatients with thyroid dysfunction are being taught about their disease. One patient is on levothyroxine (Synthroid) and states that he does not understand the reason. The patient tells the group that he takes the medication inconsistently. The nurse should: A. Tell the patient to go to his doctor B. Talk to the patient after class C. Re-adjust the teaching to emphasize correct medication administration D. Tell the class that this is incorrect and suggest that the patient has individual class sessions

(*continued*)

TABLE 1.5 Example Questions Using Bloom's Taxonomy ***(continued)***

Level of Bloom's Revised Taxonomy	NCLEX-RN® Type of Multiple-Choice Question
Evaluating **EXERCISE 1.4**	A patient who is taking levothyroxine (Synthroid) tells the nurse that he feels very anxious and has occasional palpitations. Which action by the nurse would be appropriate? A. Checking the patient's laboratory results B. Taking the patient's blood pressure C. Palpating the patient's thyroid D. Administering the patient's antianxiety medication
Analyzing **EXERCISE 1.5**	The nurse is assessing a patient who has been taking levothyroxine (Synthroid) for 5 weeks. The patient's heart rate is 90 beats per minute, weight has decreased 4 lb, T3 and T4 have increased. Which action by the nurse would be appropriate? A. Hold the medication B. Request a repeat T3 and T4 C. Assess the blood pressure D. Administer the medication
Applying **EXERCISE 1.6**	A patient taking levothyroxine (Synthroid) tells the nurse that he feels well and some days cannot remember whether he took his medication. The nurse should: A. Tell the patient to come off the medication B. Tell the patient to take his medication every day C. Tell the patient this is not an appropriate way to take any medication D. Help the patient to develop a system to remember to take the medication
Understanding **EXERCISE 1.7**	The nurse provides discharge instructions for a patient who is taking levothyroxine (Synthroid). Which of these statements, if made by the patient, would indicate correct understanding of the medication? A. "I will discontinue the medication when my symptoms improve." B. "I will take the medicine each day before breakfast and at bedtime." C. "I will feel more energetic after taking the medication for a few weeks." D. "I will probably gain some weight while taking this medicine."
Remembering **EXERCISE 1.8**	The nurse is administering levothyroxine (Synthroid) to a patient with hypothyroidism. The nurse recognizes that the medication is prescribed to: A. Replace the thyroid hormone B. Stimulate the thyroid gland C. Block the stimulation of the thyroid gland D. Decrease the chances of thyrotoxicosis

The answer can be found on page 19

Another approach that is often used to decide how to answer a question is Maslow's theory of the hierarchy of needs, as shown in Figure 1.1 (Maslow, 1943). Exercise 1.9 is an NCLEX-RN type of question that can be answered by applying Maslow's theory.

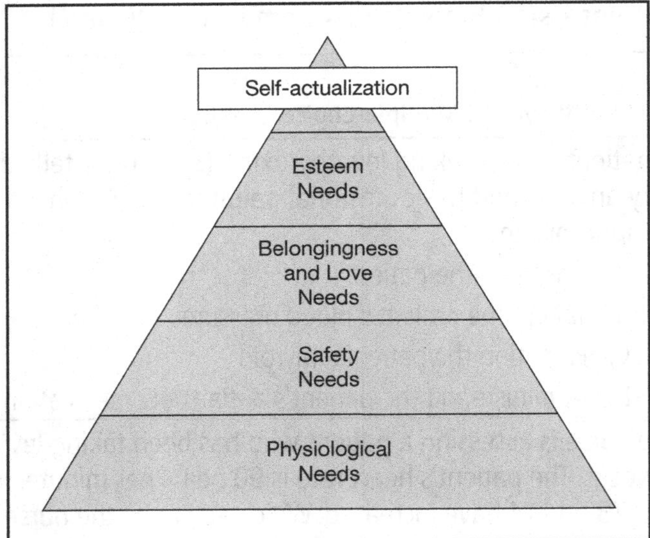

FIGURE 1.1 Maslow's hierarchy of needs.

EXERCISE 1.9 Multiple-choice:

The nurse is caring for a patient who is 35 weeks pregnant and was admitted to the emergency department (ED) with placental abruption. Which of the following actions would be most appropriate?

A. Infuse normal saline 0.9% intravenous (IV) at 150 mL/hr
B. Administer morphine 2 mg IV
C. Tell the patient that you will sit with her until her family arrives
D. Ask the patient whether she would like you to call the clergy

The answer can be found on page 21

To pass the NCLEX-RN exam, you will have to answer a minimum of 60 questions at the set competency level. Some students can accomplish this in 75 questions (60 at the set competency level plus 15 pretest questions). If you answer 265 questions, a final ability estimate is computed to determine whether you are successful. If you run out of time and have not completed all 265 questions, you can still pass if you have answered the last 60 questions at the set competency level. Approximately 1.3 minutes are allocated for each question, but we all know that some questions take a short time to answer, whereas others, including math questions, may take longer.

The NCLEX-RN exam now comprises several different types of questions, including hot spots, fill in the blank(s), drag-and-drop, order response, and select all that apply or multiple-choice questions. These are referred to as alternative types of questions and have been added to better assess your critical thinking. This book offers plenty of practice with such questions. Examples of the *select all that apply* type of question are shown in Exercises 1.10 and 1.11.

EXERCISE 1.10 Select all that apply:

The nurse is reviewing data collected from a patient who is being treated for hypothyroidism. Which information indicates that the patient has had a positive outcome?

A. Sleeps 8 hours each night, waking up to go to the bathroom once
B. Has bowel movements two times a week while on a high-fiber diet
C. Gained 10 lb since the initial clinic visit 6 weeks ago
D. Was promoted at work because of increased work production
E. Walks 2 miles within 30 minutes before work each morning

The answer can be found on page 21

EXERCISE 1.11 Select all that apply:

The hospital is expecting to receive survivors of a disaster. The charge nurse is directed to provide a list of patients for possible discharge. Which of the following patients would be placed on the list?

A. A patient who was admitted 3 days ago with urosepsis; white blood cell count is 5.4 $mm^3/\mu L$
B. A patient who was admitted 2 days ago after an acetaminophen overdose; creatinine is 2.1 mg/dL
C. A patient who was admitted with stable angina and had two stents placed in the left anterior descending coronary artery 24 hours ago
D. A patient who was admitted with an upper gastrointestinal bleed and had an endoscopic ablation 48 hours ago; hemoglobin is 10.8 g/dL

The answer can be found on page 22

An example of an NCLEX-RN *fill in the blank* question is provided in Exercise 1.12.

EXERCISE 1.12 Fill in the blanks:

The nurse is calculating the client's total intake and output to determine whether he has a positive or negative fluid balance. The intake includes the following:

1,200 mL intravenous (IV) D5NSS
200 mL of vancomycin IV
Two 8-oz glasses of juice
One 4-oz cup of broth
One 6-oz cup of water

On being emptied, the Foley bag was found to contain 350 mL of urine.
What would the nurse document? ________________; ________________; ________________.

The answer can be found on page 22

Drag and drop questions are specific to the computer because the student uses his or her mouse or touch pad to place items in order. A *hot spot* refers to moving the mouse or the touch pad to a specific point on a diagram. An example of an NCLEX-RN hot-spot question is provided in Exercise 1.13.

EXERCISE 1.13 Hot spot:

The nurse assesses a patient who has a possible brain tumor. The patient has difficulty coordinating voluntary muscle movement and balance. Which area of the brain is affected? (Please place an X at the appropriate spot.)

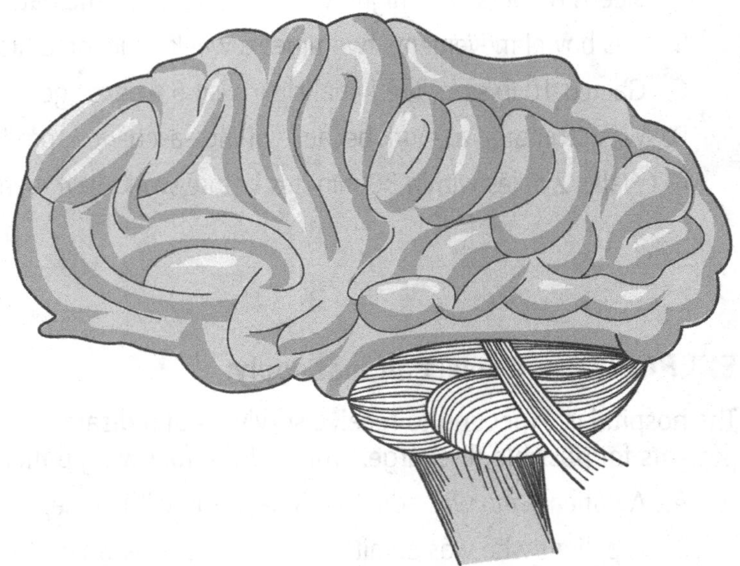

The answer can be found on page 22

An example of an *ordering* NCLEX-RN question is found in Exercise 1.14.

EXERCISE 1.14 Ordering:

The nurse is inserting an indwelling urinary catheter into a female patient. Place the steps in priority order:

_____ Ask the patient to bear down
_____ Don clean gloves and wash the perineal area
_____ Place the client in a dorsal recumbent position
_____ Advance the catheter 1.2 in. (2.5–5 cm)
_____ Inflate the balloon and pull back gently
_____ Retract the labia with the nondominant hand
_____ Use forceps with the dominant hand to cleanse the perineal area
_____ Place drapes on the bed and over the perineal area
_____ Apply sterile gloves
_____ Advance the catheter 2 to 3 in. (5–7 cm) until urine drains
_____ Test balloon, lubricate catheter, place antiseptic on cotton balls

The answer can be found on page 23

An example of an NCLEX-RN *exhibit-format* question is provided in Exercise 1.15.

EXERCISE 1.15 Exhibit-format:

A 52-year-old female patient admitted to the emergency department (ED) has had nausea and vomiting for 3 days and abdominal pain that is unrelieved after vomiting.

Skin: Pale, cool; patient shivering

Respiration: Respiratory rate (RR): 30 breaths per minute, lungs clear, SaO_2: 90

Cardiovascular (CV) system: RRR (regular rate and rhythm) with mitral regurgitation; temperature: 95°F (35°C), blood pressure (BP): 96/60 mmHg, heart rate (HR): 132 beats per minute (bpm) and weak

Extremities: +4 pulses, no edema of lower extremities

Gastrointestinal (GI) system: Hyperactive bowel sounds; vomited 100 mL of bile-colored fluid, positive abdominal tenderness

Genitourinary (GU) system: Foley inserted, no urine drained

- Hemoglobin: 10.6 g/dL
- Hematocrit: 39%
- White blood cells: 8.0 mm^3
- Sodium: 150 mEq/L
- Potassium: 7.0 mEq/L
- Blood urea nitrogen: 132 mg/dL
- Creatinine: 8.2 mg/dL
- Serum amylase: 972
- Serum lipase: 1,380
- Arterial blood gas pH: 7.0
- pO_2: 90 mmHg
- pCO_2: 39 mmHg
- HCO_3: 17 mEq/L

After reviewing the patient's assessment findings and laboratory reports, the nurse determines that the priority for the plan of care should focus on:

A. Metabolic acidosis and oliguria
B. Respiratory acidosis and dyspnea
C. Metabolic alkalosis related to vomiting
D. Respiratory alkalosis resulting from abdominal pain

The answer can be found on page 23

Another strategy to use in studying for the NCLEX-RN exam is to become familiar with the organization of the test. The test plan covers the four basic categories of client needs, including a safe and effective care environment, health promotion and maintenance, psychosocial integrity, and physiologic integrity. The following questions are designed to test your grasp of providing a "safe and effective environment" through the way you manage patient care, which is an important aspect of your role and responsibility as a licensed RN. This concept applies to what you should do as an RN as well as the tasks you can delegate to nonlicensed personnel working with you. Exercises 1.16 and 1.17 offer examples of questions based on the RN's responsibility for managing safe and effective patient care.

EXERCISE 1.16 Multiple-choice:

After returning from a hip replacement, a patient with diabetes mellitus type I is lethargic, flushed, and feeling nauseous. Vital signs are blood pressure (BP): 108/78 mmHg, heart rate (HR): 100 beats per minute (bpm), respiratory rate (RR): 24 breaths per minute and deep. What is the next action the nurse should take?

A. Notify the physician
B. Check the patient's glucose
C. Administer an antiemetic
D. Change the intravenous (IV) infusion rate

The answer can be found on page 24

Exercise 1.17 Multiple-choice:

The nurse is assigned to care for a patient with pneumonia. Which task can be delegated to the unlicensed assistive personnel by the RN?

A. Teaching a patient how to use the inhaler
B. Listening to the patient's lungs
C. Checking the results of the patient's blood work
D. Counting the patient's respiratory rate

The answer can be found on page 24

Yet another strategy to use in analyzing NCLEX-RN questions is to assess the negative/positive balance of the question. For a positive question, select the option that is correct; for a negative question, select the option that is incorrect. Examples of NCLEX-RN questions with positive and negative answers are shown in Table 1.6.

TABLE 1.6 Questions With Positive and Negative Answers

Positive NCLEX-RN® Type of Question Stem	Negative NCLEX-RN Type of Question Stem
Which statement by the client *indicates an understanding* of the medication side effects?	Which statement by the client *indicates a need for further teaching* about the medication side effects?

Therapeutic communication is one of the long-enduring basics of nursing care. As RNs, we provide therapy, not only through what we do but also through what and how we communicate with patients and families. Therapeutic communication is not what you would use in everyday conversation because it is designed to be more purposeful. Therapeutic communication is nonjudgmental, direct, truthful, empathetic, and informative (Potter & Perry, 2016). Communication and documentation are among the important threads integrated throughout the NCLEX-RN exam. An example of an NCLEX-RN question based on therapeutic communication is shown in Exercise 1.18.

EXERCISE 1.18 Multiple-choice:

An 11-year-old boy with acute lymphocytic leukemia (ALL) has been diagnosed with his second relapse following successful remissions after chemotherapy and radiation. The patient asks, "Am I going to die?" Which response by the nurse would be most helpful to the patient?

A. "Let's talk about this after I speak with your parents."
B. "Can you tell me why you feel this way?"
C. "You will need to discuss this with the oncologist."
D. "You sound like you'd like to talk about it."

The answer can be found on page 24

What Should I Know About NCLEX?

NCLEX is a computer adaptive test (CAT), meaning that it is customized to each candidate taking it. The test will have 75 to 265 questions. Fifteen pretest questions are included, which means that they do not count toward your score. The test is called *adaptive* because when you answer a question correctly, the following question will be at a higher level. Therefore, a candidate who passes NCLEX-RN with 75 questions is able to answer high-level questions correctly and remain above the passing standard set by the NCSBN (2016) for safe practice.

If the candidate answers a question incorrectly, a question is provided that is at the same level or a lower level. A candidate must stay above the passing standard to be successful. The test ends when the candidate has a score that is clearly above or clearly below the passing standard.

The candidate will be allowed up to 6 hours to complete the test. If the candidate runs out of time, the "rule of 60" applies. This means that the candidate will be successful if the competency level for the last 60 questions was above the passing standard. Some candidates have failed the NCLEX because of "rapid guessing." Therefore, it is important to take your time in reading and answering questions.

To summarize, the test is complete when one of the three following situations has occurred:

1. It is determined that the candidate is above or below the passing standard with 95% confidence.
2. A total of 265 questions have been completed.
3. The 6 hours provided to complete the test have passed.

The questions in the NCLEX test bank are divided into client-need categories. These categories reflect the percentages effective April 2016:

1. Safe and effective care environment
   - Management of care (17%–23%)
   - Safety and infection control (9%–15%)
2. Health promotion and maintenance (6%–12%)
3. Psychosocial integrity (6%–12%)
4. Physiologic integrity
   - Basic care and comfort (6%–12%)
   - Pharmacological and parenteral therapy (12%–18%)
   - Reduction of risk potential (9%–15%)
   - Physiologic adaptation (11%–17%)

Your test will be designed so that you are asked the specified percentage of questions for each category.

Scheduling the Test

1. The applicant's credentials are submitted to the state board of nursing for approval to test.
2. Test fees must be paid.
3. The applicant is provided with an authorization to test (ATT) code number.
4. The candidate is responsible for scheduling an appointment to test. First-time candidates are given an appointment within 30 days. Schedule a time that is best for you. Do you feel more alert in the morning or would a late-afternoon appointment be better for you?

Before Test Day

Go to the site so you know exactly where it is and how long it will take you to get there on time.

Test Day

Arrive at the site early; you may forfeit your appointment if you are 30 minutes late. Bring valid identification and ATT.

Preparation for Exam Day

'Twas the Night Before Testing

As the big day approaches, you should stop studying early in the day and spend time relaxing by doing something you enjoy, such as visiting a friend, going out to eat, or watching a movie. Participating in a physical activity is a good idea because it will help you get a good night's sleep. However, before you go to bed, organize everything you need and set two alarms so that you have plenty of time in the morning and arrive at the testing site slightly early, without rushing. Most important, go to bed early.

The Day of Testing

Start your day as you always do but make sure you eat good, nutritious meals. Make sure you know where the testing site is and plan two different routes. Dress comfortably in layers to accommodate variations in room temperature. Have your ID handy and, most importantly, *think positively!*

Last-Minute Test Tips

- Improve your score by:
  - Reading the question and *all* answer choices before making a selection
  - Making sure you understand what the question is asking
  - Taking your time to be sure you have answered all questions as best as you can
- Be in charge of how you use your time by:
  - Pacing yourself—avoid rapid guessing or spending too much time on any one question
  - Doing your best and then moving on
  - Wearing a watch and keeping track of your time
- Wear earplugs if you become distracted easily.
- Do not change your answers unless you are uncertain about your first answer choice.
- Answer every question. If you do not know the answer, make the most intelligent guess you can.
- As you answer the questions, eliminate choices that you know are incorrect.

- If you can eliminate two wrong answers, your chance of choosing the correct answer has improved.
- Find key words or phrases in the question that will help you choose the correct answer.
- Be sure you are responding to the question that is being asked.
- In using scratch paper or an eraser board for a math question, make sure you copy the answer correctly.
- Remember that you are not expected to know everything; standardized exams have higher level questions that will challenge the limits of your knowledge.

International Nurses Seeking Licensure in the United States

1. CGFNS International™ can provide information that will help you to fulfill all of the requirements for eligibility to take the NCLEX. Access the website at www.cgfns.org.
2. CGFNS International will review your credentials, including your secondary and nursing education.
3. A qualifying examination is administered that will test your general nursing knowledge. This examination is one of the requirements needed to obtain a visa to work in the United States. Nurses who have the CGFNS International certification have a higher rate of success on NCLEX-RN than nurses who have not been tested.
4. The Test of English as a Foreign Language (TOEFL) is also required before taking the NCLEX to ensure that you have an adequate understanding of the English language.
5. A visa can be administered by the International Commission on Healthcare Professions (ICHP), a division of CGFNS International. This information is also given on the website.

Standards of Practice

The Standards of Practice offer guidelines that encompass the knowledge, skills, and judgment required to provide safe and effective care. They also discuss the need to engage in scholarship, service, and leadership. The Standards and Scope of Practice were developed by the American Nurses Association (ANA) in order to ensure competency and establish standards whereby care can be measured. This protects the public and encourages professional nurses to take responsibility for their actions. Review the information on the website (www.nursingworld.org) to gain a better understanding of nursing as a profession in the United States (ANA, 2015).

The standards include the following:

Six Standards of Practice

1. Assessment
2. Diagnosis
3. Outcome identification
4. Planning
5. Implementation
6. Evaluation

Nine Standards of Professional Performance

1. Quality of practice
2. Education
3. Professional practice evaluation
4. Collegiality
5. Collaboration
6. Ethics
7. Research
8. Resource utilization
9. Leadership

Tips for Success

1. Research medical terminology used in the United States. Terms such as *epistaxis* (nose bleed), *lochia* (drainage from the vagina after delivery), and *erythema* (redness)—and many others—are used in NCLEX questions. It is impossible to respond accurately without an understanding of the terminology.
2. Medications used in the United States differ from those used in other countries. Schedule time to study medications, as pharmacology content consists of 12% to 18% of the NCLEX exam. Both the generic and brand names are provided on the NCLEX exam.
3. In the United States, the nursing process is the framework for providing care for patients. The nursing process also serves to teach students how to organize information relating to patient care and decision making; it provides a structure to help students learn how to organize their clinical thinking and care planning. Familiarize yourself with the nursing process and use this concept while studying.

4. Nurses are part of the health care team; therefore, nurses collaborate with professionals from other health care disciplines, such as physicians, respiratory therapists, physical therapists, and nutritionists.
5. Nurses are expected to be assertive and to question prescriptions written by physicians or other primary care providers if such prescriptions do not mesh with the guidelines for what is normally prescribed. This process helps to safeguard the patient. However, such assertive behavior may not be acceptable in some countries. Thus, even though it may seem uncomfortable to select an answer describing such an action, remember that such assertiveness is expected from RNs in the United States.
6. Patients who are being treated for drug or alcohol abuse may be referred to group therapy sessions. During these sessions, patients talk with other patients who have similar problems. In some countries, it is inappropriate to discuss this type of behavior outside of the family.
7. In the United States, a nurse is expected to maintain eye contact in communicating with patients. Eye contact indicates that you are focused on the patient and listening to him or her. This is important because it helps to build a trusting relationship between nurse and patient.
8. Technology is used in many aspects of health care. It is, therefore, important to understand the use of equipment such as cardiac monitors, ventilators, wound vacuum-assisted closure (VAC), suction equipment, peritoneal dialysis, pulmonary artery pressure monitoring, intracranial pressure monitoring, and fetal monitoring.
9. Focus your attention on information provided by the patient, such as reports of pain, weakness, edema, cough, dizziness, and nausea. These may be clues that there is a complication related to the patient's disease. Know the clinical manifestations pointing to a complication. It is important to recognize a complication early so that treatment can be initiated promptly.
10. Teaching the patient and assisting the patient to make appropriate decisions is also within the scope of practice of the RN. It is also the right of the patients to refuse care.

Plan for Academic Success

Prepare for the NCLEX-RN examination by reviewing content and questions to build your confidence. This review book provides you with a unique format that will help you envision what it would be like to actually work as an RN in the clinical area.

Answers

EXERCISE 1.1 Multiple-choice:

The physician orders the insertion of a catheter into the patient's abdomen for peritoneal dialysis. In preparing a preoperative teaching plan for this patient, the nurse would initially:

A. Invite the patient's family to join the preoperative teaching session—NO; you have not asked the patient whether this is his or her preference.

B. Ask the physician what information was already discussed with the patient—NO; the nurse needs to independently evaluate teaching needs.

C. Assess the patient's knowledge and understanding about the procedure—**YES; assessment is the first step of the nursing process.**

D. Have the operative permit signed and then institute the teaching plan—NO; the physician obtains the consent for surgery.

EXERCISE 1.2 Multiple-choice:

The nurse is caring for a client who has returned from surgery after a below-the-knee amputation of the right lower extremity. What would the nurse assess first?

A. Temperature—NO; this is important but it is not A, B, or C (in the mnemonic).

B. Tissue perfusion—**YES; C = circulation (in the mnemonic).**

C. Pain—NO; this is important but it is not A, B, or C (in the mnemonic).

D. Orientation—NO; this is important but it is not A, B, or C (in the mnemonic).

TABLE 1.5 Example Questions Using Bloom's Taxonomy

Level of Bloom's Revised Taxonomy	NCLEX-RN® Type of Multiple-Choice Question
Creating EXERCISE 1.3	A group of outpatients with thyroid dysfunction are being taught about their disease. One patient is on levothyroxine (Synthroid) and states that he does not understand the reason. The patient tells the group that he takes the medication inconsistently. The nurse should: A. Tell the patient to go to his doctor—NO; this is an understanding issue. B. Talk to the patient after class—NO; there may be others in the class who do not understand. C. Re-adjust the teaching to emphasize correct medication administration—**YES; there may be others in the class who do not understand**. D. Tell the class that this is incorrect and suggest that the patient has individual class sessions—NO; this would put the patient "on the spot."

(continued)

TABLE 1.5 Example Questions Using Bloom's Taxonomy ***(continued)***

Level of Bloom's Revised Taxonomy	NCLEX-RN® Type of Multiple-Choice Question
Evaluating **EXERCISE 1.4**	A patient who is taking levothyroxine (Synthroid) tells the nurse that he feels very anxious and has occasional palpitations. Which action by the nurse would be appropriate? A. Checking the patient's laboratory results—**YES; this will show you the thyroid hormone levels.** B. Taking the patient's blood pressure—NO; this is not an assessment contributed solely to thyroid dysfunction. C. Palpating the patient's thyroid—NO; this is usually enlarged in hypothyroidism. D. Administering the patient's antianxiety medication—NO; this may just mask symptoms of thyroid dysfunction.
Analyzing **EXERCISE 1.5**	The nurse is assessing a patient who has been taking levothyroxine (Synthroid) for 5 weeks. The patient's heart rate is 90 beats per minute, weight has decreased 4 lb, T3 and T4 have increased. Which action by the nurse would be appropriate? A. Hold the medication—NO; the medication would be held for tachycardia, angina, and insomnia. The heart rate is normal since it is less than 100 beats per minute. Weight loss and increasing T3 and T4 are positive outcomes. B. Request a repeat T3 and T4—NO; this is already known. C. Assess the blood pressure—NO; this is not an assessment contributed solely to thyroid dysfunction. D. Administer the medication—**YES; administer the medication and continue to assess the patient.**
Applying **EXERCISE 1.6**	A patient taking levothyroxine (Synthroid) tells the nurse that he feels well and some days cannot remember whether he took his medication. The nurse should: A. Tell the patient to come off the medication—NO; the patient needs the medication for proper thyroid function. B. Tell the patient to take his medication every day—NO, this alone will not help him remember. C. Tell the patient this is not an appropriate way to take any medication—NO; this will just shut off therapeutic communication. D. Help the patient to develop a system to remember to take the medication—**YES; use a calendar system or pillbox system to help him remember.**

(continued)

TABLE 1.5 Example Questions Using Bloom's Taxonomy ***(continued)***

Level of Bloom's Revised Taxonomy	NCLEX-RN® Type of Multiple-Choice Question
Understanding EXERCISE 1.7	The nurse provides discharge instructions for a patient who is taking levothyroxine (Synthroid). Which of these statements, if made by the patient, would indicate correct understanding of the medication? A. "I will discontinue the medication when my symptoms improve."—NO; patient's should not self-regulate medication. B. "I will take the medicine each day before breakfast and at bedtime."—NO; levothyroxine (Synthroid) is taken once a day. C. "I will feel more energetic after taking the medication for a few weeks."—**YES; this is an expected therapeutic outcome.** D. "I will probably gain some weight while taking this medicine."—NO; this is not a side effect.
Remembering EXERCISE 1.8	The nurse is administering levothyroxine (Synthroid) to a patient with hypothyroidism. The nurse recognizes that the medication is prescribed to: A. Replace the thyroid hormone—**YES; this is what levothyroxine does.** B. Stimulate the thyroid gland—NO; this is not its action. C. Block the stimulation of the thyroid gland—NO; this is not its action. D. Decrease the chances of thyrotoxicosis—NO; this is not its action.

EXERCISE 1.9 Multiple-choice:

The nurse is caring for a patient who is 35 weeks pregnant and was admitted to the emergency department (ED) with placental abruption. Which of the following actions would be most appropriate?

A. Infuse normal saline 0.9% intravenous (IV) at 150 mL/hr—**YES; the patient needs fluid replacement.**
B. Administer morphine 2 mg IV—NO; but this would be the second priority.
C. Tell the patient that you will sit with her until her family arrives—NO; the patient is in danger of hemorrhaging.
D. Ask the patient whether she would like you to call the clergy—NO; this may be beneficial later, after her physiologic need for fluid has been resolved.

EXERCISE 1.10 Select all that apply:

The nurse is reviewing data collected from a patient who is being treated for hypothyroidism. Which information indicates that the patient has had a positive outcome?

A. Sleeps 8 hours each night, waking up to go to the bathroom once—**YES; hypothyroidism causes severe fatigue; 8 hours of sleep and waking up once are normal.**
B. Has bowel movements two times a week while on a high-fiber diet—NO; this may be constipation.
C. Gained 10 lb since the initial clinic visit 6 weeks ago—NO; this is not an expected outcome.
D. Was promoted at work because of increased work production—**YES; energy levels are expected to increase.**
E. Walks 2 miles within 30 minutes before work each morning—**YES; energy levels are expected to increase.**

EXERCISE 1.11 Select all that apply:

The hospital is expecting to receive survivors of a disaster. The charge nurse is directed to provide a list of patients for possible discharge. Which of the following patients would be placed on the list?

A. A patient who was admitted 3 days ago with urosepsis; white blood cell count is 5.4 mm³/µL—**YES; this patient has a normal white blood cell (WBC) count and could be discharged.**

B. A patient who was admitted 2 days ago after an acetaminophen overdose; creatinine is 2.1 mg/dL—NO; this patient has a high creatinine level and needs monitoring.

C. A patient who was admitted with stable angina and had two stents placed in the left anterior descending coronary artery 24 hours ago—**YES; patients who have not had a myocardial infarction (MI) but have had stents placed normally are discharged in 24 hours.**

D. A patient who was admitted with an upper gastrointestinal bleed and had an endoscopic ablation 48 hours ago; hemoglobin is 10.8 g/dL—**YES; the patient has no active bleeding and the hemoglobin is stable.**

EXERCISE 1.12 Fill in the blanks:

The nurse is calculating the client's total intake and output to determine whether he has a positive or negative fluid balance. The intake includes the following:

1,200 mL intavenous (IV) D5NSS

200 mL of vancomycin IV

Two 8-oz glasses of juice

One 4-oz cup of broth

One 6-oz cup of water

On being emptied, the Foley bag was found to contain 350 mL of urine.
What would the nurse document?

Total intake: 2,180 mL

Total output: –350 mL

Positive fluid balance: 1,830 mL

EXERCISE 1.13 Hot spot:

The nurse assesses a patient who has a possible brain tumor. The patient has difficulty coordinating voluntary muscle movement and balance. Which area of the brain is affected? (Please place an X at the appropriate spot.)

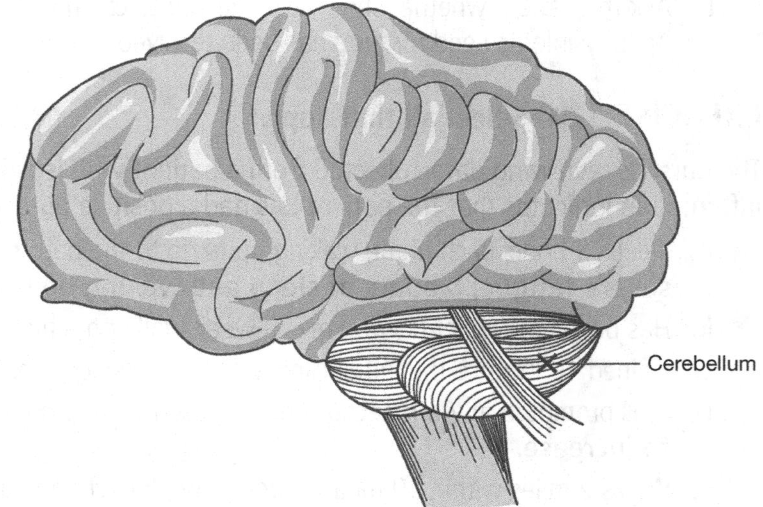

EXERCISE 1.14 Ordering:

The nurse is inserting an indwelling urinary catheter into a female patient. Place the steps in priority order:

8 Ask the patient to bear down
2 Don clean gloves and wash the perineal area
1 Place the client in a dorsal recumbent position
10 Advance the catheter 1.2 in. (2.5–5 cm)
11 Inflate the balloon and pull back gently
6 Retract the labia with the nondominant hand
7 Use forceps with the dominant hand to cleanse the perineal area
3 Place drapes on the bed and over the perineal area
4 Apply sterile gloves
9 Advance the catheter 2 to 3 in. (5–7 cm) until urine drains
5 Test balloon, lubricate catheter, place antiseptic on cotton balls

The sterile gloves are usually packaged under the drapes. Therefore, the drapes can be appropriately placed to set up a sterile field and drape the patient by touching their outer corners. The gloves are usually donned after the drapes are in place. It is not incorrect to place sterile gloves on before draping.

EXERCISE 1.15 Exhibit-format:

A 52-year-old female patient admitted to the emergency department (ED) has had nausea and vomiting for 3 days and abdominal pain that is unrelieved after vomiting.

Skin: Pale, cool; patient shivering

Respiration: Respiratory rate (RR): 30 breaths per minute, lungs clear, SaO_2: 90

Cardiovascular (CV) system: RRR (regular rate and rhythm) with mitral regurgitation; temperature: 95°F (35°C), blood pressure (BP): 96/60 mmHg, heart rate (HR): 132 beats per minute (bpm) and weak

Extremities: +4 pulses, no edema of lower extremities

Gastrointestinal (GI) system: Hyperactive bowel sounds; vomited 100 mL of bile-colored fluid, positive abdominal tenderness

Genitourinary (GU) system: Foley inserted, no urine drained

- Hemoglobin: 10.6 g/dL
- Hematocrit: 39%
- White blood cells: 8.0 mm^3
- Sodium: 150 mEq/L
- Potassium: 7.0 mEq/L
- Blood urea nitrogen: 132 mg/dL
- Creatinine: 8.2 mg/dL
- Serum amylase: 972
- Serum lipase: 1,380
- Arterial blood gas pH: 7.0
- pO_2: 90 mmHg
- pCO_2: 39 mmHg
- HCO_3: 17 mEq/L

After reviewing the patient's assessment findings and laboratory reports, the nurse determines that the priority for the plan of care should focus on:

A. Metabolic acidosis and oliguria—**YES; the pH and HCO_3 are decreased and the patient has no urine output.**

B. Respiratory acidosis and dyspnea—NO; the lungs are clear and there is no other indication of respiratory acidosis.

C. Metabolic alkalosis related to vomiting—NO; the pH is low.

D. Respiratory alkalosis resulting from abdominal pain—NO; the pH is low and the pCO_2 is normal.

EXERCISE 1.16 Multiple-choice:

After returning from a hip replacement, a patient with diabetes mellitus type I is lethargic, flushed, and feeling nauseous. Vital signs are blood pressure (BP): 108/78 mmHg, heart rate (HR): 100 beats per minute (bpm), respiratory rate (RR): 24 breaths per minute and deep. What is the next action the nurse should take?

A. Notify the physician—NO; the nurse needs to further assess.

B. Check the patient's glucose—**YES; these are signs of hypoglycemia.**

C. Administer an antiemetic—NO; this will not help.

D. Change the intravenous (IV) infusion rate—NO; this will not help.

EXERCISE 1.17 Multiple-choice:

The nurse is assigned to care for a patient with pneumonia. Which task can be delegated to the unlicensed assistive personnel by the RN?

A. Teaching a patient how to use the inhaler—NO; an RN must do initial patient teaching.

B. Listening to the patient's lungs—NO; an RN must do an initial assessment.

C. Checking the results of the patient's blood work—NO; an RN must interpret lab results.

D. Counting the patient's respiratory rate—**YES; unlicensed personnel can obtain vital signs.**

EXERCISE 1.18 Multiple-choice:

An 11-year-old boy with acute lymphocytic leukemia (ALL) has been diagnosed with his second relapse following successful remissions after chemotherapy and radiation. The patient asks, "Am I going to die?" Which response by the nurse would be most helpful to the patient?

A. "Let's talk about this after I speak with your parents."—NO; this is not responding to the patient.

B. "Can you tell me why you feel this way?"—NO; although this is not a completely wrong answer; it is more directive and may intimidate a child.

C. "You will need to discuss this with the oncologist."—NO; this is not responding to the patient's question and is not at his developmental level.

D. "You sound like you'd like to talk about it."—**YES; this is using "probing" to help the patient to dialogue.**

Resources

American Nurses Association. (2015). *Nursing: Scope and standards of practice* (3rd ed.). Washington, DC: American Nurses Publishing.

Bloom, B., Englehart, M., Furst, E., Hill, W., & Drathwohl, D. (Eds). (1956). *Taxonomy of educational objectives.* New York, NY: Longmans, Green.

Brancato, V. (2007). Teaching for the learner. In B. Moyer & R. A. Wittmann-Price (Eds.), *Nursing education: Foundations of practice excellence*. Philadelphia, PA: F. A. Davis.

Felder, R. M., & Soloman, B. A. (1998). Learning styles and strategies. Retrieved from http://www2.ncsu.edu/unity/lockers/users/f/felder/public/ILSdir/styles.htm

Fleming, N. (2001). VARK: A guide to learning styles. Retrieved from http://www.vark-learn.com/english/page.asp?p=categories

Fleming, N. D., & Mills, C. (1992). *Not another inventory, rather a catalyst for reflection: To improve the academy.* San Francisco, CA: Jossey-Bass.

Maslow, A. H. (1943). A theory of human motivation. *Psychological Review, 50*(4), 370–396.

National Council of State Boards of Nursing (NCSBN). (2016). NCLEX examinations. Retrieved from https://www.ncsbn.org/nclex.htm

Potter A. G., & Perry, P. A. (2016). *Fundamentals of nursing.* Philadelphia, PA: Mosby.

Thompson, B. (2009). Test introduction and construction. In R. A. Wittmann-Price & M. Godshall (Eds.), *Certified nurse educator (CNE) review manual.* New York, NY: Springer Publishing.

CHAPTER 2

Medical–Surgical Nursing

PART I: Nursing Care of the Patient With a Cardiovascular Disorder

Karen K. Gittings and Brenda Reap Thompson

UNFOLDING CASE STUDY 1: Ruth Marie

Ruth Marie is a 68-year-old White female. While shopping at the mall with her daughter, she saw a health fair being advertised; it had healthy snacks available and free blood pressure (BP) screening. The nurse took her BP and told her that it was 164/96 mmHg. This was the first time Ruth Marie was told that her BP was elevated.

EXERCISE 2.1 Select all that apply:

Ruth Marie asks the nurse, "What causes high blood pressure?" The nurse explains that risk factors for primary hypertension (HTN) are:

A. Obesity
B. Narrowing of the aorta
C. Alcohol consumption
D. Sodium retention
E. Sleep apnea
F. Cigarette smoking

The answer can be found on page 119

eRESOURCE

To reinforce your understanding of the causes of high blood pressure, consult Medscape on your mobile device. [Pathway: Medscape ➔ select "Conditions" ➔ enter "Hypertension" in the search field ➔ select "Hypertension" ➔ select and review "Practice Essentials" and "Epidemiology."]

A few weeks later, Ruth Marie went to her primary care provider (PCP) and had her BP taken again. She was diagnosed with HTN and prescribed an angiotensin-converting enzyme (ACE) inhibitor and a thiazide diuretic. She was also placed on the DASH (Dietary Approaches to Stop Hypertension) diet.

EXERCISE 2.2 Multiple-choice:

Which statement made by Ruth Marie indicates an understanding of the low-sodium diet?

A. "I can still drink two glasses of tomato juice every morning."
B. "I will eat a few slices of cheese every day because it has protein."
C. "When I am too tired to cook, I will eat prepared frozen meals."
D. "I will begin eating cooked cereal for breakfast."

The answer can be found on page 119

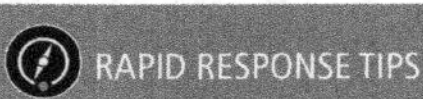
RAPID RESPONSE TIPS

DASH diet for hypertension

The DASH diet involves drinking more water and increasing one's intake of dietary fiber to decrease blood pressure. Daily intake should include the following:

- Grains: 7 to 8 servings
- Vegetables: 4 to 5 servings
- Fruits: 4 to 5 servings
- Low-fat or fat-free dairy foods: 2 to 3 servings
- Meat: 2 or fewer servings
- Nuts, seeds, dry beans: 4 to 5 servings per week

This increases fiber, calcium, potassium, and protein in the diet with decreased calories from fat.

eRESOURCE

To supplement your understanding of the DASH diet and patient teaching, consult Epocrates Online. [Pathway: https://online.epocrates.com ➔ select "Patient Resources" ➔ select "Cardiology & Vascular" ➔ scroll down to "Hypertension" ➔ scroll down to "Your Guide To Lowering Your Blood Pressure With DASH" and review content.]

Ruth Marie also had an EKG; her heart rate was 88 beats per minute (bpm) and regular and there were no abnormal findings.

EXERCISE 2.3 Multiple-choice:

The nurse can determine whether the patient's heart rate is regular by looking at the EKG rhythm strip and measuring the:

A. Distance from R wave to R wave
B. Distance from P wave to Q wave
C. Height of the R wave
D. Height of the T wave

The answer can be found on page 119

eRESOURCE

To practice interpreting EKGs, visit:

- EKG Library: http://goo.gl/fKVd
- Play ECG [EKG] Simulator: http://goo.gl/icSgp

Ruth Marie was very compliant and began walking short distances each morning. At her next office visit, her BP was 134/84 mmHg. She reported that she sometimes felt slightly light-headed. She was instructed by the nurse to sit on the side of her bed for a few minutes before getting up. During the head-to-toe assessment, it was also determined that Ruth Marie had peripheral venous disease of the lower extremities.

EXERCISE 2.4 Fill in the blanks:

Indicate which assessment findings are related to venous diseases by placing a V, or to arterial disease by placing an A where appropriate.

____ Capillary refill greater than 3 seconds
____ Pain with exercise
____ Lower leg edema
____ Cool to touch
____ Pallor with elevation
____ Bronze-brown pigment
____ Thickened, brittle nails
____ Frequent pruritus
____ Thin, shiny, dry skin
____ Absent pulses

The answer can be found on page 120

Even though her EKG was normal at rest, Ruth Marie was scheduled for a stress test because of vague chest pain with activity and positive risk factors. She will also have a lipid profile drawn and her risk factors will be reviewed.

EXERCISE 2.5 List:

Use the list on the right-hand side to categorize the risk factors for coronary artery disease (CAD):

Modifiable	Risk Factors
1. ________	A. Obesity
2. ________	B. Serum lipids: elevated triglycerides and cholesterol, decreased high-density lipoproteins (HDL)
3. ________	
4. ________	C. Race
5. ________	D. Family history
Nonmodifiable	E. Hypertension
1. ________	F. Tobacco use
2. ________	G. Physical inactivity
3. ________	H. Age

The answer can be found on page 120

---

eRESOURCE

To reinforce your understanding of the risk factors for CAD, consult Medscape on your mobile device. [Pathway: Medscape → select "Conditions" → enter "Coronary Artery Disease" in the search field → select "Risk Factors for Coronary Artery Disease" and review content.]

The nurse looked at Ruth Marie's laboratory results and interviewed her about her risk factors. Here are the results:

- Triglycerides and cholesterol were elevated; the high-density lipoproteins were decreased.
- BP was elevated, but is currently controlled with medication.
- The patient does not smoke.
- The patient did not exercise most of her life, but remained active around the house.
- The patient is within the normal weight range for her height.
- The patient is a 68-year-old White female, which means that she is at increased risk.
- The patient's mother had cardiac disease.

Ruth Marie is started on fenofibrate (TriCor), a drug that lowers blood lipids.

eRESOURCE

To learn more about adverse effects and precautions related to fenofibrate, refer to Epocrates:

- On mobile device. [Pathway: Epocrates → select "Drugs" → enter "Fenofibrate" in the search field → select "Fenofibrate" again → view "Adverse Reactions" and "Contraindications/ Cautions."]
- Online. [Pathway: http://online.epocrates.com → enter "Fenofibrate" in the search field → select "Fenofibrate" again → view "Adverse Reactions" and "Contraindications/Cautions."]

A week after her visit, Ruth Marie had a stress test with nuclear imaging that indicated cardiac ischemia. She had some chest discomfort during the stress test, which was 6 on a scale of 1 to 10. The pain was relieved with rest; otherwise she would have received nitroglycerin (NTG) 1/150 mg. Ruth Marie is scheduled for a cardiac catheterization. A few days after the stress test, Ruth Marie states she is having palpitations and feeling heaviness in her chest. She was therefore taken to the emergency department (ED). On admission, her BP was 170/96 mmHg, pulse was 180, respiration was 24, and SaO_2 (oxygen saturation) was 90%.

EXERCISE 2.6 **Multiple-choice:**

The following are prescribed orders for Ruth Marie. Which order should the nurse question?

A. Nasal oxygen 2 L
B. Aspirin (ASA) 81 mg enteric-coated orally, stat
C. Portable chest x-ray
D. Nitroglycerin (NTG) 1/150 mg sublingual, stat

The answer can be found on page 120

The EKG shows supraventricular tachycardia at a rate of 180 beats/min.

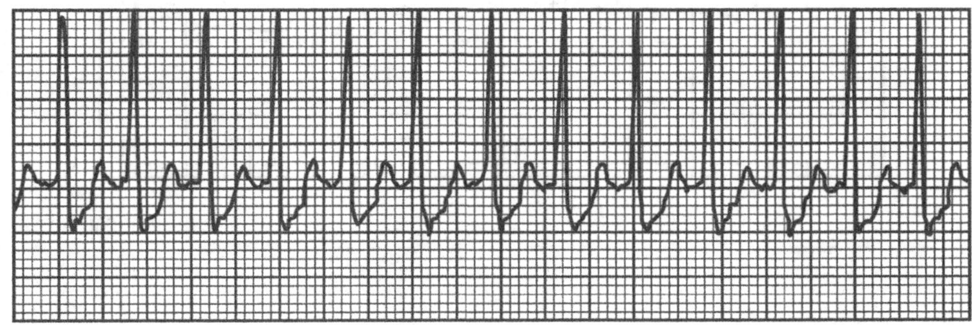

EXERCISE 2.7 Multiple-choice:

In preparing to administer adenosine (Adenocard), the nurse prioritizes which intervention?

A. Inserting an intravenous (IV) line in the nondominant hand
B. Calling anesthesia to sedate the patient
C. Placing a defibrillator with pacing capability at the patient's bedside
D. Mixing the adenosine in 50 mL of D_5W (5% dextrose and water)

The answer can be found on page 121

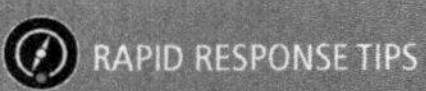

Adenosine (Adenocard)

Monitor the patient closely while administering the intravenous (IV) medication because bradycardia, hypotension, and dyspnea may be observed.

While the medication is being administered, the nurse runs a rhythm strip in order to assess for possible side effects. The rhythm strip is also used for documentation on the chart.

After the medication was administered, Ruth Marie's cardiac rate slowed. The EKG was then analyzed.

EXERCISE 2.8 Hot spot:

Indicate the area on the cardiac rhythm strip that demonstrates acute myocardial infarction (MI).

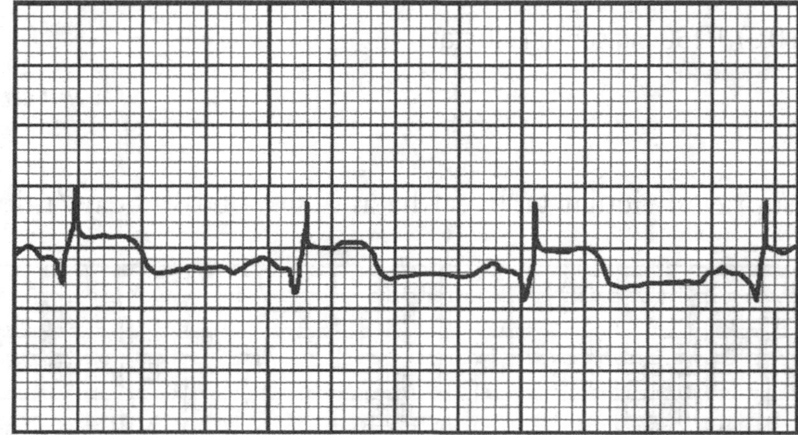

The answer can be found on page 121

EXERCISE 2.9 Select all that apply:

The EKG indicates myocardial injury in leads V_2 to V_4. The nurse understands that the patient should be observed for:

A. First-degree block
B. Third-degree block

C. Bradydysrhythmias
D. Heart failure
E. Ventricular dysrhythmias
F. Cardiogenic shock

The answer can be found on page 121

---

eRESOURCE

To reinforce your knowledge about EKG interpretation, view:

- *Intro EKG Interpretation Part 1*: http://youtu.be/ex1k_MPF-w4
- *Intro EKG Interpretation Part 2*: http://youtu.be/ecTM2O940mg

EXERCISE 2.10 Calculation:

Ruth Marie is prescribed a nitroglycerin (NTG) drip of 50 mg in 250 mL D_5W. The order is to infuse at 100 mcg/min. What flow rate in milliliters per hour would be needed to deliver this amount?

The answer can be found on page 121

---

eRESOURCE

Use MedCalc to verify your answer. [Pathway: www.medcalc.com select "Fluids/Electrolytes" → select "IV Rate" and enter information into fields.]

Ruth Marie is being prepared for cardiac catheterization. Acetylcysteine is ordered to be administered in citrus juice.

EXERCISE 2.11 Multiple-choice:

Ruth Marie drinks the medication and asks the nurse why it was prescribed. Which statement by the nurse would be appropriate?

A. "It helps to keep your airway clear during the procedure."
B. "It is used to protect your kidneys from the contrast."
C. "It will help you to breathe slowly and relax."
D. "It is used to keep the heart rate regular."

The answer can be found on page 122

The right femoral area is the site used for the cardiac catheterization and angioplasty.

The cardiac catheterization showed multiple blockages in the left anterior descending artery. At angioplasty, the placement of three stents produced a positive outcome for coronary revascularization.

EXERCISE 2.12 Select all that apply:

The nurse is caring for Ruth Marie after the percutaneous revascularization procedure. Which action is appropriate?

A. Check the pulses of the affected extremity
B. Check the color of the affected extremity
C. Encourage the patient to increase fluid intake
D. Encourage the patient to ambulate with assistance
E. Keep the head of the bed elevated at least 30°
F. Assess for bleeding or hematoma at the catheter insertion site

The answer can be found on page 122

EXERCISE 2.13 Multiple-choice:

The charge nurse is making assignments for the following shift. Ruth Marie is 2 hours post-revascularization with heparin and nitroglycerin (NTG) infusion. Her vital signs are stable, but a hematoma has developed at the catheter insertion site. It would be most appropriate to assign this patient to:

A. A recently graduated RN who started orientation 2 days ago
B. An experienced RN who recently transferred to the unit from the post-anesthesia care unit (PACU)
C. A licensed practical nurse (LPN) who has been working on the unit for 1 year
D. An RN who was pulled for the shift from a genitourinary (GU)/renal unit

The answer can be found on page 122

A few hours after Ruth Marie returns from the cardiac catheterization, the nurse notes the following rhythm on the cardiac monitor:

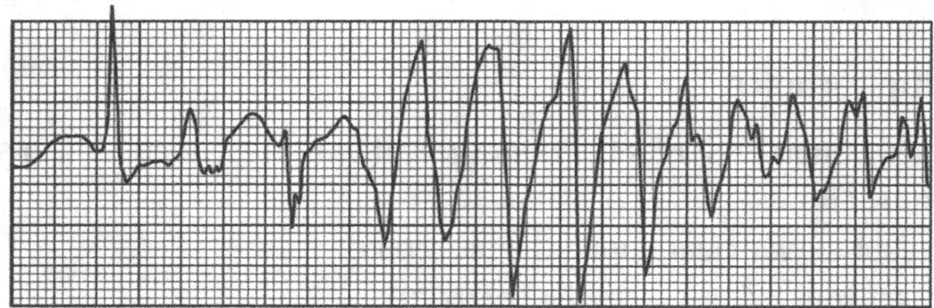

EXERCISE 2.14 Multiple-choice:

Which action would the nurse take first?

A. Call a code
B. Obtain the code cart
C. Check the patient
D. Turn on the defibrillator

The answer can be found on page 123

The nurse found that an electrode became disconnected. It was replaced, and the patient was in normal sinus rhythm (NSR).

EXERCISE 2.15 Fill in the blanks:

The nurse is reviewing medications with Ruth Marie. What should the nurse teach the patient about taking nitroglycerin (NTG) 1/150 sublingually?

____

____

____

____

____

The answer can be found on page 123

eRESOURCE

To reinforce your understanding of what the nurse should include in patient teaching, consult:

- PocketRx on you mobile device. [Pathway: PocketRx → select "Search" → select "Drugs" tab → enter "Nitroglycerin" → select "Nitroglycerin sl tablet" scroll down and select "Patient Information."]
- Epocrates Online. [Pathway: http://online.epocrates.com → select "Drugs" tab → enter "Nitroglycerin" → select "Nitroglycerin" again → select "Patient Education" and review material.]

Today Ruth Marie is being discharged from the hospital; her status is post-acute anterior MI with stent placement.

EXERCISE 2.16 Multiple-choice:

In preparing the patient for discharge, which intervention can be delegated to the unlicensed assistive personnel (UAP)?

A. Review activity instructions given by the MD
B. Arrange for a follow-up appointment with the cardiologist
C. Removal of the hemostatic dressing and application of a new dressing
D. Measurement of the predischarge vital signs

The answer can be found on page 123

Three months later, Ruth Marie is admitted following a second acute MI. She is currently exhibiting signs and symptoms of heart failure.

EXERCISE 2.17 Matching:

Indicate which assessment findings are related to right-sided or left-sided heart failure.

Column A	Column B
A. Right-sided heart failure	_______ Anasarca
B. Left-sided heart failure	_______ Jugular venous distention
	_______ Edema of lower extremities
	_______ Dyspnea
	_______ Hepatomegaly
	_______ Dry, hacking cough
	_______ Restlessness, confusion
	_______ Right-upper-quadrant pain
	_______ Crackles on auscultation of lungs
	_______ Weight gain
	_______ S3 and S4 heart sounds
	_______ Pink, frothy sputum

The answer can be found on page 123

eRESOURCE

To reinforce your understanding of heart failure, consult Medscape on your mobile device. [Pathway: Medscape ➔ select "Conditions" ➔ enter "Heart Failure" in the search field ➔ select "Heart Failure" ➔ select "Clinical Presentation" and review content.]

The nurse receives the following orders for Ruth Marie:

- 12-lead EKG
- Portable chest x-ray (PCXR)
- Echocardiogram
- Basic metabolic panel (BMP), troponin, and B-type natriuretic peptide (BNP)

EXERCISE 2.18 Exhibit-format:

12-lead EKG—Atrial fibrillation with a ventricular rate of 170

Portable chest x-ray (PCXR)—Congestion with Kerley B lines noted

Echocardiogram—Ejection fraction (EF) of 40%

B-type natriuretic peptide (BNP)—720 pg/mL

After receiving further orders from the MD, the nurse understands that the priority intervention is to:

A. Keep the head of the bed elevated greater than 30°
B. Obtain the patient's weight before giving the diuretic

C. Insert a Foley catheter for hourly input and output (I&O)
D. Administer medication to slow the heart rate

The answer can be found on page 124

After a bolus of diltiazem (Cardizem) 15 mg is given to slow the heart rate, Ruth Marie's BP falls to 84/50 mmHg. She is complaining of midsternal chest pain of seven on a scale of 1 to 10. The decision is made to perform cardioversion.

EXERCISE 2.19 Select all that apply:

Identify which interventions are a priority for the patient undergoing emergent cardioversion:

A. Verify that the defibrillator is in sync mode
B. Monitor the patient's airway and breathing
C. Keep the patient NPO (nothing orally) for at least 4 hours
D. Confirm that suction is set up and ready for use
E. Call anesthesia to intubate the patient before the procedure
F. Perform frequent assessment of vital signs

The answer can be found on page 124

eRESOURCE

To reinforce your understanding of cardioversion, consult Medscape on your mobile device. [Pathway: Medscape → select "Procedures" → enter "Cardioversion" into the search field → select "Defibrillation and Cardioversion" and review content.]

Ruth Marie was successfully cardioverted, but remains hypotensive and in acute heart failure. An order is received to begin a dobutamine drip at 5 mcg/kg/min. Ruth Marie will be transferred to the coronary care unit when a bed is assigned.

EXERCISE 2.20 Calculation:

A dobutamine drip is ordered to be started at 5 mcg/kg/min. The medication is mixed at 500 mg in 500 mL of fluid. If the patient weighs 176 lb, what flow rate in milliliters per hour would be needed to deliver this amount?

The answer can be found on page 124

eRESOURCE

Use MedCalc to verify your answer. [Pathway: www.medcalc.com select "Fluids/Electrolytes" → select "IV Rate" and enter information into fields.]

KEY TAKEAWAY POINTS

Hypertension

- Defined as a blood pressure (BP) of 140/90 mmHg or higher
- Diagnosis as defined by the Seventh Report of Joint National Committee (JNC 7) is based on the average of two or more BP measurements taken during two or more visits/contacts with a health care provider.
- Primary or essential hypertension (HTN) occurs when there is no identified cause; occurs in 95% of patients diagnosed with HTN.
- Secondary HTN, diagnosed in 5% of patients, is a high BP secondary to an identified cause.
- There are typically no signs or symptoms of HTN until organ damage has occurred.
- Treatment begins with lifestyle modifications, including the Dietary Approaches to Stop Hypertension (DASH) diet, and pharmacologic therapy.
- The goal for diabetic patients is a BP of less than 130/80 mmHg.

Coronary Artery Disease

- Risk factors are either modifiable or nonmodifiable.
- Factors that cannot be controlled are age, gender, race, and family history.
- Modifiable risk factors include diabetes, HTN, smoking, obesity, physical activity, and high cholesterol.
- Classic signs of myocardial ischemia include chest pain, shortness of breath, extreme fatigue, diaphoresis, nausea, and vomiting.
- Women, diabetic patients, and the elderly frequently do not exhibit the typical signs and symptoms.
- Treatment is aimed at modifying those risk factors that can be controlled.

Myocardial Infarction

- Myocardial infarction (MI) occurs when an area of the myocardium is permanently destroyed, usually as a result of a ruptured atherosclerotic plaque and subsequent occlusion of a coronary artery caused by a thrombus.
- *Acute coronary syndrome* is the term used to identify the continuum that exists between unstable angina and an acute MI.
- The most common presenting symptom in those having an acute MI is chest pain that occurs suddenly and continues despite rest and medication.
- Myocardial injury is seen on the EKG as ST segment elevation (greater than 1 mm above the isoelectric line).
- A pathological Q wave (0.04 seconds or longer, 25% of the R-wave depth, or did not previously exist) represents myocardial necrosis.

(*continued*)

- Troponin I and T levels are laboratory markers specific for myocardial injury; levels increase in 3 to 4 hours and return to normal in 1 to 3 weeks.
- Medical management includes MONA: morphine, oxygen, nitrates, and aspirin.
- The goal is to restore blood supply to the myocardium through thrombolytic therapy, percutaneous coronary interventions, or coronary artery revascularization.

Heart Failure

- Systolic heart failure, which is an alteration in ventricular contraction, is characterized by a weak heart muscle.
- Diastolic heart failure is characterized by a stiff and noncompliant heart muscle, which makes it difficult for the ventricle to fill.
- A normal EF is 55% to 65%; this decreases with systolic heart failure, but may remain normal with diastolic failure.
- Major risk factors are age, male gender, HTN, left ventricular hypertrophy, MI, valvular heart disease, and obesity.
- Signs and symptoms relate to whether the failure is left sided or right sided.
- Diagnostic evaluation includes a chest x-ray, EKG, echocardiogram, laboratory tests, and right-sided heart catheterization.
- Lifestyle changes that are recommended include dietary sodium restriction, control of fluid intake, avoidance of smoking and alcohol use, weight reduction, and exercise.
- Ace inhibitors, beta-blockers, diuretics, and digitalis are routinely prescribed for systolic heart failure; medications for diastolic failure depend on the cause.

Dysrhythmias

- Dysrhythmias, also called *arrhythmias*, cause disturbances of the heart rate, rhythm, or both.
- Sinus dysrhythmias occur at the sinus node; they do not generally require treatment unless the patient becomes symptomatic.
- Atrial dysrhythmias arise from the atria and often result in rapid heart rates.
- Atrial fibrillation is a rapid, disorganized rhythm that causes a loss of atrial kick, resulting in a reduction in cardiac output by 25% to 30%.
- Patients in atrial fibrillation for longer than 48 hours should be anticoagulated before attempting cardioversion to minimize the risk of an embolus.
- Ventricular dysrhythmias arise from the ventricles and can be deadly for the patient.
- Ventricular fibrillation causes ineffective quivering of the ventricles resulting in no appreciable cardiac output.
- Cardioversion can be done electively or emergently for dysrhythmias such as atrial flutter, atrial fibrillation, or supraventricular tachycardia (SVT).

(*continued*)

- Cardioversion is timed or synchronized to deliver the energy on the QRS complex or during ventricular depolarization; energy delivered on the vulnerable T wave could lead to ventricular fibrillation.
- Defibrillation is done emergently for pulseless ventricular tachycardia or ventricular fibrillation; synchronization is not required.

PART II: Nursing Care of the Patient With a Pulmonary Disorder

Nina Russell and Brenda Reap Thompson

UNFOLDING CASE STUDY 2: Max

Jeannette is a new nurse on a medical–surgical care unit. Mark, her preceptor, asks her to assess the patient's lungs.

EXERCISE 2.21 Hot spot:

Indicate where the nurse should place the stethoscope in order to auscultate for the following:

A. Bronchial breath sounds
B. Vesicular breath sounds
C. Bronchovesicular breath sounds

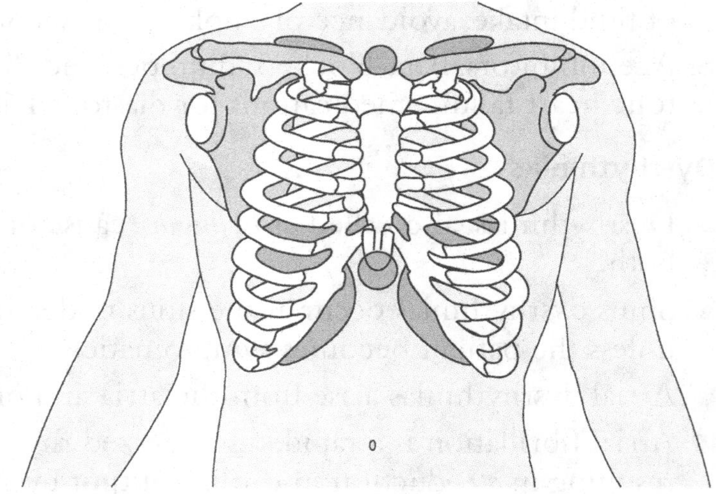

The answer can be found on page 125

eRESOURCE

To hear samples of lung sounds go to:

- *Vesicular—Normal*: http://goo.gl/ZN2bfD
- *Vesicular—Diminished*: http://goo.gl/iMjcBJ
- *Bronchial*: http://goo.gl/W0inZw
- *Bronchovesicular:* http://goo.gl/0laTwY

eRESOURCE

To reinforce your understanding of the assessment of the pulmonary system as well as the auscultation of lung sounds, consult the online *Merck Manual.* [Pathway: www.merckmanuals.com/professional ➔ select "Medical Topics" ➔ select "Pulmonary Disorders" ➔ select "Approach to the Pulmonary Patient" and review content.]

It is important for Jeannette to understand why different masks are used.

EXERCISE 2.22 Matching:

Match the reason for oxygen delivery in Column A to the method of oxygenation in Column B:

Column A	Column B
A. Rarely used; may be used to deliver oxygen for a patient who has a wired jaw	_______ Partial rebreather mask
B. Delivers fixed prescribed oxygen rates	_______ Nonrebreather mask
C. Reservoir bag has a one-way valve that prevents exhaled air from entering the reservoir; it allows for larger concentrations of oxygen to be inhaled from the reservoir bag	_______ Face tent
D. Reservoir bag connected to the mask collects one third of the patient's exhaled air; carbon dioxide is used as a respiratory stimulant	_______ Venturi mask

The answer can be found on page 125

eRESOURCE

To reinforce your understanding of oxygen delivery and the methods utilized, review:

- *Clinical Guidelines (Nursing)*: http://goo.gl/7jQrlh
- American Thoracic Society's, *Oxygen Delivery Methods*: http://goo.gl/slVAzx

Jeanette and Mark complete an admission assessment for a 22-year-old patient named Max. Max has possible tuberculosis (TB). He is homeless and has been living in a shelter since he lost his job last year.

EXERCISE 2.23 Select all that apply:

Which clinical manifestations are consistent with active tuberculosis (TB)?

A. Dyspnea
B. Night sweats
C. Fatigue
D. Low-grade fevers
E. Productive bloody sputum

F. Unexplained weight loss
G. Anorexia
H. Wheezing

The answer can be found on page 125

---

eRESOURCE

To reinforce your understanding of the clinical presentation of active TB, consult Univadis. [Pathway ➔ www.univadis.com ➔ select "References" ➔ enter "TB" into the search field ➔ select "Tuberculosis (TB)" ➔ select "Symptoms and Signs" and review content.]

The health care provider orders a Mantoux skin test (tuberculin test) to be performed intradermally.

EXERCISE 2.24 Multiple-choice:

Which statement is accurate regarding the Mantoux skin test?

A. A positive Mantoux test confirms active tuberculosis (TB)
B. The test is read within 24 hours of placement
C. An induration of 10 mm or greater indicates a positive skin test
D. An induration of 15 mm in immunocompromised patients is considered a positive test

The answer can be found on page 126

---

eRESOURCE

To learn more about this procedure, listen to/watch the Centers for Disease Control pod/vodcast:

- Audio only: http://goo.gl/6g2wtE
- Video: http://goo.gl/8rAcxJ

Max had a positive skin test and, therefore, precautions are indicated. Jeannette collects a sputum specimen to test for acid-fast bacilli (AFB).

EXERCISE 2.25 Multiple-choice:

Which statement by a student nurse needs follow-up regarding precautions for a patient with possible tuberculosis (TB)?

A. "The patient will be isolated in a negative pressure room."
B. "The nurse will wear a high-efficiency particulate air (HEPA) mask."
C. "The airborne isolation sign will be placed at the entrance to the patient's room."
D. "The patient will wear a N95 mask when leaving the room."

The answer can be found on page 126

Max is diagnosed with TB and placed on a multimedication regimen.

EXERCISE 2.26 Multiple-choice:

Which instruction will the nurse give the patient in regard to rifampin (Rifadin)?

A. The medication may turn your urine red-orange.
B. The medication may cause short-term memory loss.
C. The medication should be taken with food.
D. The medication may increase your appetite.

The answer can be found on page 126

---

eRESOURCE

To supplement your understanding of patient education for rifampin, refer to Epocrates Online. [Pathway: http://online.epocrates.com ➔ enter "Rifampin" in the search field ➔ select "Rifampin" again ➔ select "Patient Education" and view content.]

Later that day, Max tells the nurse that he would like to go back to the shelter as soon as possible because he does not like being in the hospital. He has been taking his medication for 2 weeks and is feeling better.

EXERCISE 2.27 Multiple-choice:

Which statement by the nurse is correct?

A. "You will be discharged when you stop coughing up secretions."
B. "Discharge will depend on the results of the chest x-ray."
C. "Most patients are discharged after taking their medication for 48 hours."
D. "Patients are discharged after three negative acid-fast bacilli (AFB) smears."

The answer can be found on page 126

Max is ready to be discharged. Jeannette and Mark complete the discharge teaching.

EXERCISE 2.28 Multiple-choice:

Which of the following statements indicate that the patient understands appropriate care measures?

A. "One medication can be substituted for another because they all fight infection."
B. "A sputum specimen will need to be collected every 2 to 4 weeks indefinitely."
C. "Medication will need to be taken for a 6- to 12-month duration."
D. "A standardized mask will need to be worn until medication therapy is completed."

The answer can be found on page 127

---

eRESOURCE

To reinforce your understanding of the treatment of TB, consult the online *Merck Manual*. [Pathway: www.merckmanuals.com/professional ➔ select "Medical Topics" ➔ select "Communicable

Diseases" → enter "TB" into the search field → select "Tuberculosis (TB)" → select "Treatment" and review content.]

UNFOLDING CASE STUDY 3: Dean

Tanya, a nurse working in the ED, assesses Dean, a 19-year-old who was hurt while playing football with his friends. Dean began to complain of dyspnea and pain in the left rib area after being tackled.

EXERCISE 2.29 Fill in the blanks:

Name four causes of a closed pneumothorax.

1. __________
2. __________
3. __________
4. __________

The answer can be found on page 127

EXERCISE 2.30 Fill in the blanks:

Name two causes of an open pneumothorax.

1. __________
2. __________

The answer can be found on page 127

The assessment findings are as follows—BP: 137/84 mmHg, pulse: 106, respiration rate (RR): 36, and pulse oximeter: 94%. Dean is sent to radiology for a chest x-ray.

Tanya understands that various complications can arise from a thoracic injury.

EXERCISE 2.31 Matching:

Match the manifestation in Column A to the complication in Column B:

Column A	Column B
A. Muffled distant heart sounds, hypotension	______ Flail chest
B. Deviation of the trachea, air hunger	______ Hemothorax
C. Paradoxical movement of the chest wall	______ Tension pneumothorax
D. Shock, dullness on percussion	______ Cardiac tamponade

The answer can be found on page 127

eRESOURCE

To reinforce your understanding of the causes and treatment of pneumothorax, consult the online *Merck Manual*. [Pathway: www.merckmanuals.com/professional → select "Medical Topics" → select "Pulmonary Disorders" → enter "Pneumothorax" into the search field → review content related to pneumothorax, traumatic pneumothorax, open pneumothorax, and tension pneumothorax.]

The x-ray confirms that Dean has a fractured left rib, but no pneumothorax is noted.

EXERCISE 2.32 Select all that apply:

Which findings will the nurse anticipate in a patient suffering from a fractured rib?

A. Pain during inspiration
B. Shallow, rapid respirations
C. Crackles to bilateral lower lobes
D. Splinting or guarding the chest

The answer can be found on page 127

Dean is advised to take analgesics as ordered to provide relief and facilitate adequate respirations.

eRESOURCE

To reinforce your understanding of the clinical presentation associated with a rib fracture, consult Medscape on your mobile device. [Pathway: Medscape → select "Conditions" → enter "Rib Fracture" in the search field → select and review "Clinical Presentation."]

UNFOLDING CASE STUDY 4: Mr. Williams

Jeannette is assessing Mr. Williams, who was recently diagnosed with chronic obstructive pulmonary disease (COPD). Mr. Williams states that he has smoked for 20 years and is employed by a chemical company. He also says that there were no safety regulations at the plant until 5 years ago.

EXERCISE 2.33 Fill in the blanks:

What are the differences between chronic bronchitis and emphysema?

Chronic bronchitis: ______________________________

____

____

Emphysema: ______________________________

____

____

The answer can be found on page 128

EXERCISE 2.34 List:

Identify which clinical manifestations are related to chronic obstructive pulmonary disease (COPD) and which are related to asthma.

A. Onset is at 40 to 50 years of age
B. Dyspnea is always experienced during exercise
C. Clinical symptoms are intermittent from day to day
D. There is frequent sputum production
E. Weight loss is characteristic
F. There is a history of allergies, rhinitis, and eczema
G. Disability worsens progressively

COPD	Asthma
________________	________________
________________	________________

The answer can be found on page 128

eRESOURCE

To reinforce your understanding of the symptomology of COPD, consult Medscape on your mobile device. [Pathway: Medscape ➔ select "Conditions" ➔ enter "COPD" in the search field ➔ select "COPD" ➔ select and review "Overview" and "Clinical Presentation."]

Jeannette notes that the patient is orthopneic, has a nonproductive cough, and has an increased anteroposterior (AP) diameter.

EXERCISE 2.35 Multiple-choice:

The nurse's findings are most consistent with which diagnosis?

A. Tuberculosis (TB)
B. Chronic obstructive pulmonary disease (COPD)
C. Pneumonia
D. Congestive heart failure (CHF)

The answer can be found on page 128

Jeannette observes that the patient is on a Venturi mask. The patient's wife asks Jeannette, "Why does my husband have this mask instead of a nasal cannula like he does at home?"

EXERCISE 2.36 Multiple-choice:

Which statement by the nurse demonstrates understanding of oxygen delivery via Venturi mask?

A. "Using a Venturi mask will prevent the nasal mucosa from drying and reduce coughing."
B. "The Venturi mask provides a low-flow oxygen delivery system."
C. "The Venturi mask provides a consistent, precise concentration of oxygen to maintain respiratory drive."
D. "The Venturi mask is a high-flow system that flushes the expired carbon dioxide out of the mask preventing further retention."

The answer can be found on page 128

eRESOURCE

To reinforce your understanding of oxygen delivery and the methods used, review:

- *Clinical Guidelines (Nursing)*: http://goo.gl/7jQrlh
- American Thoracic Society's *Oxygen Delivery Methods*: http://goo.gl/sIVAzx

Mr. Williams is at increased risk of complications from COPD.

EXERCISE 2.37 Matching:

Match the associated factors in Column A to the complication in Column B:

Column A	Column B
A. Fever, increased cough, dyspnea	_______ Cor pulmonale
B. Occurs in patients who have chronic retention of CO_2	_______ Acute respiratory failure or corticosteroid therapy
C. Occurs in patients who discontinue use of a bronchodilator	_______ Peptic ulcer disease
D. Administration of benzodiazepines, sedatives, narcotics	
E. Crackles are audible in the bases of the lungs	

The answer can be found on page 129

eRESOURCE

To reinforce your understanding of the symptomology of COPD, consult Medscape on your mobile device. [Pathway: Medscape → select "Conditions" → enter "COPD" in the search field → select "COPD" → select and review "Follow-up" → select "Complications" and review content.]

PART III: Nursing Care of the Patient With Renal Disease

Karen K. Gittings and Brenda Reap Thompson

UNFOLDING CASE STUDY 5: Fran

Fran, a 36-year-old mother of three, has had two urinary tract infections (UTIs) over the past few years, both occurred during pregnancy. She now has symptoms of a UTI again. Medical history includes:

Allergy: penicillin

Lifestyle: cigarette smoking—1.5 packs/day since age 16 years

Alcoholic beverages: beer on weekends
Past medical history: eczema on arms and legs, frequent UTIs

The nurse at the clinic understands that clinical manifestations are related to the location of the UTI.

EXERCISE 2.38 Matching:

Match the clinical manifestations in Column A with the types of urinary tract infections (UTI) in Column B:

Column A	Column B
A. Flank pain, fever, vomiting	____ Pyelonephritis
B. Urgency, painful bladder, frequency	____ Glomerulonephritis
C. Purulent discharge, dysuria, urgency	____ Urethritis
D. Hematuria, proteinuria, elevated creatinine	____ Interstitial cystitis

The answer can be found on page 129

Fran has interstitial cystitis. The nurse instructs Fran to drink more fluid because this will dilute the urine and make the bladder less irritable. It will also increase the frequency of urination, which will help to flush out bacteria. The nurse also instructs Fran to apply a heating pad to the suprapubic area at the lowest setting. Finally, the nurse discusses dietary changes that may prevent bladder irritation.

eRESOURCE

To reinforce your understanding of the treatment and management of interstitial cystitis, consult Medscape on your mobile device. [Pathway: Medscape ➔ enter "Cystitis" in the search field ➔ select "Interstitial Cystitis" ➔ select and review "Treatment & Management."]

EXERCISE 2.39 Select all that apply:

The nurse is providing Fran with information about bladder irritants. Fran would be instructed to avoid:

A. Caffeine
B. Alcohol
C. Milk
D. Chocolate
E. Spicy foods
F. Legumes

The answer can be found on page 129

eRESOURCE

To reinforce your understanding of foods that are bladder irritants, consult Medscape on your mobile device. [Pathway: Medscape ➔ enter "Cystitis" in the search field ➔ select "Interstitial Cystitis" ➔ select "Treatment & Management" ➔ select and review "Dietary Therapy."]

The nurse understands that UTIs can cause symptoms related to the emptying or storage of urine.

EXERCISE 2.40 **Fill in the blanks:**

What four questions would the nurse ask to determine whether Fran has problems with urinary emptying?

1. ______________________________
2. ______________________________
3. ______________________________
4. ______________________________

What four questions would the nurse ask to determine whether Fran has problems with urinary storage?

1. ______________________________
2. ______________________________
3. ______________________________
4. ______________________________

The answer can be found on page 129

Since Fran has had three UTIs, it would be important to teach her health-promotion activities that could decrease the incidence of infection.

EXERCISE 2.41 **Select all that apply:**

What health-promotion activities could the nurse teach the patient?

A. Empty the bladder every 6 hours
B. Evacuate the bowel regularly
C. Wipe the perineal area from front to back
D. Urinate before and after intercourse
E. Drink cranberry juice daily
F. Shower rather than bathe in the tub

The answer can be found on page 130

EXERCISE 2.42 Hot spot:

What area would the nurse percuss to assess for kidney infection?

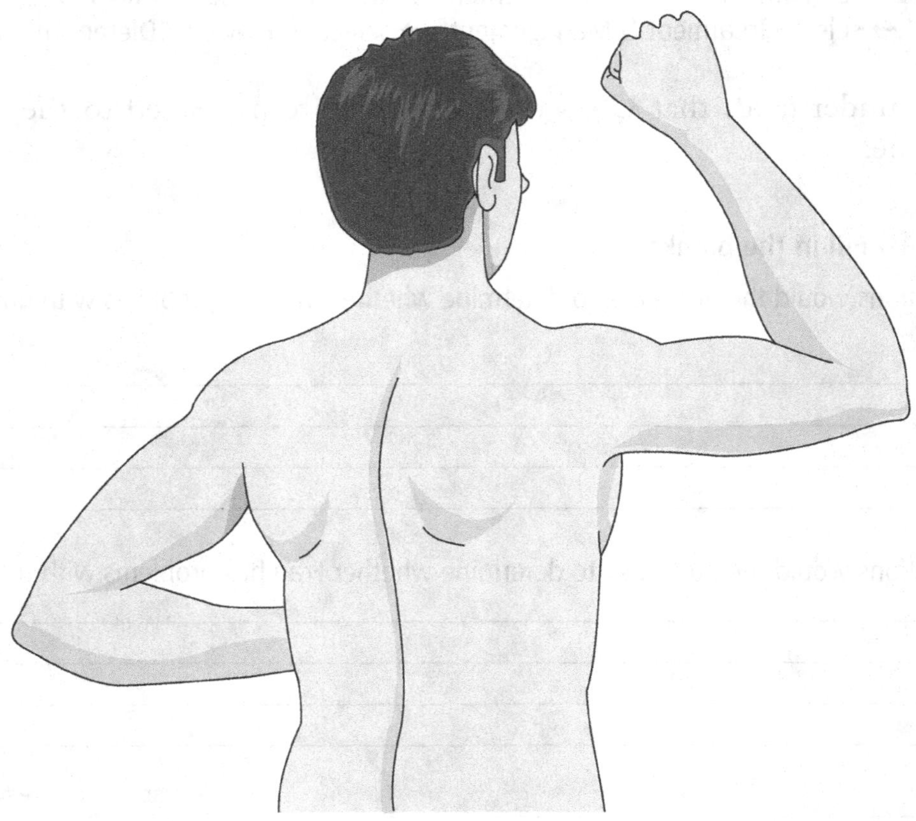

The answer can be found on page 130

eRESOURCE

To reinforce your understanding of the clinical presentation of a kidney infection (acute pyelonephritis), consult:

- Epocrates Online. [Pathway: http://online.epocrates.com ➔ select "Diseases" ➔ select "Nephrology" ➔ select "Acute Pyelonephritis" ➔ review content under "Basics" and "Diagnosis."]
- Medscape on your mobile device. [Pathway: Medscape ➔ enter "Pyelonephritis" in the search field ➔ select "Acute Pyelonephritis" ➔ select "Overview" and review content.]

Six months after her visit, Fran is taken to the ED in the middle of the night with nausea, vomiting, hematuria, and abdominal pain. Her skin is cool and moist. She said that she had been out in the sun doing yard work for the previous 2 days. A renal ultrasound indicates that she has urinary calculi.

EXERCISE 2.43 Select all that apply:

Fran asks the nurse what causes urinary calculi. Which of the following answers from the nurse are correct?

A. Low fluid intake
B. Decreased uric acid levels
C. Warm climate
D. Family history for renal calculi
E. Immobility
F. Frequent urination

The answer can be found on page 131

eRESOURCE

To learn more about factors contributing to the formation of renal calculi, refer to:

- Epocrates Online. [Pathway: http://online.epocrates.com → select "Diseases" → enter "Renal Calculi" into the search field → select "Risk Factors" and review content.]
- *Merck Manual.* [Pathway: www.merckmanuals.com → select "Medical Topics" → select "Genitourinary Disorders" → enter "Renal Calculi" into the search field → select "Renal Calculi" → review "Etiology" and "Pathophysiology."]

Intense colicky pain may be present when the stone is passing down the ureter. Lithotripsy is sometimes recommended to break up the stones if they are too large to pass. Hematuria is common after lithotripsy. A stent is usually inserted to facilitate passage of the stones and decrease stenosis. The stents are removed after about 2 weeks because they pose an increased risk of infection. The ultrasound results can determine whether the stones are small enough to pass through the ureter into the bladder.

KEY TAKEAWAY POINTS

Urinary Tract Infections (UTIs)

- Upper UTIs (pyelonephritis, renal abscesses, interstitial nephritis) are less common, but may be more severe than lower UTIs (cystitis, prostatitis, and urethritis).
- In most hospital-acquired UTIs, the cause is frequently instrumentation of the urinary tract or catheterization.
- Clinical manifestations include dysuria, burning on urination, frequency, urgency, nocturia, incontinence, hematuria, and suprapubic or pelvic pain.
- Diagnosis is made by urine culture and sensitivity (C&S).
- Medical treatment involves antibiotics; pyelonephritis usually requires a longer course of treatment.

(continued)

- Preventive measures include showers rather than tub baths, females cleaning from front to back, liberal intake of fluids, avoidance of urinary tract irritants (coffee, tea, colas, alcohol), void every 2 to 3 hours and after intercourse, and acidify the urine with vitamin C or cranberry juice.

Renal Calculi

- Stones form more often in dehydrated persons.
- Clinical manifestations depend on the location of the stone, presence of obstruction, infection, and edema, but can include pain and discomfort, hematuria, nausea, vomiting, and diarrhea.
- Diagnosis is made by x-rays of the kidneys, ureters, and bladder (KUB); ultrasound; or urography/pyelography.
- Medical treatment involves opioid analgesics and stone removal.
- Most patients can pass a stone 0.5 to 1 cm in diameter; larger stones can be removed through ureteroscopy, extracorporeal shock wave lithotripsy (ESWL), or endourologic methods.
- Urine should be strained and stones sent for analysis; calcium-based stones are the most common.

Preventive measures for all stone types include increasing fluid intake to avoid dehydration, drinking two glasses of water at bedtime, maintaining a urine output of greater than 2 L/d, and possible diet restrictions based on stone type.

UNFOLDING CASE STUDY 6: Joe

Joe, 62 years old, has a history of smoking and is being examined for a bladder tumor. Bladder cancer is most common in men 60 to 70 years of age and is three times more common in men than in women.

EXERCISE 2.44 Fill in the blanks:

What information in Joe's history suggests an increased risk for bladder cancer?

____

____

____

The answer can be found on page 131

EXERCISE 2.45 Select all that apply:

Identify risk factors associated with bladder cancer:

A. Contaminated drinking water

B. Dehydration

C. Recurrent or chronic urinary tract infections (UTIs)
D. Exposure to environmental carcinogens
E. Diabetes
F. Pelvic radiation therapy

The answer can be found on page 131

The clinical manifestations of bladder cancer are intermittent hematuria that is not accompanied by pain, frequency, and urgency.

eRESOURCE

To reinforce your understanding of the clinical manifestations of bladder cancer, refer to Epocrates Online. [Pathway: http://online.epocrates.com ➔ select "Diseases" ➔ enter "Bladder Cancer" into the search field ➔ select "Risk Factors" and review content.]

Cystoscopy will be scheduled to determine whether the tumor in the bladder is cancer. Most bladder cancers are superficial; that is, they do not invade the wall of the bladder. These tumors respond well to treatment; however, the risk of recurrence is high. Before cystoscopy, the nurse checks to make sure that the patient has completed the consent form. Joe states that the procedure was explained to him and that he has no additional questions.

EXERCISE 2.46 Select all that apply:

What are the responsibilities of the nurse when the patient returns from cystoscopy?

A. Monitor for bright-red blood in the urine
B. Encourage the patient to change position slowly
C. Irrigate the catheter daily
D. Provide warm sitz baths
E. Monitor for signs of urinary tract infection (UTI)
F. Strain all urine for stones

The answer can be found on page 131

After the procedure, Joe is told that treatment is necessary but also that the tumor is superficial and small. Joe is scheduled for a transurethral resection of the tumor followed by intravesical administration of bacillus Calmette–Guérin (BCG).

EXERCISE 2.47 Multiple-choice:

Joe is receiving his first treatment with Bacillus Calmette–Guérin (BCG). It is evident that further teaching is needed when Joe states:

A. "I will have to have a catheter inserted to receive the treatment."
B. "I will need to retain this solution for 1.5 to 2 hours before voiding."
C. "I should drink large amounts of fluid before and during the treatment."
D. "I should change my position every 30 to 45 minutes during the treatment."

The answer can be found on page 131

KEY TAKEAWAY POINTS

Bladder Cancer

- Risk factors are cigarette smoking; exposure to environmental carcinogens; recurrent or chronic urinary tract infections; bladder stones; high urinary pH; high cholesterol intake; pelvic radiation therapy; and cancers in the colon, prostate, or rectum of males.
- The most common symptom is painless gross hematuria; changes in voiding or urine may also occur.
- Diagnosis is made by cystoscopy and biopsy.
- Simple, superficial tumors can be removed by transurethral resection or fulguration; invasive or multiple tumors require a cystectomy, removal of the bladder.
- Bacillus Calmette–Guérin, which is an attenuated live strain of *Mycobacterium bovis,* is an effective treatment for recurrent bladder cancer; it works by enhancing the body's immune response.

UNFOLDING CASE STUDY 7: Sarah

Rachel, a recent graduate from nursing school, is trying to provide safe and effective care for patients. Lynn, her mentor, is very helpful and understanding. However, Rachel must make many independent decisions because the unit is so busy.

EXERCISE 2.48 Multiple-choice:

Rachel has received reports on four patients. Which patient should be assessed first?

A. Sarah—blood pressure (BP): 88/60 mmHg, pulse: 124, respiratory rate (RR): 30; had a 100-mL urine output for more than 8 hours.
B. Coleen—temperature: 101°F (38.3°C); has blood in the urine with each void.
C. Theresa—blood urea nitrogen (BUN): 36 mg/dL, creatinine: 0.8 mg/dL; vomited 200 mL of undigested food 6 hours earlier.
D. Tyra—BP: 112/78 mmHg, pulse: 88, respiratory rate (RR): 24; is on diuretics and became slightly dizzy when getting up to void.

The answer can be found on page 132

The progress notes state that Sarah was vomiting for 5 days before admission. Her IV became dislodged 12 hours earlier, and she refuses to have it reinserted as she thought she would be able to tolerate liquids by mouth. She felt nauseous, so she drank only small sips of fluid.

EXERCISE 2.49 Fill in the blanks:

After reading Sarah's laboratory results in the left column, complete the laboratory interpretation in the middle column and the intervention in the right column.

Laboratory Results	Laboratory Interpretation	Intervention
Creatinine: 2.8 mg/dL (normal: 0.5–1.5)	____________________	____________________
Hemoglobin: 9.8 g/dL (normal adult women: 12–16 g/dL)	____________________	____________________
Hematocrit: 38% (normal: 38%–42%)	____________________	____________________
Serum potassium: 5.6 mEq/L (normal: 3.5–5.0 mEq/L)	____________________	____________________
Arterial blood gases (ABGs): pH: 7.32 (normal: 7.35–7.45) HCO_3: 19 (normal: 22–26) $PaCO_2$: 37 (normal: 35–45)	____________________	____________________

The answer can be found on page 132

eRESOURCE

To reinforce your understanding of laboratory studies relevant to dehydration, refer to Medscape on your mobile device. [Pathway: Medscape → select "Conditions"→ select "Dehydration" → select "Workup" → review "Laboratory Studies."]

Sarah is diagnosed with acute renal failure (ARF) related to dehydration. The health care provider (HCP) explains to Sarah the seriousness of her condition and the necessary treatment.

EXERCISE 2.50 Multiple-choice:

As her intravenous (IV) is being inserted, Sarah asks again why her kidneys are not working well. The nurse's best response is:

A. "This has occurred because you declined to have your IV reinserted."
B. "This has occurred because of damage to the glomeruli of the kidneys."
C. "Dehydration has decreased blood flow to the kidneys, resulting in damage."
D. "The high heart rate you are experiencing is detrimental to the kidneys."

The answer can be found on page 133

eRESOURCE

To reinforce your understanding of the causes and the clinical presentation of acute renal failure, refer to Epocrates Online. [Pathway: http://online.epocrates.com → under the "Diseases" tab, enter "Renal Failure" in the search field → select "Acute Renal Failure" → review "Highlights," "Basics," and "Diagnosis."]

EXERCISE 2.51 Matching:

Match the categories of acute renal failure (ARF) in Column A with the different causes of ARF in Column B:

Column A	Column B
A. Prerenal ARF	_______ Hemorrhage
B. Intrarenal ARF	_______ Heart failure
C. Postrenal ARF	_______ Radiopaque contrast agents
	_______ Calculi
	_______ Myoglobinuria
	_______ Benign prostatic hyperplasia
	_______ Nasogastric (NG) suction
	_______ Sepsis
	_______ Vomiting, diarrhea
	_______ Tumors
	_______ Acute pyelonephritis
	_______ Nonsteroidal anti-inflammatory drugs (NSAIDs)

The answer can be found on page 133

Sarah remains acutely ill. Her most recent labs are:

Laboratory Results	Arterial blood gases (ABGs):
Creatinine: 3.6 mg/dL	pH: 7.30
Hemoglobin: 9.6 g/dL	HCO_3: 17
Hematocrit: 38%	$PaCO_2$: 30
Serum potassium: 5.9 mEq/L	

EXERCISE 2.52 Multiple-choice:

After reviewing the laboratory results, the nurse prepares to call the health care provider (HCP). What is a priority for the nurse to communicate to the HCP?

A. Potassium: 5.9 mEq/L
B. Creatinine: 3.6 mg/dL
C. pH: 7.30
D. Hemoglobin: 9.6 g/dL

The answer can be found on page 134

eRESOURCE

To reinforce your understanding of laboratory studies relevant to acute renal failure, refer to Medscape on your mobile device. [Pathway: Medscape ➔ select "Conditions"➔ enter "Renal Failure" into the search field ➔ select "Acute Renal Failure Complications" and review content.]

RAPID RESPONSE TIPS

Situation, background, assessment, and recommendation

The situation, background, assessment and recommendation (SBAR) technique has been recognized as the best practice for standardized communication in health care by The Joint Commission. The SBAR technique provides an effective method for standardizing communication and bridging gaps in situations such as hand-offs, patient transfers, critical communications, and telephone calls. SBAR promotes quality and patient safety by improving communication efficiency and accuracy.

- *S*ituation—The patient has abnormal lab values.
- *B*ackground—The patient was admitted with a 5-day history of vomiting and she is now in ARF.
- *A*ssessment—Her lab values are as follows: potassium 5.9 mEq/L, creatinine 3.6 mg/dL, and pH 7.30.
- *R*ecommendation—I suggest a consult with nephrology and a line placement for dialysis; consider administering Kayexalate.

KEY TAKEAWAY POINTS

Acute Renal Failure (ARF)

- ARF is the abrupt loss of kidney function over a period of hours to days, but it is usually reversible.
- The major categories are prerenal caused by hypoperfusion, intrarenal caused by parenchymal damage, and postrenal caused by obstruction; acute tubular necrosis is the most common cause of ARF in hospitalized patients.
- Clinical manifestations include olguria (less than 500 mL urine output/d) or anuria (less than 50 mL urine output/d); increased creatinine, BUN, and other nitrogenous waste products; hyperkalemia; metabolic acidosis; calcium and phosphorous imbalances; fluid volume excess; failing blood pressure regulation; and anemia.
- Preventive measures include providing adequate hydration, preventing/treating hypotension promptly, monitoring urine output in hospitalized patients, monitoring renal function, preventing/treating infections promptly, catheter care with removal of catheter as soon as possible, and monitoring drug levels of nephrotoxic medications (such as gentamicin).

(*continued*)

- Medical treatment includes identifying the underlying cause, treating fluid and electrolyte imbalances, and hemodialysis if needed.
- Nutritional therapy includes a high-carbohydrate diet with restriction of foods high in protein, potassium, and phosphorous.

PART IV: Nursing Care of the Patient With a Musculoskeletal Disorder

Nina Russell and Brenda Reap Thompson

UNFOLDING CASE STUDY 8: Kayla

Kayla, a 55-year-old female, has been overweight her entire life. She was admitted to the orthopedic unit earlier in the day for a knee replacement (arthroplasty) and has been allowed nothing by mouth since midnight. While going through her preoperative checklist, the nurse finds that Kayla's complete blood count (CBC) is within normal limits (WNL); urinalysis is negative for a UTI; and her electrolytes, BUN, and creatinine are normal. Kayla's outpatient chest x-ray and EKG are normal. Kayla is a nonsmoker. She has a past medical history of HTN and has taken her BP medication this morning with a sip of water as instructed. Kayla is anxious, because she has never had surgery. It was also decided preoperatively that she would do her rehabilitation in an inpatient facility owing to her obesity and history of immobility.

Following surgery, Kayla is taken to the post-anesthesia care unit (PACU) for 2 hours and is now on the orthopedic floor.

EXERCISE 2.53 Ordering:

Place the postoperative nursing care issues in priority order from 1 to 6:

_______ Administer pain medication
_______ Monitor input and output (I&O)
_______ Monitor for deep vein thrombosis (DVT)
_______ Start continuous passive range of motion (ROM) to prevent contractures
_______ Facilitate early ambulation
_______ Monitor for bleeding at the site

The answer can be found on page 134

Kayla is doing well on postoperative day 1. Repeat blood work has been ordered to include a CBC, electrolytes, BUN, and creatinine. The nurse is reviewing Kayla's vital signs as well as her input and output (I&O) for the previous 8 hours.

EXERCISE 2.54 Multiple-choice:

Which finding will the nurse report to the health care provider (HCP)?

A. Blood urea nitrogen (BUN): 22 mg/dL
B. Blood pressure (BP): 108/72 mmHg
C. Urine output: 30 mL/hr
D. Hemoglobin: 12.8 g/dL

The answer can be found on page 134

Kayla's lab work, vital signs, and urine output are WNL. A nutritionist is consulted to help her lose weight to ensure surgical success.

On the second postoperative day, Kayla complains of pain in the unaffected leg and points to her calf. The nurse notes that the calf is warm and tender to palpation. A Doppler study of the extremity is ordered. It is positive for deep vein thrombosis (DVT). The nurse notifies the HCP and obtains an order for a heparin drip.

eRESOURCE

To reinforce your understanding of the clinical presentation of deep vein thrombosis (DVT) and associated treatment, refer to Medscape on your mobile device. [Pathway: Medscape → select "Conditions"→ enter "DVT" into the search field → select "DVT" and review content.]

EXERCISE 2.55 Multiple-choice:

The prescriber's order calls for heparin infusion at 1,800 units/hr. The label on the intravenous (IV) bag reads: Heparin 10,000 units in 500 mL D_5W. How many mL/hr will deliver the correct dose?

A. 120 mL/hr
B. 90 mL/hr
C. 85 mL/hr
D. 73 mL/hr

The answer can be found on page 134

---

eRESOURCE

To verify your answer, consult MedCalc. [Pathway: www.medcalc.com → select "Fluids/Electrolytes" → select "IV Rate" and enter information into fields.]

eRESOURCE

To reinforce your understanding of heparin, refer to Epocrates Online. [Pathway: http://online.epocrates.com → under the "Drugs" tab, enter "Heparin" in the search field → select "Heparin" → review "Adult Dosing," "Adverse Reactions," and "Safety/Monitoring."]

The nurse understands that Kayla is at risk for a pulmonary embolism (PE) secondary to the DVT.

EXERCISE 2.56 Select all that apply:

Which clinical manifestations are associated with a pulmonary embolus?

A. Bradycardia
B. Dyspnea
C. Back pain
D. Diaphoresis
E. Anxiety
F. Tachypnea

The answer can be found on page 135

---

eRESOURCE

To reinforce your understanding of the clinical presentation of a pulmonary embolism, refer to Medscape on your mobile device. [Pathway: Medscape ➔ select "Conditions" ➔ enter "Pulmonary Embolism" into the search field ➔ select "Pulmonary Embolism" and review content.]

The heparin drip has been initiated, and Kayla is resting comfortably. The nurse understands that bleeding precautions must be initiated for patients on heparin therapy.

EXERCISE 2.57 Select all that apply:

Which of the following constitute bleeding precautions?

A. Hemoccult all stool
B. Give all meds via intramuscular (IM) route
C. Limit blood draws
D. Use an electric razor

The answer can be found on page 135

EXERCISE 2.58 Multiple-choice:

Which medication would the nurse administer as the antidote to heparin?

A. Vitamin K
B. Protamine sulfate
C. Aspirin
D. Erythropoietin

The answer can be found on page 135

UNFOLDING CASE STUDY 9: Rebecca

Rebecca, a 20-year-old female, is admitted to the orthopedic floor with a compound femur fracture secondary to a skiing accident. She is complaining of severe pain rated at nine out of 10. The orthopedic surgeon determines that Rebecca's fracture requires open reduction and internal fixation (ORIF). She is taken to the operating room, where her bone is pinned and an immobilizer is placed on her leg.

EXERCISE 2.59 Multiple-choice:

What is the priority nursing diagnosis for a patient with an open reduction and internal fixation (ORIF)?

A. Risk for constipation
B. Risk for infection
C. Activity intolerance
D. Risk for injury

The answer can be found on page 135

eRESOURCE

To reinforce your understanding of the surgical procedure, refer to Medscape on your mobile device. [Pathway: Medscape → select "Conditions"→ enter "Open Reduction" into the search field → select "Open Reduction and Internal Fixation" and review content.]

Rebecca is doing well on postoperative day 1. The nurse prepares to assist Rebecca out of bed for the first time since her surgery.

EXERCISE 2.60 Multiple-choice:

Before assisting a patient with open reduction and internal fixation (ORIF) in ambulation for the first time, the nurse will:

A. Review the postoperative orders for weight-bearing status
B. Use a mechanical lift to transfer from bed to chair
C. Administer pain medication 3 hours before ambulation
D. Encourage patient to empty bladder to minimize interruption

The answer can be found on page 135

Rebecca is happy that she does not need traction. She will be sent home in a wheelchair with an immobilizer. She will need to follow up with the orthopedic outpatient center in a week.

UNFOLDING CASE STUDY 10: Boylan

Boylan, a 78-year-old war veteran, is seen in the outpatient orthopedic center. He has had type 1 diabetes mellitus for a long time and suffers from peripheral vascular disease. He is scheduled for a right above-the-knee amputation (AKA) and has been admitted to the medical inpatient unit.

EXERCISE 2.61 Fill in the blank:

In caring for a patient with an amputation, the nurse should place a ________________ at the bedside for emergency use.

The answer can be found on page 136

---

eRESOURCE

To reinforce your understanding of this surgical procedure and its postoperative care, refer to Medscape on your mobile device. [Pathway: Medscape ➔ select "Conditions"➔ enter "Amputation" into the search field ➔ select "Amputation of the Lower Extremity" and review content, particularly, "Postoperative Details."]

Boylan's surgery went well and, after a short time in the PACU, he is admitted to the orthopedic floor. The nurse understands that Boylan, like all surgical patients, is at risk for complications, particularly given his history of type 1 diabetes mellitus.

EXERCISE 2.62 Select all that apply:

To reduce the patient's risk for surgical complications, the nurse will:

A. Monitor blood glucose levels
B. Encourage use of an incentive spirometer every 2 hours
C. Administer insulin as prescribed
D. Assess heart and lung sounds
E. Administer metformin (Glucophage)
F. Mark dressing if any bleeding occurs

The answer can be found on page 136

EXERCISE 2.63 Select all that apply:

During the first 24 hours following a right above-the-knee amputation (AKA), the nurse will:

A. Place the patient in the Trendelenburg position
B. Monitor vital signs and surgical site
C. Elevate the amputated limb with pillows

D. Monitor input and output (I&O)
E. Administer pain medication as needed
F. Keep amputated limb flat on the bed

The answer can be found on page 136

EXERCISE 2.64 Multiple-choice:

In patients with diabetes mellitus, the nurse understands to monitor for which complication?

A. Edema of the stump
B. Mild erythema of the incision
C. Separation of the surgical wound edges
D. Bleeding to surgical stump dressing

The answer can be found on page 136

---

eRESOURCE

To reinforce your understanding of considerations for diabetic patients following surgery, refer to Medscape on your mobile device. [Pathway: Medscape → select "Conditions"→ enter "Diabetes" into the search field → select "Type 1 Diabetes Mellitus" → select "Treatment & Management" → select "Glycemic Control During Serious Medical Illness and Surgery" and review content.]

After his amputation, the nurse offers Boylan a number of instructions. She explains that after healing is complete and the residual limb is well molded, he will be fitted with a prosthesis.

EXERCISE 2.65 Multiple-choice:

The nurse determines that teaching has been effective when the patient says:

A. "I should lie on my abdomen for 30 minutes three to four times a day."
B. "I should change the shrinker bandage when it becomes soiled or stretched out."
C. "I should use lotion on the stump to prevent drying and cracking of the skin."
D. "I should elevate the limb on a pillow most of the day to decrease swelling."

The answer can be found on page 136

Postoperatively, the nurse monitors Boylan's left foot carefully with tests such as angiography, ankle-brachial indexes, Doppler ultrasound, and transcutaneous oxygen pressures. Boylan receives pain medication for occasional phantom limb pain. He is attending physical therapy to strengthen his upper body and improve circulation in the left leg.

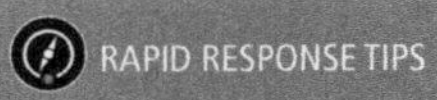

Bandaging of an above-the-knee amputation (AKA)

Use figure-eight bandaging of an AKA amputation to promote shaping and molding for a prosthesis.

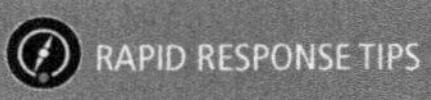

Patient teaching

In order to minimize edema, teach the patient who had a below-the-knee amputation (BKA) to avoid dangling the residual limb over the bedside.

UNFOLDING CASE STUDY 11: Michelle

Michelle, age 66 years, regularly seeks treatment at the outpatient orthopedic clinic for osteoarthritis of the hands and spinal osteoporosis.

EXERCISE 2.66 Select all that apply:

Risk factors for osteoporosis include:

A. Postmenopausal female
B. History of smoking
C. Asian ethnicity
D. Male older than 60 years
E. History of strength-training exercises
F. Sedentary lifestyle

The answer can be found on page 137

EXERCISE 2.67 Multiple-choice:

What is the leading cause of osteoporosis?

A. Progesterone deficiency
B. Vitamin D deficiency
C. Folic acid deficiency
D. Estrogen deficiency

The answer can be found on page 137

eRESOURCE

To reinforce your understanding of the causes of osteoarthritis, refer to Medscape on your mobile device. [Pathway: Medscape ➔ select "Conditions"➔ enter "Osteoarthritis" into the search field ➔ select "Osteoarthritis"➔ select "Introduction" and review content.]

Treatment for osteoporosis is aimed at preserving bone mass, preventing fractures, maintaining function, and decreasing pain. Michelle is prescribed medications for the management of her osteoporosis and osteoarthritis.

EXERCISE 2.68 Multiple-choice:

Which instructions will the nurse include in teaching about alendronate (Fosamax)?

A. Take with food and a full glass of water
B. Take at bedtime with a full glass of water
C. Take before breakfast and remain upright for 30 minutes after ingestion
D. Lie down for at least 30 minutes after ingestion

The answer can be found on page 137

Michelle asks the nurse about any adverse effects associated with Fosamax.

EXERCISE 2.69 Multiple-choice:

When teaching about adverse effects, a patient taking alendronate (Fosamax) should be instructed to report:

A. Dysphagia
B. Poor appetite
C. Insomnia
D. Tinnitus

The answer can be found on page 137

---

eRESOURCE

To reinforce your understanding of alendronate, refer to Epocrates Online. [Pathway: http://online.epocrates.com ➔ under the "Drugs" tab, enter "Alendronate" in the search field ➔ select "Fosamax" ➔ review "Adult Dosing," "Adverse Reactions," "Safety/Monitoring," and "Patient Education."]

In addition to medication, the nurse discusses lifestyle modification with Michelle to minimize further damage and maintain optimal function.

EXERCISE 2.70 Select all that apply:

For patients with osteoporosis, lifestyle modification includes:

A. Regular, weight-bearing exercise
B. Intake of calcium-rich foods
C. Altering home environment for safety
D. Routine bedrest to prevent pain

The answer can be found on page 137

Michelle reports being upset when the osteoarthritis in her hands prevents her from knitting or crocheting.

EXERCISE 2.71 Select all that apply:

Which interventions will minimize the pain and inflammation commonly associated with osteoarthritis?

A. Encourage adequate sleep each night
B. Encourage regular rest periods throughout the day
C. Splint hands to immobilize acutely inflamed joints
D. Use Tylenol (acetaminophen) as needed for pain
E. Promote regular physical activity
F. Avoid warm packs at all times

The answer can be found on page 138

---

eRESOURCE

To reinforce your understanding of the treatment and management of osteoarthritis, refer to Medscape on your mobile device. [Pathway: Medscape → select "Conditions" → enter "Osteoarthritis" into the search field → select "Osteoarthritis" → select "Treatment & Management" and review content.]

Michelle is prescribed glucosamine sulfate and Tylenol (acetaminophen) as needed for pain or discomfort.

EXERCISE 2.72 Multiple-choice:

The action of glucosamine sulfate is to:

A. Rebuild cartilage in the joint
B. Decrease inflammation of the joint
C. Stabilize the joint
D. Provide a heat effect to the joint

The answer can be found on page 138

She will return for follow-up in 1 month to evaluate for side effects and tolerance of glucosamine sulfate.

eRESOURCE

To reinforce your understanding of glucosamine sulfate, refer to Epocrates Online. [Pathway: http://online.epocrates.com → under the "Drugs" tab, enter "Glucosamine Sulfate" in the search field → select "Glucosamine Sulfate" → review "Cautions" and "Adverse Reactions."]

PART V: Nursing Care of the Patient With a Neurological Disorder

Nina Russell and Brenda Reap Thompson

UNFOLDING CASE STUDY 12: Martha

The nurse on a medical unit is providing care for 32-year-old Martha Newman, who has multiple sclerosis (MS). She was diagnosed after she gave birth to a healthy baby girl 5 years earlier.

EXERCISE 2.73 Select all that apply:

How is multiple sclerosis (MS) diagnosed?

A. History and physical examination
B. MRI
C. Bone scan
D. Electroencephalogram (EEG)

The answer can be found on page 138

EXERCISE 2.74 Multiple-choice:

In patients with multiple sclerosis (MS), the MRI scan reveals:

A. Multiple bright white lesions
B. Increased cerebral spinal fluid
C. Narrowing of the fourth ventricle
D. Several petechial hemorrhages

The answer can be found on page 138

EXERCISE 2.75 **Select all that apply:**

Which clinical manifestations are associated with multiple sclerosis (MS)?

A. Weakness
B. Fatigue
C. Vertigo
D. Visual disturbances
E. Paresthesia
F. Muscle spasms
G. Headache
H. Pain
I. Impaired memory
J. Depression

The answer can be found on page 138

eRESOURCE

To supplement your understanding of the clinical presentation associated with multiple sclerosis (MS), refer to the *Merck Manual*. [Pathway: www.merckmanuals.com ➔ select "Medical Topics"➔ select "Neurologic Disorders" ➔ enter "MS" into the search field ➔ select "Multiple Sclerosis (MS)" ➔ review "Pathophysiology" and "Signs and Symptoms."]

Martha tells the nurse that she has really been struggling with fatigue. She asks about ways to help increase her energy level.

EXERCISE 2.76 **Select all that apply:**

Which strategies for alleviating fatigue should the nurse provide a patient with multiple sclerosis (MS)?

A. Avoid environments with extremely cold temperatures
B. Maintain an adequate sleep regimen
C. Discontinue medication during periods of extreme fatigue
D. Uphold a routine exercise regimen
E. Avoid alcohol and tobacco products
F. Consume fresh fruits and vegetables daily

The answer can be found on page 139

eRESOURCE

To reinforce your understanding of symptom management for multiple sclerosis (MS), refer to Medscape on your mobile device. [Pathway: Medscape ➔ select "Conditions"➔ enter "MS" into the search field ➔ select "Multiple Sclerosis (MS)" select "Treatment & Management" ➔ select "Symptom Management" and review content.]

As part of the discharge-teaching plan, the nurse tells Martha that at times performing physical activity may become difficult; however, water therapy is an excellent alternative to promote physical activity. The nurse also advises Martha to review the information on the MS society's website. She is scheduled for a follow-up in the MS clinic.

UNFOLDING CASE STUDY 13: Margaret

Margaret, a 44-year-old female, accompanied by her husband, presents to the emergency room with complaints of dizziness, blurred vision, numbness and weakness of the right arm, and slurred speech. According to her husband, the patient's symptoms began about 20 to 30 minutes ago.

EXERCISE 2.77 Multiple-choice:

Which physician order should the nurse anticipate?

A. Obtain a CT of the head, stat
B. Initiate heparin drip per protocol
C. Administer aspirin 325 mg orally, stat
D. Administer atropine 2 mg intravenous (IV), stat

The answer can be found on page 139

EXERCISE 2.78 Select all that apply:

Identify risk factors for ischemic stroke:

A. Hypertension (HTN)
B. Diabetes mellitus
C. Smoking
D. Sickle cell anemia
E. High cholesterol
F. Depression

The answer can be found on page 139

eRESOURCE

To reinforce your understanding of the risk factors associated with ischemic stroke as well as treatment, refer to Epocrates Online. [Pathway: http://online.epocrates.com → under the "Diseases" tab, enter "Ischemic Stroke" in the search field → select "Ischemic Stroke" → review content, particularly "Risk Factors" and "Treatment."]

The HCP orders an EKG. Margaret's husband questions the purpose for the EKG.

EXERCISE 2.79 Multiple-choice:

Which statement depicts the nurse's comprehension of factors that contribute to ischemic strokes?

A. "The symptoms indicate that a pacemaker may be necessary."
B. "It is routine for patients older than the age of 40 years to have an EKG completed as a precaution."
C. "It is to check for an irregular heart rhythm, which may contribute to a stroke."
D. "To determine whether management of a heart attack will be necessary."

The answer can be found on page 139

No intracranial hemorrhage is noted on the CT and the HCP orders reteplase (Retavase) to be administered.

EXERCISE 2.80 Select all that apply:

Which are absolute contraindications to reteplase (Retavase)?

A. 51 years of age
B. Systolic blood pressure (BP): 188 mmHg
C. Currently on Coumadin with a prothrombin time (PT) of 49 seconds and an international normalized ratio (INR) of 2.5
D. Platelet count of 51,000

The answer can be found on page 140

---

eRESOURCE

To reinforce your understanding of reteplase, refer to Epocrates Online. [Pathway: http://online.epocrates.com ➔ under the "Drugs" tab, enter "Reteplase" in the search field ➔ select "Reteplase" ➔ review content, particularly "Adult Dosing," "Adverse Reactions," and "Safety/Monitoring."]

After receiving reteplase (Retavase), Margaret is transferred to the intensive care unit for close observation of hemodynamic status, including monitoring for signs of bleeding, monitoring vital signs every 15 minutes, and hourly neurological checks.

UNFOLDING CASE STUDY 14: Mr. Rodriguez

Mr. Rodriquez, a 52-year-old patient who was diagnosed with Parkinson's disease 4 years ago, arrives for a routine follow-up with his PCP. His wife joins him for this particular visit, because she has noticed that her husband is having difficulty swallowing.

EXERCISE 2.81 Select all that apply:

Which clinical manifestations are associated with Parkinson's disease?

A. Mask-like expression
B. Decline in intellect

C. Pill rolling
D. Cogwheel movement
E. Shuffling gate
F. Micrographia
G. Drooling
H. Aphasia
I. Tremor
J. Dysphonia

The answer can be found on page 140

EXERCISE 2.82 Select all that apply:

Complications commonly found in a patient with Parkinson's disease include:

A. Depression
B. Diarrhea
C. Dyskinesia
D. Dysphagia
E. Dementia
F. Dysphonia

The answer can be found on page 140

---

eRESOURCE

To reinforce your understanding of the clinical presentation and complications associated with Parkinson's disease, refer to:

- Medscape on your mobile device. [Pathway: Medscape ➔ select "Conditions"➔ enter "Parkinson's" into the search field ➔ select "Parkinson's Disease" and review content.]
- Epocrates Online. [Pathway: http://online.epocrates.com ➔ under the "Diseases" tab, enter "Parkinson" in the search field ➔ select "Parkinson Disease" ➔ review "Content," particularly "Complications."]

As a result of his dysphagia, Mr. Rodriguez and his wife receive instruction regarding diet modification as well as using a specific technique for swallowing.

EXERCISE 2.83 Multiple-choice:

Which diet is recommended for a patient with Parkinson's disease who is having difficulty swallowing?

A. Pureed food with thin liquids
B. Semisolid food with thick liquids
C. Solid food with thick liquids
D. Semisolid food with thin liquids

The answer can be found on page 140

EXERCISE 2.84 Ordering:

Place the swallowing technique for a patient with Parkinson's disease in the correct order from 1 to 3:

_______ Close lips and teeth
_______ Lift the tongue up and back to swallow
_______ Place semisolid food on the tongue

The answer can be found on page 141

EXERCISE 2.85 Select all that apply:

Which nursing interventions will support nutritional intake in a patient with Parkinson's disease?

A. Drinking fluids after swallowing food
B. Cutting food into bite-sized pieces
C. Providing six small meals each day
D. Increasing time allotted to eat meals

The answer can be found on page 141

As Mr. Rodriguez does not exhibit any clinical manifestations of dyskinesia, the HCP renews his prescription of levodopa–carbidopa (Sinemet) and a follow-up appointment is scheduled.

eRESOURCE

To reinforce your understanding of levodopa, refer to Epocrates Online. [Pathway: http://online.epocrates.com ➔ under the "Drugs" tab, enter "Levodopa" in the search field ➔ select "Sinemet" ➔ review "Adult Dosing," "Adverse Reactions," and "Safety/Monitoring."]

EXERCISE 2.86 Select all that apply:

Clinical manifestations of dyskinesia that are associated with long-term use of Sinemet include:

A. Facial grimaces
B. Sleep disturbances
C. Jerking movement of extremities
D. Smacking movements
E. Hallucinations
F. Involuntary jerking of the trunk

The answer can be found on page 141

---

eRESOURCE

To reinforce your understanding of dyskinesia, refer to Medscape on your mobile device. [Pathway: Medscape ➔ select "Conditions"➔ enter "Dyskinesia" into the search field ➔ select "Tardive Dyskinesia" and review content.]

UNFOLDING CASE STUDY 15: Jessica

Jessica, a 23-year-old college student, is admitted to the hospital with an unconfirmed diagnosis of myasthenia gravis (MG) and requires diagnostic work-up.

EXERCISE 2.87 Multiple-choice:

Which is a clinical manifestation associated with myasthenia gravis (MG)?

A. Cogwheel rigidity
B. Loss of coordination
C. Intermittent periods of visual disturbance
D. Progressive weakness throughout the day
E. Ascending paralysis

The answer can be found on page 141

EXERCISE 2.88 Multiple-choice:

Myasthenia gravis (MG) is confirmed by:

A. Positive Brudzinski's sign
B. Positive Kernig's sign
C. Positive edrophonium (Tensilon) test
D. Positive sweat chloride test

The answer can be found on page 141

eRESOURCE

To reinforce your understanding of myasthenia gravis, refer to Medscape on your mobile device. [Pathway: Medscape → select "Conditions"→ enter "Myasthenia Gravis" into the search field → select "Myasthenia Gravis" and review content.]

The nurse tells Jessica that a Tensilon test will be performed and explains the purpose and findings of the examination.

EXERCISE 2.89 Multiple-choice:

Which medication should be readily available during the Tensilon test?

A. Epinephrine
B. Atropine
C. Narcan
D. Amiodarone

The answer can be found on page 142

EXERCISE 2.90 Multiple-choice:

Which patient response to the administration of Tensilon confirms the diagnosis of myasthenia gravis (MG)?

A. Symptom improvement of just the ptosis
B. Rapid but brief improvement of symptoms
C. Prolonged improvement of symptoms
D. Brief exaggeration of symptoms

The answer can be found on page 142

eRESOURCE

To reinforce your understanding of how myasthenia gravis is diagnosed, refer to the *Merck Manual*. [Pathway: www.merckmanuals.com ➔ select "Medical Topics"➔ select "Neurologic Disorders" ➔ enter "Myasthenia Gravis" into the search field ➔ select "Myasthenia Gravis" ➔ select "Diagnosis" and review content regarding the traditional anticholinesterase test.]

Jessica is diagnosed with MG and begins pyridostigmine bromide (Mestinon) therapy. The nurse explains the many factors that can exacerbate the disease and about the prevention of a myasthenic crisis.

EXERCISE 2.91 Select all that apply:

Precipitating factors for myasthenic crisis include:

A. Physical overexertion
B. Emotional stress
C. Taking excess medication
D. Omitting a dose of medication
E. Pregnancy
F. Influenza

The answer can be found on page 142

Jessica is discharged from the hospital and is scheduled to follow up with her neurologist in 2 weeks.

UNFOLDING CASE STUDY 16: Fernando

Fernando, a 22-year-old male, presents to the emergency room following a motor vehicle accident. He was unrestrained and had no passengers in the vehicle. Currently, he is on a backboard and has a cervical collar in place.

EXERCISE 2.92 Multiple-choice:

Which does the nurse assess first?

A. Level of consciousness and orientation
B. Heart rate (HR) and blood pressure (BP)
C. Muscle strength and reflexes
D. Airway patency and breathing pattern

The answer can be found on page 142

Fernando is alert with his eyes open; answers questions without any difficulty; and is oriented to person, place, and time. There are multiple abrasions and bruises on his face. He is unable to move or feel his upper or lower extremities. The nurse uses the Glasgow Coma Scale to determine the extent of neurological injury.

eRESOURCE

Use Medscape's Glasgow Coma Scale to enter the data given in the text to determine Fernando's score. [Pathway: Medscape → select "Calculators"→ enter "Glasgow" into the search field → select "Glasgow Coma Scale" and enter aforementioned data.]

EXERCISE 2.93 Multiple-choice:

Using the aforementioned Glasgow Coma Scale, which score does the nurse assign to this patient?

A. Score of 15
B. Score of 3
C. Score of 10
D. Score of 6

The answer can be found on page 142

EXERCISE 2.94 Multiple-choice:

What is the minimum score possible on the Glasgow Coma Scale?

A. 3
B. 4
C. 6
D. 8

The answer can be found on page 143

EXERCISE 2.95 Multiple-choice:

What is the maximum score possible on the Glasgow Coma Scale?

A. 13
B. 15
C. 9
D. 20

The answer can be found on page 143

A CT scan is ordered and confirms a C2 spinal injury. Multiple abrasions and bruises are noted on his face; however, the CT scan of the head is negative. The provider has written orders for an IV bolus followed by a continuous infusion of methylprednisolone. The patient weighs 155 lb.

EXERCISE 2.96 Calculation:

Order: 30 mg/kg intravenous (IV) bolus to be given over 15 minutes

Calculate the bolus dose: ___________________

The answer can be found on page 143

EXERCISE 2.97 Calculation:

The prescriber's order calls for methylprednisolone intravenous (IV) infusion of 5.4 mg/kg/hr for 23 hours to begin 45 minutes after the bolus dose. The label on the IV bag reads: Methylprednisolone 100 mg/ 50 mL D_5W. How many mL/hr will deliver the correct dose?

A. 190 mL/hr
B. 125 mL/hr
C. 140 mL/hr
D. 150 mL/hr

The answer can be found on page 143

---

eRESOURCE

To verify your answer, consult MedCalc. [Pathway: www.medcalc.com ➔ select "Fluids/Electrolytes" ➔ select "IV Rate" and enter information into fields.]

Fernando is admitted to the trauma-surgical intensive care unit (ICU) for close observation.

EXERCISE 2.98 Select all that apply:

Which is true regarding the administration of methylprednisolone to a patient with a spinal cord injury?

A. Methylprednisolone should be given within the first 8 hours following injury.
B. Methylprednisolone is associated with adverse effects such as hypoglycemia.
C. Methylprednisolone increases the risk of infection and stress ulcers.
D. Methylprednisolone is only indicated in patients with severe hypotension and bradycardia.

The answer can be found on page 143

---

eRESOURCE

To supplement your understanding of the clinical presentation associated with MS, refer to the *Merck Manual.* [Pathway: www.merckmanuals.com → select "Medical Topics"→ select "Neurologic Disorders" → enter "Spinal Cord Injury" into the search field → select "Spinal Trauma" → Select "Treatment" and review "Immediate Care."]

EXERCISE 2.99 Select all that apply:

Acute complications that may occur following a spinal cord injury include:

A. Neurogenic shock
B. Deep vein thrombosis (DVT)
C. Pneumonia
D. Myocardial infarction (MI)
E. Respiratory failure
F. Autonomic dysreflexia

The answer can be found on page 144

The nurse understands that patients are at risk for seizures after sustaining a head injury and prepares to initiate seizure precautions.

EXERCISE 2.100 Select all that apply:

Which of the following constitute seizure precautions?

A. Maintain bed in low position
B. Keep side rails up and padded
C. Keep bright lights on to easily visualize the patient
D. Ensure suction is available at the bedside
E. Keep a tongue depressor at the bedside to use as a bite guard
F. Maintain a low-stimulus environment

The answer can be found on page 144

The new graduate nurse asks the charge nurse about a positive Babinski sign on a patient following a cervical spine injury.

EXERCISE 2.101 Multiple-choice:

Which statement regarding a positive Babinski reflects the nurse's comprehension of spinal cord injuries?

A. "A positive Babinski is a good sign indicating adequate spinal cord perfusion."
B. "A positive Babinski is a normal neurological finding in all age groups."
C. "A positive Babinski indicates injury to nerves innervating muscles involved in voluntary movement."
D. "A positive Babinski is a sign of nervous system excitation requiring implementation of seizure precautions."

The answer can be found on page 144

eRESOURCE

To supplement your understanding of the evaluation of a neurologic patient, refer to the *Merck Manual*. [Pathway: www.merckmanuals.com ➔ select "Medical Topics"➔ select "Neurologic Disorders" ➔ enter "Babinski" into the search field ➔ select "Evaluation of a Neurologic Patient" ➔ scroll down and read section on "Reflexes" and review content (be sure to view video, *How to Test Reflexes*).]

EXERCISE 2.102 Select all that apply:

Which interventions minimize the risk of deep vein thrombosis (DVT) in a patient with an acute spinal injury?

A. Anticoagulation
B. Range of motion (ROM) exercises
C. Antiembolism stockings
D. Pneumatic compression devices
E. Antiplatelet medication
F. Hydration

The answer can be found on page 144

eRESOURCE

To reinforce your understanding of the clinical presentation of a DVT, refer to Medscape on your mobile device. [Pathway: Medscape ➔ select "Conditions"➔ enter "DVT" into the search field ➔ select "DVT" and review content.]

Fernando will be transferred to a rehabilitation facility that specializes in spinal cord injuries once medically stable.

PART VI: Nursing Care of the Patient With an Endocrine Disorder

Karen K. Gittings and Brenda Reap Thompson

UNFOLDING CASE STUDY 17: Maria

The nurse is caring for Maria, who was admitted to the hospital with diabetic ketoacidosis (DKA). Maria had a virus for 3 days before hospitalization.

EXERCISE 2.103 Fill in the blanks:

Name four clinical features of diabetic ketoacidosis (DKA).

1. ______________________________
2. ______________________________
3. ______________________________
4. ______________________________

The answer can be found on page 145

eRESOURCE

To reinforce your understanding of the clinical presentation of a DKA, refer to Epocrates Online. [Pathway: http://online.epocrates.com ➔ under the "Diseases" tab, enter "Diabetic Ketoacidosis" in the search field ➔ select "Diabetic Ketoacidosis" ➔ review "Highlights," "Basics," and "Diagnosis."]

Colin, the nurse, assesses Maria frequently. The characteristics of DKA and hyperglycemic hyperosmolar nonketotic syndrome (HHNS) are very similar, but it is important to differentiate between the two.

EXERCISE 2.104 Matching:

Indicate whether each characteristic in Column B is associated with diabetic ketoacidosis (DKA) or hyperglycemic hyperosmolar nonketotic syndrome (HHNS), mentioned in Column A:

Column A	Column B
A. DKA	________ More common in type 1 diabetes
B. HHNS	________ Often caused by omission of insulin
	________ Onset is usually over several days
	________ Acidotic with pH less than 7.30

(*continued*)

Column A	Column B
	_______ Plasma bicarbonate levels normal
	_______ Often caused by physiologic stress
	_______ Absence of serum and urine ketones
	_______ Kussmaul respirations
	_______ Serum osmolality greater than 350 mOsm/L

The answer can be found on page 145

eRESOURCE

To reinforce your understanding of the characteristics associated with DKA and HHNS, refer to Epocrates Online. [Pathway: http://online.epocrates.com ➔ under the "Diseases" tab, enter "Diabetic Ketoacidosis" in the search field ➔ select "Diabetic Ketoacidosis" ➔ select "Differential Diagnosis" and review content.]

EXERCISE 2.105 Select all that apply:

The nurse understands that the initial treatment for Maria would include:

A. Administering oxygen
B. Establishing an intravenous (IV) line
C. Administering 0.9% normal saline (NS) IV
D. Infusing neutral protamine Hagedorn (NPH) insulin
E. Monitoring potassium levels closely
F. Encouraging intake of Gatorade

The answer can be found on page 145

EXERCISE 2.106 Multiple-choice:

The nurse reviews the laboratory reports from blood samples drawn 1 hour after the administration of intravenous (IV) insulin. What would the nurse expect?

A. Hyponatremia
B. Hypercalcemia
C. Hypoglycemia
D. Hypokalemia

The answer can be found on page 145

eRESOURCE

To reinforce your understanding of the treatment for DKA, refer to Epocrates Online. [Pathway: http://online.epocrates.com ➔ under the "Diseases" tab, enter "Diabetic Ketoacidosis" in the search field ➔ select "Diabetic Ketoacidosis" ➔ select "Tx Details" under the "Treatment Tab" and review content.]

Maria is feeling better within 24 hours. The nurse begins to explain to her how to prevent this occurrence in the future.

EXERCISE 2.107 Select all that apply:

Which sick-day rules should the nurse include in the teaching?

A. Continue eating regular meals if possible
B. Increase the intake of noncaloric fluids
C. Take insulin as prescribed
D. Check glucose once daily
E. Test for ketones if glucose is greater than 240 mg/dL
F. Report moderate ketones to the health care provider (HCP)

The answer can be found on page 146

---

eRESOURCE

To reinforce your understanding of DKA, refer to Epocrates Online. [Pathway: http://online.epocrates.com ➔ under the "Diseases" tab, enter "DKA" in the search field ➔ select "Diabetic Ketoacidosis" ➔ Under the Treatment tab, select "Prevention" and review content.]

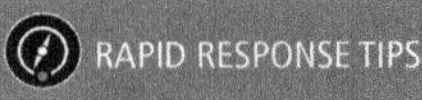

Manifestations of diabetes mellitus

Macrovascular complications occur from early-onset atherosclerosis, causing:

- Cardiovascular disease
- Cerebrovascular disease
- Peripheral vascular disease

Microvascular complications occur from thickening of the vessel membranes in the capillaries and arterioles, causing problems with:

- Vision (retinopathy)
- Kidneys (nephropathy)

EXERCISE 2.108 Multiple-choice:

The night charge nurse is making assignments for the following day shift. The plan is for Maria to be discharged home. It would be best to assign Maria to:

A. An experienced RN pulled from another medical unit
B. A new-graduate RN who has been on the unit for 1 week
C. An experienced RN who has just been transferred from the operating room
D. A licensed practical nurse (LPN) who has been on the unit for 3 months

The answer can be found on page 146

EXERCISE 2.109 Matching:

Match the information in Column A with the disease alteration in Column B (an option may be used more than once):

Column A	Column B
A. Older than 35 years of age	________Type 1 diabetes mellitus
B. Overweight	________Type 2 diabetes mellitus
C. Polyphagia	
D. Sudden weight loss	
E. Younger than 30 years of age	
F. May be controlled by diet	
G. Polyuria	
H. Polydipsia	

The answer can be found on page 146

KEY TAKEAWAY POINTS

Diabetes Mellitus

- Characteristics of type 1 diabetes include an onset of usually less than 30 years of age, thin at diagnosis with recent weight loss, little or no insulin production, needs insulin for life, and ketosis prone (DKA).
- Characteristics of type 2 diabetes include an onset at any age although many type 2 diabetics are older than 30 years of age, usually obese at diagnosis, problem with either decreased amount of insulin or insulin resistance, treatment focuses on weight loss and oral antidiabetic agents, ketosis is uncommon (HHNS).
- Risk factors include a family history, obesity, ethnicity, age, HTN, dyslipidemia, and history of gestational diabetes or delivery of babies weighing more than 9 lb.

(*continued*)

- The classic clinical manifestations are the three Ps: polyuria, polydipsia, and polyphagia. Others include fatigue, vision changes, wounds that will not heal, and recurrent infections.
- Criteria for diagnosis include symptoms of diabetes plus a casual plasma glucose greater than or equal to 200 mg/dL or a fasting plasma glucose greater than or equal to 126 mg/dL.
- Management focuses on nutrition, exercise, monitoring, medication, and education.
- Insulin regimens can be conventional or intensive. The intensive regimen is beneficial in reducing the risk of long-term complications, but increases the risk of hypoglycemia because of tight blood sugar controls.
- Hypoglycemia is a potentially deadly complication. Early symptoms include sweating, tachycardia, palpitations, and anxiety. As the blood sugar falls further, central nervous system (CNS) symptoms develop, which can significantly impair the patient.
- Treatment of hypoglycemia involves administration of 15 g of a fast-acting concentrated source of carbohydrate.
- The primary features of DKA are hyperglycemia, ketosis, dehydration, electrolyte loss, and acidosis.
- DKA can occur when diabetic patients are sick and stop taking their insulin. "sick-day rules" are designed to minimize the risk of DKA occurring.
- Treatment of DKA focuses on treating the hyperglycemia and correcting dehydration, electrolyte loss, and acidosis.
- HHNS is similar to DKA except there is no ketosis and pH and bicarbonate levels are normal.
- Long-term complications from diabetes are categorized as macrovascular and microvascular complications.

UNFOLDING CASE STUDY 18: Lisa

Lisa has been feeling extremely nervous and has come to the clinic for an evaluation. She is 34 years old, has three children, and works full time. The laboratory results indicate that she has hyperthyroidism. The most common cause of hyperthyroidism is Graves' disease.

EXERCISE 2.110 Select all that apply:

Which health alterations can cause hyperthyroidism?

A. Toxic nodular goiter
B. Thyroiditis
C. Cancer of the tongue

D. Thyroid cancer
E. Hyperfunction of the adrenal glands
F. Exogenous iodine intake

The answer can be found on page 147

EXERCISE 2.111 Matching:

Match the clinical manifestations in Column A with the disease alteration in Column B:

Column A	Column B
A. Palpitations	________ Hyperthyroidism
B. Increased respiratory rate	________ Hypothyroidism
C. Dry, sparse, coarse hair	
D. Anemia	
E. Diaphoresis	
F. Muscle wasting	
G. Enlarged, scaly tongue	
H. Decreased breathing capacity	
I. Muscle aches and pains	
J. Diarrhea	
K. Slow, slurred speech	
L. Fine tremors of fingers	
M. Exophthalmos	
N. Intolerance to cold	

The answer can be found on page 147

eRESOURCE

To supplement your understanding of the causes as well as the signs and symptoms associated with hyperthyroidism, refer to the *Merck Manual*. [Pathway: www.merckmanuals.com/professional ➔ enter "Hyperthyroidism"➔ select "Hyperthyroidism" ➔ select and review "Etiology" and "Symptoms and Signs."]

Two days after being diagnosed with Graves' disease, Lisa presents to the emergency room with palpitations, chest pain, and extreme anxiety. Her BP is elevated and the EKG shows a rhythm of sinus tachycardia with a rate of 134. Lisa states that she has been very anxious since being told of her diagnosis.

EXERCISE 2.112 Multiple-choice:

Lisa is being admitted with the diagnosis of thyrotoxic crisis. When making a room assignment for this patient, the charge nurse knows it would be best to assign:

A. A room in which the roommate is not infected
B. A room that is directly across from the nursing station
C. A private room
D. A room in which the roommate is very pleasant and talkative

The answer can be found on page 147

---

eRESOURCE

To supplement your understanding of thyrotoxic crisis, refer to Medscape on your mobile device. [Pathway: Medscape ➔ enter "Thyrotoxic" into the search field ➔ select "Thyrotoxicosis Imaging" and review content in "Overview."]

KEY TAKEAWAY POINTS

Thyroid Disorders

- The most common cause of hypothyroidism in adults is Hashimoto's disease, which occurs when the immune system attacks the thyroid gland.
- Thyroid deficiency can affect all body functions.
- Clinical manifestations include fatigue, hair loss, brittle nails, dry skin, and constipation. Later symptoms are progressively worse and include subdued emotional responses, cold intolerance, weight gain, bradycardia, and hypotension. Myxedema coma is the most extreme stage of hypothyroidism.
- Normal metabolism is restored by replacing the missing hormone with synthetic hormone. Dosages are based on serum thyroid-stimulating hormone (TSH) levels.
- The most common cause of hyperthyroidism is the autoimmune disorder Graves' disease.
- Symptoms of hyperthyroidism may occur after an emotional shock, stress, or infection.
- Clinical manifestations include nervousness, irritability, palpitations, rapid HR, elevated BP, heat intolerance, excessive perspiration, weight loss, tremors of the hands and tongue, and exophthalmos. Thyroid storm is an abrupt onset of severe hyperthyroidism.
- Management involves several options, including radioactive iodine-131 therapy, antithyroid drug therapy, or thyroidectomy.

UNFOLDING CASE STUDY 19: Marilyn

Marilyn, age 70 years, has been taking corticosteroids intermittently for many years to treat rheumatoid arthritis. These high amounts of corticosteroids can cause many physiological and psychological changes; in Marilyn's case, they have caused Cushing's disease.

EXERCISE 2.113 Select all that apply:

Which of the following clinical manifestations are present in Cushing's disease?

A. Buffalo hump
B. Hypovolemia
C. Weight loss
D. Hyperpigmentation of skin
E. Moon face
F. Muscle wasting in the extremities
G. Purple striae on the abdomen

The answer can be found on page 148

eRESOURCE

To supplement your understanding of Cushing's disease, refer to the *Merck Manual.* [Pathway: www.merckmanuals.com/professional → enter "Cushing"→ select "Cushing Disease" → select and review "Etiology" and "Symptoms and Signs."]

The treatment of Cushing's disease is related to the cause, which may be a tumor of the pituitary or adrenal gland or excessive secretion of adrenocorticotropic hormone (ACTH) from carcinoma of the lung. Some patients may need surgery to remove the tumor that is causing these symptoms. In Marilyn's case, Cushing's has developed as a result of long-term corticosteroid use.

EXERCISE 2.114 Multiple-choice:

In order to manage Cushing's disease, the health care provider (HCP) recommends:

A. Discontinuing the corticosteroid therapy immediately
B. Weaning her off the corticosteroid medication slowly
C. Using the corticosteroid only as needed for severe pain
D. Administering the corticosteroid before bedtime

The answer can be found on page 148

EXERCISE 2.115 Select all that apply:

Select the information that should be included in the teaching session for this patient.

A. Keep a medical identification device with you
B. Keep a list of medications and doses with you

C. Increase the sodium in your diet
D. Avoid exposure to infection
E. Hold the medication if side effects occur
F. Monitor for excessive weight gain

The answer can be found on page 148

Musculoskeletal changes can occur with Cushing's disease, which may result in kyphosis and compression fractures of the vertebrae.

EXERCISE 2.116 Multiple-choice:

In order to prevent injuries, it is a priority to teach the patient to:

A. Increase protein in his or her diet
B. Begin an aerobics exercise class
C. Use assistive devices as much as possible
D. Establish a protective environment

The answer can be found on page 148

KEY TAKEAWAY POINTS

Cushing's Disease

- Although overproduction of endogenous corticosteroids can lead to Cushing's, it is more commonly caused by chronic use of synthetic corticosteroid medications.
- Clinical manifestations include central-type obesity, fatty buffalo hump in the neck area, moon face, thin skin, muscle wasting, retention of sodium and water, weight gain, hyperglycemia, virilization in females, and changes in mood and mental activity.
- Treatment is directed at the cause.
- To minimize the risk of Cushing's, corticosteroids are best taken around 8:00 a.m., in the lowest dose possible, for the shortest period of time.
- Corticosteroids should never be abruptly stopped because of the risk of causing adrenal insufficiency.

UNFOLDING CASE STUDY 20: Isabella

Isabella is admitted to the hospital in Addisonian crisis. She has a history of Addison's disease.

EXERCISE 2.117 Multiple-choice:

After Isabella arrives on the unit, the nursing team begins the admission process. What role can be delegated to the licensed practical nurse (LPN)?

A. Perform the initial physical assessment
B. Obtain the patient's weight
C. Hang a new bag of intravenous (IV) fluids
D. Educate the patient on the plan of care

The answer can be found on page 149

EXERCISE 2.118 Fill in the blanks:

What three hormones does the adrenal cortex produce and what is their primary function?

1. ____________________
2. ____________________
3. ____________________

The answer can be found on page 149

EXERCISE 2.119 Matching:

Match the hormones in Column A with the related clinical manifestations of deficiency in Column B:

Column A	Column B
A. Mineralocorticoids	_______ Hypovolemia, hyperkalemia, hypoglycemia, and decreased muscle size
B. Glucocorticoids	_______ Decreased cardiac output, anemia, depression, and confusion
C. Androgen	_______ Decreased heart size, decreased muscle tone, weight loss, and skin hyperpigmentation

The answer can be found on page 149

Isabella states that she was taking her medications as prescribed and she does not understand why she had this problem.

EXERCISE 2.120 Fill in the blanks:

List four causes of Addisonian crisis.

1. ______________________
2. ______________________
3. ______________________
4. ______________________

The answer can be found on page 149

eRESOURCE

To supplement your understanding of Addison's disease and its causes, refer to Medscape on your mobile device. [Pathway: Medscape ➔ enter "Addison's" into the search field ➔ select "Addison Disease" and review content in "Overview."]

The nurse explains that hormone replacement will always be needed, but the doses of medication must be increased when there are events that cause psychological or physical stress.

EXERCISE 2.121 Select all that apply:

Which symptoms would indicate that Isabella is in Addisonian crisis?

A. Hypertension (HTN)
B. Bradycardia
C. Dehydration
D. Hyperkalemia
E. Nausea and vomiting
F. Weakness

The answer can be found on page 149

eRESOURCE

To reinforce your understanding of the treatment for Addisonian crisis, refer to Medscape on your mobile device. [Pathway: Medscape ➔ enter "Addison's" into the search field ➔ select "Addison Disease" and review content in "History" and "Treatment & Management."]

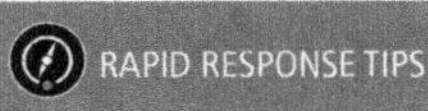

Addisonian crisis

The collaborative care includes:

- Restoring fluid volume deficit with normal saline 0.9% IV
- Administering hydrocortisone replacement
- Monitoring and treating hyperkalemia and hypoglycemia
- Evaluating vital signs and cardiac rhythm frequently to assess for fluid volume deficit and hyperkalemia

UNFOLDING CASE STUDY 21: Gabriel

Gabriel had a craniotomy to remove a benign brain tumor. Two days after surgery, he began putting out copious amounts of very dilute urine. He was subsequently diagnosed with diabetes insipidus (DI) and transferred back to the intensive care unit. On arrival, Gabriel is hypotensive, tachycardic, and complaining of intense thirst.

EXERCISE 2.122 Multiple-choice:

After receiving transfer orders on Gabriel, the nurse knows that the priority intervention is to:

A. Draw all laboratory tests before starting any treatment
B. Administer fluid-replacement therapy
C. Fill up the patient's water pitcher as requested
D. Obtain the patient's baseline weight

The answer can be found on page 150

EXERCISE 2.123 Fill in the blank:

Which type of diabetes insipidus (DI) does Gabriel have? Explain.

____

____

The answer can be found on page 150

EXERCISE 2.124 Select all that apply:

Which clinical manifestations would be present in a patient with diabetes insipidus (DI)?

A. Polydipsia
B. Polyuria
C. Urine output less than 100 mL in 24 hours
D. Specific gravity less than 1.005
E. Weight loss
F. Hypertension (HTN)

The answer can be found on page 150

eRESOURCE

To reinforce your understanding of the manifestation of DI, refer to Medscape on your mobile device. [Pathway: Medscape ➔ enter "Diabetes" into the search field ➔ select "Diabetes Insipidus" and review content in "Introduction" and "Clinical Presentation."]

The patient's BP remains low and the urine output continues to increase. Gabriel is feeling very weak.

EXERCISE 2.125 Select all that apply:

The nurse understands that appropriate treatment for a patient with diabetes insipidus (DI) includes:

A. Titrating intravenous (IV) fluids to replace urine output
B. Administering thiazide diuretics
C. Initiating a low-sodium diet
D. Administering desmopressin acetate (DDAVP)
E. Monitoring a strict input and output (I&O)
F. Allowing the patient to drink as desired

The answer can be found on page 150

eRESOURCE

To reinforce your understanding of the manifestation of DI, refer to Medscape on your mobile device. [Pathway: Medscape → enter "Diabetes" into the search field → select "Diabetes Insipidus" and review content in "Treatment & Management."]

KEY TAKEAWAY POINTS

Diabetes Insipidus

- DI is characterized by a deficiency of antidiuretic hormone (ADH ; vasopressin).
- The three types are neurogenic, nephrogenic, and psychogenic.
- An output of very large amounts of dilute urine can quickly lead to a fluid volume deficit.
- Other signs and symptoms are related to the fluid volume deficit that results; these include weight loss, poor skin turgor, dry mucous membranes, increased HR, and hypotension.
- The patient experiences an intense thirst and may drink up to 20 L/d. Limiting the fluid intake will not alter the high volume loss of urine.
- Medical management includes identifying and correcting the cause if possible, ensuring adequate fluid replacement, and administering desmopressin, which is synthetic vasopressin.

PART VII: Nursing Care of the Patient With a Gastrointestinal Disorder

Karen K. Gittings, Ruth A. Wittmann-Price, and Brenda Reap Thompson

UNFOLDING CASE STUDY 22: Jonathan

Donna works in the gastrointestinal (GI) lab, in which many endoscopies (with contrast dye) and scope procedures are done.

EXERCISE 2.126 Matching:

Match the names of the procedures in Column A with the interventions in Column B:

Column A	Column B
A. Bronchoscopy	____ Visualizes the bile duct system of the liver and gall bladder
B. Colonoscopy	____ Visualizes anus, rectum, and sigmoid colon
C. Cystoscopy	____ Visualizes the oropharynx, esophagus, stomach, and duodenum
D. Esophagogastroduodenoscopy (EGD)	____ Visualizes the urethra, bladder, prostate, and ureters
E. Endoscopic retrograde cholangiopancreatography (ERCP)	____ Visualizes the anus, rectum, and colon
F. Sigmoidoscopy	____ Visualizes the larynx, trachea, bronchi, and alveoli

The answer can be found on page 151

Jonathan comes to the clinic and receives preprocedure instructions for a colonoscopy.

EXERCISE 2.127 Select all that apply:

Which factors does the nurse consider while giving Jonathan instructions for his endoscopic examination?

A. Age
B. Medications
C. Allergies
D. Transportation
E. Previous radiographic examinations
F. Language and cultural barriers

The answer can be found on page 151

eRESOURCE

To reinforce your understanding of the procedure, refer to Medscape on your mobile device. [Pathway: Medscape → select "Procedures"→ enter "Colonoscopy" into the search field → select "Colonoscopy" and review content.]

EXERCISE 2.128 Multiple-choice:

When a new-graduate nurse asks about obtaining consent for the procedure, the nurse's best response is:

A. "Since the physician has already obtained informed consent, we will get the patient to sign the consent."
B. "Yes, we get consent when the patient comes for preprocedure instructions."

C. "We need to wait until the physician is in the room to get the patient to sign the consent."
D. "We usually wait until a family member is present before obtaining consent."

The answer can be found on page 151

One of Donna's main nursing interventions for patients during their procedure is to position them correctly to reduce the incidence of complications.

EXERCISE 2.129 Matching:

Match the tests in Column A with the correct positions in Column B (you may use positions more than once):

Column A	Column B
A. Bronchoscopy	____ Knee–chest
B. Colonoscopy	____ Lithotomy
C. Cystoscopy	____ Supine
D. Esophagogastroduodenoscopy (EGD)	____ Left side, knees to chest
E. Endoscopic retrograde cholangiopancreatography (ERCP)	
F. Sigmoidoscopy	

The answer can be found on page 152

EXERCISE 2.130 Multiple-choice:

After completing preprocedure teaching about the colonoscopy, the nurse knows that Jonathan requires further instruction when he states:

A. "I need to stop eating 8 hours before the test is scheduled."
B. "I need to make sure that someone is with me to drive me home."
C. "I will be able to resume my normal diet after the procedure."
D. "I will only have to take a mild laxative the evening before the procedure."

The answer can be found on page 152

EXERCISE 2.131 Fill in the blanks:

List the two tests that require bowel preparations, such as laxatives and GoLYTELY.

1. ____________________
2. ____________________

The answer can be found on page 152

eRESOURCE

To reinforce your understanding of GoLytely, refer to Epocrates Online. [Pathway: http://online.epocrates.com → under the "Drugs" tab, enter "GoLytely" in the search field → select "GoLytely" → review content.]

EXERCISE 2.132 Select all that apply:

Jonathan is in the endoscopy room ready for his procedure. Identify the final safety checks that must be completed by the nurse:

A. Confirm the correct patient and procedure
B. Have resuscitative equipment available
C. Confirm that an oral airway has been inserted
D. Position the patient in the supine position with head of bed at 30°
E. Review the patient's allergies before administering medications
F. Have suctioning equipment ready for use

The answer can be found on page 152

During the procedure, Jonathan's respiration rate is 18 breaths per minute, BP is 130/90 mmHg, and pulse is 88 beats per minute. Postprocedure, Donna takes his vital signs every 15 minutes to check for complications.

EXERCISE 2.133 Matching:

Match the symptoms in Column A with the possible causes in Column B:

Column A	Column B
A. Difficult to arouse, slow respirations, may be hypoxic	____ Aspiration
B. Cool, clammy skin, low blood pressure (BP), tachycardia	____ Perforation
C. Dyspnea, tachypnea, tachycardia, and possible fever	____ Oversedation
D. Chest or abdominal pain, nausea, vomiting, and abdominal distention	____ Hemorrhage

The answer can be found on page 153

Jonathan's colonoscopy is significant for large obstructive polyps; he needs reparative surgery and a temporary ostomy or opening from his GI tract to bypass the surgical repair. By the end of the week, he is admitted to the surgical unit following a colon resection with colostomy placement.

EXERCISE 2.134 Multiple-choice:

After taking Jonathan to his new room, the post-anesthesia care unit (PACU) nurse hands off care to the nurse on the surgical unit. What would be most important for the PACU nurse to communicate?

A. Estimated blood loss during the procedure was 160 mL.
B. Vital signs were stable during the operative and recovery phases.
C. The patient vomited twice while in the PACU.
D. The patient's family is on the way to the room.

The answer can be found on page 153

Jonathan is upset about the surgery and does not like to "wear the bag." He also complains about leakage from the bag and the nurse checks the seal, because the drainage can cause ulceration of the surrounding skin. Jonathan has a good support system; he has been married for 30 years and tomorrow he and his wife will participate in discharge teaching. The next day the nurse goes over the discharge-teaching list.

EXERCISE 2.135 Matching:

Match the discharge topics in Column A with the appropriate teaching issues in Column B:

Column A	Column B
Discharge Topic	**Teaching**
A. Normal skin appearance of the stoma	_____ Empty frequently
B. Skin barriers and creams	_____ Empty when the bag is ¼ full
C. Emptying ostomy bag	_____ Limited drainage
D. Dietary changes	_____ Abdominal bloating
E. Signs of obstruction	_____ Allow patient to verbalize
F. Sexual concerns	_____ Provide patient with suggestions
	_____ Use to protect the skin
	_____ Allow them to dry before placing bag on
	_____ Pink
	_____ Moist
	_____ Avoid foods that cause odor, such as fish, eggs, and leafy vegetables
	_____ Avoid gas-forming foods such as beer, dairy, and corn

The answer can be found on page 153

KEY TAKEAWAY POINTS

Endoscopic Procedures

- Endoscopic procedures allow direct visualization of the GI, respiratory, or urinary tracts.
- Preprocedure instructions and postprocedure care are specific to the procedures being done.
- Sedation is given to reduce anxiety and diminish the patient's memory of the procedure, which can be uncomfortable.
- Patients are NPO preprocedure to minimize vomiting and the risk of aspiration.
- Lower GI procedures require a bowel prep in order to visualize the tract.
- After the procedure, patients should be closely monitored for airway, breathing, circulation, and any signs of complications.
- Beginning at the age of 50 years, a colonoscopy is recommended every 10 years to screen for colorectal cancer.

Colostomies

- A colostomy is created as a temporary or permanent fecal diversion.
- The stoma should be beefy red or pink in appearance; a dark-brown, black, or purplish color could be suggestive of compromised circulation.
- The consistency of the stool output is related to the placement of the colostomy; stool is increasingly solid the closer to the sigmoid colon and rectum.
- Ileostomies, which divert stool from the small bowel, produce more loose/liquid output than colostomies.
- Appliances are usually changed every 5 to 7 days or when leaking.
- Emptying the appliance when one quarter to one third full minimizes the chances of the bag pulling loose from the skin.
- Patients can usually follow a regular diet, although avoiding foods that produce gas (dairy, corn), cause odor (fish, eggs), or are hard to digest (popcorn, seeds) is recommended.

UNFOLDING CASE STUDY 23: Ranesha

Thomas, the nurse, is admitting Ranesha, who is well known to the GI inpatient unit because she often has ascites. Ranesha, although rehabilitated now, has a long history of alcoholism.

EXERCISE 2.136 Multiple-choice:

When admitting Ranesha to the unit, what task can the nurse delegate to the unlicensed assistive personnel (UAP)?

A. List her home medications
B. Measure her input and output (I&O)
C. Assess for edema
D. Measure her abdominal girth

The answer can be found on page 154

On admission, Thomas assesses Ranesha's respiratory status and finds that she is dyspneic with a peripheral pulse oximetry level of 88%. Thomas calls Ranesha's PCP and sets up the procedure room for a paracentesis.

EXERCISE 2.137 Multiple-choice:

One of the major complications that can occur postparacentesis is:

A. Polycythemia
B. Low white blood cells (WBCs)
C. Hypovolemia
D. Hypervolemia

The answer can be found on page 154

Thomas assesses Ranesha and takes her weight; he measures her abdominal girth and has her void before the paracentesis is started. The paracentesis drains 1 L of fluid from Ranesha's abdomen, which should decrease her weight by 1 kg (2.2 lb).

eRESOURCE

To reinforce your understanding of the procedure, refer to Medscape on your mobile device. [Pathway: Medscape → select "Procedures"→ enter "Paracentesis" into the search field → select "Paracentesis" and review content.]

After the procedure, the PCP orders an electrolyte study. Thomas knows the normal lab values and compares them with Ranesha's blood work.

EXERCISE 2.138 Matching:

Match the lab tests in Column A with the normal values in Column B:

Column A	Column B
A. Albumin	___ 10 to 20 mg/dL
B. Protein	___ 0.6 to 1.5 mg/dL
C. Glucose	___ 70 to 100 mg/dL
D. Amylase	___ 3.5 to 5.0 g/dL
E. Blood urea nitrogen (BUN)	___ 53 to 123 units/L
F. Creatinine	___ 6.0 to 8.0 g/dL

The answer can be found on page 154

eRESOURCE

To reinforce your understanding of normal lab values, refer to Epocrates Online. [Pathway: http://online.epocrates.com ➔ under the "Tables" tab, select "Lab Reference" ➔ select "Lab Values: Normal Adult" ➔ review content.]

Thomas assesses Ranesha for the signs of hypovolemia.

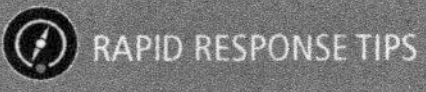

Clinical manifestations of hypovolemia

- Tachycardia
- Hypotension
- Pallor
- Diaphoresis
- Dizziness

Two other complications for which Thomas assesses Ranesha during the night include:

- Bladder perforation
  - Hematuria
  - Oliguria
  - Lower abdominal pain
- Peritonitis
  - Sharp abdominal pain
  - Fever
  - Vomiting
  - Hypoactive bowel sounds

Ranesha does well after the procedure; Thomas notices a little leakage from the insertion site and places a sterile gauze on it. Ranesha reports feeling better because she finds it easier to breathe.

KEY TAKEAWAY POINTS

Ascites

- The exact cause of ascites is unknown, but it is believed that failure of the liver to metabolize aldosterone, sodium and water retention, and decreased albumin contribute to its development.
- Clinical manifestations include increased abdominal girth, weight gain, swelling of the lower extremities, and dyspnea.

(*continued*)

- Management includes dietary restriction of sodium and diuretics; spironolactone (Aldactone) combined with furosemide (Lasix) has been found to be most effective.
- A paracentesis is done to remove fluid that is causing the patient significant problems, such as respiratory distress; this is only a temporary solution as ascites can rapidly recur.
- After the procedure, the patient should be monitored for bleeding or excessive drainage from the puncture site, elevated temperature, change in mental status, and signs of hypovolemia or electrolyte shifts.

UNFOLDING CASE STUDY 24: Elin

Thomas now turns his attention to his other patients on the unit. Another patient, Elin, had her call bell light on twice during this time and Jed, the nursing assistant, has responded but reports to Thomas that Elin is still uncomfortable with "severe indigestion." Thomas reads her medical record and finds that this patient was admitted with gastroesophageal reflux disease (GERD). Thomas knows that GERD can cause esophageal spasms from inflammation.

EXERCISE 2.139 Select all that apply:

Select all the nursing interventions that may help Elin's pain.

A. Offer her a cup of tea
B. Position her flat
C. Administer an antacid
D. Position her on the right side
E. Provide additional pillows
F. Encourage her to remain upright after eating

The answer can be found on page 154

eRESOURCE

To supplement your understanding of the clinical presentation associated with GERD, refer to the *Merck Manual*. [Pathway: www.merckmanuals.com → select "Medical Topics" → select "GERD" → select "Gastroesophageal Reflux Disease (GERD)" → review "Pathophysiology" and "Signs & Symptoms."]

Elin is scheduled for inpatient surgery the following day because her endoscopy showed Barrett's esophagus from persistent GERD and she has an intolerance of medications. She is scheduled for a fundoplication, which repositions the fundus of the stomach to decrease the chance of reflux. Elin does well postoperatively but has complaints of constipation.

eRESOURCE

To reinforce your understanding of the clinical presentation of Barrett's esophagus, refer to Medscape on your mobile device. [Pathway: Medscape ➔ select "Conditions"➔ enter "Barrett" into the search field ➔ select "Barrett esophagus" and review content.]

EXERCISE 2.140 Select all that apply:

To decrease Elin's problems with constipation, the nurse encourages her to:

A. Avoid frequent use of laxatives
B. Decrease fluids
C. Increase fiber in her diet
D. Decrease her level of physical activity
E. Minimize the use of opioids for pain control
F. Discuss any home remedies that have worked in the past

The answer can be found on page 155

EXERCISE 2.141 Select all that apply:

What breakfast would you encourage Elin to order?

A. Bran cereal
B. Yogurt
C. Fresh fruit
D. White toast

The answer can be found on page 155

KEY TAKEAWAY POINTS

Gastroesophageal Reflux Disease

- Excessive reflux may result from an incompetent lower esophageal sphincter, pyloric stenosis, or a motility disorder.
- Clinical manifestations include pyrosis (burning), dyspepsia (indigestion), regurgitation, dysphagia, and esophagitis.
- A low-fat diet is recommended with avoidance of caffeine, tobacco, beer, milk, carbonated beverages, and peppermint or spearmint.
- Other management strategies include avoiding eating or drinking 2 hours before bedtime, elevating the head of the bed on 6- to 8-in. blocks, and maintaining a normal body weight.
- Medications that may be used include antacids, H_2 receptor antagonists, proton pump inhibitors, and prokinetic agents.

UNFOLDING CASE STUDY 25: Christian

Christian, a 32-year-old executive, was admitted yesterday for peptic ulcer disease (PUD). An esophagogastroduodenoscopy (EGD) in the clinic confirmed a gastric ulcer, and he is being worked up for *Helicobacter pylori*, a major causative agent of PUD.

EXERCISE 2.142 Multiple-choice:

At change of shift report, a new nurse, who is unfamiliar with *H. pylori*, asks whether the patient should be in isolation. Her preceptor's best response would be:

A. "If the patient starts vomiting, we should put him in contact isolation."
B. "As long as he has started treatment with antibiotics, isolation is not necessary."
C. "Standard precautions are all that are needed in this case."
D. "By the end of our shift, I want you to be able to tell me all about *H. pylori*."

The answer can be found on page 155

Christian's history includes a high-stress job and frequent headaches on the job. He takes NSAIDs frequently. Thus, his history is typical for a patient with PUD. He reports bloating, fullness, and nausea 30 to 60 minutes after meals. Christian is prescribed medication and lifestyle changes and will be discharged and monitored.

eRESOURCE

To reinforce your understanding of the clinical presentation of PUD, refer to Medscape on your mobile device. [Pathway: Medscape ➔ select "Conditions"➔ enter "PUD" into the search field select "PUD" and review content.]

EXERCISE 2.143 Multiple-choice:

During discharge teaching, the nurse sees that Christian understands his instructions when he states:

A. "I will eat large meals three times a day."
B. "I will find a relaxation technique such as yoga."
C. "I can still drink all the iced tea that I want."
D. "I can have a few glasses of wine with dinner."

The answer can be found on page 156

Christian is prescribed four medications to start before his return visit to the GI clinic in 2 weeks.

EXERCISE 2.144 Matching:

Match the medications in Column A with the indications in Column B:

Column A	Column B
A. Bismuth	___ Inhibits *H. pylori*
B. Metronidozole and tetracycline	___ Protects the healing gastric ulcer
C. Antacids	___ Hyposecretory medication that inhibits the proton pump
D. Sucralfate (Carafate)	___ Neutralizes gastric acid

The answer can be found on page 156

Three months later, Christian is seen in the ED for severe gastric pain, a rigid abdomen, and hyperactive bowel sounds with rebound tenderness. A perforation is suspected and he is taken to the operating room. A gastrojejunostomy (Billroth II procedure) is done to remove the lower portion of the ulcerated stomach.

EXERCISE 2.145 Select all that apply:

What are some important postoperative nursing interventions for Christian?

A. Keep supine postoperatively
B. Monitor bowel sounds
C. Turn, cough, and breathe deeply
D. Monitor input and output (I&O)
E. Teach about dumping syndrome
F. Encourage liquids with meals

The answer can be found on page 156

KEY TAKEAWAY POINTS

Peptic Ulcer Disease

- Peptic ulcers can occur in the esophagus, stomach, or duodenum, although a duodenal ulcer is most common.
- Research has shown that peptic ulcers result from infection with *H. pylori*, a Gram-negative bacteria acquired through ingestion of food and water.
- Clinical manifestations include a dull, aching pain or burning in the midepigastric or back area, pyrosis (heartburn), vomiting, and bleeding.
- Duodenal ulcers cause pain hours after a meal, frequently wake a person up at night, and are relieved by eating.

(continued)

- Gastric ulcers are often aggravated by the ingestion of food, so pain may occur ½ to 1 hour after eating a meal.
- The goal of treatment is to eradicate *H. pylori* and manage gastric acidity.
- Management includes lifestyle changes and pharmacologic therapy; surgical options are a last resort.
- Complications include hemorrhage, perforation and/or penetration, and pyloric obstruction.

Gastric Surgery

- Following gastric surgery, patients must be monitored closely to ensure that they receive optimal nutrition.
- Dumping syndrome commonly occurs following a gastric surgery in which only a small gastric remnant is connected to the jejunum through a large opening; symptoms can be managed through various strategies.
- Vitamin and mineral deficiencies also occur, especially vitamin B_{12}, as intrinsic factor is lost with significant gastric surgeries.
- Patients require extensive education about their diet after gastric surgery.

UNFOLDING CASE STUDY 26: Simon

Christian understands his discharge instructions, and adjusts well after returning home. He later returns to the GI clinic for his 2-week checkup. Donna is the RN assessing patients. Just as Donna ushers him into the room, her certified nursing assistant (CNA) comes in and asks her to come quickly to the waiting room. There, Simon, age 21 years, is doubled over with right-lower-quadrant pain and severe rebound tenderness over McBurney's point.

EXERCISE 2.146 Hot spot:

Place a mark on McBurney's point.

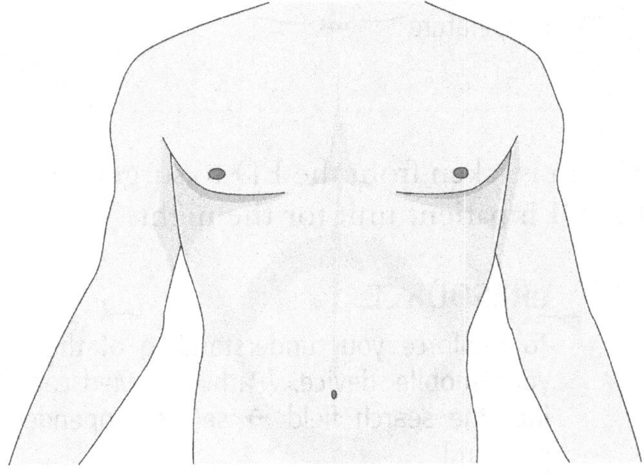

The answer can be found on page 156

eRESOURCE

To supplement your understanding of the clinical presentation associated with acute abdominal pain, refer to the *Merck Manual*. [Pathway: www.merckmanuals.com → select "Medical Topics" enter "Abdominal Pain" into the search field → select "Acute Abdominal Pain" → review content and images.]

Donna asks the administrative manager to call the transport ambulance and have Simon taken immediately to the ED for a suspected ruptured appendix. She phones ahead to notify the ED staff of the direct admission and her assessment. Donna also draws Simon's blood to expedite the admission process, because it all goes to the same lab through a pneumatic tube system.

EXERCISE 2.147 Select all that apply:

Identify the priority interventions for the patient admitted with acute appendicitis:

A. Prepare the patient for surgery
B. Maintain NPO (nothing orally) status
C. Administer an enema preoperatively
D. Insert an intravenous (IV) catheter and begin IV fluids
E. Notify the surgeon if the pain becomes more diffuse
F. Insert a nasogastric (NG) tube

The answer can be found on page 157

EXERCISE 2.148 Multiple-choice:

What other assessment is important to rule out peritonitis as a complication of a ruptured appendix?

A. Blood pressure (BP)
B. Pulse
C. Respiration
D. Temperature

The answer can be found on page 157

Simon is taken from the ED to surgery, and an appendectomy is done. He is admitted to the GI inpatient unit for the night.

eRESOURCE

To reinforce your understanding of the perioperative care for Simon, refer to Medscape on your mobile device. [Pathway: Medscape → select "Conditions"→ enter "Appendectomy" into the search field → select "Appendectomy" → select "Periprocedural Care" and review content.]

On the following day, Simon is being prepared for discharge. He has a postoperative appointment for the clinic, but he suddenly starts vomiting. Thomas, the nurse, notifies the physician, who orders the placement of an NG tube.

EXERCISE 2.149 Hot spot:

Trace on the diagram how you should measure a nasogastric (NG) tube:

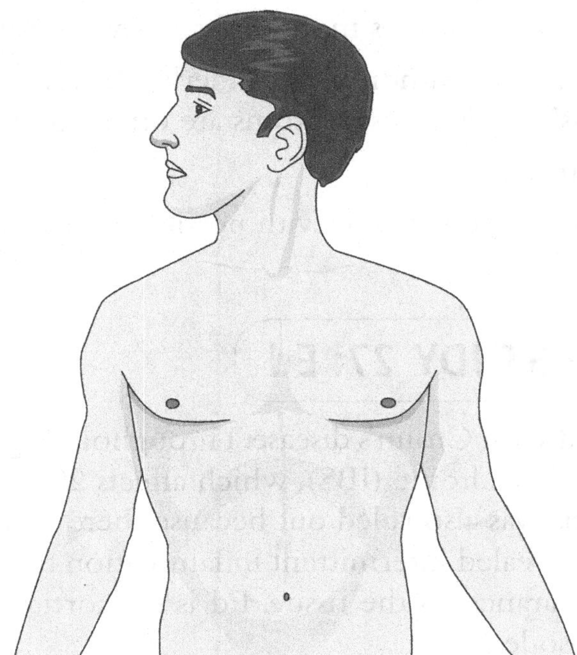

The answer can be found on page 157

EXERCISE 2.150 Multiple-choice:

What is considered the most accurate method for verifying placement of the nasogastric (NG) tube?

A. Aspiration of stomach contents
B. Bolus of air and listen for the gurgle as injected
C. Check the pH of aspirated contents
D. X-ray verification

The answer can be found on page 158

Thomas attached the NG tube to suction to remove any further gastric contents. The orders are to keep Simon NPO for at least 24 hours before discontinuing the tube and providing fluids orally.

KEY TAKEAWAY POINTS

Appendicitis

- When the appendix is kinked or occluded, inflammation occurs; rupture usually occurs within 24 hours of the onset of pain.
- Pain may begin in the periumbilical area and then localizes to the right lower quadrant; pain that changes and becomes more diffuse may indicate rupture.
- Although appendicitis is uncommon in the elderly, it carries a higher risk of perforation because the classic signs and symptoms are often absent.
- Treatment is immediate surgery.
- The major complication is perforation with possible resultant peritonitis.

UNFOLDING CASE STUDY 27: Ed

Ed was recently diagnosed with Crohn's disease. Throughout high school, it was thought that he had irritable bowel syndrome (IBS), which affects 20% of Americans. When Ed was admitted, diverticulitis was also ruled out because there was no acute inflammation on colonoscopy. The test revealed intermittent inflammation throughout the bowel with a classic cobblestone appearance to the tissue. Ed is on corticosteroids to decrease the current inflammatory episode.

EXERCISE 2.151 Matching:

Indicate whether each characteristic in Column B is associated with Crohn's disease or ulcerative colitis, as mentioned in Column A:

Column A	Column B
A. Crohn's	___ Mucosal ulceration
B. Ulcerative colitis	___ Occurs in rectum, descending colon
	___ Discontinuous lesions
	___ Severe diarrhea 10 to 20 times a day
	___ Minimal bleeding
	___ Occurs in ileum, ascending colon
	___ Bleeding is common

The answer can be found on page 158

Ed is taught dietary control for his Crohn's disease and discharged with a return appointment to the GI clinic.

eRESOURCE

To reinforce your understanding of Crohn's disease, refer to Epocrates Online. [Pathway: http://online.epocrates.com → under the "Diseases" tab, enter "Crohn's Disease" in the search field → select "Crohn's Disease" → review content.]

EXERCISE 2.152 Select all that apply:

Select the types of foods recommended for patients with Crohn's disease.

A. High calorie
B. Low calorie
C. High protein
D. High fiber
E. High fat
F. Low fat

The answer can be found on page 158

KEY TAKEAWAY POINTS

Inflammatory Bowel Disease

- Although Crohn's disease and ulcerative colitis differ in some of their characteristics and clinical manifestations, the management for both is quite similar.
- The cause of inflammatory bowel disease (IBD) is unknown, but it is thought to be triggered by environmental agents; NSAIDs have been found to exacerbate IBD.
- Crohn's disease usually occurs in the ileum or ascending colon, ulcerations are discontinuous giving a "cobblestone" appearance, bleeding is uncommon, and diarrhea is less severe than with ulcerative colitis.
- Ulcerative colitis spreads diffusely in the rectum and descending colon, bleeding is much more common, and diarrhea is often severe.
- Treatment focuses on reducing inflammation, suppressing the immune response, resting the bowel, preventing complications, and improving quality of life.
- A low-residue, high-protein, high-calorie diet with supplemental vitamins is recommended.
- Several medications are used such as corticosteroids and immunomodulators.
- Surgery is indicated when other measures have failed to relieve the symptoms of IBD and quality of life is poor.

UNFOLDING CASE STUDY 28: Polly

Polly is examined by Donna, the nurse working at the clinic. Polly came to the clinic because she had an attack (not her first)—which she describes as right-upper-quadrant (RUQ) pain after dinner. Polly is 3 months postpartum with her sixth child. An RUQ ultrasound finds the gallbladder to be edematous with several stones present.

EXERCISE 2.153 Multiple-choice:

After being diagnosed with cholelithiasis, Polly has many questions. Donna provides education on her disease process, but it is evident that Polly needs further instruction when she states:

A. "These painful attacks are often precipitated by a fatty meal."
B. "If the pain does not resolve, it could indicate that the stone is obstructed."
C. "I won't have to be in the hospital long if I am able to have a laparoscopic cholecystectomy."
D. "If I can withstand the painful episodes, eventually the stones will dissolve."

The answer can be found on page 158

---

eRESOURCE

To reinforce your understanding of the causes of cholelithiasis, refer to Medscape on your mobile device. [Pathway: Medscape → select "Conditions" → enter "Cholelithiasis" into the search field → select "Gallstones (Cholelithiasis)" → select "Etiology" and review content.]

Polly is counseled on dietary management. She would like to avoid a cholecystectomy if possible because of child-care issues.

EXERCISE 2.154 Select all that apply:

Select the foods that would be appropriate for Polly.

A. Beans
B. Eggs
C. Ice cream
D. Chicken
E. Apple
F. Bacon

The answer can be found on page 159

Polly returns to the ED with pain 2 weeks later and is admitted for an open cholecystectomy. After surgery, she has a Penrose drain at the surgical site. This allows fluid to drain into the dressing on the abdomen.

EXERCISE 2.155 Fill in the blanks:

Two other kinds of drainage tubes used postoperatively are described. Fill in the names.

1. It is a tube with a bulb at the end that is compressed to produce gentle suction at the surgical site.

   ____

2. It is a tube with a spring-activated device that is compressed to produce gentle suction at the surgical site.

   ____

The answer can be found on page 159

eRESOURCE

To reinforce your understanding of the open cholecystectomy procedure, refer to Medscape on your mobile device. [Pathway: Medscape select "Conditions" → enter "Open Cholecystectomy" into the search field and review content.]

KEY TAKEAWAY POINTS

Gallbladder Disease

- Cholecystitis can exist without stones, but 90% of the people with acute cholecystitis also have cholelithiasis (stones).
- Risk factors include obesity, females, rapid weight loss or frequent changes in weight, estrogen therapy, and family history.
- There are two major types of stones; one is comprised primarily of pigment and the second cholesterol.
- Symptoms are related to the gallbladder disease itself or obstruction of the bile passages.
- Ursodeoxycholic acid (UDCA) has been used to successfully dissolve small cholesterol-based stones.
- Laparoscopic cholecystectomies have decreased the surgical risks, length of hospital stay, and recovery period.

UNFOLDING CASE STUDY 29: Erik

Erik, another patient in the clinic, visits frequently, sometimes more than once in a single week. He too has a history of alcoholism. He complains of epigastric pain that radiates to his back and left shoulder. It normally starts after eating, and he experiences nausea and vomiting. Donna assesses him, and finds that he is slightly jaundiced; she also notes two other unusual signs, discolorations, on Erik.

EXERCISE 2.156 Hot spot:

Place the marks where you would find the discoloration of Turner's sign and Cullen's sign.

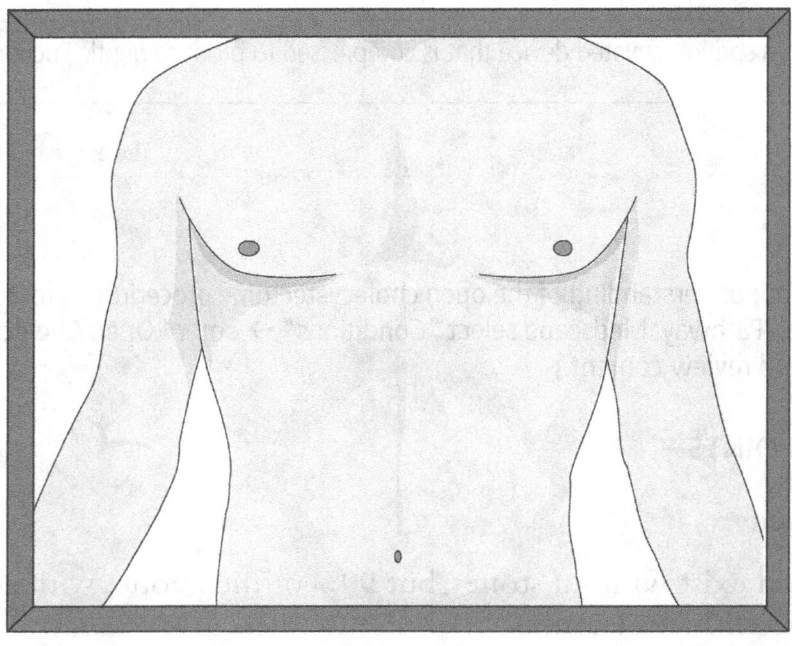

The answer can be found on page 159

Donna draws labs on Erik and finds the following:

- Decreased serum calcium and magnesium
- Elevated serum bilirubin and liver enzymes
- Elevated WBCs

Erik is admitted to the GI unit and an NG tube is inserted. He is given total parenteral nutrition (TPN), analgesics, and anticholinergics. Other types of tubes may also be used for long-term feedings.

EXERCISE 2.157 Matching:

Match the names of the tubes in Column A with the identifying information in Column B:

Column A	Column B
A. Percutaneous endoscopic gastrostomy (PEG) tube	___ Placed in the esophagus to stop bleeding of esophageal varices; it has an aspiration port.
B. Percutaneous endoscopic jejunostomy (PEJ) tube	___ Small-bore silicone nasogastric (NG) tube that has a weighted tip and is inserted with a guide wire for feeding.
C. Miller–Abbott tube	___ Tube placed endoscopically into the jejunum of the small bowel for long-term feeding.
D. Levin tube	___ Tube placed endoscopically into the stomach for long-term feeding.
E. Salem sump	___ Large-bore NG tube with two lumens; one attached to suction to promote drainage and one to allow airflow to the gastric mucosa.
F. Dobhoff tube	___ Two-lumen nasointestinal tube used to treat bowel obstructions; it is tungsten weighted at the end and has a lumen for drainage.
G. Cantor tube	___ Single-lumen nasointestinal tube used to treat bowel obstructions; it has a mercury-filled balloon at the end.
H. T-tube	___ Large-bore NG tube with one lumen attached to a low-suction pump for gastric decompression.
I. Sengstaken–Blakemore tube	___ Tube inserted into the common bile duct to drain bile.
J. Minnesota tube	___ Tube placed in the esophagus to stop bleeding of esophageal varices; it has three lumens.

The answer can be found on page 160

UNFOLDING CASE STUDY 30: Malcolm

Malcolm, age 44 years, is also a regular visitor in the clinic. He is a reformed drug abuser with hepatitis C and is now trying to decrease the effects of the hepatitis.

EXERCISE 2.158 Matching:

Match the types of hepatitis in Column A with the transmission and risk factors in Column B:

Column A	Column B
A. Hepatitis A (HAV)	___ Coinfection usually exists with HBV and is transmitted by drug use.
B. Hepatitis B (HBV)	___ Blood transmission by drug use and sexual contact.
C. Hepatitis C (HCV)	___ Oral–fecal route by ingestion of contaminated food or water.
D. Hepatitis D (HDV)	___ Oral–fecal route; very severe in pregnant women.
E. Hepatitis E (HEV)	___ Blood transmission by drug use, sexual contact, or by health care workers.

The answer can be found on page 161

eRESOURCE

To reinforce your understanding of the clinical presentation of a PE, refer to Medscape on your mobile device. [Pathway: Medscape → select "Conditions"→ enter "Hepatitis C" into the search field → select "Treatment & Management" and review content.]

Malcolm's liver enzymes are elevated. His alanine aminotransferase (ALT) is above 20 (normal is 8–20 units/L) and the aspartate aminotransferase (AST) is 60 (normal is 5–40 units/L). His alkaline phosphatase (ALP) is also elevated (normal is 42–128 units/L).

eRESOURCE

To reinforce your understanding of the liver function tests, refer to WebMD on your mobile device. [Pathway: WebMD → enter "Liver Function Tests" into the search field → select "Liver Function Tests" and review content.]

He is admitted to the inpatient GI unit for a liver biopsy, bed rest, and nutritional counseling. All the patients who are admitted to the GI inpatient unit are followed closely in the clinic after they are discharged.

EXERCISE 2.159 Multiple-choice:

In preparing to send Malcolm for a liver biopsy, the nurse prioritizes:

A. Make him NPO (nothing orally) after midnight
B. Start intravenous (IV) fluids before the procedure

C. Check for the results of coagulation tests
D. Obtain a consent for a blood transfusion

The answer can be found on page 161

eRESOURCE

To reinforce your understanding of the periprocedural care for a patient undergoing a liver biopsy, refer to Medscape on your mobile device. [Pathway: Medscape select "Conditions" ➔ enter "Liver Biopsy" into the search field ➔ select "Periprocedural Care" and review content.]

KEY TAKEAWAY POINTS

Hepatitis

- Hepatitis is a systemic viral infection that causes inflammation and necrosis of liver cells.
- HAV and HEV are very similar.
- HBV, HCV, and HDV carry a high risk for chronic liver disease.
- Vaccinations are available for HAV and HBV.
- The focus is on prevention.

PART VIII: Nursing Care of Patients With Infectious Diseases

Nina Russell and Brenda Reap Thompson

UNFOLDING CASE STUDY 31: Ada

Ada, a 23-year-old female, presents to the emergency room with complaints of a fever and rash that began about 2 days ago on her face, but has now progressed to cover most of her body. She recently travelled to India to visit family and returned 4 days ago. Ada never attended public school and did not receive her childhood immunizations. She is suspected of having measles (rubeola) and measles immunoglobulin M (IgM) and immunoglobulin G (IgG) antibodies are ordered.

EXERCISE 2.160 Select all that apply:

Clinical manifestations of measles include:

A. Low-grade fever
B. Cough
C. Koplik spots
D. Runny nose
E. Red, watery eyes
F. Rash that begins on the face and spreads to the trunk and extremities

The answer can be found on page 161

Ada's test results are positive for both IgG and IgM antibodies, confirming that she does have measles.

EXERCISE 2.161 Select all that apply:

Which of the following is accurate regarding measles?

A. Incubation period of 7 to 14 days
B. Contagious 4 days before to 4 days after rash appears
C. Verbal report of vaccination is acceptable evidence of immunity
D. More severe in the immunocompromised
E. Reportable communicable disease
F. Supportive treatment to alleviate symptoms

The answer can be found on page 161

---

eRESOURCE

To supplement your understanding of the clinical presentation associated with measles, refer to the *Merck Manual.* [Pathway: www.merckmanuals.com/professional → enter "Measles" into the search field → select "Measles" → review "Overview," "Pathophysiology," "Symptoms and Signs," and "Treatment."]

Ada likely contracted measles in India and may have infected others. The case should be reported to the Centers for Disease Control and Prevention (CDC) as well as the local health department for appropriate follow-up and disease containment. Hospital personnel need to use proper isolation precautions to prevent the dissemination of measles.

EXERCISE 2.162 Select all that apply:

The proper isolation precautions for measles:

A. Contact
B. Airborne
C. Droplet
D. Standard

The answer can be found on page 162

EXERCISE 2.163 Multiple-choice:

Which infection would require airborne precautions?

A. Varicella (chickenpox)
B. Anthrax
C. *Neisseria meningitides* (meningococcal infection)
D. *Haemophilus influenzae* type b

The answer can be found on page 162

EXERCISE 2.164 Select all that apply:

Airborne precautions include:

A. Airborne infection isolation room (AIIR)
B. N95 respirator
C. Door closed
D. Disposable dishes

The answer can be found on page 162

The nurse in the ED who completed Ada's initial assessment before it was determined that Ada had measles (rubeola) was never immunized for measles and never contracted the virus.

EXERCISE 2.165 Fill in the blanks:

The nurse who was never immunized for measles should be instructed to:

____

or

____

The answer can be found on page 162

The nurse will be excluded from duty to prevent spread of the virus.

eRESOURCE

To reinforce your understanding of measles and the pathophysiology of the disease, refer to Medscape on your mobile device. [Pathway: Medscape → enter "Measles" into the search field → select "Measles" and review content focusing primarily on the content under "Introduction."]

After caring for the patient, the nurse will remove personal protective equipment (PPE) in the designated area carefully to avoid self-contamination.

EXERCISE 2.166 Ordering:

Place the steps for doffing personal protective equipment (PPE) in the correct order from 1 to 4:

_______ Unfasten neck of gown, then waist ties; pull gown down from each shoulder.

_______ Take elastic band of N95 respirator from behind the head, discard by holding the band.

_______ Grab outside of glove with opposite gloved hand and peel off; hold removed glove in hand while pulling the second glove inside out over the first glove.

_______ Remove the face shield by touching the clean earpieces or headband.

The answer can be found on page 162

The nurses are discussing precautions used to prevent the transmission of infection. A student nurse states that she is not sure when to use standard precautions.

EXERCISE 2.167 Select all that apply:

Standard precautions are used to:

A. Start an intravenous (IV) line
B. Care for a patient with *Clostridium difficile*
C. Empty a urinary catheter
D. Change a patient's bed that is soiled with drainage
E. Administer medication down a gastrostomy tube
F. Change a dressing 24 hours after surgery

The answer can be found on page 163

It is important to follow up with anyone who may have been exposed to measles. Individuals without adequate medical documentation of immunization, such as vaccination, laboratory titers, or a history of measles infection, should receive the measles, mumps, and rubella (MMR) vaccine or the measles immune globulin.

eRESOURCE

To reinforce your understanding of the treatment of the disease, refer to Medscape on your mobile device. [Pathway: Medscape → enter "Measles" into the search field → select "Measles" and review content under "Treatment & Management."]

UNFOLDING CASE STUDY 32: Layla

Layla, a 32-year-old female, presents to the ED with complaints of ongoing cough, nasal congestion, and myalgia that began about 24 hours ago and is progressively getting worse. She has no significant past medical history and takes no routine medications. Vital signs: Temperature, 101.8°F; BP, 120/74 mmHg; HR, 86; RR, 18; oxygen saturation, 96% on room air.

EXERCISE 2.168 Select all that apply:

To minimize the risk of infection to others, the triage nurse would:

A. Provide the patient with tissues to cover the mouth and nose
B. Direct the patient to discard the tissues promptly after use
C. Place the patient before the other patients waiting for treatment
D. Instruct the patient to apply a surgical mask
E. Seat the patient 3 feet away from other patients
F. Educate the patient to wash his or her hands after contact with secretions

The answer can be found on page 163

Layla's symptoms are indicative of influenza and a rapid flu test is ordered.

EXERCISE 2.169 Select all that apply:

Signs and symptoms of influenza include:

A. Fever
B. Myalgia
C. Nonproductive cough
D. Malaise
E. Productive cough
F. Nasal congestion and sore throat

The answer can be found on page 163

Layla's nasopharyngeal test is positive for influenza A. She asks about how the flu virus is spread and is concerned about infecting others.

EXERCISE 2.170 Select all that apply:

Influenza can be contracted by:

A. Contact with virus-contaminated blood
B. Contact with virus-contaminated surfaces
C. Close proximity of a virus-infected person who coughs
D. Close proximity of a virus-infected person who sneezes

The answer can be found on page 163

Layla will not be admitted and is discharged home on antiviral medication and given instructions on minimizing potential exposure to family members, friends, co-workers, and so on.

EXERCISE 2.171 Multiple-choice:

What isolation precautions are required for the inpatient or outpatient management of patients with influenza?

A. Contact
B. Airborne
C. Droplet
D. Standard

The answer can be found on page 164

The nurse is providing Layla with discharge teaching regarding ways to prevent transmission of the flu to others inside and outside of the home.

EXERCISE 2.172 Select all that apply:

To minimize potential exposure of noninfected individuals to influenza, patient education would include:

A. Do not share eating utensils or linens
B. Avoid public places for 48 hours
C. Wear surgical mask while coughing
D. Cover nose and mouth to cough and sneeze
E. Wash hands with soap and water
F. Disinfect all contaminated surfaces

The answer can be found on page 164

---

eRESOURCE

To supplement your understanding of the clinical presentation associated with influenza and associated treatment, refer to the *Merck Manual.* [Pathway: www.merckmanuals.com/professional ➔ enter "influenza" into the search field ➔ select "Influenza" ➔ review "Epidemiology," "Symptoms and Signs," and "Treatment."]

Layla is given a prescription for the antiviral Tamiflu (oseltamivir) and asks the nurse how the medication works.

EXERCISE 2.173 Multiple-choice:

Which statement by the nurse demonstrates correct teaching about the antiviral drug Tamiflu?

A. "It is used to treat, not prevent, influenza."
B. "It is only active against influenza type A virus."
C. "It should be started within 48 hours of symptom onset."
D. "It should never be given to a pregnant patient."

The answer can be found on page 164

Layla is encouraged to drink plenty of fluids, rest, and take Tylenol (acetaminophen) as needed for fever or muscle aches. The nurse also stresses the importance of yearly influenza vaccines.

eRESOURCE

To reinforce your understanding of Tamiflu, refer to Epocrates Online. [Pathway: http://online.epocrates.com → under the "Drugs" tab, enter "Tamiflu" in the search field → select "Tamiflu" → review "Adult Dosing," "Adverse Reactions," "Safety/Monitoring," and "Patient Education."]

Answers

EXERCISE 2.1 Select all that apply:

Ruth Marie asks the nurse, "What causes high blood pressure?" The nurse explains that risk factors for primary hypertension (HTN) are:

A. Obesity—**YES; this increases the risk of primary HTN.**
B. Narrowing of the aorta—NO; this is a cause of secondary HTN.
C. Alcohol consumption—**YES; this increases the risk of primary HTN.**
D. Sodium retention—**YES; this increases the risk of primary HTN.**
E. Sleep apnea—NO; this is a cause of secondary HTN.
F. Cigarette smoking—NO; this does not increase the risk of HTN, but, coupled with HTN, it increases the risk of heart disease.

EXERCISE 2.2 Multiple-choice:

Which statement made by Ruth Marie indicates an understanding of the low-sodium diet?

A. "I can still drink two glasses of tomato juice every morning."—NO; canned foods are high in sodium and should be restricted.
B. "I will eat a few slices of cheese every day because it has protein."—NO; cheese, tomatoes, canned foods, and prepared frozen dinners are high in sodium and should be restricted.
C. "When I am too tired to cook, I will eat prepared frozen meals."—NO; prepared frozen dinners are high in sodium and should be restricted.
D. "I will begin eating cooked cereal for breakfast."—**YES; cooked cereal is low in sodium.**

EXERCISE 2.3 Multiple-choice:

The nurse can determine whether the patient's heart rate is regular by looking at the EKG rhythm strip and measuring the:

A. Distance from R wave to R wave—**YES; this is used to determine whether the heart rate is regular.**
B. Distance from the P wave to Q wave—NO; this does not provide a total cycle to evaluate.

C. Height of the R wave—NO; this does not provide a total cycle to evaluate.
D. Height of the T wave—NO; this does not provide a total cycle to evaluate.

EXERCISE 2.4 Fill in the blanks:

Indicate which assessment findings are related to venous disease by placing a V, or to arterial disease by placing an A where appropriate.

A Capillary refill less than 3 seconds
A Pain with exercise
V Lower leg edema
A Cool to touch
A Pallor with elevation
V Bronze-brown pigment
A Thickened, brittle nails
V Frequent pruritus
A Thin, shiny, dry skin
A Absent pulses

EXERCISE 2.5 List:

Use the list on the right-hand side to categorize the risk factors for coronary artery disease (CAD):

Modifiable	Risk Factors
1. **A**	A. Obesity
2. **B**	B. Serum lipids: elevated triglycerides and cholesterol, decreased high-density lipoproteins (HDL)
3. **E**	C. Race
4. **F**	D. Family history
5. **G**	E. Hypertension
Nonmodifiable	F. Tobacco use
1. **C**	G. Physical inactivity
2. **D**	H. Age
3. **H**	

EXERCISE 2.6 Multiple-choice:

The following are prescribed orders for Ruth Marie. Which order should the nurse question?

A. Nasal oxygen 2 L—NO; the additional oxygen is needed at this time.
B. Aspirin (ASA) 81 mg enteric-coated orally, stat—**YES; ASA 325 mg is usually prescribed, with instructions to chew and swallow.**
C. Portable chest x-ray—NO; portable chest x-ray is prescribed so the patient can remain in the ED for observation.
D. Nitroglycerin (NTG) 1/150 mg sublingual, stat—NO; this is the usual prescribed dose for patients with chest pain.

EXERCISE 2.7 Multiple-choice:

In preparing to administer adenosine (Adenocard), the nurse prioritizes which intervention?

A. Inserting an intravenous (IV) line in the nondominant hand—NO; the IV should be inserted into a vein in close proximity to the heart, such as the antecubital vein.
B. Calling anesthesia to sedate the patient—NO; this is not necessary for administration of adenosine.
C. Placing a defibrillator with pacing capability at the patient's bedside—**YES; bradycardia, hypotension, and sinus arrest may occur, but are usually short-lived because of the drug's short duration of action.**
D. Mixing the adenosine in 50 mL of D_5W (5% dextrose and water)—NO; the adenosine should be given via rapid IV push over 1 to 2 seconds.

EXERCISE 2.8 Hot spot:

Indicate the area on the cardiac rhythm strip that demonstrates acute myocardial infarction (MI).

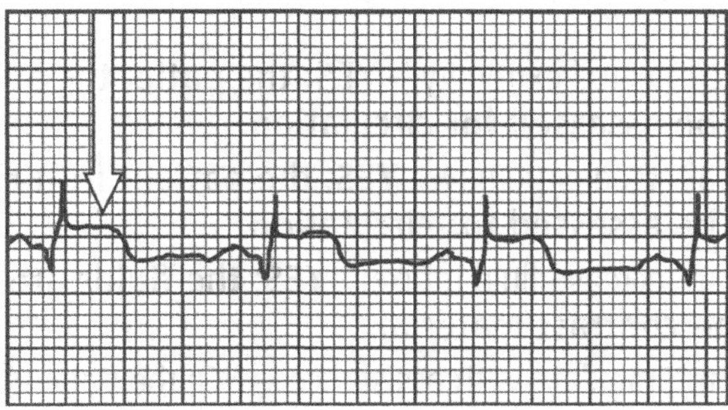

EXERCISE 2.9 Select all that apply:

The EKG indicates myocardial injury in leads V_2 to V_4. The nurse understands that the patient should be observed for:

A. First-degree block—NO.
B. Third-degree block—**YES; EKG changes in V_2 to V_4 indicate an anterior myocardial infarction (MI).**
C. Bradydysrhythmias—NO; this is more common with inferior MIs.
D. Heart failure—**YES; this occurs more often with anterior MIs.**
E. Ventricular dysrhythmias—**YES; this can occur with any MI.**
F. Cardiogenic shock—**YES; this can occur after a large anterior MI.**

EXERCISE 2.10 Calculation:

Ruth Marie is prescribed a nitroglycerin (NTG) drip of 50 mg in 250 mL D_5W. The order is to infuse at 100 mcg/min. What flow rate in milliliters per hour would be needed to deliver this amount?

100 mcg/min × 60 minute = 6,000 mcg/hr
Convert mcg to mg 1,000 mcg = 1 mg
6,000 mcg/hr = 6 mg/hr
Calculate the flow rate in milliliters per hour
50 mg: 250 mL = 6 mg: *x* mL
50*x*/50 = 1,500/50
***x* = 30 mL/hr**

EXERCISE 2.11 Multiple-choice:

Ruth Marie drinks the medication and asks the nurse why it was prescribed. Which statement by the nurse would be appropriate?

A. "It helps to keep your airway clear during the procedure." —NO; this is not the reason.
B. "It is used to protect your kidneys from the contrast." —**YES; Mucomyst is administered orally to patients at increased risk for renal failure prior to procedures that include the use of contrast.**
C. "It will help you to breathe slowly and relax." —NO; this is not the action of the medication.
D. "It is used to keep the heart rate regular." —NO; this is not the action of the medication.

EXERCISE 2.12 Select all that apply:

The nurse is caring for Ruth Marie after the percutaneous revascularization procedure. Which action is appropriate?

A. Check the pulses of the affected extremity—**YES; the patient is at risk of emboli and therefore the extremity must be assessed for circulation.**
B. Check the color of the affected extremity—**YES; the patient is at risk of emboli and therefore the extremity must be assessed for circulation.**
C. Encourage the patient to increase fluid intake—**YES; the fluids are increased to help the patient eliminate the contrast material.**
D. Encourage the patient to ambulate with assistance—NO; the patient is initially on bedrest until hemostasis is achieved.
E. Keep the head of the bed elevated at least 30°—NO; the head of the bed is kept flat or less than 30° immediately following the procedure.
F. Assess for bleeding or hematoma at the catheter insertion site—**YES; this should be done with the pulse and temperature checks.**

EXERCISE 2.13 Multiple-choice:

The charge nurse is making assignments for the following shift. Ruth Marie is 2 hours post-revascularization with heparin and nitroglycerin (NTG) infusion. Her vital signs are stable, but a hematoma has developed at the catheter insertion site. It would be most appropriate to assign this patient to:

A. A recently graduated RN who started orientation 2 days ago—NO; the new RN likely does not have the knowledge to manage this patient with intravenous (IV) drips and a new hematoma.
B. An experienced RN who recently transferred to the unit from the post-anesthesia care unit (PACU)—**YES; this RN would have experience in managing IV drips and performing cardiovascular checks, as well as in managing bleeding.**
C. A licensed practical nurse (LPN) who has been working on the unit for 1 year—NO; this patient has developed a complication and should not be assigned to the LPN.
D. An RN who was pulled for the shift from a genitourinary (GU)/renal unit—NO; this RN would not have the expertise needed.

EXERCISE 2.14 Multiple-choice:

Which action would the nurse take first?

A. Call a code—NO; not before assessing the patient.
B. Obtain the code cart—NO; not before assessing the patient.
C. Check the patient—**YES; the nurse would assess the patient first, because an electrode may be causing interference. In this case, the patient was brushing her teeth.**
D. Turn on the defibrillator—NO; not before assessing the patient.

EXERCISE 2.15 Fill in the blanks:

The nurse is reviewing medications with Ruth Marie. What should the nurse teach the patient about taking nitroglycerin (NTG) 1/150 sublingually?

1. **Place the tablet under your tongue if you have chest discomfort.**
2. **Take one tablet every 5 minutes times three doses if needed.**
3. **Call the ambulance if chest pain is not relieved by the first dose of NTG.**
4. **The drug may lose potency 3 to 6 months after the bottle has been opened.**
5. **Always store the tablets in the original bottle.**

EXERCISE 2.16 Multiple-choice:

In preparing the patient for discharge, which intervention can be delegated to the unlicensed assistive personnel (UAP)?

A. Review activity instructions given by the MD—NO; discharge instructions should be given by the licensed nurse.
B. Arrange for a follow-up appointment with the cardiologist—NO; this can be done by the unit secretary.
C. Removal of the hemostatic dressing and application of a new dressing—NO; this should be done by the licensed nurse; the patient has a hematoma so this needs to be assessed.
D. Measurement of the predischarge vital signs—**YES; this is a role for the unlicensed assistive personnel (UAP).**

EXERCISE 2.17 Matching:

Indicate which assessment findings are related to right-sided or left-sided heart failure.

Column A	Column B	
A. Right-sided heart failure	**A**	Anasarca
B. Left-sided heart failure	**A**	Jugular venous distention
	A	Edema of lower extremities
	B	Dyspnea
	A	Hepatomegaly
	B	Dry, hacking cough
	B	Restlessness, confusion
	A	Right-upper-quadrant pain
	B	Crackles on auscultation of lungs
	A	Weight gain
	B	S3 and S4 heart sounds
	B	Pink, frothy sputum

EXERCISE 2.18 Exhibit-format:

12-lead EKG—Atrial fibrillation with a ventricular rate of 170

Portable chest x-ray (PCXR)—Congestion with Kerley B lines noted

Echocardiogram—Ejection fraction (EF) of 40%

B-type natriuretic peptide (BNP)—720 pg/mL

After receiving further orders from the MD, the nurse understands that the priority intervention is to:

A. Keep the head of the bed elevated greater than 30°—NO; this will help with shortness of breath, but the patient was hypotensive.
B. Obtain the patient's weight before giving the diuretic—NO; this is not the priority when the patient is in distress.
C. Insert a Foley catheter for hourly input and output (I&O)—NO; this may not be necessary if the patient stabilizes.
D. Administer medication to slow the heart rate—**YES; slowing the heart rate makes the heart not work as hard. The patient may convert to a sinus rhythm, which would help with the heart failure.**

EXERCISE 2.19 Select all that apply:

Identify which interventions are a priority for the patient undergoing emergent cardioversion:

A. Verify that the defibrillator is in sync mode—**YES; this is essential to time the delivery of the energy current.**
B. Monitor the patient's airway and breathing—**YES; this is important during any procedure, but especially if the patient receives any sedation.**
C. Keep the patient NPO (nothing orally) for at least 4 hours—NO; ideally, the patient would be NPO, but in an emergent situation, this is not a priority.
D. Confirm that suction is set up and ready for use—**YES; this is important in the event the patient begins vomiting, especially if he or she were not nothing by mouth (NPO) before the procedure.**
E. Call anesthesia to intubate the patient before the procedure—NO; this is not required for this procedure, although if time permits, conscious sedation should be administered.
F. Perform frequent assessment of vital signs—**YES; the patient should be monitored closely during and after the procedure.**

EXERCISE 2.20 Calculation:

A dobutamine drip is ordered to be started at 5 mcg/kg/min. The medication is mixed at 500 mg in 500 mL of fluid. If the patient weighs 176 lb, what flow rate in milliliters per hour would be needed to deliver this amount?

24 mL/hr

EXERCISE 2.21 Hot spot:

Indicate where the nurse should place the stethoscope in order to auscultate for the following:

A. Bronchial breath sounds
B. Vesicular breath sounds
C. Bronchovesicular breath sounds

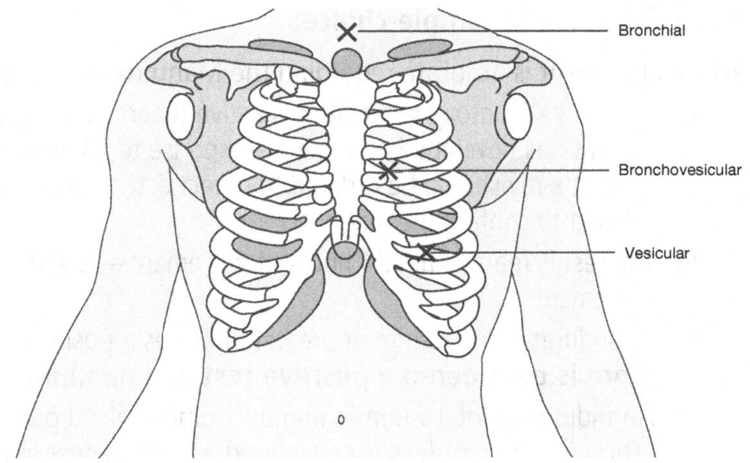

EXERCISE 2.22 Matching:

Match the reason for oxygen delivery in Column A to the method of oxygenation in Column B:

Column A	Column B
A. Rarely used; may be used to deliver oxygen for a patient who has a wired jaw	D Partial rebreather mask
B. Delivers fixed prescribed oxygen rates	C Nonrebreather mask
C. Reservoir bag has a one-way valve that prevents exhaled air from entering the reservoir; it allows for larger concentrations of oxygen to be inhaled from the reservoir bag	A Face tent
D. Reservoir bag connected to the mask collects one third of the patient's exhaled air; carbon dioxide is used as a respiratory stimulant	B Venturi mask

EXERCISE 2.23 Select all that apply:

Which clinical manifestations are consistent with active tuberculosis (TB)?

A. Dyspnea—**YES; this is a late sign.**
B. Night sweats—**YES; this is a definite symptom.**
C. Fatigue—**YES; this is a definite symptom.**
D. Low-grade fevers—**YES; this is a definite symptom.**
E. Productive bloody sputum—**YES; this is a late sign but only occurs in 10%; a dry cough or mucopurulent sputum is common.**
F. Unexplained weight loss—**YES; this is a definite symptom.**
G. Anorexia—**YES; this is a definite symptom.**
H. Wheezing—NO; this is not normally a symptom.

EXERCISE 2.24 Multiple-choice:

Which statement is accurate regarding the Mantoux skin test?

A. A positive Mantoux test confirms active tuberculosis (TB)—NO; a positive TB skin test indicates that a patient has developed an immune response to TB; it does not confirm active disease; a chest x-ray should be ordered to detect active lesions in the lung; an acid-fast bacilli (AFB) culture is needed to confirm the diagnosis.

B. The test is read within 24 hours of placement—NO; this test should be read 48 to 72 hours following placement.

C. An induration of 10 mm or greater indicates a positive skin test—**YES; induration of 10 mm or more is considered a positive test in nonimmunocompromised patients.**

D. An induration of 15 mm in immunocompromised patients is considered a positive test—NO; induration of 5 mm or less is considered a positive test in immunocompromised patients.

EXERCISE 2.25 Multiple-choice:

Which statement by a student nurse needs follow-up regarding precautions for a patient with possible tuberculosis (TB)?

A. "The patient will be isolated in a negative pressure room."—NO; this is correct because patients with active disease need to be in a negative pressure room.

B. "The nurse will wear a high-efficiency particulate air (HEPA) mask."—NO; this is correct practice to prevent the nurse from breathing in the active TB particles.

C. "The airborne isolation sign will be placed at the entrance to the patient's room."—NO; it is appropriate that the airborne precaution sign should be visible so that the proper protective equipment may be donned.

D. "The patient will wear a N95 mask when leaving the room."—**YES; follow-up is needed because the patient should wear a surgical mask when leaving the room to prevent the active TB particles from being released**.

EXERCISE 2.26 Multiple-choice:

Which instruction will the nurse give the patient in regard to rifampin (Rifadin)?

A. The medication may turn your urine red-orange.—**YES; rifampin may turn your urine, stools, saliva, sputum, sweat, and tears a red-orange color; the effect is harmless.**

B. The medication may cause short-term memory loss.—NO; this is not a side effect of rifampin.

C. The medication should be taken with food.—NO; rifampin should be taken 1 hour before or 2 hours after a meal.

D. The medication may increase your appetite.—NO; medication may cause gastrointestinal (GI) upset.

EXERCISE 2.27 Multiple-choice:

Which statement by the nurse is correct?

A. "You will be discharged when you stop coughing up secretions."—NO.

B. "Discharge will depend on the results of the chest x-ray."—NO.

C. "Most patients are discharged after taking their medication for 48 hours."—NO.

D. "Patients are discharged after three negative acid-fast bacilli (AFB) smears."—**YES; the patient is considered noninfectious after three negative AFB smears.**

EXERCISE 2.28 Multiple-choice:

Which of the following statements indicate that the patient understands appropriate care measures?

A. "One medication can be substituted for another because they all fight infection."—NO.

B. "A sputum specimen will need to be collected every 2 to 4 weeks indefinitely."—NO; once the patient is noninfectious, regular sputum collections are not warranted.

C. "Medication will need to be taken for a 6- to 12-month duration."—**YES; medication therapy is needed for 6 to 12 months.**

D. "A standardized mask will need to be worn until medication therapy is completed."—NO; after three negative AFB smears, the patient is not infectious and no mask is needed.

EXERCISE 2.29 Fill in the blanks:

Name four causes of a closed pneumothorax.

1. **Injury during the insertion of a subclavian catheter**
2. **Rupture of blebs in the lung, which is common when a patient has chronic obstructive pulmonary disease (COPD)**
3. **Injury to the lung from broken ribs**
4. **Injury from mechanical ventilation with positive-end-expiratory pressure**

EXERCISE 2.30 Fill in the blanks:

Name two causes of an open pneumothorax.

1. **Stab wound**
2. **Gunshot wound**

EXERCISE 2.31 Matching:

Match the manifestation in Column A to the complication in Column B:

Column A	Column B
A. Muffled distant heart sounds, hypotension	C Flail chest
B. Deviation of the trachea, air hunger	D Hemothorax
C. Paradoxical movement of the chest wall	B Tension pneumothorax
D. Shock, dullness on percussion	A Cardiac tamponade

EXERCISE 2.32 Select all that apply:

Which findings will the nurse anticipate in a patient suffering from a fractured rib?

A. Pain during inspiration—**YES; pain when patient breathes in.**

B. Shallow, rapid respirations—**YES; pain during respiration results in rapid, shallow breathing.**

C. Crackles to bilateral lower lobes—NO; not associated with a fractured rib; common in congestive heart failure (CHF).

D. Splinting or guarding the chest—**YES; chest rise and fall results in splinting or guarding.**

EXERCISE 2.33 Fill in the blanks:

What are the differences between chronic bronchitis and emphysema?

Chronic bronchitis: **Chronic bronchitis is the presence of a chronic cough for 3 months in 2 consecutive years.**

Emphysema: **Emphysema is enlargement of the air sacs with destruction of the walls.**

EXERCISE 2.34 List:

Identify which clinical manifestations are related to chronic obstructive pulmonary disease (COPD) and which are related to asthma.

A. Onset is at 40 to 50 years of age
B. Dyspnea is always experienced during exercise
C. Clinical symptoms are intermittent from day to day
D. There is frequent sputum production
E. Weight loss is characteristic
F. There is a history of allergies, rhinitis, and eczema
G. Disability worsens progressively

COPD

A. **Onset is at 40 to 50 years of age**
B. **Dyspnea is always experienced during exercise**
D. **There is frequent sputum production**
E. **Weight loss is characteristic**
G. **Disability worsens progressively**

Asthma

C. **Clinical symptoms are intermittent from day to day**
F. **There is a history of allergies, rhinitis, and eczema**

EXERCISE 2.35 Multiple-choice:

The nurse's findings are most consistent with which diagnosis?

A. Tuberculosis (TB)—NO.
B. Chronic obstructive pulmonary disease (COPD)—**YES.**
C. Pneumonia—NO.
D. Congestive heart failure (CHF)—NO.

EXERCISE 2.36 Multiple-choice:

Which statement by the nurse demonstrates understanding of oxygen delivery via a Venturi mask?

A. "Using a Venturi mask will prevent the nasal mucosa from drying and reduce coughing."—NO.
B. "The Venturi mask provides a low-flow oxygen delivery system."—NO; a Venturi mask is a high-flow oxygen delivery system.
C. "The Venturi mask provides a consistent, precise concentration of oxygen to maintain respiratory drive."—**YES; a Venturi mask delivers a consistent concentration of oxygen.**

D. "The Venturi mask is a high-flow system that flushes the expired carbon dioxide out of the mask preventing further retention."—NO.

EXERCISE 2.37 Matching:

Match the associated factors in Column A to the complication in Column B:

Column A	Column B
A. Fever, increased cough, dyspnea	**E** Cor pulmonale
B. Occurs in patients who have chronic retention of CO_2	**A, C, D** Acute respiratory failure or corticosteroid therapy
C. Occurs in patients who discontinue use of a bronchodilator	**B** Peptic ulcer disease
D. Administration of benzodiazepines, sedatives, narcotics	
E. Crackles are audible in the bases of the lungs	

EXERCISE 2.38 Matching:

Match the clinical manifestations in Column A with the types of urinary tract infections (UTI) in Column B:

Column A	Column B
A. Flank pain, fever, vomiting	**A** Pyelonephritis
B. Urgency, painful bladder, frequency	**D** Glomerulonephritis
C. Purulent discharge, dysuria, urgency	**C** Urethritis
D. Hematuria, proteinuria, elevated creatinine	**B** Interstitial cystitis

EXERCISE 2.39 Select all that apply:

The nurse is providing Fran with information about bladder irritants. Fran would be instructed to avoid:

A. Caffeine—**YES.**
B. Alcohol—**YES.**
C. Milk—NO.
D. Chocolate—**YES.**
E. Spicy foods—**YES.**
F. Legumes—NO.

EXERCISE 2.40 Fill in the blanks:

What four questions would the nurse ask to determine whether Fran has problems with urinary emptying?

1. **Do you have difficulty starting the urinary stream?**
2. **Do you have pain during urination?**

3. **Do you have urinary dribbling after you urinate?**
4. **Do you feel like you did not completely empty your bladder after you urinate?**

What four questions would the nurse ask to determine whether Fran has problems with urinary storage?

1. **Do you urinate small quantities more often than every 2 hours?**
2. **Do you find that you have to urinate immediately?**
3. **Do you urinate before you can get to the bathroom?**
4. **Do you wake up more than once during the night to urinate?**

EXERCISE 2.41 Select all that apply:

What health-promotion activities could the nurse teach the patient?

A. Empty the bladder every 6 hours—NO; evacuate the bladder every 3 to 4 hours.
B. Evacuate the bowel regularly—**YES; avoid constipation.**
C. Wipe the perineal area from front to back—**YES.**
D. Urinate before and after intercourse—**YES; this helps to expel bacteria.**
E. Drink cranberry juice daily—**YES; this acidifies the urine.**
F. Shower rather than bathe in the tub—**YES; tub baths increase the chance of bacteria entering the urinary tract.**

EXERCISE 2.42 Hot spot:

What area would the nurse percuss to assess for kidney infection?

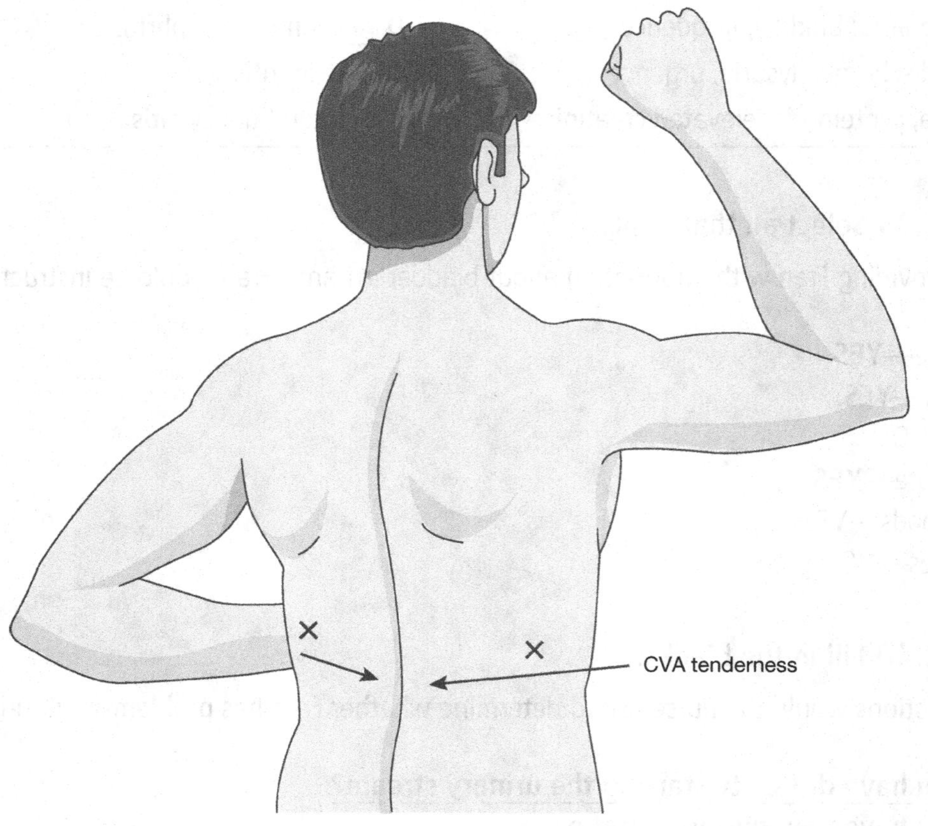

EXERCISE 2.43 Select all that apply:

Fran asks the nurse what causes urinary calculi. Which of the following answers from the nurse are correct?

A. Low fluid intake—**YES; it causes a concentrated, decreased urine output.**
B. Decreased uric acid levels—NO; increased uric acid levels cause urinary calculi.
C. Warm climate—**YES; it increases the risk of dehydration.**
D. Family history for renal calculi—**YES; family history is a known risk factor.**
E. Immobility—**YES; immobility causes stasis of urine.**
F. Frequent urination—NO; this actually helps to flush the urinary system.

EXERCISE 2.44 Fill in the blanks:

What information in Joe's history suggests an increased risk for bladder cancer?

Age, gender, and cigarette smoking.

EXERCISE 2.45 Select all that apply:

Identify risk factors associated with bladder cancer:

A. Contaminated drinking water—**YES; levels of arsenic in drinking water are related to the area where you live and whether water is from a well or public system.**
B. Dehydration—NO; this is more associated with renal calculi.
C. Recurrent or chronic urinary tract infections (UTIs)—**YES.**
D. Exposure to environmental carcinogens—**YES; such as dyes, rubber, leather, or paint.**
E. Diabetes—NO.
F. Pelvic radiation therapy—**YES.**

EXERCISE 2.46 Select all that apply:

What are the responsibilities of the nurse when the patient returns from cystoscopy?

A. Monitor for bright-red blood in the urine—**YES; this is a complication, but burning on urination and pink-tinged urine are expected findings.**
B. Encourage the patient to change position slowly—**YES; because orthostatic hypotension is common after the procedure.**
C. Irrigate the catheter daily—NO; irrigating a catheter may cause infection.
D. Provide warm sitz baths—**YES; warm sitz baths and analgesics will be offered to promote comfort.**
E. Monitor for signs of urinary tract infection (UTI)—**YES; most hospital-acquired urinary tract infections (UTIs) follow instrumentation of the urinary tract.**
F. Strain all urine for stones—NO; this is appropriate for the patient with renal calculi.

EXERCISE 2.47 Multiple-choice:

Joe is receiving his first treatment with Bacillus Calmette–Guérin (BCG). It is evident that further teaching is needed when Joe states:

A. "I will have to have a catheter inserted to receive the treatment."—NO; a small catheter is inserted and the solution is infused via gravity.

B. "I will need to retain this solution for 1.5 to 2 hours before voiding."—NO; this is accurate.
C. "I should drink large amounts of fluid before and during the treatment."—**YES; fluids should be encouraged after the patient has voided out the solution to further flush the medication from the bladder.**
D. "I should change my position every 30 to 45 minutes during the treatment."—NO; this helps to ensure the solution contacts all areas of the bladder.

EXERCISE 2.48 Multiple-choice:

Rachel has received reports on four patients. Which patient should be assessed first?

A. Sarah—blood pressure (BP): 88/60 mmHg, pulse: 124, respiratory rate (RR): 30; had a 100-mL urine output for more than 8 hours.**—YES; the urine output of less than 30 mL/hr and the vital signs are indications of renal failure (prerenal category), and the patient needs immediate treatment.**
B. Coleen—temperature: 101°F (38.3°C); has blood in the urine with each void.—NO; these are symptoms of cystitis.
C. Theresa—blood urea nitrogen (BUN): 36 mg/dL, creatinine: 0.8 mg/dL; vomited 200 mL of undigested food 6 hours earlier.—NO; the BUN is elevated (normal is 10–20 mg) and the creatinine is normal. The patient may be dehydrated but renal function is normal.
D. Tyra—BP: 112/78 mmHg, pulse: 88, respiratory rate (RR): 24; is on diuretics and became slightly dizzy when getting up to void.—NO; diuretics may be decreasing her BP, so she will have to stand up slowly. However, her vital signs are normal.

EXERCISE 2.49 Fill in the blanks:

After reading Sarah's laboratory result in the left column, complete the laboratory interpretation in the middle column and the intervention in the right column.

Laboratory Results	Laboratory Interpretation	Intervention
Creatinine: 2.8 mg/dL (normal: 0.5–1.5)	**Renal failure from dehydration**	**Administer intravenous (IV) fluids; monitor urine output, blood urea nitrogen (BUN), and creatinine**
Hemoglobin: 9.8 g/dL (normal adult women: 12–16 g/dL)	**Anemia may be from various causes such as reduction of erythropoietin production or iron deficiency. More testing is necessary to determine the cause of anemia.**	**Encourage patient to increase intake of foods such as green leafy vegetables, whole-wheat bread, and beef.** **Instruct patient to change positions slowly when sitting or standing.**

(*continued*)

Laboratory Results	Laboratory Interpretation	Intervention
Hematocrit: 38% (normal: 38%–42%)	**Dehydration from vomiting; elevated in comparison to the hemoglobin**	**Monitor vital signs; administer intravenous (IV) fluids**
Serum potassium: 5.6 mEq/L (normal: 3.5–5.0 mEq/L)	**Hyperkalemia related to renal failure**	**Assess cardiac monitor for dysrhythmias; monitor electrolytes**
Arterial blood gases (ABGs): pH: 7.32 (normal: 7.35–7.45) HCO_3: 19 (normal: 22–26) $PaCO_2$: 37 (normal: 35–45)	**Metabolic acidosis:** **pH decreased** **HCO_3 decreased**	**Administer IV fluids; observe for Kussmaul respirations as respiratory rate (RR) increases to compensate; observe for mental confusion and gastrointestinal (GI) symptoms.**

EXERCISE 2.50 Multiple-choice:

As her intravenous (IV) is being inserted, Sarah asks again why her kidneys are not working well. The nurse's best response is:

A. "This has occurred because you declined to have your IV reinserted."—NO; this is a judgmental statement.

B. "This has occurred because of damage to the glomeruli of the kidneys."—NO; this would be an explanation for an intrarenal cause.

C. "Dehydration has decreased blood flow to the kidneys, resulting in damage."—**YES; this is an accurate explanation for a prerenal cause.**

D. "The high heart rate you are experiencing is detrimental to the kidneys."—NO; the high heart rate (HR) is in response to the low blood pressure (BP) and may actually be helping to perfuse the kidneys.

EXERCISE 2.51 Matching:

Match the categories of acute renal failure (ARF) in Column A with the different causes of ARF in Column B:

Column A	Column B
A. Prerenal ARF	A Hemorrhage
B. Intrarenal ARF	A Heart failure
C. Postrenal ARF	B Radiopaque contrast agents
	C Calculi
	B Myoglobinuria

(*continued*)

Column A	Column B
	C Benign prostatic hyperplasia
	A Nasogastric (NG) suction
	A Sepsis
	A Vomiting, diarrhea
	C Tumors
	B Acute pyelonephritis
	B Nonsteroidal anti-inflammatory drugs (NSAIDs)

EXERCISE 2.52 Multiple-choice:

After reviewing the laboratory results, the nurse prepares to call the health care provider (HCP). What is a priority for the nurse to communicate to the HCP?

A. Potassium: 5.9 mEq/L—**YES; this is the most life threatening of the abnormal labs.**
B. Creatinine: 3.6 mg/dL—NO; this needs close monitoring but is not immediately life threatening.
C. pH: 7.30—NO; this needs to be monitored, but is not as critical as the high potassium.
D. Hemoglobin: 9.6 g/dL—NO; this is not life threatening.

EXERCISE 2.53 Ordering:

Place the postoperative nursing care issues in priority order from 1 to 6:

3 Administer pain medication
4 Monitor input and output (I&O)
2 Monitor for deep vein thrombosis (DVT)
5 Start continuous passive range of motion (ROM) to prevent contractures
6 Facilitate early ambulation
1 Monitor for bleeding at the site

EXERCISE 2.54 Multiple-choice:

Which finding will the nurse report to the health care provider (HCP)?

A. Blood urea nitrogen (BUN): 22 mg/dL—NO.
B. Blood pressure (BP): 108/72 mmHg—NO.
C. Urine output: 30 mL/hr—**YES.**
D. Hemoglobin: 12.8 g/dL—NO.

EXERCISE 2.55 Multiple-choice:

The prescriber's order calls for heparin infusion at 1,800 units/hr. The label on the intravenous (IV) bag reads: Heparin 10,000 units in 500 mL D_5W. How many mL/hr will deliver the correct dose?

A. 120 mL/hr—NO.
B. 90 mL/hr—**YES.**

C. 85 mL/hr—NO.
D. 73 mL/hr—NO.

EXERCISE 2.56 Select all that apply:

Which clinical manifestations are associated with a pulmonary embolus?

A. Bradycardia—NO.
B. Dyspnea—**YES.**
C. Back pain—NO.
D. Diaphoresis—**YES.**
E. Anxiety—**YES.**
F. Tachypnea—**YES.**

EXERCISE 2.57 Select all that apply:

Which of the following constitute bleeding precautions?

A. Hemoccult all stool—**YES.**
B. Give all meds via intramuscular (IM) route—NO; avoid or minimize injections.
C. Limit blood draws—**YES.**
D. Use an electric razor—**YES.**

EXERCISE 2.58 Multiple-choice:

Which medication would the nurse administer as the antidote to heparin?

A. Vitamin K—NO; this is used for patients on Coumadin therapy.
B. Protamine sulfate—**YES.**
C. Aspirin—NO.
D. Erythropoietin—NO.

EXERCISE 2.59 Multiple-choice:

What is the priority nursing diagnosis for a patient with an open reduction and internal fixation (ORIF)?

A. Risk for constipation—NO.
B. Risk for infection—**YES; surgical incision site increases the risk of infection and osteomyelitis.**
C. Activity intolerance—NO.
D. Risk for injury—NO.

EXERCISE 2.60 Multiple-choice:

Before assisting a patient with open reduction and internal fixation (ORIF) in ambulation for the first time, the nurse will:

A. Review the postoperative orders for weight-bearing status—**YES; postoperative orders for ORIF patients differ; therefore, the nurse needs to check before ambulating the patient.**
B. Use a mechanical lift to transfer from bed to chair—NO; mechanical lifts are typically not needed.

C. Administer pain medication 3 hours before ambulation—NO; pain medication should be given approximately 30 minutes before activity.
D. Encourage patient to empty bladder to minimize interruption—NO; does not impact mobilization,

EXERCISE 2.61 **Fill in the blank:**

In caring for a patient with an amputation, the nurse should place a **tourniquet** at the bedside for emergency use.

EXERCISE 2.62 **Select all that apply:**

To reduce the patient's risk for surgical complications, the nurse will:

A. Monitor blood glucose levels—**YES.**
B. Encourage use of an incentive spirometer every 2 hours—**YES.**
C. Administer insulin as prescribed—**YES.**
D. Assess heart and lung sounds—**YES.**
E. Administer metformin (Glucophage)—NO; this is withheld until labs indicate normal renal function, and metformin is only prescribed to patients with type 2 diabetes mellitus.
F. Mark dressing if any bleeding occurs—**YES.**

EXERCISE 2.63 **Select all that apply:**

During the first 24 hours following a right above-the-knee amputation (AKA), the nurse will:

A. Place the patient in the Trendelenburg position—NO.
B. Monitor vital signs and surgical site—**YES.**
C. Elevate the amputated limb with pillows—**YES.**
D. Monitor input and output (I&O)—**YES.**
E. Administer pain medication as needed—**YES.**
F. Keep amputated limb flat on the bed—NO; the limb is kept elevated for the first 24 hours.

EXERCISE 2.64 **Multiple-choice:**

In patients with diabetes mellitus, the nurse understands to monitor for which complication?

A. Edema of the stump—NO; this is not specific to diabetics.
B. Mild erythema of the incision—NO; not specific to diabetics.
C. Separation of the surgical wound edges—**YES; diabetes impairs wound healing.**
D. Bleeding to surgical stump dressing—NO; not specific to diabetes.

EXERCISE 2.65 **Multiple-choice:**

The nurse determines that teaching has been effective when the patient says:

A. "I should lie on my abdomen for 30 minutes three to four times a day."—**YES; this will prevent hip flexion contractures.**
B. "I should change the shrinker bandage when it becomes soiled or stretched out."—NO; the shrinker bandage should be changed daily.

C. "I should use lotion on the stump to prevent drying and cracking of the skin."—NO; lotion should not be placed on the limb.
D. "I should elevate the limb on a pillow most of the day to decrease swelling."—NO; this would cause flexion contractures.

EXERCISE 2.66 Select all that apply:

Risk factors for osteoporosis include:

A. Postmenopausal female—**YES; secondary to estrogen deficiency.**
B. History of smoking—**YES.**
C. Asian ethnicity—**YES.**
D. Male older than 60 years—**YES.**
E. History of strength-training exercises—NO.
F. Sedentary lifestyle—**YES.**

EXERCISE 2.67 Multiple-choice:

What is the leading cause of osteoporosis?

A. Progesterone deficiency—NO; this is not a factor.
B. Vitamin D deficiency—NO; vitamin D deficiency causes rickets.
C. Folic acid deficiency—NO; folic acid deficiency causes spinal defects in the fetus.
D. Estrogen deficiency—**YES; osteoporosis is caused by a postmenopausal estrogen deficit.**

EXERCISE 2.68 Multiple-choice:

Which instructions will the nurse include in teaching about alendronate (Fosamax)?

A. Take with food and a full glass of water—NO; take without food.
B. Take at bedtime with a full glass of water—NO; take in the morning.
C. Take before breakfast and remain upright for 30 minutes after ingestion—**YES; this prevents esophagitis.**
D. Lie down for at least 30 minutes after ingestion—NO; remain upright to prevent esophagitis.

EXERCISE 2.69 Multiple-choice:

When teaching about adverse effects, a patient taking alendronate (Fosamax) should be instructed to report:

A. Dysphagia—**YES; this is indicative of esophagitis.**
B. Poor appetite—NO.
C. Insomnia—NO.
D. Tinnitus—NO.

EXERCISE 2.70 Select all that apply:

For patients with osteoporosis, lifestyle modification includes:

A. Regular, weight-bearing exercise—**YES.**
B. Intake of calcium-rich foods—**YES.**

C. Altering home environment for safety—**YES.**
D. Routine bedrest to prevent pain—NO; regular physical activity is recommended except during periods of acute pain.

EXERCISE 2.71 Select all that apply:

Which interventions will minimize the pain and inflammation commonly associated with osteoarthritis?

A. Encourage adequate sleep each night—**YES.**
B. Encourage regular rest periods throughout the day—**YES.**
C. Splint hands to immobilize acutely inflamed joints—**YES.**
D. Use Tylenol (acetaminophen) as needed for pain—**YES.**
E. Promote regular physical activity—**YES.**
F. Avoid warm packs at all times—NO; warm packs or warm soaks are recommended to promote circulation and maintain mobility as well as flexibility of joints.

EXERCISE 2.72 Multiple-choice:

The action of glucosamine sulfate is to:

A. Rebuild cartilage in the joint—**YES.**
B. Decrease inflammation of the joint—NO; corticosteroid injections decrease inflammation.
C. Stabilize the joint—NO; this drug does not have this action.
D. Provide a heat effect to the joint—NO; this drug does not have this action.

EXERCISE 2.73 Select all that apply:

How is multiple sclerosis (MS) diagnosed?

A. History and physical examination—**YES.**
B. MRI—**YES.**
C. Bone scan—NO.
D. Electroencephalogram (EEG)—NO.

EXERCISE 2.74 Multiple-choice:

In patients with multiple sclerosis (MS), the MRI scan reveals:

A. Multiple bright white lesions—**YES; there are multiple bright white or dark lesions depending on the type of MRI scan used.**
B. Increased cerebral spinal fluid—NO.
C. Narrowing of the fourth ventricle—NO.
D. Several petechial hemorrhages—NO.

EXERCISE 2.75 Select all that apply:

Which clinical manifestations are associated with multiple sclerosis (MS)?

A. Weakness—**YES.**
B. Fatigue—**YES.**

C. Vertigo—**YES.**
D. Visual disturbances—**YES.**
E. Paresthesia—**YES.**
F. Muscle spasms—**YES.**
G. Headache—NO.
H. Pain—**YES.**
I. Impaired memory—**YES.**
J. Depression—**YES.**

EXERCISE 2.76 Select all that apply:

Which strategies for alleviating fatigue should the nurse provide a patient with multiple sclerosis (MS)?

A. Avoid environments with extremely cold temperatures—NO.
B. Maintain an adequate sleep regimen—**YES.**
C. Discontinue medication during periods of extreme fatigue—NO.
D. Uphold a routine exercise regimen—**YES.**
E. Avoid alcohol and tobacco products—**YES.**
F. Consume fresh fruits and vegetables daily—**YES.**

EXERCISE 2.77 Multiple-choice:

Which physician order should the nurse anticipate?

A. Obtain a CT of the head, stat—**YES; a CT of the head is ordered to rule out intracranial hemorrhage as a window of opportunity is still open to administer reteplase (Retavase).**
B. Initiate heparin drip per protocol—NO; not indicated.
C. Administer aspirin 325 mg orally, stat—NO; not indicated.
D. Administer atropine 2 mg intravenous (IV), stat—NO; not indicated.

EXERCISE 2.78 Select all that apply:

Identify risk factors for ischemic stroke:

A. Hypertension (HTN)—**YES.**
B. Diabetes mellitus—**YES.**
C. Smoking—**YES.**
D. Sickle cell anemia—**YES.**
E. High cholesterol—**YES.**
F. Depression—NO.

EXERCISE 2.79 Multiple-choice:

Which statement depicts the nurse's comprehension of factors that contribute to ischemic strokes?

A. "The symptoms indicate that a pacemaker may be necessary."—NO.
B. "It is routine for patients older than the age of 40 years to have an EKG completed as a precaution."—NO.

C. "It is to check for an irregular heart rhythm, which may contribute to a stroke."—**YES; atrial fibrillation can cause clot formation contributing to a stroke. The EKG is obtained to evaluate the patient for atrial fibrillation.**
D. "To determine whether management of a heart attack will be necessary."—NO.

EXERCISE 2.80 Select all that apply:

Which are absolute contraindications to reteplase (Retavase)?

A. 51 years of age—NO; not relevant.
B. Systolic blood pressure (BP): 188 mmHg—**YES; a systolic BP greater than 185 mmHg is an absolute contraindication.**
C. Currently on Coumadin with a prothrombin time (PT) of 49 seconds and an international normalized ratio (INR) of 2.5—**YES; a PT greater than 45 seconds regardless of being on Coumadin is an absolute contraindication.**
D. Platelet count of 51,000—**YES; a platelet count less than 100,000 is an absolute contraindication.**

EXERCISE 2.81 Select all that apply:

Which clinical manifestations are associated with Parkinson's disease?

A. Mask-like expression—**YES.**
B. Decline in intellect—NO.
C. Pill rolling—**YES.**
D. Cogwheel movement—**YES.**
E. Shuffling gate—**YES.**
F. Micrographia—**YES.**
G. Drooling—**YES.**
H. Aphasia—NO.
I. Tremor—**YES.**
J. Dysphonia—**YES.**

EXERCISE 2.82 Select all that apply:

Complications commonly found in a patient with Parkinson's disease include:

A. Depression—**YES; depression is common secondary to their condition.**
B. Diarrhea—NO; constipation is a not a common complaint with Parkinson's disease.
C. Dyskinesia—**YES; involuntary spontaneous movements.**
D. Dysphagia—**YES; difficulty in swallowing.**
E. Dementia—**YES; found in 20% to 40% of patients with Parkinson's disease.**
F. Dysphonia—**YES; soft, slurred speech.**

EXERCISE 2.83 Multiple-choice:

Which diet is recommended for a patient with Parkinson's disease who is having difficulty swallowing?

A. Pureed food with thin liquids—NO.
B. Semisolid food with thick liquids—**YES; easiest to swallow.**

C. Solid food with thick liquids—NO.
D. Semisolid food with thin liquids—NO.

EXERCISE 2.84 Ordering:

Place the swallowing technique for a patient with Parkinson's disease in the correct order from 1 to 3:

__2__ Close lips and teeth
__3__ Lift the tongue up and back to swallow
__1__ Place semisolid food on the tongue

EXERCISE 2.85 Select all that apply:

Which nursing interventions will support nutritional intake in a patient with Parkinson's disease?

A. Drinking fluids after swallowing food—NO; this will cause aspiration, particularly with dysphagia.
B. Cutting food into bite-sized pieces—**YES; this helps prevent aspiration.**
C. Providing six small meals each day—**YES; improves digestion.**
D. Increasing time allotted to eat meals—**YES; prevents choking and improves digestion.**

EXERCISE 2.86 Select all that apply:

Clinical manifestations of dyskinesia that are associated with long-term use of Sinemet include:

A. Facial grimaces—**YES.**
B. Sleep disturbances—NO.
C. Jerking movement of extremities—**YES.**
D. Smacking movements—**YES.**
E. Hallucinations—NO.
F. Involuntary jerking of the trunk—**YES.**

EXERCISE 2.87 Multiple-choice:

Which is a clinical manifestation associated with myasthenia gravis (MG)?

A. Cogwheel rigidity—NO.
B. Loss of coordination—NO.
C. Intermittent periods of visual disturbances—NO.
D. Progressive weakness throughout the day—**YES.**
E. Ascending paralysis—NO.

EXERCISE 2.88 Multiple-choice:

Myasthenia gravis (MG) is confirmed by:

A. Positive Brudzinski's sign—NO.
B. Positive Kernig's sign—NO.
C. Positive edrophonium (Tensilon) test—**YES.**
D. Positive sweat chloride test—NO.

EXERCISE 2.89 Multiple-choice:

Which medication should be readily available during the Tensilon test?

A. Epinephrine—NO.
B. Atropine—**YES; this is a cholinergic antagonist that, if needed, can counteract the effects of Tensilon.**
C. Narcan—NO.
D. Amiodarone—NO.

EXERCISE 2.90 Multiple-choice:

Which patient response to the administration of Tensilon confirms the diagnosis of myasthenia gravis (MG)?

A. Symptom improvement of just the ptosis—NO.
B. Rapid but brief improvement of symptoms—**YES; Tensilon increases muscle strength with a peak effect in 30 seconds and lasts for a few minutes.**
C. Prolonged improvement of symptoms—NO.
D. Brief exaggeration of symptoms—NO.

EXERCISE 2.91 Select all that apply:

Precipitating factors for myasthenic crisis include:

A. Physical overexertion—**YES; results in muscle fatigue.**
B. Emotional stress—**YES; this stresses the immune system.**
C. Taking excess medication—NO; this results in a cholinergic crisis.
D. Omitting a dose of medication—**YES; crisis is often caused by undermedication.**
E. Pregnancy—**YES; stresses the immune system.**
F. Influenza—**YES; stress on the immune system.**

EXERCISE 2.92 Multiple-choice:

Which does the nurse assess first?

A. Level of consciousness and orientation—NO.
B. Heart rate (HR) and blood pressure (BP)—NO.
C. Muscle strength and reflexes—NO.
D. Airway patency and breathing pattern—**YES; first priority for a patient with a possible spinal cord injury is assessment of respiratory status and airway patency. All other choices should be performed after airway and breathing are assessed.**

EXERCISE 2.93 Multiple-choice:

Using the aforementioned Glasgow Coma Scale, which score does the nurse assign to this patient?

A. Score of 15—NO.
B. Score of 3—NO.
C. Score of 10—**YES.**
D. Score of 6—NO.

EXERCISE 2.94 Multiple-choice:

What is the minimum score possible on the Glasgow Coma Scale?

A. 3—**YES.**
B. 4—NO.
C. 6—NO.
D. 8—NO.

EXERCISE 2.95 Multiple-choice:

What is the maximum score possible on the Glasgow Coma Scale?

A. 13—NO.
B. 15—**YES.**
C. 9—NO.
D. 20—NO.

EXERCISE 2.96 Calculation:

Order: 30 mg/kg intravenous (IV) bolus to be given over 15 minutes

Calculate the bolus dose: **2,100 mg**

EXERCISE 2.97 Calculation:

The prescriber's order calls for methylprednisolone intravenous (IV) infusion of 5.4 mg/kg/hr for 23 hours to begin 45 minutes after the bolus dose. The label on the IV bag reads: Methylprednisolone 100 mg/ 50 mL D_5W. How many mL/hr will deliver the correct dose?

A. 190 mL/hr—**YES.**
B. 125 mL/hr—NO.
C. 140 mL/hr—NO.
D. 150 mL/hr—NO.

EXERCISE 2.98 Select all that apply:

Which is true regarding the administration of methylprednisolone to a patient with a spinal cord injury?

A. Methylprednisolone should be given within the first 8 hours following injury.—**YES; methylprednisolone is a corticosteroid that should be administered ASAP or within 8 hours of a spinal cord injury to alleviate edema and facilitate spinal cord perfusion.**
B. Methylprednisolone is associated with adverse effects such as hypoglycemia.—NO; hyperglycemia is an adverse effect.
C. Methylprednisolone increases the risk of infection and stress ulcers.—**YES; this drug increases the risk of infection and gastrointestinal (GI) bleed from stress ulcer formation.**
D. Methylprednisolone is only indicated in patients with severe hypotension and bradycardia.—NO; not indicated for hypotension or bradycardia.

EXERCISE 2.99 Select all that apply:

Acute complications that may occur following a spinal cord injury include:

A. Neurogenic shock—**YES.**
B. Deep vein thrombosis (DVT)—**YES.**
C. Pneumonia—**YES.**
D. Myocardial infarction (MI)—NO.
E. Respiratory failure—**YES.**
F. Autonomic dysreflexia—**YES.**

EXERCISE 2.100 Select all that apply:

Which of the following constitute seizure precautions?

A. Maintain bed in low position—**YES.**
B. Keep side rails up and padded—**YES.**
C. Keep bright lights on to easily visualize the patient—NO; lights should be low.
D. Ensure suction is available at the bedside—**YES.**
E. Keep a tongue depressor at the bedside to use as a bite guard—NO; should not be used.
F. Maintain a low-stimulus environment—**YES.**

EXERCISE 2.101 Multiple-choice:

Which statement regarding a positive Babinski reflects the nurse's comprehension of spinal cord injuries?

A. "A positive Babinski is a good sign indicating adequate spinal cord perfusion."—NO.
B. "A positive Babinski is a normal neurological finding in all age groups."—NO.
C. "A positive Babinski indicates injury to nerves innervating muscles involved in voluntary movement."—**YES; a positive Babinski indicates an injury along the pyramidal (descending spinal) tract; the descending pyramidal tracts are the pathways by which motor signals are sent from the brain to the lower motor neurons that directly innervate muscles to produce voluntary movement. This may be transient because of edema, or permanent, indicating paralysis.**
D. "A positive Babinski is a sign of nervous system excitation requiring implementation of seizure precautions."—NO.

EXERCISE 2.102 Select all that apply:

Which interventions minimize the risk of deep vein thrombosis (DVT) in a patient with an acute spinal injury?

A. Anticoagulation—**YES.**
B. Range of motion (ROM) exercises—**YES.**
C. Antiembolism stockings—**YES.**
D. Pneumatic compression devices—**YES.**
E. Antiplatelet medication—NO; not helpful in preventing venous thrombi.
F. Hydration—**YES.**

EXERCISE 2.103 Fill in the blanks:

Name four clinical features of diabetic ketoacidosis (DKA).

1. **Hyperglycemia**
2. **Ketosis**
3. **Acidosis**
4. **Dehydration**

EXERCISE 2.104 Matching:

Indicate whether each characteristic in Column B is associated with diabetic ketoacidosis (DKA) or hyperglycemic hyperosmolar nonketotic syndrome (HHNS), mentioned in Column A:

Column A	Column B	
A. DKA	A	More common in type 1 diabetes
B. HHNS	A	Often caused by omission of insulin
	B	Onset is usually over several days
	A	Acidotic with pH less than 7.30
	B	Plasma bicarbonate levels normal
	B	Often caused by physiologic stress
	B	Absence of serum and urine ketones
	A	Kussmaul respirations
	B	Serum osmolality greater than 350 mOsm/L

EXERCISE 2.105 Select all that apply:

The nurse understands that the initial treatment for Maria would include:

A. Administering oxygen—**YES; it is important because of acidosis.**
B. Establishing an intravenous (IV) line—**YES; regular insulin is given intravenously.**
C. Administering 0.9% normal saline (NS) IV—**YES; for treatment of dehydration.**
D. Infusing neutral protamine Hagedorn (NPH) insulin—NO; regular insulin is administered.
E. Monitoring potassium levels closely—**YES; potassium levels may be low related to osmotic diuresis or high related to hydrogen shifts that occur with acidemia.**
F. Encouraging intake of Gatorade.—NO; Gatorade has a high sugar content.

EXERCISE 2.106 Multiple-choice:

The nurse reviews the laboratory reports from blood samples drawn 1 hour after the administration of intravenous (IV) insulin. What would the nurse expect?

A. Hyponatremia—NO; insulin does not cause low sodium.
B. Hypercalcemia—NO; insulin does not increase calcium in the blood.
C. Hypoglycemia—NO; insulin brings the serum glucose to normal slowly.
D. Hypokalemia—**YES; insulin moves potassium into the cells causing hypokalemia.**

EXERCISE 2.107 Select all that apply:

Which sick-day rules should the nurse include in the teaching?

A. Continue eating regular meals if possible—**YES; this will maintain normal insulin and glucose levels.**
B. Increase the intake of noncaloric fluids—**YES; the body's metabolism increases during sickness, and fluids are needed to prevent dehydration.**
C. Take insulin as prescribed—**YES; the routine doses should be maintained.**
D. Check glucose once daily—NO; check glucose levels every 4 hours.
E. Test for ketones if glucose is greater than 240 mg/dL—**YES; ketones are another indicator of poor control.**
F. Report moderate ketones to the health care provider (HCP)—**YES; this will prevent severe diabetic ketoacidosis (DKA).**

EXERCISE 2.108 Multiple-choice:

The night charge nurse is making assignments for the following day shift. The plan is for Maria to be discharged home. It would be best to assign Maria to:

A. An experienced RN pulled from another medical unit—**YES; an experienced medical nurse should have the knowledge to provide discharge teaching for a diabetic patient.**
B. A new-graduate RN who has been on the unit for 1 week—NO; this new nurse may lack the knowledge about the discharge process and the in-depth instructions needed.
C. An experienced RN who has just been transferred from the operating room—NO; this nurse is probably unfamiliar with the discharge process.
D. A licensed practical nurse (LPN) who has been on the unit for 3 months—NO; extensive discharge teaching should be handled by the RN.

EXERCISE 2.109 Matching:

Match the information in Column A with the disease alteration in Column B (an option may be used more than once):

Column A	Column B	
A. Older than 35 years of age	C, D, E, G, H	Type 1 diabetes mellitus
B. Overweight	A, B, C, F, G, H	Type 2 diabetes mellitus
C. Polyphagia		
D. Sudden weight loss		
E. Younger than 30 years of age		
F. May be controlled by diet		
G. Polyuria		
H. Polydipsia		

EXERCISE 2.110 Select all that apply:

Which health alterations can cause hyperthyroidism?

A. Toxic nodular goiter—**YES; there is a noticeable goiter present.**
B. Thyroiditis—NO; the thyroid is not infected.
C. Cancer of the tongue—NO; this is not a cause.
D. Thyroid cancer—**YES; this is a cause.**
E. Hyperfunction of the adrenal glands—NO; this affects kidney function.
F. Exogenous iodine intake—**YES; the thyroid is sensitive to iodine.**

EXERCISE 2.111 Matching:

Match the clinical manifestations in Column A with the disease alterations in Column B:

Column A	Column B
A. Palpitations	**A, B, E, F, J, L, M** Hyperthyroidism
B. Increased respiratory rate	**C, D, G, H, I, K, N** Hypothyroidism
C. Dry, sparse, coarse hair	
D. Anemia	
E. Diaphoresis	
F. Muscle wasting	
G. Enlarged, scaly tongue	
H. Decreased breathing capacity	
I. Muscle aches and pains	
J. Diarrhea	
K. Slow, slurred speech	
L. Fine tremors of fingers	
M. Exophthalmos	
N. Intolerance to cold	

EXERCISE 2.112 Multiple-choice:

Lisa is being admitted with the diagnosis of thyrotoxic crisis. When making a room assignment for this patient, the charge nurse knows it would be best to assign:

A. A room in which the roommate is not infected—NO; infection status is not relevant.
B. A room that is directly across from the nursing station—NO; this may be too noisy or busy of an area for this patient.
C. A private room—**YES; emotional hyperexcitability, irritability, and apprehension are common in patients with hyperthyroidism, so a private room would be less stimulating.**
D. A room in which the roommate is very pleasant and talkative—NO; this may be overstimulating for this patient.

EXERCISE 2.113 Select all that apply:

Which of the following clinical manifestations are present in Cushing's disease?

A. Buffalo hump—**YES; there are deposits of adipose tissue in the shoulder area.**
B. Hypovolemia—NO; that is common in Addison's disease.
C. Weight loss—NO; there is weight gain.
D. Hyperpigmentation of skin—NO; hyperpigmentation is a clinical manifestation of Addison's disease.
E. Moon face—**YES; the face is fuller.**
F. Muscle wasting in the extremities—**YES; the muscle is affected.**
G. Purple striae on the abdomen—**YES; this is common.**

EXERCISE 2.114 Multiple-choice:

In order to manage the Cushing's disease, the health care provider (HCP) recommends:

A. Discontinuing the corticosteroid therapy immediately—NO; corticosteroids should never be stopped abruptly.
B. Weaning her off the corticosteroid medication slowly—**YES; this is to prevent adrenal insufficiency.**
C. Using the corticosteroid only as needed for severe pain—NO; this medication is not for as needed use.
D. Administering the corticosteroid before bedtime—NO; this could actually contribute to Cushing's. Corticosteroids are best given around 8:00 a.m.

EXERCISE 2.115 Select all that apply:

Select the information that should be included in the teaching session for this patient.

A. Keep a medical identification device with you—**YES; this is a safety issue.**
B. Keep a list of medications and doses with you—**YES; this is a safety issue.**
C. Increase the sodium in your diet—NO; hypernatremia is common.
D. Avoid exposure to infection—**YES; there is an increased risk for infection.**
E. Hold the medication if side effects occur—NO; this medication should be weaned off and not stopped abruptly.
F. Monitor for excessive weight gain—**YES; sodium and water retention can occur leading to weight gain. Appetite may also increase.**

EXERCISE 2.116 Multiple-choice:

In order to prevent injuries, it is a priority to teach the patient to:

A. Increase protein in his or her diet—NO; this may help minimize muscle wasting, but is not the priority.
B. Begin an aerobics exercise class—NO; the patient should be encouraged to begin gentle exercise such as yoga.
C. Use assistive devices as much as possible—NO; the patient should be encouraged to remain as independent as possible.
D. Establish a protective environment—**YES; a safe home environment is important in preventing falls.**

EXERCISE 2.117 Multiple-choice:

After Isabella arrives on the unit, the nursing team begins the admission process. What role can be delegated to the licensed practical nurse (LPN)?

A. Perform the initial physical assessment—NO; this should be done by the RN.
B. Obtain the patient's weight—NO; this can be delegated to the unlicensed assistive personnel (UAP).
C. Hang a new bag of intravenous (IV) fluids—**YES; this is within the scope of practice of the LPN.**
D. Educate the patient on the plan of care—NO; this should be done by the RN.

EXERCISE 2.118 Fill in the blanks:

What three hormones does the adrenal cortex produce and what is their primary function?

1. **Mineralocorticoids—cause increased sodium absorption in exchange for excretion of potassium or hydrogen ions.**
2. **Glucocorticoids—influence glucose metabolism, inhibit the inflammatory response to tissue injury, and suppress allergic manifestations.**
3. **Androgens—effects similar to the male sex hormones.**

EXERCISE 2.119 Matching:

Match the hormones in Column A with the related clinical manifestations of deficiency in Column B:

Column A	Column B	
A. Mineralocorticoids	B	Hypovolemia, hyperkalemia, hypoglycemia, and decreased muscle size
B. Glucocorticoids	A	Decreased cardiac output, anemia, depression, and confusion
C. Androgens	C	Decreased heart size, decreased muscle tone, weight loss, and skin hyperpigmentation

EXERCISE 2.120 Fill in the blanks:

List four causes of Addisonian crisis.

1. **Sepsis**
2. **Trauma**
3. **Stress**
4. **Steroid withdrawal**

EXERCISE 2.121 Select all that apply:

Which symptoms would indicate that Isabella is in Addisonian crisis?

A. Hypertension (HTN)—NO; in Addisonian crisis, she would have hypotension.
B. Bradycardia—NO; in Addisonian crisis, she would have a weak rapid pulse.

C. Dehydration—NO; dehydration is not usually a symptom.
D. Hyperkalemia—**YES; increased potassium is a common symptom.**
E. Nausea and vomiting—**YES; this is a common symptom.**
F. Weakness—**YES; weakness is experienced.**

EXERCISE 2.122 Multiple-choice:

After receiving transfer orders on Gabriel, the nurse knows that the priority intervention is to:

A. Draw all laboratory tests before starting any treatment—NO; this is not the priority.
B. Administer fluid-replacement therapy—**YES; it is important to begin fluid replacement immediately because the patient is hypotensive and tachycardic.**
C. Fill up the patient's water pitcher as requested—NO; the patient should be permitted to drink when stable, but this is not the priority.
D. Obtain the patient's baseline weight—NO; this can be done when the patient is more stable.

EXERCISE 2.123 Fill in the blanks:

Which type of diabetes insipidus (DI) does Gabriel have? Explain.

Central (neurogenic) DI—This results from destruction of the posterior pituitary gland, resulting in a lack of vasopressin. Causes include head trauma, brain tumors, surgery or irradiation to the pituitary gland, or infections.

EXERCISE 2.124 Select all that apply:

Which clinical manifestations would be present in a patient with diabetes insipidus (DI)?

A. Polydipsia—**YES; there is increased thirst.**
B. Polyuria—**YES; there is increased urination.**
C. Urine output less than 100 mL in 24 hours—NO; it is increased.
D. Specific gravity less than 1.005—**YES; it is more dilute than normal. Urine output is greater than 5 L in 24 hours, making urine very dilute.**
E. Weight loss—**YES; this can occur with excessive fluid loss.**
F. Hypertension (HTN)—NO; hypotension is more likely with a fluid volume deficit.

EXERCISE 2.125 Select all that apply:

The nurse understands that appropriate treatment for a patient with diabetes insipidus (DI) includes:

A. Titrating intravenous (IV) fluids to replace urine output—**YES; fluid replacement is important.**
B. Administering thiazide diuretics—**YES; thiazide diuretics are given to patients with nephrogenic DI because they slow the glomerular filtration rate, allowing the kidneys to absorb water.**
C. Initiating a low-sodium diet—**YES; a low-sodium diet is also used to treat nephrogenic DI.**
D. Administering desmopressin acetate (DDAVP)—**YES; because it helps to decrease output.**
E. Monitoring a strict input and output (I&O)—**YES; this is important in monitoring fluid-replacement therapy.**
F. Allowing the patient to drink as desired—**YES; this will help the patient to stay hydrated.**

EXERCISE 2.126 Matching:

Match the names of the procedures in Column A to the interventions in Column B:

Column A	Column B	
A. Bronchoscopy	E	Visualizes the bile duct system of the liver and gall bladder
B. Colonoscopy	F	Visualizes anus, rectum, and sigmoid colon
C. Cystoscopy	D	Visualizes the oropharynx, esophagus, stomach, and duodenum
D. Esophagogastroduodenoscopy (EGD)	C	Visualizes the urethra, bladder, prostate, and ureters
E. Endoscopic retrograde cholangiopancreatography (ERCP)	B	Visualizes the anus, rectum, and colon
F. Sigmoidoscopy	A	Visualizes the larynx, trachea, bronchi, and alveoli

EXERCISE 2.127 Select all that apply:

Which factors does the nurse consider while giving Jonathan instructions for his endoscopic examination?

A. Age—**YES; instructions may need to be repeated or explained in more detail if the patient is elderly.**
B. Medications—**YES; some medications may need to be discontinued for 48 hours before a procedure.**
C. Allergies—**YES; allergies need to be documented for each patient.**
D. Transportation—**YES; patients require transportation after procedures because of the sedation.**
E. Previous radiographic examinations—**YES; complications during or after procedures are important to document.**
F. Language and cultural barriers—**YES; an interpreter may be necessary if there is a language barrier.**

EXERCISE 2.128 Multiple-choice:

When a new-graduate nurse asks about obtaining consent for the procedure, the nurse's best response is:

A. "Since the physician has already obtained informed consent, we will get the patient to sign the consent."—**YES; the physician obtains informed consent; the nurse witnesses the patient's signature.**
B. "Yes, we get consent when the patient comes for preprocedure instructions."—NO; the physician obtains informed consent.
C. "We need to wait until the physician is in the room to get the patient to sign the consent."—NO; this is not required.
D. "We usually wait until a family member is present before obtaining consent."—NO; this is not necessary as long as the patient is competent.

EXERCISE 2.129 Matching:

Match the tests in Column A with the correct positions in Column B (you may use positions more than once):

Column A	Column B	
A. Bronchoscopy	F	Knee–chest
B. Colonoscopy	C	Lithotomy
C. Cystoscopy	A, D, E	Supine
D. Esophagogastroduodenoscopy (EGD)	B	Left side, knees to chest
E. Endoscopic retrograde cholangiopancreatography (ERCP)		
F. Sigmoidoscopy		

EXERCISE 2.130 Multiple-choice:

After completing preprocedure teaching about the colonoscopy, the nurse knows that Jonathan requires further instruction when he states:

A. "I need to stop eating 8 hours before the test is scheduled."—NO; this is correct; patients are usually instructed to stop intake at 12 midnight.

B. "I need to make sure that someone is with me to drive me home."—NO; this is required because of the sedation.

C. "I will be able to resume my normal diet after the procedure."—NO; the patient is usually able to resume their normal diet after they have recovered.

D. "I will only have to take a mild laxative the evening before the procedure."—**YES; this procedure requires a thorough bowel cleansing, which involves more than a mild laxative.**

EXERCISE 2.131 Fill in the blanks:

List the two tests that require bowel preparations, such as laxatives and GoLYTELY.

1. **Colonoscopy**
2. **Sigmoidoscopy**

EXERCISE 2.132 Select all that apply:

Jonathan is in the endoscopy room ready for his procedure. Identify the final safety checks that must be completed by the nurse:

A. Confirm the correct patient and procedure—**YES; this is referred to as a "time-out."**

B. Have resuscitative equipment available—**YES; as sedation is used, it will be important to have this equipment available in the event problems occur.**

C. Confirm that an oral airway has been inserted—NO; this is inserted with esophagogastroduodenoscopy (EGD).

D. Position the patient in the supine position with head of bed at 30°—NO; the patient should be positioned on his or her left side.

E. Review the patient's allergies before administering medications—**YES.**

F. Have suctioning equipment ready for use—**YES; this is in the event vomiting occurs with sedation.**

EXERCISE 2.133 Matching:

Match the symptoms in Column A with the possible causes in Column B:

Column A	Column B
A. Difficult to arouse, slow respirations, may be hypoxic	C Aspiration
B. Cool, clammy skin, low blood pressure (BP), tachycardia	D Perforation
C. Dyspnea, tachypnea, tachycardia, and possible fever	A Oversedation
D. Chest or abdominal pain, nausea, vomiting, and abdominal distention	B Hemorrhage

EXERCISE 2.134 Multiple-choice:

After taking Jonathan to his new room, the post-anesthesia care unit (PACU) nurse hands off care to the nurse on the surgical unit. What would be most important for the PACU nurse to communicate?

A. Estimated blood loss during the procedure was 160 mL.—NO; this is not a large amount to be concerned with.
B. Vital signs were stable during the operative and recovery phases.—NO; this is understood if not stated otherwise.
C. The patient vomited twice while in the PACU.—**YES; this was a side effect of anesthesia. The patient needs to be monitored for further vomiting because this increases the risk of aspiration.**
D. The patient's family is on the way to the room.—NO; this is not the most important.

EXERCISE 2.135 Matching:

Match the discharge topics in Column A with the appropriate teaching issues in Column B:

Column A	Column B
Discharge Topic	**Teaching**
A. Normal skin appearance of the stoma	C Empty frequently
B. Skin barriers and creams	D Empty when the bag is ¼ full
C. Emptying ostomy bag	E Limited drainage
D. Dietary changes	F Abdominal bloating
E. Signs of obstruction	F Allow patient to verbalize
F. Sexual concerns	F Provide patient with suggestions
	B Use to protect the skin
	C Allow them to dry before placing bag on
	A Pink

(*continued*)

Column A	Column B
Discharge Topic	**Teaching**
	A Moist
	D Avoid foods that cause odor, such as fish, eggs, and leafy vegetables
	E Avoid gas-forming foods such as beer, dairy, and corn

EXERCISE 2.136 Multiple-choice:

When admitting Ranesha to the unit, what task can the nurse delegate to the unlicensed assistive personnel (UAP)?

A. List her home medications—NO, this is the responsibility of the licensed nurse.
B. Measure her input and output (I&O)—**YES; this is within the scope of the UAP.**
C. Assess for edema—NO; this should be done by the RN.
D. Measure her abdominal girth—NO; this should be done by the RN while completing the assessment.

EXERCISE 2.137 Multiple-choice:

One of the major complications that can occur postparacentesis is:

A. Polycythemia—NO; this is not a problem.
B. Low white blood cells (WBCs)—NO; this by itself is not a concern.
C. Hypovolemia—**YES; hypovolemia is a major concern because the fluid removed is protein enriched and can cause an intravascular-to-extravascular fluid shift.**
D. Hypervolemia—NO; the shift is from intravascular fluid.

EXERCISE 2.138 Matching:

Match the lab tests in Column A with the normal values in Column B:

Column A	Column B	
A. Albumin	E	10 to 20 mg/dL
B. Protein	F	0.6 to 1.5 mg/dL
C. Glucose	C	70 to 100 mg/dL
D. Amylase	A	3.5 to 5.0 g/dL
E. Blood urea nitrogen (BUN)	D	53 to 123 units/L
F. Creatinine	B	6.0 to 8.0 g/dL

EXERCISE 2.139 Select all that apply:

Select all the nursing interventions that may help Elin's pain.

A. Offer her a cup of tea—NO; she should stay away from caffeinated beverages, fatty and fried food, spicy food, tomatoes, citrus, alcohol, and peppermint because they all relax the lower esophageal sphincter (LES) and increase the problem of gastroesophageal reflux disease (GERD).

B. Position her flat—NO; these patients should be positioned sitting up to decrease stress on the LES.
C. Administer an antacid—**YES; antacids, such as aluminum hydroxide, neutralize the stomach acid. Other drugs that are used for GERD are histamine receptor antagonists such as ranitidine (Zantac), famotidine (Pepcid), and cimetidine (Tagamet). Proton pump inhibitors, another class of drugs, including pantoprazole (Protonix), omeprazole (Prilosec), and lansoprazole (Prevacid), are also used to suppress gastric acid.**
D. Position her on the right side—NO; positioning will not decrease the pain.
E. Provide additional pillows—**YES; this helps to reduce symptoms.**
F. Encourage her to remain upright after eating—**YES; she should also refrain from eating or drinking 2 hours before bedtime.**

EXERCISE 2.140 Select all that apply:

To decrease Elin's problems with constipation, the nurse encourages her to:

A. Avoid frequent use of laxatives—**YES; the use of laxatives increases the chance for constipation.**
B. Decrease fluids—NO; increasing fluids helps constipation.
C. Increase fiber in her diet—**YES; fiber increases bowel motility.**
D. Decrease her level of physical activity—NO; increasing activity will decrease constipation.
E. Minimize the use of opioids for pain control—**YES; constipation is a side effect of opioids.**
F. Discuss any home remedies that have worked in the past—**YES; some patients have success with prune juice or other safe remedies.**

EXERCISE 2.141 Multiple-choice:

What breakfast would you encourage Elin to order?

A. Bran cereal—**YES; this is high in fiber.**
B. Yogurt—NO; this is not high in fiber.
C. Fresh fruit—**YES; this is high in fiber.**
D. White toast—NO; this is not high in fiber.

EXERCISE 2.142 Multiple-choice:

At change of shift report, a new nurse, who is unfamiliar with *H. pylori*, asks whether the patient should be in isolation. Her preceptor's best response would be:

A. "If the patient starts vomiting, we should put him in contact isolation."—NO; this is not necessary.
B. "As long as he has started treatment with antibiotics, isolation is not necessary."—NO; isolation is not necessary.
C. "Standard precautions are all that are needed in this case."—**YES; there are no special precautions for H. pylori.**
D. "By the end of our shift, I want you to be able to tell me all about *H. pylori*."—NO, this does not answer the new nurse's question.

EXERCISE 2.143 Multiple-choice:

During discharge teaching, the nurse sees that Christian understands his instructions when he states:

A. "I will eat large meals three times a day."—NO; small frequent meals are better.
B. "I will find a relaxation technique such as yoga."—**YES; he needs a way to relax.**
C. "I can still drink all the iced tea that I want."—NO; caffeine is a gastric irritant.
D. "I can have a few glasses of wine with dinner."—NO; alcohol consumption is not encouraged.

EXERCISE 2.144 Matching:

Match the medications in Column A with the indications in Column B.

Column A	Column B	
A. Bismuth	B	Inhibits *H. pylori*
B. Metronidozole and tetracycline	D	Protects the healing gastric ulcer
C. Antacids	A	Hyposecretory medication that inhibits the proton pump
D. Sucralfate (Carafate)	C	Neutralizes gastric acid

EXERCISE 2.145 Select all that apply:

What are some important postoperative nursing interventions for Christian?

A. Keep supine postoperatively—NO; semi-Fowler's is more comfortable and decreases stress on the operative site.
B. Monitor bowel sounds—**YES; it is important to note that there is return of bowel sounds.**
C. Turn, cough, and breathe deeply—**YES; this is important for the respiratory status of all postoperative patients.**
D. Monitor input and output (I&O)—**YES; it is important to monitor I&O for absorption evaluation.**
E. Teach about dumping syndrome—**YES; gastric surgery poses the risk of dumping syndrome, which is characterized by vertigo, diaphoresis, tachycardia, and palpitations.**
F. Encourage liquids with meals—NO; eliminate liquids 1 hour before and after meals to decrease dumping syndrome, which is the effect of chyme entering the small intestine all at once after a meal.

EXERCISE 2.146 Hot spot:

Place a mark on McBurney's point.

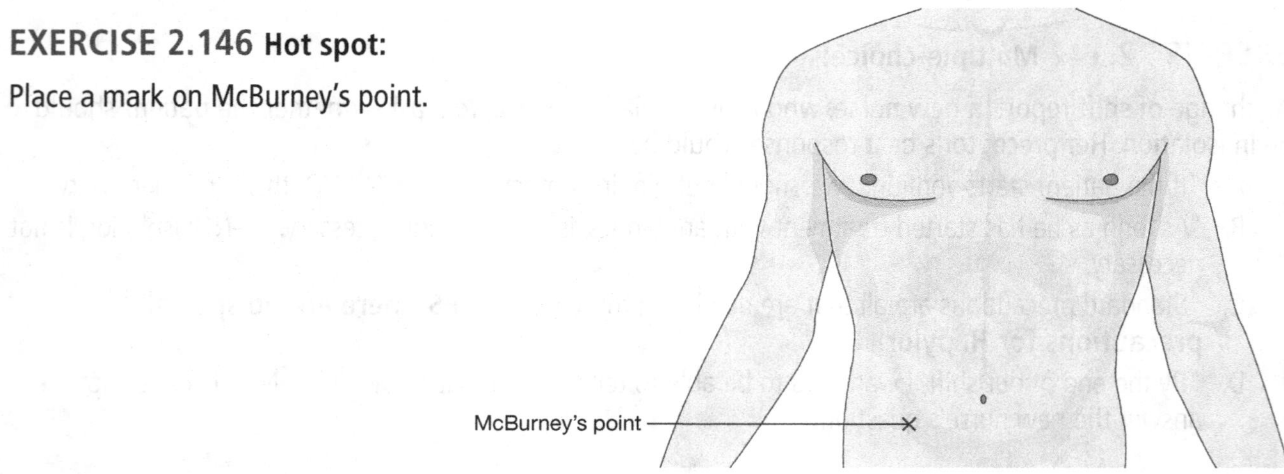

EXERCISE 2.147 Select all that apply:

Identify the priority interventions for the patient admitted with acute appendicitis:

A. Prepare the patient for surgery—**YES; this is the primary treatment.**
B. Maintain NPO (nothing orally) status—**YES; the patient has an acute abdomen and will require surgery.**
C. Administer an enema preoperatively—NO; this increases the risk of perforation.
D. Insert an intravenous (IV) catheter and begin IV fluids—**YES; the patient will be going to surgery.**
E. Notify the surgeon if the pain becomes more diffuse—**YES; this could indicate that perforation has occurred.**
F. Insert a nasogastric (NG) tube—NO; this is not routine, but would be inserted in the operating room if necessary.

EXERCISE 2.148 Multiple-choice:

What other assessment is important to rule out peritonitis as a complication of a ruptured appendix?

A. Blood pressure (BP)—NO; this may be affected, but it is not the most important vital sign for infection.
B. Pulse—NO; this may be affected, but it is not the most important vital sign for infection.
C. Respiration—NO; this may be affected, but it is not the most important vital sign for infection.
D. Temperature—**YES; a temperature of 101°F or higher is common with peritonitis.**

EXERCISE 2.149 Hot spot:

Trace on the diagram how you should measure a nasogastric (NG) tube:

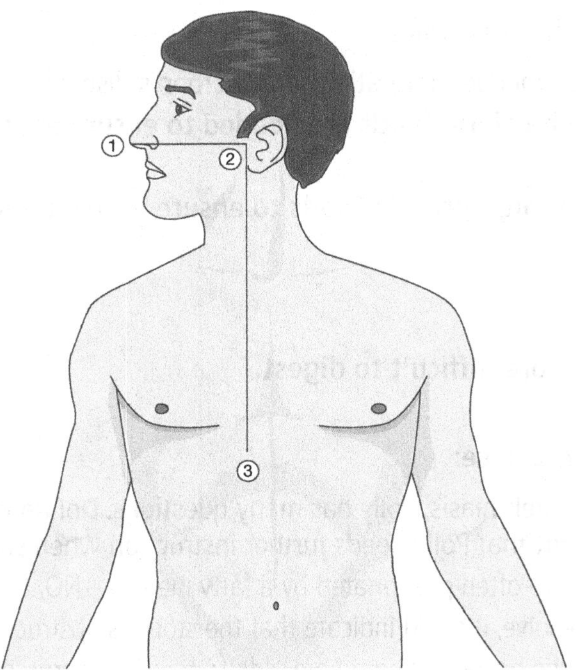

EXERCISE 2.150 Multiple-choice:

What is considered the most accurate method for verifying placement of the nasogastric (NG) tube?

A. Aspiration of stomach contents—NO; this supports proper placement, but is not the most accurate.
B. Bolus of air and listen for the gurgle as injected—NO; this is not considered an accurate method.
C. Check the pH of aspirated contents—NO; pH can be affected by certain medications.
D. X-ray verification—**YES; this is the most accurate method and should be used for initial verification after new tube insertions.**

EXERCISE 2.151 Matching:

Indicate whether each characteristic in Column B is associated with Crohn's disease or ulcerative colitis, as mentioned in Column A:

Column A	Column B	
A. Crohn's	B	Mucosal ulceration
B. Ulcerative colitis	B	Occurs in rectum, descending colon
	A	Discontinuous lesions
	B	Severe diarrhea 10 to 20 times a day
	A	Minimal bleeding
	A	Occurs in ileum, ascending colon
	B	Bleeding is common

EXERCISE 2.152 Select all that apply:

Select the types of foods recommended for patients with Crohn's disease.

A. High calorie—**YES; high-calorie foods are needed to ensure enough nutrients are ingested.**
B. Low calorie—NO.
C. High protein—**YES; eat high-protein foods to ensure enough nutrients for gastrointestinal (GI) repair.**
D. High fiber—NO.
E. High fat—NO.
F. Low fat—**YES; fat is more difficult to digest.**

EXERCISE 2.153 Multiple-choice:

After being diagnosed with cholelithiasis, Polly has many questions. Donna provides education on her disease process, but it is evident that Polly needs further instruction when she states:

A. "These painful attacks are often precipitated by a fatty meal."—NO; this is true.
B. "If the pain does not resolve, it could indicate that the stone is obstructed."—NO; this is true.
C. "I won't have to be in the hospital long if I am able to have a laparoscopic cholecystectomy."—NO, length of stay is shorter with a laparoscopic procedure.
D. "If I can withstand the painful episodes, eventually the stones will dissolve."—**YES; the stones will not spontaneously dissolve.**

EXERCISE 2.154 **Select all that apply:**

Select the foods that would be appropriate for Polly:

A. Beans—NO; this is gas forming and should be avoided.
B. Eggs—NO; they are high in cholesterol and should be avoided.
C. Ice cream—NO; this contains too much fat.
D. Chicken—**YES; this is low in calories and fat.**
E. Apple—**YES; this is low in calories and fat.**
F. Bacon—NO; this also contains too much fat.

EXERCISE 2.155 **Fill in the blanks:**

Two other kinds of drainage tubes used postoperatively are described below. Fill in the names.

1. It is a tube with a bulb at the end that is compressed to produce gentle suction at the surgical site.
   Jackson–Pratt
2. It is a tube with a spring-activated device that is compressed to produce gentle suction at the surgical site.
   Hemovac

EXERCISE 2.156 **Hot spot:**

Place the marks where you would find the discoloration of Turner's sign and Cullen's sign.

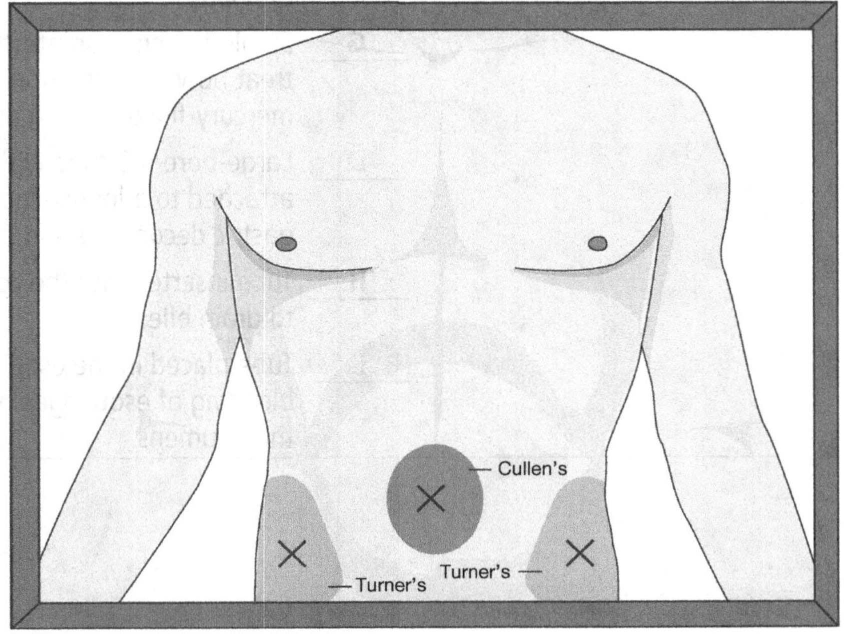

EXERCISE 2.157 Matching:

Match the names of the tubes in Column A with the identifying information in Column B:

Column A	Column B	
A. Percutaneous endoscopic gastrostomy (PEG) tube	J	Placed in the esophagus to stop bleeding of esophageal varices; it has an aspiration port.
B. Percutaneous endoscopic jejunostomy (PEJ) tube	F	Small-bore silicone nasogastric (NG) tube that has a weighted tip and is inserted with a guide wire for feeding.
C. Miller–Abbott tube	B	Tube placed endoscopically into the jejunum of the small bowel for long-term feeding.
D. Levin tube	A	Tube placed endoscopically into the stomach for long-term feeding.
E. Salem sump	E	Large-bore NG tube with two lumens; one attached to suction to promote drainage and one to allow airflow to the gastric mucosa.
F. Dobhoff tube	C	Two-lumen nasointestinal tube used to treat bowel obstructions; it is tungsten weighted at the end and has a lumen for drainage.
G. Cantor tube	G	Single-lumen nasointestinal tube used to treat bowel obstructions; it has a mercury-filled balloon at the end.
H. T-tube	D	Large-bore NG tube with one lumen attached to a low-suction pump for gastric decompression.
I. Sengstaken–Blakemore tube	H	Tube inserted into the common bile duct to drain bile.
J. Minnesota tube	I	Tube placed in the esophagus to stop bleeding of esophageal varices; it has three lumens.

EXERCISE 2.158 Matching:

Match the types of hepatitis in Column A with the transmission and risk factors in Column B:

Column A	Column B	
A. Hepatitis A (HAV)	D	Coinfection usually exists with HBV and is transmitted by drug use.
B. Hepatitis B (HBV)	C	Blood transmission by drug use and sexual contact.
C. Hepatitis C (HCV)	A	Oral–fecal route by ingestion of contaminated food or water.
D. Hepatitis D (HDV)	E	Oral–fecal route; very severe in pregnant women.
E. Hepatitis E (HEV)	B	Blood transmission by drug use, sexual contact, or by health care workers.

EXERCISE 2.159 Multiple-choice:

In preparing to send Malcolm for a liver biopsy, the nurse prioritizes:

A. Make him NPO (nothing orally) after midnight—NO; NPO is not required.
B. Start intravenous (IV) fluids before the procedure—NO; this is not required.
C. Check for the results of coagulation tests—**YES; this is very important because many patients with liver disease have clotting defects.**
D. Obtain a consent for a blood transfusion—NO; this is not necessary unless the patient needs transfusion.

EXERCISE 2.160 Select all that apply:

Clinical manifestations of measles include:

A. Low-grade fever—NO; fever is high, often greater than 104°F.
B. Cough—**YES.**
C. Koplik spots—**YES; tiny white spots with bluish-white centers in the mouth.**
D. Runny nose—**YES.**
E. Red, watery eyes—**YES.**
F. Rash that begins on the face and spreads to the trunk and extremities—**YES.**

EXERCISE 2.161 Select all that apply:

Which of the following is accurate regarding measles?

A. Incubation period of 7 to 14 days—**YES.**
B. Contagious 4 days before to 4 days after rash appears—**YES.**
C. Verbal report of vaccination is acceptable evidence of immunity—NO; acceptable evidence of immunity requires valid medical documentation of vaccination, lab titers, or previous infection.
D. More severe in the immunocompromised—**YES.**

E. Reportable communicable disease—**YES.**
F. Supportive treatment to alleviate symptoms—**YES; treatment aims to improve symptoms and prevent complications.**

EXERCISE 2.162 Select all that apply:

The proper isolation precautions for measles:

A. Contact—NO.
B. Airborne—**YES.**
C. Droplet—NO.
D. Standard—**YES.**

EXERCISE 2.163 Multiple-choice:

Which infection would require airborne precautions?

A. Varicella (chickenpox)—**YES.**
B. Anthrax—NO; contact is used for cutaneous anthrax; standard is used for pulmonary anthrax.
C. *Neisseria meningitides* (meningococcal infection)—NO; droplet precautions are used.
D. *Haemophilus influenzae* type b—NO; droplet precautions are used.

EXERCISE 2.164 Select all that apply:

Airborne precautions include:

A. Airborne infection isolation room (AIIR)—**YES.**
B. N95 respirator—**YES.**
C. Door closed—**YES.**
D. Disposable dishes—NO; soap and water for cleaning dishes is appropriate.

EXERCISE 2.165 Fill in the blanks:

The nurse who was never immunized for measles should be instructed to:

Obtain postexposure vaccine (MMR)

or

Obtain immune globulin

EXERCISE 2.166 Ordering:

Place the steps for doffing personal protective equipment (PPE) in the correct order from 1 to 4:

3 Unfasten neck of gown, then waist ties; pull gown down from each shoulder.
4 Take elastic band of N95 respirator from behind the head, discard by holding the band.
1 Grab outside of glove with opposite gloved hand and peel off; hold removed glove in hand while pulling the second glove inside out over the first glove.
2 Remove the face shield by touching the clean earpieces or headband.

EXERCISE 2.167 Select all that apply:

Standard precautions are used to:

A. Start an intravenous (IV) line—**YES; gloves provide protection against blood-borne pathogens.**

B. Care for a patient with *Clostridium difficile*—NO; use contact precautions.

C. Empty a urinary catheter—**YES; gloves and goggles protect against splashes on the skin and eyes.**

D. Change a patient's bed that is soiled with drainage—**YES; gloves protect against bacteria.**

E. Administer medication down a gastrostomy tube—**YES; gloves and goggles protect against gastric drainage or splashes in the eyes.**

F. Change a dressing 24 hours after surgery—NO; sterile procedure would be used to protect the patient, whereas standard precautions protect the health care worker.

EXERCISE 2.168 Select all that apply:

To minimize the risk of infection to others, the triage nurse would:

A. Provide the patient with tissues to cover the mouth and nose—**YES; to decrease transmission.**

B. Direct the patient to discard the tissues promptly after use—**YES; to decrease transmission.**

C. Place the patient before the other patients waiting for treatment—NO; this patient would not be the highest priority because there are no respiratory complications noted.

D. Instruct the patient to apply a surgical mask—**YES; to decrease transmission.**

E. Seat the patient 3 feet away from other patients—**YES; to decrease transmission.**

F. Educate the patient to wash his or her hands after contact with secretions—**YES; to decrease transmission.**

EXERCISE 2.169 Select all that apply:

Signs and symptoms of influenza include:

A. Fever—**YES.**

B. Myalgia—**YES.**

C. Nonproductive cough—**YES.**

D. Malaise—**YES.**

E. Productive cough—NO; nonproductive cough is noted in influenza.

F. Nasal congestion and sore throat—**YES.**

EXERCISE 2.170 Select all that apply:

Influenza can be contracted by:

A. Contact with virus-contaminated blood—NO.

B. Contact with virus-contaminated surfaces—**YES.**

C. Close proximity of a virus-infected person who coughs—**YES.**
D. Close proximity of a virus-infected person who sneezes—**YES.**

EXERCISE 2.171 Multiple-choice:

What isolation precautions are required for the inpatient or outpatient management of patients with influenza?

A. Contact—NO.
B. Airborne—NO.
C. Droplet—**YES.**
D. Standard—NO.

EXERCISE 2.172 Select all that apply:

To minimize potential exposure of noninfected individuals to influenza, patient education would include:

A. Do not share eating utensils or linens—**YES; influenza-infected patients should not share utensils or linens.**
B. Avoid public places for 48 hours—NO; to prevent transmission, infected adults should avoid noninfected individuals for 7 days after becoming ill.
C. Wear surgical mask while coughing—NO; surgical masks should be worn at all times (unless eating) to prevent transmission to others in the home as well as transfer to objects.
D. Cover nose and mouth to cough and sneeze—**YES; to prevent transmission.**
E. Wash hands with soap and water—**YES; to prevent transmission.**
F. Disinfect all contaminated surfaces—**YES; to prevent transmission.**

EXERCISE 2.173 Multiple-choice:

Which statement by the nurse demonstrates correct teaching about the antiviral drug Tamiflu?

A. "It is used to treat, not prevent, influenza."—NO; Tamiflu is used for the treatment of influenza and the prevention of influenza in those exposed to the virus.
B. "It is only active against influenza type A virus."—NO; Tamiflu is active against influenza type A and type B.
C. "It should be started within 48 hours of symptom onset."—**YES; Tamiflu provides the greatest clinical benefit when initiated within 48 hours of symptom or illness onset.**
D. "It should never be given to a pregnant patient."—NO; Tamiflu is the preferred antiviral treatment in pregnancy.

Resources

Altman, R. D. (2012). Osteoarthritis (OA). Retrieved from http://www.merckmanuals.com/professional/musculoskeletal-and-connective-tissue-disorders/joint-disorders/osteoarthritis-oa

American Thoracic Society. (n.d.). Oxygen delivery methods. Retrieved from http://www.thoracic.org/copd-guidelines/for-health-professionals/exacerbation/inpatient-oxygen-therapy/oxygen-delivery-methods.php

Apatoff, B. R. (2014). Multiple sclerosis. Retrieved from http://www.merckmanuals.com/professional/neurologic-disorders/demyelinating-disorders/multiple-sclerosis-ms

Bolster, M. B. (2012). Osteoporosis. Retrieved from http://www.merckmanuals.com/professional/musculoskeletal-and-connective-tissue-disorders/osteoporosis/osteoporosis

Centers for Disease Control and Prevention. (2015). Influenza (flu). Retrieved from http:// www.cdc.gov/flu/index.htm

Centers for Disease Control and Prevention. (2015). Measles (Rubeola): For healthcare professionals. Retrieved from http://www.cdc.gov/measles/hcp/index.html

Gonzalez-Usigli, H. A., & Espay, A. (2013). Parkinson disease. Retrieved from http://www.merckmanuals.com/professional/neurologic-disorders/movement-and-cerebellar-disorders/parkinson-disease

Jauch, E. C., Saver, J. L., Adams, H. P., Bruno, A., Connors, J. J., Demaerschalk, B. M., . . . Khatri, P. (2013). AHA/AHA guideline: Guidelines for the early management of patients with acute ischemic stroke: A guideline for health care professionals from the American Heart Association/American Stroke Association. *Stroke, 44,* 870–947.

Lechtzin, N. (2013). Evaluation of the pulmonary patient. Retrieved from http://www.merckmanuals.com/professional/pulmonary-disorders/approach-to-the-pulmonary-patient/evaluation-of-the-pulmonary-patient

Moroz, A. (2013). Leg amputation rehabilitation. Retrieved from http://www.merckmanuals.com/professional/special-subjects/rehabilitation/leg-amputation-rehabilitation

Rubin, M. (2014). Myasthenia gravis. Retrieved from http://www.merckmanuals.com/professional/neurologic-disorders/peripheral-nervous-system-and-motor-unit-disorders/myasthenia-gravis

Tapson, V. F. (2015). Pulmonary embolism (PE). Retrieved from http://www.merckmanuals.com/professional/pulmonary-disorders/pulmonary-embolism-pe/pulmonary-embolism-pe

Weiser, T. G. (2014). Overview of thoracic trauma. Retrieved from http://www.merckmanuals.com/professional/injuries-poisoning/thoracic-trauma/overview-of-thoracic-trauma

Wilberger, J. E., & Dupre, D.A. (2013). Spinal trauma. Retrieved from http://www.merckmanuals.com/professional/injuries-poisoning/spinal-trauma/spinal-trauma

Wise, R. A. (2014). Chronic obstructive pulmonary disease (COPD). Retrieved from http://www.merckmanuals.com/professional/pulmonary-disorders/chronic-obstructive-pulmonary-disease-and-related-disorders/chronic-obstructive-pulmonary-disease-copd

CHAPTER 3

Mental Health Nursing

Roseann V. Regan and Roberta Waite

The nurse is the instrument.—Author unknown

UNFOLDING CASE STUDY 1: Angelique

Angelique, age 18 years, has recently demonstrated a change in behavior and has difficulty concentrating. She is HIV positive. Angelique came to the outpatient clinic because she was not feeling well. She states that she does not know what's wrong and is reluctant to "open up" during her visit. The nurse understands that in order to help Angelique, the nurse must obtain her trust.

EXERCISE 3.1 Matching:

What strategies either facilitate or impede trust in a therapeutic communication process in the nurse–patient relationship?

Match the elements of a therapeutic relationship in Column A with the nursing interventions in Column B:

Column A	Column B
A. Respect	_____ Giving recognition to the person's worth
B. Empathy	_____ Being honest about feelings
C. Positive self-regard	_____ Honoring the person's dignity
D. Genuineness	_____ Trying to understand the person's view
E. Confidentiality	_____ Fulfilling promises and being reliable
F. Self-awareness	_____ Knowing one's own attitudes and feelings
G. Trust	_____ Keeping information private
H. Acceptance	_____ Meeting the person where he or she is

The answer can be found on page 214

EXERCISE 3.2 Matching:

Match the therapeutic or nontherapeutic communication techniques in Column A with the nurse statements in Column B:

Column A	Column B
A. Sympathy	____ "Don't worry; you will get your boyfriend back."
B. Asking why	____ "I felt differently when I was in the hospital."
C. False reassurance	____ "Why are you nervous?"
D. Giving advice	____ "You should quit your job."
E. Seeking clarification	____ "What happened before you got upset?"
F. Exploring	____ "Are you telling me you felt angry when you didn't get your raise?"
G. Broad opening	____ "How are you doing?"
H. Countertransference	____ "Stop interrupting me! You're just like my sister!"

The answer can be found on page 215

EXERCISE 3.3 Fill in the blanks:

Fill in the blanks using the following list:

Sympathy
Asking why
False reassurance
Giving advice
Seeking clarification
Exploring
Broad opening
Countertransference

Therapeutic communication includes: ____________________

Nontherapeutic communication includes: ____________________

The answer can be found on page 215

eRESOURCE

To reinforce your understanding of therapeutic communication, refer to Nursing Planet. [Pathway: http://nursingplanet.com ➔ select "Mental Health Nursing" ➔ scroll down to the "Assessment & Evaluation" section and select "Therapeutic Communication" and review the content.]

EXERCISE 3.4 Select all that apply:

Setting boundaries for patients is done in order to accomplish which of the following?

A. Setting rules of behavior that guide interaction with others
B. Allowing a patient and nurse to connect safely in a therapeutic relationship based on the patient's needs
C. Making sure the patient does not influence other patients
D. Helping us control the impact others have on us as well as our impact on others
E. Helping families of patients better understand the diagnosis

The answer can be found on page 215

After the assessment, the nurse identifies that Angelique complains of having a lack of energy, which has persisted for several weeks. Neither Angelique's self-report nor her laboratory results reflect current or recent substance use.

EXERCISE 3.5 Select all that apply:

Angelique expresses a loss of interest and pleasure in activities and believes her life is going nowhere and looks bleak. She also says that she does not feel like getting out of bed in the morning and has no interest in sleeping or eating. What symptoms will the nurse report?

A. Echolalia, apathy, delusions
B. Obsessions, compulsions, hypersomnia
C. Perseveration, somatization, dissociation
D. Anergia, anhedonia, insomnia
E. Hopelessness, helplessness, negativism

The answer can be found on page 216

EXERCISE 3.6 Exhibit-format:

Angelique sees an advanced practice registered nurse (APRN) who records the following findings:

Patient states that she is tired all the time and sleeps a lot.

Patient has lost 5 lb in 2 months and lacks concentration. She has difficulty finishing a thought process. The APRN understands that these manifestations may indicate a diagnosis of:

A. Obsessive-compulsive behavior
B. Depression
C. Personality disorder
D. Addiction

The answer can be found on page 216

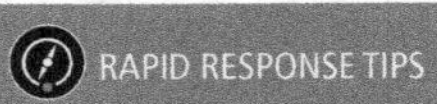

Risk factors versus protective factors

From a health perspective, *risk factors* are things that increase a person's chance of getting a disorder. *Protective factors* are things that decrease the chance of getting a disorder.

EXERCISE 3.7 Matching:

Identify risk factors and protective factors for depression. Use the letter in Column A to indicate whether the attribute is a risk or protective factor in Column B:

Column A	Column B
A. Being female	_____ Risk factor
B. Having a depressed parent	_____ Protective factor

The answer can be found on page 216

EXERCISE 3.8 Select all that apply:

What are accepted "truths" about suicide?

A. Asking about it gives the patient the idea
B. Only some depressed patients are at risk
C. Asking gives the patient permission to talk about it
D. History of attempts increases risk
E. A plan increases risk
F. It is a rational decision

The answer can be found on page 216

Psychiatric History

Angelique had her first depressive episode when she was 15 years old, after the death of her mother. She received family support but did not take any medication and was not involved in traditional counseling services. Recently, Angelique, now 18 years old, discovered that she is HIV positive; this occurred roughly on the anniversary of her mother's passing. Nurses must understand that suicidal tendencies are increased around the anniversary dates of the death of a significant other or family member and also when individuals are diagnosed with a chronic or disabling medical illness, such as HIV. This is of particular importance if the individual experiences significant hopelessness and social stigma.

eRESOURCE

To reinforce your understanding of the clinical presentation of depression, refer to Medscape on your mobile device. [Pathway: Medscape → enter "Depression" into the search field → select "Depression" and review content.]

EXERCISE 3.9 True/False:

Facts about suicide:

A. Suicide is one of the top 10 causes of death among all age groups.

______ True

______ False

B. Suicide is the third leading cause of death among 15- to 24-year-olds.

______ True

______ False

C. White people are twice as likely to die by suicide as non-White people.

______ True

______ False

D. White men commit more than 70% of all U.S. suicides.

______ True

______ False

E. The number of elderly suicides is decreasing.

______ True

______ False

F. The ethnic groups with the highest suicide rates are Asians and Blacks.

______ True

______ False

G. Decreased serotonin levels play a role in suicidal behavior.

______ True

______ False

H. The person who is suicidal often has the desire to be free of pain and to be saved.

______ True

______ False

The answer can be found on page 217

EXERCISE 3.10 Fill in the blanks:

Word list:

- Directly
- Suicide plan
- Family history
- Secrecy
- Confidentiality
- Lethality
- Coping

Suicide assessment:

- Ask ___________ about suicidal thoughts/behavior.
- Identify whether the person has a ______________.
- Explore whether the person has a _______________ of suicide.
- Do not swear to __________.
- Discuss the limits of ________________.
- Suicidal intent and ___________.
- Assess the person's _________ potential.

The answer can be found on page 217

Most suicide attempts are expressions of extreme distress, not bids for attention. Suicidal behavior develops along a continuum.

EXERCISE 3.11 Matching:

Match the definitions in Column A with the terms in Column B:

Column A	Column B
A. The beginning of the suicide continuum is the process of contemplating suicide or the methods used without acting on these thoughts. At this point, the patient might not talk about these thoughts unless he or she is pressed.	_____ Ideation
B. The act of intentionally killing oneself may follow prior attempts, but about 30% of those who commit suicide are believed to have done so on their first attempt. Suicide results when the person can see no other option for relief from unbearable emotional or physical pain.	_____ Suicide gesture
	_____ Suicide attempt
	_____ Suicide

(*continued*)

Column A	Column B
C. Taking a potentially lethal dose of medication indicates that the person wants to die and has no wish to be rescued.	
D. Actions may be taken that are not likely to be lethal, such as taking a few pills or making superficial cuts on the wrist. These suggest that the patient is ambivalent about dying or has not planned to die. He or she has the will to survive, wants to be rescued, and is experiencing a mental conflict. This act is often called a "cry for help" because the patient is struggling with unmanageable stress.	

The answer can be found on page 218

eRESOURCE

To reinforce your understanding of suicide and assessing for suicide risk, refer to Medscape on your mobile device. [Pathway: Medscape ➔ enter "Suicide" into the search field ➔ select "Suicide" and review content.]

Angelique requires inpatient psychiatric care because of her worsening condition and concerns related to her safety. She is admitted for treatment and safety measures.

EXERCISE 3.12 **Fill in the blank:**

Angelique has the right to ____________________ before health care interventions are undertaken.

The answer can be found on page 218

EXERCISE 3.13 **Select all that apply:**

Informed consent includes which of the following:

A. Adequate and accurate knowledge and information
B. An individual with legal capacity to consent
C. The understanding that it is changeable
D. Consent is given voluntarily
E. Family input

The answer can be found on page 219

EXERCISE 3.14 True/False:

Voluntary patients are considered competent unless otherwise adjudicated and therefore have the absolute right to refuse treatment, including psychotropic medications, unless they are dangerous to themselves or others.

______ True

______ False

The answer can be found on page 219

EXERCISE 3.15 Select all that apply:

Voluntary patients have the right to:

A. Refuse treatments
B. Sign a 72-hour notice to leave
C. Receive visitors
D. Use cell phone on unit
E. Refuse antianxiety medication if violent
F. Smoke cigarettes on a smoke-free unit

The answer can be found on page 219

EXERCISE 3.16 Select all that apply:

Involuntary patients have the right to:

A. Receive visitors
B. Sign a 72-hour notice to leave
C. Vote
D. Refuse antianxiety medication if calm
E. Make phone calls
F. Smoke cigarettes if the unit has accommodations for it

The answer can be found on page 219

EXERCISE 3.17 Select all that apply:

Angelique will start on a selective serotonin reuptake inhibitor (SSRI). Which would the nurse anticipate giving from this group?

A. Lithium carbonate (Lithobid)
B. Fluoxetine (Prozac)
C. Risperidone (Risperdal)
D. Paroxetine (Paxil)
E. Sertraline (Zoloft)

The answer can be found on page 220

---

eRESOURCE

To reinforce your understanding of SSRI drugs, refer to Epocrates Online. [Pathway: http://online.epocrates.com ➔ under the "Classes" column, select "Psychiatric," then under the "Psychiatric Subclasses" column, select "Selective Serotonin Reuptake Inhibitor (SSRI)" and review drugs listed under the third column. Click on each drug name to learn more about the drug.]

EXERCISE 3.18 Multiple-choice:

Antidepressant drugs, such as fluoxetine and sertraline, selectively act on:

A. Acetylcholine receptors
B. Norepinephrine receptors
C. Serotonin receptors
D. Melatonin receptors

The answer can be found on page 220

---

eRESOURCE

To reinforce your understanding of fluoxetine and sertraline, refer to Epocrates Online. [Pathway: http://online.epocrates.com ➔ under the "Drugs" tab, enter "Fluoxetine" in the search field ➔ select "Fluoxetine" ➔ review "Adult Dosing," "Pharmacology," "Adverse Reactions," and "Safety/Monitoring." Repeat with "Sertraline."]

EXERCISE 3.19 Multiple-choice:

Angelique is prescribed medication for a psychiatric disorder. After 3 days, the patient tells the nurse that she has been constipated. The nurse should instruct the patient to:

A. Eat more high-protein foods
B. Increase fiber and fluid intake
C. Take a stool softener
D. Have patience as this will subside

The answer can be found on page 220

EXERCISE 3.20 Multiple-choice:

Before administering a medication for the first time, an important assessment to make on a patient with a psychiatric disorder, like Angelique, is to determine his or her:

A. Cultural background
B. Height and weight
C. Preexisting symptoms
D. Physical stamina

The answer can be found on page 220

EXERCISE 3.21 Multiple-choice:

A major side effect of bupropion (Wellbutrin) is:

A. Seizures
B. Urinary frequency
C. Palpitations
D. Hallucinations

The answer can be found on page 220

---

eRESOURCE

To reinforce your understanding of Wellbutrin, refer to Epocrates Online. [Pathway: http://online.epocrates.com ➔ under the "Drugs" tab, enter "Wellbutrin" in the search field ➔ select "Wellbutrin" ➔ review "Adverse Reactions" and "Safety/Monitoring."]

EXERCISE 3.22 Multiple-choice:

Angelique has been prescribed the drug paroxetine (Paxil) for depression. The nurse should explain to her that selective serotonin reuptake inhibitors (SSRIs) may have a side effect of:

A. Hypertension
B. Gastrointestinal distress
C. Rigidity
D. Increased sexual desire

The answer can be found on page 221

EXERCISE 3.23 Select all that apply:

Angelique has been prescribed the drug sertraline (Zoloft), a selective serotonin reuptake inhibitor (SSRI), for depression. The nurse should teach her to report possible side effects of:

A. Sleep disturbance
B. Increased sexual desire
C. Dry mouth
D. Agranulocytosis
E. Agitation
F. Hypertension

The answer can be found on page 221

EXERCISE 3.24 Select all that apply:

According to best practices for patient teaching, the nurse must also do which of the following:

A. Give Angelique a pamphlet to read later
B. Have Angelique read the pamphlet to the nurse
C. Have Angelique do a teach-back of the possible side effects
D. Have Angelique tell the nurse what she will do (inform provider) if she has side effects
E. Document in the chart what was taught and the patient's response
F. Send the patient to pharmacy to get a medication printout

The answer can be found on page 221

EXERCISE 3.25 Select all that apply:

The nurse recognizes that more teaching is needed if Angelique says which of the following?

A. "I can stop the medication if I feel better."
B. "The depression will be gone after 1 week."
C. "If I have a side effect, I just stop the medication."
D. "I must report suicidal thoughts with or without a plan to my provider."
F. "I can take over-the-counter St. John's wort with my prescribed antidepressant."
G. "I can drink alcohol."

The answer can be found on page 221

---

eRESOURCE

To reinforce your understanding of fluoxetine and sertraline, refer to Epocrates Online. [Pathway: http://online.epocrates.com → under the "Drugs" tab, enter "Fluoxetine" in the search field → select "Fluoxetine" → review "Adverse Reactions," "Safety/Monitoring," and "Patient Education." Repeat with "Sertraline."]

UNFOLDING CASE STUDY 2: Luke

The nurse is also caring for Luke. He is 65 years old and recently lost his wife of 42 years to breast cancer. He is depressed and was referred by his son because he has lost interest in all his normal activities and his hygiene has declined.

EXERCISE 3.26 Multiple-choice:

In a hospitalized patient who has been prescribed desvenlafaxine (Pristiq), the nurse should monitor for:

A. Nausea
B. Hypertension
C. Somnolence
D. Constipation

The answer can be found on page 222

EXERCISE 3.27 Matching:

To examine differences in antidepressant therapy, match the effects in Column A to the medications in Column B:

Column A	Column B
A. SSRI (selective serotonin reuptake inhibitor)	_____ Elavil, Anafranil, Norpramin
B. MAOI (monoamine oxidase inhibitor)	_____ Zoloft, Paxil, Prozac
C. SNRI (serotonin/norepinephrine reuptake inhibitor)	_____ Cymbalta, Effexor, Pristiq
D. Tricyclic antidepressant	_____ Marplan, Parnate, Nardil

The answer can be found on page 222

EXERCISE 3.28 Matching:

Match medications in Column A to the common side effects in Column B:

Column A	Column B
A. Tofranil, Elavil, Pamelor	_____ Avoid taking decongestants and consuming foods that contain high levels of tyramine
B. Luvox, Lexapro, Zoloft	_____ Liver dysfunction occurs: yellowing of the skin or whites of the eyes, unusually dark urine, loss of appetite that lasts for several days, nausea, or abdominal pain
C. Wellbutrin, Serzone	_____ Dry mouth, constipation, bladder problems, sexual dysfunction, blurred vision
D. Nardil, Parnate, Marplan	_____ Sexual dysfunction, nausea, nervousness, insomnia, and agitation

The answer can be found on page 222

EXERCISE 3.29 Select all that apply:

Luke has been placed on phenelzine (Nardil). The teaching was successful if Luke says he will avoid foods such as:

A. Red wine
B. Bananas and raisins
C. Aged cheese
D. Liver
E. Apples
F. Pepperoni

The answer can be found on page 222

EXERCISE 3.30 True/False:

Plant and herbal remedies are natural, so they are good to take with all medications.

_____ True
_____ False

The answer can be found on page 223

---

eRESOURCE

To reinforce your understanding of phenelzine, refer to Epocrates Online. [Pathway: http://online.epocrates.com ➔ under the "Drugs" tab, enter "Phenelzine" in the search field select "Nardil" ➔ review "Adverse Reactions," "Safety/Monitoring," and "Patient Education."]

EXERCISE 3.31 Fill in the blanks:

The nurse caring for Luke knows that serotonin is a ________________ that regulates many functions, including mood, appetite, and sensory perception. With too much serotonin in the brain, a condition called *serotonin syndrome (SS)* can occur. Name four symptoms of SS: ____________, ____________, ____________, and ____________.

The answer can be found on page 223

---

eRESOURCE

To supplement your understanding of the clinical presentation associated with serotonin syndrome, refer to the *Merck Manual.* [Pathway: www.merckmanuals.com/professional ➔ enter "Serotonin Syndrome" into the search field ➔ select "Serotonin Syndrome" ➔ review the content, particularly "Symptoms and Signs," "Treatment," and "Key Points."]

EXERCISE 3.32 Multiple-choice:

Luke must also be told to check the fine print of over-the-counter (OTC) cold medication (and others) and check with his provider. Taking an monoamine oxidase inhibitor (MAOI) with such medications (if prohibited) can cause:

A. Anaphylactic shock
B. Neuroleptic malignant syndrome
C. Hypertensive crisis
D. Seizures

The answer can be found on page 223

---

eRESOURCE

To supplement your understanding of the drugs that can cause serotonin syndrome, refer to the *Merck Manual*. [Pathway: www.merckmanuals.com/professional → enter "Serotonin Syndrome" into the search field → select "Serotonin Syndrome" → select "Drugs That Can Cause Serotonin Syndrome" and review the content.]

On admission assessment, the nurse notes that Luke has a lack of energy, a lack of appetite with a 10-lb weight loss, constipation, and difficulty sleeping with early-morning awakening. Luke admits to having suicidal thoughts at times, but has no current plan.

EXERCISE 3.33 Ordering:

Place the nursing interventions in priority order from 1 to 5:

_____ Provide assistance with activities of daily living (ADL)
_____ Encourage a high-fiber nutritious diet
_____ Monitor for suicidal ideation and contract for safety
_____ Teach about medications
_____ Promote sleep hygiene

The answer can be found on page 223

Luke's son tells the nurse that he does not understand why his father does not "snap out of this" and "what is depression anyway?"

EXERCISE 3.34 Select all that apply:

What is the best response by the nurse to the son?

A. "Depression is an illness that can be treated."
B. "Depression is his choice."
C. "It is just the usual grieving response."
D. "Depression may be a chronic illness with remissions and exacerbations."
E. "Depression may have a genetic and an environmental component."

The answer can be found on page 224

Luke tells the nurse that his roommate told him he may strangle Luke if he does not do what the roommate wants.

EXERCISE 3.35 Select all that apply:

The nurse should provide for Luke's safety by:

A. Placing the roommate into four-point restraints
B. Reviewing the unit procedure on violence precautions
C. Identifying the evidence-based practice for preventing violence
D. Notifying the health team (doctor and supervisor)
E. Placing the roommate in a private room
F. Assessing the roommate for violence threat and placing on one-to-one observation

The answer can be found on page 224

The nurse is introducing interventions to help Luke effectively grieve for the loss of his wife, increase his self-esteem, and meet his needs for love and belonging (both needs on Maslow's hierarchy).

EXERCISE 3.36 Select all that apply:

The nursing interventions to meet these underlying needs might include:

A. Providing Luke an activity to create something
B. Giving Luke medications
C. Providing television in lounges
D. Developing a grief support group
E. Acknowledging Luke's achievements by displaying his works on unit
F. Encouraging family participation in Luke's activities and recovery (family teaching)

The answer can be found on page 224

Luke is about to be discharged to home and outpatient therapy. The nurse discusses these plans with Luke.

EXERCISE 3.37 Select all that apply:

Which statements by Luke would indicate movement to positive achievement of the discharge plan?

A. "I plan to attend therapy."
B. "I don't like going home to an empty house."
C. "I am going to visit my son and grandchildren."
D. "I am joining a volunteer group."
E. "I will stop my medication if too expensive."
F. "I am going to exercise at the gym."

The answer can be found on page 224

UNFOLDING CASE STUDY 1 (CONTINUED): Angelique

During Angelique's hospitalization, she presents with auditory hallucinations, hearing her mother's voice saying "join me," and visual hallucinations of mice running on the floor. These hallucinations have increased in intensity during the past week. She also exhibits fluctuations in mood and has been more irritable for about 4 days. This mood state was clearly different from her usual nondepressed mood (*euthymia*). After assessment by the health care team and obtaining Angelique's approval, she is started on a low-dose antipsychotic and a mood stabilizer.

EXERCISE 3.38 Matching:

Match the nursing interventions in Column A with the side effects of the antipsychotic medications in Column B:

Column A	Column B
A. Monitor white blood cells (WBC)	_____ Dry mouth
B. Get out of chair slowly	_____ Constipation
C. Increase fluids and fiber	_____ Photophobia
D. Use sugarless candy and sips of water	_____ Weight gain
E. Maintain low-calorie diet	_____ Agranulocytosis
F. Wear sunglasses	_____ Orthostatic hypotension
G. Get up and dress early	_____ Sedation

The answer can be found on page 225

EXERCISE 3.39 Exhibit-format:

The nurse reviews the patient data:

Vital signs (VS): Temperature: 98.2°F, respiratory rate (RR): 24 breaths per minute, heart rate (HR), 90 beats per minute (bpm), blood pressure (BP): 132/86 mmHg

Physical examination: Head symmetrical, dull affective responses, pupils equal and reactive to light and accommodation (PERLA), difficulty in fully extending arms and ataxic gait

The nurse suspects that these assessment findings are consistent with:

A. Parkinson's disease
B. Extrapyramidal side effects (EPSE)
C. Transient ischemic attack (TIA)
D. Signs of overdose

The answer can be found on page 225

EXERCISE 3.40 Select all that apply:

Which of the following is true about the atypical antipsychotics?

A. Cause fewer or no extrapyramidal side effects (EPSE)
B. Used to treat both positive and negative symptoms of schizophrenia
C. Exert both dopamine and serotonin receptor blocking action
D. Cause more EPSE
E. Treat only positive symptoms of schizophrenia

The answer can be found on page 225

---

eRESOURCE

To reinforce your understanding of extrapyramidal side effects, refer to Nursing Planet. [Pathway: http://nursingplanet.com → select "Mental Health Nursing" → scroll down to the "Psychopharmacology Reviews" section and select "Neuroleptic-Induced Extrapyramidal Symptoms" and review the content.]

EXERCISE 3.41 Select all that apply:

In teaching about the antipsychotics, the nurse would tell her to do the following:

A. Stop taking meds when you feel better
B. Report adverse effects promptly
C. Do not drink alcohol
D. Do not take over-the-counter (OTC) meds causing drowsiness
E. Do not drive or use hazardous equipment or do activities needing alertness
F. Give medication 1 week to relieve symptoms

The answer can be found on page 225

EXERCISE 3.42 Fill in the blanks:

What two neurotransmitters in the body are targeted with atypical and typical antipsychotics?

1. ______________________________
2. ______________________________

The answer can be found on page 226

EXERCISE 3.43 Matching:

Indicate whether the medication in Column A is a typical or atypical antipsychotic in Column B:

Column A	Column B
A. Chlorpromazine (Thorazine)	_____ Typical antipsychotic
B. Fluphenazine (Prolixin)	_____ Atypical antipsychotic
C. Risperidone (Risperdal)	
D. Trifluoperazine (Stelazine)	
E. Olanzapine (Zyprexa)	
F. Haloperidol (Haldol)	
G. Aripiprazole (Abilify)	
H. Thioridazine (Loxapine)	
I. Clozapine (Clozaril)	
J. Thiothixene (Navane)	
K. Ziprasidone (Geodon)	

The answer can be found on page 226

EXERCISE 3.44 Matching:

Please match the effects in Column A with the medications in Column B:

Column A	Column B
A. Fixed false beliefs strongly held in spite of invalidating evidence	_____ Chlorpromazine (Thorazine)
B. Flat affect and apathy	_____ Fluphenazine (Prolixin)
C. Reduction in the range and intensity of emotional expression	_____ Risperidone (Risperidal)
D. Reduced ability, difficulty, or inability to initiate and persist in goal-directed behavior	_____ Trifluoperazine (Stelazine)
E. Marked decrease in reaction to the immediate surrounding environment	_____ Olanzapine (Zyprexa)
F. Hallucinations and delusions	_____ Haloperidol (Haldol)
G. Poverty of speech	_____ Aripiprazole (Abilify)
H. Distortions or exaggerations of perception in any of the senses	_____ Thoridazine (Loxapine)
I. Loss of feeling or an inability to experience pleasure	_____ Clozapine (Clozaril)

The answer can be found on page 226

eRESOURCE

To reinforce your understanding of antipsychotic drugs, refer to Epocrates Online. [Pathway: http://online.epocrates.com → under the "Classes" column, select "Psychiatric," then under the "Psychiatric Subclasses" column, select "Antipsychotics, 1st Generation" and review drugs listed under the third column. Click on each drug name to learn more about the drug.]

EXERCISE 3.45 Multiple-choice:

Angelique complains of itching and dermatitis after taking a medication for a psychiatric disorder; after 3 days, the nurse should:

A. Reassure the patient
B. Offer the patient soothing lotions
C. Contact the physician
D. Offer the patient a warm tub bath

The answer can be found on page 227

UNFOLDING CASE STUDY 3: Marina

Marina, age 31 years, is being admitted as an inpatient because of a psychosis; she was first admitted at the age of 18 years. At the time of referral, it had been 2 years since Marina's last admission. Diagnosis at discharge was schizophrenia. The most prominent symptom Marina reported experiencing was auditory hallucinations with derogatory comment "you're a freak of nature" and "you'll never move on," which increased with stress. She had been prescribed ziprasidone (Geodon) for a number of years, but she was not getting the same relief recently. Marina lives in a structured facility and is in contact with the community mental health nurse.

EXERCISE 3.46 Multiple-choice:

When Marina requires larger doses of a given medication to maintain its therapeutic effect, the nurse determines that she has developed:

A. Abuse
B. Tolerance
C. Addiction
D. Allergies

The answer can be found on page 227

EXERCISE 3.47 Multiple-choice:

Which of the following atypical antipsychotic agents is associated with the most weight gain?

A. Ziprasidone (Geodon)
B. Aripiprazole (Abilify)
C. Olanzapine (Zyprexa)
D. Quetiapine (Seroquel)
E. Risperidone (Risperdal)

The answer can be found on page 227

EXERCISE 3.48 Select all that apply:

Schizophrenia spectrum includes:

A. Borderline personality
B. Schizotypal personality
C. Schizophreniform disorder
D. Schizoaffective disorder
E. Psychosis not otherwise specified

The answer can be found on page 227

EXERCISE 3.49 Select all that apply:

Which of the following is true about schizophrenia?

A. Initial symptoms most often occur in early adulthood
B. The patients usually do not need medication
C. It requires long-term treatment
D. Families require support and education
E. Cause is clearly known

The answer can be found on page 228

---

eRESOURCE

To reinforce your understanding of the clinical presentation of schizophrenia, refer to Medscape on your mobile device. [Pathway: Medscape → enter "Schizophrenia" into the search field → select "Schizophrenia" and review content.]

Marina reveals to the nurse that she does not understand English very well because it is her second language. Russian is her first. She also reveals that she is Russian Orthodox and requires certain dietary provisions.

EXERCISE 3.50 Select all that apply:

What should the nurse do to provide culturally competent care for Marina?

A. Get a family member to translate
B. Insist Marina eat what other patients eat
C. Contact a hospital-approved translator
D. Meet Marina's request for dietary consult
E. Ask Marina whether she would like to have clergy visit

The answer can be found on page 228

Marina shares with the nurse that the voices have started telling her to kill herself, but Marina tells the nurse to keep it a secret.

EXERCISE 3.51 Select all that apply:

What should the nurse do?

A. Reassure Marina she will not tell
B. Tell Marina she cannot keep it a secret
C. Notify the health team
D. Place Marina on one-to-one observation
E. Ask Marina's roommate to watch her
F. Put Marina in a seclusion room

The answer can be found on page 228

Even though extrapyramidal side effects (EPSE) are rare with atypical antipsychotics, the doctor writes a prescription for as-needed medication.

EXERCISE 3.52 Fill in the blanks:

____________________, ____________________, and ____________________ are examples of anticholinergic, antihistamine, and dopamine agonists to treat extrapyramidal side effects (EPSE).

The answer can be found on page 229

EXERCISE 3.53 Select all that apply:

What teaching should the nurse include for both Marina and her family caregiver?

A. Return for white blood cell (WBC) testing as prescribed
B. Notify provider of any infection or fever
C. Take over-the-counter (OTC) medications as she wishes
D. Call 911 if Marina has command hallucinations to hurt herself or others
E. Do teach-back to evaluate what they understood
F. Have an interpreter present

The answer can be found on page 229

EXERCISE 3.54 Select all that apply:

Please select the top-10 signs of schizophrenia:

A. Delusions (believing things that are not true)
B. Hallucinations (seeing or hearing things that are not there)
C. Depression
D. Disorganized thinking
E. Agitation
F. Mania
G. Violence
H. Using drugs and alcohol
I. Low intellect
J. Disorganized speech (e.g., frequent derailment or incoherence)
K. Grossly disorganized or catatonic behavior
L. Lack of drive or initiative
M. Social withdrawal
N. Apathy
O. Emotional unresponsiveness

The answer can be found on page 229

---

eRESOURCE

To supplement your understanding of the signs and symptoms associated with schizophrenia, refer to the *Merck Manual.* [Pathway: www.merckmanuals.com/professional → enter "Schizophrenia" into the search field → select "Schizophrenia" → review "Symptoms and Signs."]

EXERCISE 3.55 Multiple-choice:

Most drug metabolism occurs in the

A. Liver
B. Stomach
C. Brain
D. Gallbladder

The answer can be found on page 230

EXERCISE 3.56 Multiple-choice:

If Marina is prescribed a neuroleptic drug to treat a psychiatric disorder, the nurse should explain to her and her family that neuroleptic drugs are the same as:

A. Antipsychotic medications
B. Central nervous system depressants
C. Anticholinesterase inhibitors
D. Tranquilizers

The answer can be found on page 230

EXERCISE 3.57 Multiple-choice:

A patient diagnosed with schizophrenia is being treated with traditional antipsychotic medications. The nurse should explain to the patient and the patient's family that one negative symptom that may worsen during drug therapy is:

A. Insomnia
B. Social withdrawal
C. Hallucinations
D. Delusions

The answer can be found on page 230

EXERCISE 3.58 Multiple-choice:

Marina has been taking clozapine (Clozaril) for 6 weeks and visits the clinic complaining of fever, sore throat, and mouth sores. The nurse contacts the patient's physician as these symptoms are indicative of:

A. Severe anemia
B. Bacterial infection
C. Viral infection
D. Agranulocytosis

The answer can be found on page 230

EXERCISE 3.59 Matching:

Match the symptoms in Column A to the disorder in Column B:

Column A	Column B
A. Subjective or inner restlessness resulting in difficulty sitting still, leg movement, and pacing; it produces intense anxiety and fidgeting	_____ Acute dystonia
B. Tremors, mask-like face, bradykinesia, loss of facial expression, flattening of vocal inflection, stiffness, cogwheel rigidity, and reduced social functioning	_____ Akathisia
C. Neuroleptic-induced delirium	_____ Parkinsonism
D. Acute spasms of the muscles of the jaw, face, eyes, trunk, and chest	_____ Neuroleptic malignant syndrome

The answer can be found on page 231

eRESOURCE

To supplement your understanding of the treatment and management of schizophrenia, refer to Medscape on your mobile device. [Pathway: Medscape → enter "Schizophrenia" into the search field → select "Schizophrenia" and review content under the "Treatment & Management" section focusing on "Antipsychotic Pharmacotherapy."]

UNFOLDING CASE STUDY 4: José

José, age 17 years, began to isolate himself and exhibit progressively more extravagant behavior (eating in his room alone, spending more and more time staring at himself in the mirror), suspiciousness, and agitation in the year before being referred to a psychiatric department. Four months before entering the department, he consulted a psychiatric nurse practitioner, who prescribed oral haloperidol (Haldol) 2 mg/d. After several weeks of treatment, José showed increasingly unusual behavior and was subsequently brought to a psychiatric hospital. There, he was given a single dose of oral haloperidol (5 mg) and within hours began to experience fever (38.5°C/101.3°F), muscular rigidity, and increased creatine phosphokinase (CPK) levels to 1,920 IU/L, and leukocytosis (cells numbering 20,600/mL). After ruling out organic pathology (normal brain CT and cerebral spinal fluid [CSF] examination with glucose 64 mg/d, proteins 34 mg/d and no cells), this was deemed to be a case of neuroleptic malignant syndrome (NMS).

EXERCISE 3.60 Multiple-choice:

The nurse is caring for José, who has been taking haloperidol (Haldol) for 3 days. To assess José for neuroleptic malignant syndrome (NMS), the nurse should assess the patient's:

A. Blood pressure
B. Serum sodium level
C. Temperature
D. Weight

The answer can be found on page 231

EXERCISE 3.61 Multiple-choice:

Two medications that the nurse may give that are key in treating neuroleptic malignant syndrome (NMS) include:

A. Aspirin and lorazepam
B. Calcium and lithium
C. Bromocriptine (Parlodel) and dantrolene (Dantrium)
D. Lamictal (Lamotrigine) and olanzopine (Zyprexa)

The answer can be found on page 231

EXERCISE 3.62 Select all that apply:

Because neuroleptic malignant syndrome (NMS) is a life-threatening illness that may lead to rhabdomyolysis and renal failure, the nurse anticipates the following interventions:

A. Place the patient on isolation precautions
B. Hold Haldol (or other antipsychotic) and call provider
C. Call 911 and prepare for transfer
D. Admission to the intensive care unit (ICU)
E. Use cooling blanket, antipyretic, fluids, and hemodialysis at the medical hospital

The answer can be found on page 232

Because the nurse does not see this problem often (NMS is rare), she delegates the search for hospital policy and evidence-based practice in the literature to the other RN.

eRESOURCE

To supplement your understanding of the treatment and management of NMS, refer to Medscape on your mobile device. [Pathway: Medscape → enter "Neuroleptic Malignant Syndrome" into the search field → select "Neuroleptic Malignant Syndrome" and review content under the "Practice Essentials," "Clinical Presentation," and "Treatment & Management" sections.]

EXERCISE 3.63 Select all that apply:

In evaluating the intervention that was taken for meeting the Quality and Safety Education for Nurses (QSEN) standards, the nurse reviews:

A. Whether hospital procedure agrees with the literature best practices
B. Whether staff like the interventions
C. Whether staff collaborate as a team
D. Whether staff could find the procedure
E. Whether staff consider the patient response

The answer can be found on page 232

EXERCISE 3.64 Select all that apply:

What are the risk factors that place José at risk for neuroleptic malignant syndrome (NMS)?

A. Young age
B. Hispanic ethnicity
C. Male gender
D. Presence of affective illness and agitation

The answer can be found on page 232

---

eRESOURCE

To supplement your understanding of the risk factors associated with NMS, refer to Medscape on your mobile device. [Pathway: Medscape → enter "Neuroleptic Malignant Syndrome" into the search field → select "Neuroleptic Malignant Syndrome" and review content under the "Background," "Pathophysiology," "Etiology," and "Epidemiology" sections.]

EXERCISE 3.65 Select all that apply:

Which of the following statements are true of electroconvulsive therapy (ECT)?

A. Changes personality
B. Changes neurotransmitters
C. Causes a seizure
D. Uses muscle relaxant and general anesthesia
E. Always used before trying medication
F. Is given in a series of treatments

The answer can be found on page 232

EXERCISE 3.66 True/False:

A. Nurse can delegate pre- and post-electroconvulsive therapy (ECT) assessment to a mental health technician.

______True

______False

B. Patient may return to unit and sleep, then wake up confused.

______True

______False

C. Patient may complain of headache post-ECT.

______True

______False

D. Patient disorientation and short-term memory problem usually resolves within 24 hours.

______True

______False

E. Patient cannot refuse ECT.

______True

______False

F. Patient or guardian must sign an informed consent for ECT.

______True

______False

G. ECT cannot be done as an outpatient.

______True

______False

H. Nurse administers the voltage.

______True

______False

The answer can be found on page 233

---

eRESOURCE

To supplement your understanding of ECT, refer to Medscape on your mobile device. [Pathway: Medscape ➔ enter "Electroconvulsive Therapy" into the search field ➔ select "Electroconvulsive Therapy" and review content.]

José must be taught about his medication before he is discharged.

EXERCISE 3.67 Select all that apply:

The nurse would teach that Depakote:

A. Must be taken as directed
B. Is a neuroleptic
C. Is an anticonvulsant used as a mood stabilizer
D. Can be stopped abruptly
E. Abrupt withdrawal can cause a seizure

The answer can be found on page 233

José tells the nurse that he sometimes drinks alcohol to relax.

EXERCISE 3.68 Select all that apply:

What should the nurse tell him about his plan to drink alcohol?

A. Alcohol use is fine.
B. Alcohol use is not an effective way of coping.
C. Take his medication instead.
D. Do not drink alcohol with medication.
E. Practice relaxation techniques or listen to music as good coping skills.

The answer can be found on page 233

---

eRESOURCE

To reinforce your understanding of Depakote, refer to Epocrates Online. [Pathway: http://online.epocrates.com ➔ under the "Drugs" tab, enter "Depakote" in the search field ➔ select "Depakote" ➔ review "Patient Education" and "Safety/Monitoring."]

José is Hispanic. The nurse knows that in order to give culturally competent care, it is important to consider certain aspects of his culture.

EXERCISE 3.69 Select all that apply:

The nurse addresses the following:

A. Family is highly valued
B. Religion, primarily Catholic, is important
C. Health is thought to be God's will
D. Religion is not important
E. Hispanics tend to be verbally expressive

The answer can be found on page 234

José also states that he plans to spend several months of the year in Puerto Rico with his relatives there. He explains that when he is there, he goes to a folk healer who gives him "treatments" that do not include his medication.

EXERCISE 3.70 Select all that apply:

What interventions should the nurse make?

A. Forbid him from using the healer
B. Tell him to listen to the healer
C. Explain the importance of taking medication
D. Encourage family to support taking medication
E. Discuss folk customs that complement Western medicine

The answer can be found on page 234

EXERCISE 3.71 Multiple-choice:

The drug that is most successful in treating the side effect of akathisia is:

A. Carbamazepine (Tegretol)
B. Diazepam (Valium)
C. Lorazepam (Ativan)
D. Propranolol (Inderal)

The answer can be found on page 234

EXERCISE 3.72 Multiple-choice:

If José has been diagnosed with a manic disorder, the nurse anticipates that the physician will most likely prescribe:

A. Clonazepam (Klonopin)
B. Lorazepam (Ativan)
C. Imipramine (Tofranil)
D. Lithium (Lithobid)

The answer can be found on page 234

EXERCISE 3.73 Multiple-choice:

When a patient is prescribed 300 mg of oral lithium three times a day, the nurse should instruct the patient to contact the physician if he or she experiences:

A. Metallic taste
B. Urinary frequency
C. Loose stools
D. Thirst

The answer can be found on page 235

EXERCISE 3.74 Multiple-choice:

Lithium is:

A. An anticonvulsant
B. A salt
C. A nickel by-product
D. A thyroid-stimulating hormone

The answer can be found on page 235

---

eRESOURCE

To reinforce your understanding of lithium, refer to Epocrates Online. [Pathway: http://online.epocrates.com ➔ under the "Drugs" tab, enter "Lithium" in the search field ➔ select "Lithium" ➔ review content.]

EXERCISE 3.75 Multiple-choice:

The nurse is caring for a hospitalized patient who has been diagnosed with mixed mania and is not responding to lithium therapy. The nurse anticipates that the physician will most likely prescribe:

A. Tricyclic antidepressants
B. Anticonvulsants
C. Sedatives
D. Stimulants

The answer can be found on page 235

EXERCISE 3.76 True/False:

A. Lithium is contraindicated in pregnancy because of possible congenital defects.

______True

______False

B. Continuous gastrointestinal (GI) upset may be a sign of toxic reaction.

______True

______False

C. Lithium levels are not needed if the patient follows orders.

______True

______False

D. If sodium decreases, the lithium level decreases.

______True

______False

E. Full effect takes 2 to 3 weeks.

______True

______False

F. Long-term use may lead to hypothyroidism.

______True

______False

The answer can be found on page 234

UNFOLDING CASE STUDY 5: Tamara

Tamara, age 34 years, is admitted through the emergency department (ED) by her significant other. She paces constantly, has not slept well in a week, and is worried all the time. Tamara is admitted with the diagnosis of mixed mania.

EXERCISE 3.77 Multiple-choice:

The nurse is caring for Tamara who has been hospitalized with mixed mania and is to receive lamotrigine (Lamictol) as a medication. The nurse should explain to her that the target symptom of this medication is:

A. Anxiety
B. Lethargy
C. Mood stability
D. Sedation

The answer can be found on page 236

eRESOURCE

To reinforce your understanding of lamotrigine, refer to Epocrates Online. [Pathway: http://online.epocrates.com ➔ under the "Drugs" tab, enter "Lamotrigine" in the search field ➔ select "Lamotrigine" ➔ review "Adult Dosing" and "Patient Education."]

EXERCISE 3.78 True/False:

A. Normal serum levels of divalproex sodium (Depakote) are 150 to 200 mcg/mL.

_____ True

_____ False

B. The therapeutic range for serum divalproex sodium (Depakote) is 50 to 120 mcg/mL.

_____ True

_____ False

The answer can be found on page 236

eRESOURCE

To reinforce your understanding of therapeutic drug levels of Depakote, refer to Epocrates Online. [Pathway: http://online.epocrates.com ➔ under the "Drugs" tab, enter "Depakote" in the search field ➔ select "Depakote" ➔ review "Safety/Monitoring."]

EXERCISE 3.79 Multiple-choice:

A patient with mixed mania is prescribed carbamazepine (Tegretol). The nurse should instruct the patient that toxic side effects can occur if he or she concurrently takes a medication such as:

A. Lithium
B. Amoxicillin
C. Cimetidine
D. Buspirone

The answer can be found on page 236

EXERCISE 3.80 Multiple-choice:

A patient who has been taking the medication carbamazepine (Tegretol) tells the nurse that he has been continually nauseated. The nurse should explain to the patient that the nausea may be decreased if the medication is:

A. Decreased in dosage
B. Taken at bedtime
C. Supplemented with zinc
D. Taken with food

The answer can be found on page 236

EXERCISE 3.81 True/False:

Electroconvulsive therapy (ECT) is a type of somatic treatment in which an electric current is applied to the chest area through electrodes placed on the chest. The current is sufficient to induce a grand mal seizure.

_____ True

_____ False

The answer can be found on page 237

EXERCISE 3.82 Multiple-choice:

Electroconvulsive therapy (ECT) is thought to work by:

A. Decreasing dopamine levels
B. Increasing acetylcholine levels
C. Stabilizing histamine and epinephrine levels
D. Increasing norepinephrine and serotonin levels

The answer can be found on page 237

eRESOURCE

To supplement your understanding of ECT, refer to Medscape on your mobile device. [Pathway: Medscape ➔ enter "Electroconvulsive Therapy" into the search field ➔ select "Electroconvulsive Therapy" and review content.]

UNFOLDING CASE STUDY 1 (CONTINUED): Angelique

While in the hospital, Angelique attends group therapy. There are several therapeutic factors of group therapy.

EXERCISE 3.83 Matching:

Match the communication interventions between Columns A and B:

Column A	Column B
A. The nurse may enhance this by bringing attention to the progress of group members. It helps maintain the patients' faith in the therapeutic modality.	_____ Instillation of hope
B. Prevents the patient from feeling unique or different	_____ Interpersonal learning
	_____ Altruism
	_____ Imparting of information
	_____ Imitative behavior
	_____ Universality

(*continued*)

Column A	Column B
C. The act of giving, such as patients helping each other	_____ Development of socializing techniques
D. Giving information in a planned and structured manner	_____ Catharsis
E. Feedback and role playing are two methods used in group therapy to develop social skills.	_____ Existential factors
F. Patients imitate healthy behavior of other group members and the leader, which demonstrates growth.	_____ Group cohesiveness
G. Correction of interpersonal distortions is the goal.	
H. Relates to bonding in the group. The patient's role in the group influences self-esteem. Cohesive groups create positive patient results.	
I. Expression of feelings; is effective when followed by insight and learning.	
J. Emphasizes the present quality, content, subjective awareness, freedom of choice, and state of being. Examples are responsibility and recognition of mortality.	

The answer can be found on page 237

Social History

Angelique lives with her boyfriend and she will be discharged from the hospital in a few days, given the status of her psychological improvement. She is interested in developing an psychiatric advance directive and she wants assistance to develop one.

EXERCISE 3.84 Select all that apply:

Advantages of a psychiatric advance directive include:

A. An advance directive empowers the patient to make his or her treatment preferences known.
B. An advance directive will improve communication between the patient and the physician.
C. It can prevent clashes with professionals over treatment and may prevent forced treatment.
D. Having an advance directive may shorten a patient's hospital stay.

The answer can be found on page 238

EXERCISE 3.85 True/False:

A psychiatric advance directive can cover medical and surgical treatment.

_____ True

_____ False

The answer can be found on page 238

Dietary History

Angelique is slightly overweight. She feels much better and intends to change her diet and exercise activity. Given her family history of hypertension, she plans to drastically decrease the sodium in her diet and start taking a natural herbal supplement (St. John's wort) to improve her health. The psychopharmacologic medications Angelique is taking include lithium (Litobid), sertraline (Zoloft), and buspirone (Buspar).

EXERCISE 3.86 Fill in the blanks:

Name two concerns noted in the changes Angelique intends to make after discharge from the hospital.

1. ______________________________

2. ______________________________

The answer can be found on page 238

While Angelique is preparing for discharge, she asks to have a family meeting that includes not only her boyfriend but her father as well. She informs the nurse that her father speaks English but prefers using her native language, Spanish.

EXERCISE 3.87 Multiple-choice:

Having a Spanish-speaking interpreter for the father during the family meeting demonstrates:

A. Marginalizing

B. Cultural insensitivity

C. Support for the patient's recovery process

D. Assuming inferior cognition

The answer can be found on page 238

EXERCISE 3.88 True/False:

Good psychiatric nursing care involves treating all patients equally.

_____ True

_____ False

The answer can be found on page 238

EXERCISE 3.89 Select all that apply:

Patients' rights under the law include:

A. Right to treatment
B. Right to assent
C. Right to refuse treatment
D. Right to informed consent
E. Rights surrounding involuntary commitment
F. Psychiatric advance directives
G. Rights regarding seclusion and restraint

The answer can be found on page 239

The nurse taking care of Angelique is aware of the American Psychiatric Association's classifications of disorders.

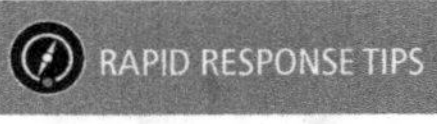

American Psychiatric Association classifications of psychiatric disorders

Axis I: Major Psychiatric Disorders
Axis II: Personality Disorders and Intellectual Disability
Axis III: Medical Conditions
Axis IV: Psychosocial/Environmental Problems
Axis V: Global Assessment of Functioning (GAF)

Angelique's case of new-onset depression, co-occurring medical illness (HIV), and the implications for proactive nursing interventions and family support are clearly indicated. Building effective rapport can promote therapeutic engagement and sharing of information, particularly as it relates to understanding what Angelique is experiencing. It also offers an opportunity for nurses to clarify any concerns or misinterpreted information. Ongoing education is relevant for both patient and family. Self-advocacy in developing a psychiatric advance directive helps give voice to Angelique's wishes. She also had the opportunity to share this with her boyfriend and other family members. It is important to note that Angelique's case illustrated the importance of cultural sensitivity as it relates to "comfort language" among family members. This means that professional nurses must be aware of patients' and their family members' language preference when receiving information, particularly when patients are bilingual and indicate that English is their second language.

UNFOLDING CASE STUDY 6: Matthew

Matthew is a 36-year-old male. He comes to the ED psychiatric crisis unit with his wife. The nurse, Dave, documents the following assessment:
Progress Note
10/2/14
1600
36-year-old male admitted to the ED psychiatric crisis unit
Vital signs: Temperature: 99.6°F, pulse: 88 bpm, respiratory rate (RR): 24 breaths per minute, blood pressure (BP): 120/80 mmHg
Patient states "I am having thoughts of killing self with my Army gun"
History of drinking every day
Last drink was 1 day ago
Blood alcohol level (BAL) equals 0

EXERCISE 3.90 Multiple-choice:

What is the nurse's priority nursing diagnosis for Matthew?

A. Ineffective individual coping
B. Alteration in thought process
C. Alteration in self-concept
D. Potential for violence (against self)

The answer can be found on page 239

EXERCISE 3.91 Multiple-choice:

The nurse initiates a verbal contract with Matthew for which of the following?

A. Safety
B. Admission
C. Monitoring
D. Drinking

The answer can be found on page 239

Matthew refuses to contract, which the nurse documents and then informs the physician of this. Dave then records Matthew's history. Matthew is a computer technician who was deployed twice to Afghanistan by his Army Reserve unit. While in combat, he saw several of his fellow soldiers get wounded or die. He states: "I only joined the reserves for some extra money to support my family." When he returned from the second deployment a couple of months ago, he started feeling very anxious around loud noises such as cars backfiring. He also has flashbacks and nightmares. He is suspicious and startled if anyone suddenly "walks up to me," even his wife and children. He has not gone to the Veterans Affairs (VA) for screening or help because "I don't trust them and it could hurt my record."

EXERCISE 3.92 Multiple-choice:

The nurse recognizes that Matthew's symptoms may be consistent with which disorder?

A. Social anxiety disorder
B. Posttraumatic stress disorder
C. Dissociative identity disorder
D. Paranoid disorder

The answer can be found on page 239

Dave decides to speak with Matthew's wife, who accompanied Matthew to the ED, to get collateral information. The wife reports that Matthew has been drinking heavily (one six-pack per day), fighting with her, arguing with his boss, and being short tempered with his children. The wife found him yesterday holding his gun while drinking. Matthew told her, "I should have died with my buddies." The family physician was called and she directed Matthew's wife to take Matthew to the ED psychiatric unit.

EXERCISE 3.93 Select all that apply:

What other nursing diagnoses can the nurse record at this point?

A. Ineffective individual coping
B. Ineffective family coping
C. Alteration in sleep pattern
D. Anxiety
E. Alteration in self-concept
F. Alteration in thought process (suicidal ideation)

The answer can be found on page 240

The physician writes the diagnoses of depression not otherwise specified (NOS, Code 311) with suicidal ideation, posttraumatic stress disorder (PTSD), and alcohol use. The physician arranges for admission to the inpatient psychiatric unit.

eRESOURCE

To supplement your understanding of posttraumatic stress disorder, refer to Medscape on your mobile device. [Pathway: Medscape → enter "Posttraumatic Stress Disorder" into the search field → select "Posttraumatic Stress Disorder" and review content.]

EXERCISE 3.94 Select all that apply:

The nurse prepares a situation, background, assessment, recommendation (SBAR) report for the psychiatric inpatient unit nurse. What information is critical to convey in terms of safety and continuity?

A. Patient admission for depression not otherwise specified (NOS) with suicidal ideation
B. Patient has plan and weapon at home (gun)
C. Patient drinks heavily, last drink 1 day ago
D. Patient refuses to contract for safety
E. Patient is a computer technician
F. Maintain on one-to-one observation until further assessment

The answer can be found on page 240

On admission to the psychiatric unit, Matthew acknowledges that he has thoughts and a plan of using his gun to kill himself. He did admit that he hid the loaded gun in the house.

EXERCISE 3.95 True/False:

Which of the following statements are true or false in reference to suicidal/homicidal patients?

A. Ask patient directly about suicidal/homicidal thoughts
______True
______False

B. Ask the family whether the patient has suicidal/homicidal thoughts
______True
______False

C. Depressed patients are not high risk
______True
______False

D. Establish a safety contract with the patient
______True
______False

E. Assume that the patient is just seeking attention
______True
______False

F. Patient is thinking rationally
______True
______False

G. Remove access to weapons
______True
______False

H. Patient's right to bear arms is primary

______True

______False

I. Duty to inform potential victim of declared threat

______True

______False

The answer can be found on page 240

The evening nurse, Karen, finds Matthew pacing and begging to be discharged. Matthew says, "Why didn't I die instead of my buddies?" He is afraid to go to sleep because of the nightmares he has of being back in the war. Karen notifies the physician that Matthew still refuses to contract for safety. Karen decides to give Matthew as-needed medication for anxiety.

EXERCISE 3.96 Select all that apply:

When the nurse goes to the medication-dispensing machine (Pyxis) for antianxiety medication, the drawer is empty. The nurse goes to another unit and takes lorazepam (Ativan) from the unit's supply. This system workaround works for the short term, but may cause a problem in the long term. Why?

A. Manager not informed
B. Supply not replaced
C. Staff continues "time-saving" short cut
D. Identification of patient may be bypassed
E. Medication amount may be incorrect
F. Hospital does not want to know as long as patient is satisfied

The answer can be found on page 241

Matthew attends therapies and takes medication for depression and anxiety and is treated for alcohol use. He attends Dual-Diagnosis Unit groups, Alcoholics Anonymous (AA) meetings, and a PTSD support group.

EXERCISE 3.97 Select all that apply:

What issues about alcohol use would indicate that the nurse and Matthew are in the working phase of the nurse–patient relationship?

A. Patient denies he has a problem with alcohol.
B. Patient identifies problems in marriage related to alcohol use.
C. Patient discusses how alcohol impairs his work.
D. Patient claims arguments with boss are definitely harassment by the boss.
E. Patient feels remorse for being impatient with his children.
F. Patient says goodbye and states he will continue Alcoholics Anonymous (AA) meetings after discharge.

The answer can be found on page 241

Matthew speaks with the health care team about discharge plans and services the VA has to offer veterans with PTSD and other disorders that often accompany it, such as anxiety, depression substance use, aggressive behavior, and homicidal and/or suicidal behavior. Matthew decides he is willing to go to outpatient VA counseling and support groups. He contracts for safety and agrees to submit his gun to his reserve unit. Because his wife has been affected, she agrees to go to Al Anon and a VA support group for military spouses. The children will attend VA and AA support groups for children.

EXERCISE 3.98 Multiple-choice:

One of the groups his wife will attend is Al Anon. Which statement by the wife demonstrates recovery and improvement in their relationship?

A. "When my husband comes home I will hide the bottles of alcohol."

B. "If he doesn't go into work, I will call and say he is sick."

C. "I will continue to be both mother and father to the children."

D. "I will take care of myself and let him manage his own responsibilities."

The answer can be found on page 241

EXERCISE 3.99 Multiple-choice:

What is the best response by the nurse when Matthew tells the same story over and over again of how his buddies died?

A. Listen and be nonjudgmental

B. Give suggestions for what he could do

C. Set limits and terminate discussion

D. Clarify and probe further

The answer can be found on page 242

EXERCISE 3.100 Multiple-choice:

Which statement by Matthew best demonstrates that he is coping better with his survivor guilt?

A. "I wish I had died instead of my buddies."

B. "I don't know why they died, they were better than me."

C. "If I had fought harder my buddies would be here."

D. "I am still here; I can help others with their memories."

The answer can be found on page 242

Matthew continues outpatient treatment at the VA. He finds their services are especially helpful because they understand his needs. He finds that his wife and children are better able to cope with him and the times he still occasionally retreats to his "man cave" to regroup. He also received a therapy dog for veterans and joined a martial arts class to channel his aggression appropriately. He goes to the VA support groups for PTSD and AA and wants to help newer veterans learn what he learned about coping.

UNFOLDING CASE STUDY 7: Sarah

Sarah is a 40-year-old woman admitted to the ED of her local community hospital. The nurse documents the following assessment:
Progress Notes
11/15/14
0100
African American female admitted with multiple facial lacerations and other blunt head trauma. Patient is confused; disoriented to person, place, and time; and is lethargic.
Assessment
Vital signs: Temperature: 98.6°F, pulse: 68 beats per minute (bpm), respiratory rate (RR): 14 breaths per minute, blood pressure (BP): 100/70 mmHg, blood alcohol level (BAL): 0.28. MRI of head is negative.
Complete physical examination is completed by the ED physician, Dr. James.

EXERCISE 3.101 Multiple-choice:

Which of the following conditions is the patient most likely experiencing?

A. Amphetamine intoxication
B. Alcohol withdrawal
C. Alcohol intoxication
D. Alcoholic dementia

The answer can be found on page 242

Sarah informs the nurse that she was drinking at a bar where a man asked her to go with him. He followed her to her car and he physically and sexually assaulted her. Sarah says her head hurts. Because of the assault, Sarah is seen by a sexual assault nurse examiner (SANE), Kathy, and by the ED crisis team.

EXERCISE 3.102 Select all that apply:

After Sarah is medically cleared, what disorder(s) is the crisis team focused on preventing?

A. Dissociative fugue
B. Borderline personality disorder
C. Acute stress disorder

D. Depression
E. Delusional disorder
F. Somatization disorder

The answer can be found on page 242

EXERCISE 3.103 Select all that apply:

Which of the following is true about rape?

A. It is never the victim's fault.
B. The victim probably provoked it.
C. Only women who lose control get raped.
D. "No" sometimes means "yes."
E. If a person is drunk, he or she cannot consent.
F. It is an act of aggression and control.

The answer can be found on page 243

---

eRESOURCE

To supplement your understanding of care for victims of sexual assault, refer to Medscape on your mobile device. [Pathway: Medscape ➔ enter "Sexual Assault" into the search field ➔ select "Sexual Assault" and review content.]

Sarah's history includes her acknowledgment that she has been drinking heavily since her divorce at the age of 28. She states that she attended an alcohol rehabilitation program but relapsed. She also states that she smokes one pack of cigarettes per day.

EXERCISE 3.104 Multiple-choice:

Considering Sarah's chronic use of alcohol, what is the most important information that the nurse should obtain and report?

A. Type of alcoholic drink
B. Time of last drink
C. Source of alcohol
D. Drinking at home alone or in a bar

The answer can be found on page 243

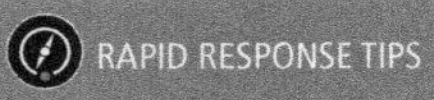

Alcohol withdrawal

At 6 to 8 hours after the last drink, the patient is at risk of signs of alcohol withdrawal. The nurse must know the signs and report them immediately to the primary care provider (PCP) for withdrawal management. If not, the patient is in danger of seizures and progression to delirium tremens (DTs) within 48–72 hours.

EXERCISE 3.105 Multiple-choice:

Which of the following would be signs of alcohol withdrawal?

A. Slurred speech, ataxia, hypothermia
B. Decreased reflexes, hypotension, drowsiness
C. Bradycardia, sedation, decreased respiration
D. Mild tremors, tachycardia, hypertension

The answer can be found on page 243

eRESOURCE

To supplement your understanding of clinical presentation and care considerations for persons withdrawing from alcohol, refer to Medscape on your mobile device. [Pathway: Medscape → enter "Delirium Tremens" into the search field → select "Delirium Tremens" and review content, focusing on "Clinical Presentation" and "Treatment & Management."]

EXERCISE 3.106 Select all that apply:

The nurse has the responsibility to foster and document the following interventions for Sarah in order to adhere to The Joint Commission (TJC) and Centers for Medicare & Medicaid Core Measures for quality and safety, which is required for accreditation and reimbursement of hospitals.

A. Median time from emergency department (ED) arrival to ED departure
B. Admit decision time to ED transfer
C. Encourage and offer a smoking-cessation program; document acceptance or refusal
D. Screen and document alcohol intoxication; document treatment acceptance or refusal
E. Refuse admission to those who refuse screening and treatment for alcohol, drugs, and tobacco use
F. Report alcohol and drug use to police

The answer can be found on page 243

EXERCISE 3.107 Select all that apply:

In the following list, which are the measures on which patients and families rate hospitals for quality?

A. Communication with doctors
B. Communication on social media
C. Communication with nurses
D. Responsiveness of hospital staff
E. Pain management
F. Medication communication
G. Pet therapy
H. Discharge information
I. Clean and quiet environment
J. Hotel accommodations

The answer can be found on page 244

Sarah is now exclaiming: "I need a drink!" She is also complaining of hand tremors.
Progress Notes
11/15/14
0700
Her nursing assessment is: Vital signs: Temperature: 98.6°F, pulse: 98 bpm, RR: 28 breaths per minute, BP: 140/90 mmHg. Patient anxious with hand tremors. Patient requesting "a drink." Patient states "I usually have a drink in the morning for my nerves." Patient exhibiting signs of alcohol withdrawal. Notified Dr. James of urgent need for withdrawal treatment.—K. Walsh, RN

EXERCISE 3.108 Matching:

Sarah is in the process of being transferred to the inpatient psychiatric unit. The nurse, Kathy, is giving a situation, background, assessment, recommendation (SBAR) report to the psychiatric inpatient nurse, Marie. Based on the aforementioned progress note, Kathy gives a report to Marie. Match the information in Column A with the parts of SBAR in column B:

Column A	Column B
A. Temperature: 98.6°F, pulse: 98 beats per minute (bpm), respiratory rate (RR): 28 breaths per minute, blood pressure (BP): 140/90 mmHg, anxious, hand tremors, 6 hours last drink	_____ Situation
B. Sarah, 40 years old, alcohol withdrawal	_____ Background
C. Needs medication for alcohol withdrawal	_____ Assessment
D. Patient states "I need a drink," "usually needed in morning to calm nerves," has been drinking heavily for 12 years	_____ Recommendation

The answer can be found on page 244

EXERCISE 3.109 Select all that apply:

The nurse anticipates that the primary care provider (PCP) may order which of the following medications for withdrawal?

A. Sertraline (Zoloft)
B. Clonidine (Catapres)
C. Lithium carbonate (Lithobid)
D. Oxazepam (Serax)
E. Propanolol (Inderal)
F. Lorazepam (Ativan)

The answer can be found on page 244

eRESOURCE

To supplement your understanding of clinical presentation and care considerations for persons withdrawing from alcohol, refer to Medscape on your mobile device. [Pathway: Medscape ➔ enter "Delirium Tremens" into the search field ➔ select "Delirium Tremens" and review content, focusing on "Medication."]

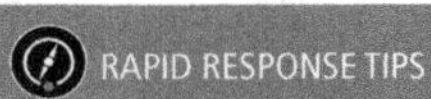

Patient safety

Patient safety is a major goal of TJC and a nursing standard. Measures include reporting deteriorating patient status as well as using SBAR to improve communication.

On the psychiatric inpatient unit, Sarah tells Marie she has been feeling depressed since her divorce and that her husband wants to take the children (ages 12, 9, and 6 years). Her ex-husband claims that Sarah is an unfit mother. Sarah tearfully tells Marie that the children are currently home alone and that she fears losing them since she has no family to help her. She also says she is afraid the man who assaulted her will do so again. Sarah admits to thoughts of suicide and that "everyone would be better off without me." Marie gives the lorazepam (Ativan) for withdrawal that the physician ordered.

EXERCISE 3.110 Ordering:

What is the nurse's priority at this time in terms of Sarah's interdisciplinary care plan? Place the following nursing diagnoses in priority order from 1 to 6:

_____ Ineffective individual coping
_____ Ineffective parenting
_____ Potential for violence (against self)
_____ Ineffective grieving
_____ Alteration in nutrition (less than requirements)
_____ Risk for injury (seizure from withdrawal)

The answer can be found on page 245

EXERCISE 3.111 Select all that apply:

The nurse implements nursing interventions for a suicidal patient. What does this include?

A. Establish a patient contract for safety
B. Place the patient in seclusion and restraints
C. Place the patient on one-to-one observation
D. Allow the patient to go off unit
E. Give the patient knitting needles in group
F. Notify physician of suicide ideation

The answer can be found on page 245

---

eRESOURCE

To reinforce your understanding of the care of the suicidal patient, refer to the *Merck Manual.* [Pathway: www.merckmanuals.com/professional → enter "Suicide" into the search field → select "Suicidal Behavior" → review "Management" and "Prevention."]

EXERCISE 3.112 Select all that apply:

Sarah has been dually diagnosed with major depression and substance use (alcohol). The medication group of first choice for depression is the selective serotonin reuptake inhibitors (SSRIs). Why?

A. They have no adverse effects
B. They have side effects such as headache, nausea, drowsiness, insomnia, and sexual dysfunction
C. They are less expensive
D. They may take up to 5 weeks for full effect
E. Suicide risk increases in the first couple of weeks
F. They may be taken with alcohol

The answer can be found on page 245

EXERCISE 3.113 Select all that apply:

Sarah is being discharged to a drug and alcohol rehabilitation program. What are the nurse's responsibilities?

A. Provide teaching about discharge plan
B. Report patient dissatisfaction with discharge plan
C. Give a situation, background, assessment, recommendation (SBAR) report to rehabilitation program
D. Consult with social services for safety of children
E. Tell the patient she may resume alcohol in future if she handles it better
F. Encourage continued participation in Alcoholics Anonymous (AA) and sexual trauma support group

The answer can be found on page 245

Sarah tells Marie that she thinks she can control her drinking if she does not have so much stress. She believes that her ex-husband and children drove her to drink and her drinking was not that bad. It was her only way to deal with her problems and that going to that bar made her drink too much.

EXERCISE 3.114 Select all that apply:

What defense mechanism(s) is Sarah using?

A. Rationalization
B. Projection
C. Minimization
D. Repression
E. Denial
F. Reaction formation

The answer can be found on page 246

After her rehabilitation program, Sarah continues her outpatient therapy and attends AA meetings and the sexual trauma survivors' group. Through social service support she receives job training and finds employment. She is able to obtain joint custody of her children because of her sobriety and is now supporting her family. She is much more hopeful about her future.

Answers

EXERCISE 3.1 Matching:

What strategies either facilitate or impede trust in a therapeutic communication process in the nurse–patient relationship?

Match the elements of a therapeutic relationship in Column A with the nursing interventions in Column B:

Column A	Column B
A. Respect	A Giving recognition to the person's worth
B. Empathy	D Being honest about feelings
C. Positive self-regard	C Honoring the person's dignity
D. Genuineness	B Trying to understand the person's view
E. Confidentiality	G Fulfilling promises and being reliable
F. Self-awareness	F Knowing one's own attitudes and feelings
G. Trust	E Keeping information private
H. Acceptance	H Meeting the person where he or she is

EXERCISE 3.2 Matching:

Match the therapeutic or nontherapeutic communication techniques in Column A with the nurse statements in Column B:

Column A	Column B
A. Sympathy	__C__ "Don't worry; you will get your boyfriend back."
B. Asking why	__A__ "I felt differently when I was in the hospital."
C. False reassurance	__B__ "Why are you nervous?"
D. Giving advice	__D__ "You should quit your job."
E. Seeking clarification	__F__ "What happened before you got upset?"
F. Exploring	__E__ "Are you telling me you felt angry when you didn't get your raise?"
G. Broad opening	__G__ "How are you doing?"
H. Countertransference	__H__ "Stop interrupting me! You're just like my sister!"

EXERCISE 3.3 Fill in the blanks:

Fill in the blanks using the following list:

Sympathy
Asking why
False reassurance
Giving advice
Seeking clarification
Exploring
Broad opening
Countertransference

Therapeutic communication includes: **seeking clarification, exploring, and broad opening**

Nontherapeutic communication includes: **sympathy, asking why, false reassurance, giving advice, and countertransference**

EXERCISE 3.4 Select all that apply:

Setting boundaries for patients is done in order to accomplish which of the following:

A. Setting rules of behavior that guide interaction with others—**YES**.

B. Allowing a patient and nurse to connect safely in a therapeutic relationship based on the patient's needs—**YES**.

C. Making sure the patient does not influence other patients—NO; patients need to build rapport with each other when they are in group sessions.

D. Helping us control the impact others have on us as well as our impact on others—**YES**.

E. Helping families of patients better understand the diagnosis—NO; this is not done for family education.

EXERCISE 3.5 Select all that apply:

Angelique expresses a loss of interest and pleasure in activities and believes her life is going nowhere and looks bleak. She also says that she does not feel like getting out of bed in the morning and has no interest in sleeping or eating. What symptoms will the nurse report?

A. Echolalia, apathy, delusions—NO; this is the repetition of words that have been said by others, lack of interest or enthusiasm, and beliefs that are clearly false.

B. Obsessions, compulsions, hypersomnia—NO; this is compulsive preoccupation with something, irresistible urge to behave in a certain way, and excessive sleepiness.

C. Perseveration, somatization, dissociation—NO; this is repetition of a particular response; the production of multiple, recurrent symptoms with no physical cause; and disconnecting from physical and emotional experiences.

D. Anergia, anhedonia, insomnia—**YES; this is the lack of energy, the inability to gain pleasure from enjoyable experiences, and the inability to sleep**.

E. Hopelessness, helplessness, negativism—NO; this is a feeling of futility and despair; feeling exposed and vulnerable; and an attitude of being skeptical, critical, or pessimistic.

EXERCISE 3.6 Exhibit-format:

Angelique sees an advanced practice registered nurse (APRN), who records the following findings:

Patient states that she is tired all the time and sleeps a lot.

Patient has lost 5 lb in 2 months and lacks concentration. She has difficulty finishing a thought process. The APRN understands that these manifestations may indicate a diagnosis of:

A. Obsessive-compulsive behavior—NO; this is not the usual manifestation of "doing things" that are repetitive.

B. Depression—**YES; these are manifestations of depression.**

C. Personality disorder—NO; there are no attention-getting mechanisms noted.

D. Addiction—NO; there is no indication of chemical impairment.

EXERCISE 3.7 Matching:

Identify risk factors and protective factors for depression. Use the letter in Column A to indicate whether the attribute is a risk or protective factor in Column B:

Column A	Column B
A. Being female	**A, B** Risk factor
B. Having a depressed parent	_____ Protective factor

EXERCISE 3.8 Select all that apply:

What are accepted "truths" about suicide?

A. Asking about it gives the patient the idea—NO; asking about suicide does not "plant the seed" in the person's mind.

B. Only some depressed patients are at risk—NO; depression is a risk factor for suicide.

C. Asking gives the patient permission to talk about it—**YES; those who are suicidal are often relieved that someone has allowed them to unburden themselves.**

D. History of attempts increases risk—**YES; each attempt a person makes increases his or her likelihood of committing suicide.**

E. A plan increases risk—**YES; the majority of suicides are attempted after planning the act.**

F. It is a rational decision—**YES; people do not usually want to die, but they may not see another option.**

EXERCISE 3.9 True/False:

Facts about suicide:

A. Suicide is one of the top 10 causes of death among all age groups.

__X__ True

B. Suicide is the third leading cause of death among 15- to 24-year-olds.

__X__ True

C. White people are twice as likely to die by suicide as non-White people.

__X__ True

D. White men commit more than 70% of all U.S. suicides.

__X__ True

E. The number of elderly suicides is decreasing.

__X__ False

F. The ethnic groups with the highest suicide rates are Asians and Blacks.

__X__ False

G. Decreased serotonin levels play a role in suicidal behavior.

__X__ True

H. The person who is suicidal often has the desire to be free of pain and to be saved.

__X__ True

EXERCISE 3.10 Fill in the blanks:

Word list:

Directly
Suicide plan
Family history
Secrecy
Confidentiality
Lethality
Coping

Suicide assessment:

Ask **directly** about suicidal thoughts/behavior.

Identify whether the person has a **suicide plan**.

Explore whether the person has a **family history** of suicide.

Do not swear to **secrecy**.

Discuss the limits of **confidentiality**.

Suicidal intent and **lethality**.

Assess the person's **coping** potential.

EXERCISE 3.11 Matching:

Match the definitions in Column A with the terms in Column B:

Column A	Column B
A. The beginning of the suicide continuum is the process of contemplating suicide or the methods used without acting on these thoughts. At this point, the patient might not talk about these thoughts unless he or she is pressed.	**A** Ideation
B. The act of intentionally killing oneself may follow prior attempts, but about 30% of those who commit suicide are believed to have done so on their first attempt. Suicide results when the person can see no other option for relief from unbearable emotional or physical pain.	**D** Suicide gesture
C. Taking a potentially lethal dose of medication indicates that the person wants to die and has no wish to be rescued.	**C** Suicide attempt
D. Actions may be taken that are not likely to be lethal, such as taking a few pills or making superficial cuts on the wrist. These suggest that the patient is ambivalent about dying or has not planned to die. He or she has the will to survive, wants to be rescued, and is experiencing a mental conflict. This act is often called a "cry for help" because the patient is struggling with unmanageable stress.	**B** Suicide

EXERCISE 3.12 Fill in the blank:

Angelique has the right to **informed consent** before health care interventions are undertaken.

EXERCISE 3.13 Select all that apply:

Informed consent includes which of the following:

A. Adequate and accurate knowledge and information—**YES**.
B. An individual with legal capacity to consent—**YES**.
C. The understanding that it is changeable—NO; informed consent is a signed legal document.
D. Consent is given voluntarily—**YES**.
E. Family input—NO; the patient is the one who must consent.

EXERCISE 3.14 True/False:

Voluntary patients are considered competent unless otherwise adjudicated and therefore have the absolute right to refuse treatment, including psychotropic medications, unless they are dangerous to themselves or others.

__X__ True

EXERCISE 3.15 Select all that apply:

Voluntary patients have the right to:

A. Refuse treatments—**YES; voluntary patients are considered competent unless otherwise adjudicated and, therefore, have the right to refuse treatment.**
B. Sign a 72-hour notice to leave—**YES; voluntary patients are considered competent unless otherwise adjudicated and, therefore, have the right to sign a 72-hour notice to leave.**
C. Receive visitors—**YES; voluntary patients are considered competent unless otherwise adjudicated and, therefore, have the right to receive visitors.**
D. Use cell phone on unit—**YES; voluntary patients are considered competent unless otherwise adjudicated and, therefore, have the right to use cell phone on the unit.**
E. Refuse antianxiety medication if violent—NO; voluntary patients do not have the right to refuse treatment if they are dangerous to themselves or others.
F. Smoke cigarettes on a smoke-free unit—NO; smoking is not allowed for anyone on a smoke-free unit.

EXERCISE 3.16 Select all that apply:

Involuntary patients have the right to:

A. Receive visitors—**YES; involuntary patients retain the right to have visitors.**
B. Sign a 72-hour notice to leave—NO; involuntary patients may not discharge themselves.
C. Vote—**YES; involuntary patients retain the right to vote.**
D. Refuse antianxiety medication if calm—**YES; involuntary patients have the right to refuse treatment, including medications, unless they are incapable of giving consent.**
E. Make phone calls—**YES; involuntary patients retain the right to communicate, including making phone calls.**
F. Smoke cigarettes if unit has accommodations for it—NO; all health care facilities are smoke free.

EXERCISE 3.17 Select all that apply:

Angelique will start on a selective serotonin reuptake inhibitor (SSRI). Which would the nurse anticipate giving from this group?

A. Lithium carbonate (Lithobid)—NO; it is an anticonvulsant.
B. Fluoxetine (Prozac)—NO; it is an antipsychotic drug.
C. Risperidone (Risperdal)—NO; it is an antipsychotic drug.
D. Paroxetine (Paxil)—**YES; it is an antidepressant (SSRI).**
E. Sertraline (Zoloft)—**YES; it is an antidepressant (SSRI).**

EXERCISE 3.18 Multiple-choice:

Antidepressant drugs, such as fluoxetine and sertraline, selectively act on:

A. Acetylcholine receptors—NO; this deals with motor dysfunction.
B. Norepinephrine receptors—NO; Cymbalta and Effexor are selective serotonin/norepinephrine reuptake inhibitors.
C. Serotonin receptors—**YES; they are both serotonin reuptake inhibitors (SSRIs).**
D. Melatonin receptors—NO; melatonin is a hormone.

EXERCISE 3.19 Multiple-choice:

Angelique is prescribed medication for a psychiatric disorder. After 3 days, the patient tells the nurse that she has been constipated. The nurse should instruct the patient to:

A. Eat more high-protein foods—NO; this tends to be constipating.
B. Increase fiber and fluid intake—**YES; this will help the patient to have a bowel movement.**
C. Take a stool softener—NO; try natural foods first before taking additional medication.
D. Have patience as this will subside—NO; it has already been 3 days . . . do not "wait and see."

EXERCISE 3.20 Multiple-choice:

Before administering a medication for the first time, an important assessment to make on a patient with a psychiatric disorder, like Angelique, is to determine his or her:

A. Cultural background—NO; this usually does not produce physiological problems.
B. Height and weight—NO; medications are ordered based on weight so this should have already been done.
C. Preexisting symptoms—**YES; a baseline is needed to evaluate outcomes.**
D. Physical stamina—NO; this is usually not the only assessment needed.

EXERCISE 3.21 Multiple-choice:

A major side effect of bupropion (Wellbutrin) is:

A. Seizures—**YES; it is known to cause seizures, especially in certain groups of people.**
B. Urinary frequency—NO; this is a minimal problem that affects 2% of users.
C. Palpitations—NO; heart palpitations are not a side effect of buproprion.
D. Hallucinations—NO; this only occurs with an overdose of buproprion.

EXERCISE 3.22 Multiple-choice:

Angelique has been prescribed the drug paroxetine (Paxil) for depression. The nurse should explain to her that selective serotonin reuptake inhibitors (SSRIs) may have a side effect of:

A. Hypertension—NO; they are associated with postural hypotension.

B. Gastrointestinal distress—**YES; they can cause nausea, disturbances in appetite, and diarrhea.**

C. Rigidity—NO; tremors are a side effect, not rigidity.

D. Increased sexual desire—NO; they decrease libido.

EXERCISE 3.23 Select all that apply:

Angelique has been prescribed the drug sertraline (Zoloft), a selective serotonin reuptake inhibitor (SSRI), for depression. The nurse should teach her to report possible side effects of:

A. Sleep disturbance—**YES; insomnia is a side effect.**

B. Increased sexual desire—NO; sexual dysfunction is a side effect.

C. Dry mouth—**YES; dry mouth is a side effect.**

D. Agranulocytosis—NO; this is not a side effect.

E. Agitation—**YES; agitation is a side effect.**

F. Hypertension—NO; chest pain and palpitations are side effects.

EXERCISE 3.24 Select all that apply:

According to best practices for patient teaching, the nurse must also do which of the following:

A. Give Angelique a pamphlet to read later—NO; this may not be read.

B. Have Angelique read the pamphlet to the nurse—NO; this is not therapeutic.

C. Have Angelique do a teach-back of the possible side effects—**YES.**

D. Have Angelique tell the nurse what she will do (inform provider) if she has side effects—**YES.**

E. Document in the chart what was taught and the patient's response—**YES.**

F. Send the patient to pharmacy to get a medication printout—NO; the nurse should review with the patient.

EXERCISE 3.25 Select all that apply:

The nurse recognizes that more teaching is needed if Angelique says which of the following?

A. "I can stop the medication if I feel better."—**YES.**

B. "The depression will be gone after 1 week."—**YES.**

C. "If I have a side effect, I just stop the medication."—**YES.**

D. "I must report suicidal thoughts with or without a plan to my provider."—NO.

E. "I can take over-the-counter St. John's wort with my prescribed antidepressant."—**YES.**

F. "I can drink alcohol."—**YES.**

EXERCISE 3.26 Multiple-choice:

In a hospitalized patient who has been prescribed desvenlafaxine (Pristiq), the nurse should monitor for:

A. Nausea—NO; this is a side effect but not the most important side effect listed.
B. Hypertension—**YES; this listed side effect is the most important to monitor, think about the ABCs (airway, breathing, circulation) of patient care.**
C. Somnolence—NO; this is a side effect but not the most important one listed.
D. Constipation—NO; this is a side effect but not the most important one listed.

EXERCISE 3.27 Matching:

To examine differences in antidepressant therapy, match the effects in Column A to the medications in Column B:

Column A	Column B
A. SSRI (selective serotonin reuptake inhibitor)	__A__ Elavil, Anafranil, Norpramin
B. MAOI (monoamine oxidase inhibitor)	__B__ Zoloft, Paxil, Prozac
C. SNRI (serotonin/norepinephrine reuptake inhibitor)	__D__ Cymbalta, Effexor, Pristiq
D. Tricyclic antidepressant	__C__ Marplan, Parnate, Nardil

EXERCISE 3.28 Matching:

Match medications in Column A to the common side effects in Column B:

Column A	Column B
A. Tofranil, Elavil, Pamelor	__D__ Avoid taking decongestants and consuming foods that contain high levels of tyramine
B. Luvox, Lexapro, Zoloft	__C__ Liver dysfunction occurs: yellowing of the skin or whites of the eyes, unusually dark urine, loss of appetite that lasts for several days, nausea, or abdominal pain
C. Wellbutrin, Serzone	__A__ Dry mouth, constipation, bladder problems, sexual dysfunction, blurred vision
D. Nardil, Parnate, Marplan	__B__ Sexual dysfunction, nausea, nervousness, insomnia, and agitation

EXERCISE 3.29 Select all that apply:

Luke has been placed on phenelzine (Nardil). The teaching was successful if Luke says he will avoid foods such as:

A. Red wine—**YES; avoid because it contains tyramine.**
B. Bananas and raisins—**YES; avoid because they contain tyramine.**

C. Aged cheese—**YES; avoid because it contains tyramine.**

D. Liver—**YES; avoid because it contains tyramine.**

E. Apples—NO; unless overripe; overripe fruit contains tyramine.

F. Pepperoni—**YES; avoid because it contains tyramine.**

EXERCISE 3.30 True/False:

Plant and herbal remedies are natural, so they are good to take with all medications.

__X__ **False; the herb St. John's wort (*Hypericum perforatum*) is primarily used to treat mild to moderate depression. It is possible that it might raise serotonin levels too high, causing a dangerous condition called *serotonin syndrome*.**

EXERCISE 3.31 Fill in the blanks:

The nurse caring for Luke knows that serotonin is a __**neurotransmitter**__ that regulates many functions, including mood, appetite, and sensory perception. With too much serotonin in the brain, a condition called *serotonin syndrome (SS)* can occur. Name four symptoms of SS:

Symptoms include restlessness, hallucinations, loss of coordination, fast heartbeat, rapid changes in blood pressure, increased body temperature, overactive reflexes, nausea, vomiting, and diarrhea.

EXERCISE 3.32 Multiple-choice:

Luke must also be told to check the fine print of over-the-counter (OTC) cold medication (and others) and check with his provider. Taking an monoamine oxidase inhibitor (MAOI) with such medications (if prohibited) can cause:

A. Anaphylactic shock—NO; this is not a side effect of MAOIs.

B. Neuroleptic malignant syndrome—NO; this is not a side effect of MAOIs.

C. Hypertensive crisis—**YES; this is a side effect of an MAOI drug–drug interaction.**

D. Seizures—NO; this is not a side effect of MAOIs.

EXERCISE 3.33 Ordering:

Place the nursing interventions in priority order from 1 to 5:

__5__ Provide assistance with activities of daily living (ADL); **fatigue is a common side effect, so the patient may need extra assistance.**

__4__ Encourage a high-fiber nutritious diet; **constipation is a common side effect, so a high-fiber diet can assist the patient in avoiding constipation.**

__1__ Monitor for suicidal ideation and contract for **safety; safety is a number-one priority.**

__2__ Teach about medications; **the patient needs to know what side effects to report.**

__3__ Promote sleep hygiene; **promoting sleep is very important because sleep disturbances are a common side effect.**

EXERCISE 3.34 Select all that apply:

What is the best response by the nurse to the son?

A. "Depression is an illness that can be treated."—**YES.**

B. "Depression is his choice."—NO; depression is a condition not a patient's choice.

C. "It is just the usual grieving response."—NO; it is more than "normal grieving."

D. "Depression may be a chronic illness with remissions and exacerbations."—**YES.**

E. "Depression may have a genetic and an environmental component."—**YES.**

EXERCISE 3.35 Select all that apply:

The nurse should provide for Luke's safety by:

A. Placing the roommate into four-point restraints—NO.

B. Reviewing the unit procedure on violence precautions—**YES.**

C. Identifying the evidence-based practice for preventing violence—**YES.**

D. Notifying the health team (doctor and supervisor)—**YES.**

E. Placing the roommate in a private room—NO.

F. Assessing the roommate for violence threat and placing on one-to-one observation—**YES.**

EXERCISE 3.36 Select all that apply:

The nursing interventions to meet these underlying needs might include:

A. Providing Luke an activity to create something—**YES.**

B. Giving Luke medications—NO.

C. Providing television in lounges—**YES.**

D. Developing a grief support group—**YES.**

E. Acknowledging Luke's achievements by displaying his works on unit—**YES.**

F. Encouraging family participation in Luke's activities and recovery (family teaching)—**YES.**

EXERCISE 3.37 Select all that apply:

Which statements by Luke would indicate movement to positive achievement of the discharge plan?

A. "I plan to attend therapy."—**YES.**

B. "I don't like going home to an empty house."—NO.

C. "I am going to visit my son and grandchildren."—**YES.**

D. "I am joining a volunteer group."—**YES.**

E. "I will stop my medication if too expensive."—**YES.**

F. "I am going to exercise at the gym."—**YES.**

EXERCISE 3.38 Matching:

Match the nursing interventions in Column A with the side effects of the antipsychotic medications in Column B:

Column A	Column B
A. Monitor white blood cells (WBC)	D Dry mouth
B. Get out of chair slowly	C Constipation
C. Increase fluids and fiber	F Photophobia
D. Use sugarless candy and sips of water	E Weight gain
E. Maintain low-calorie diet	A Agranulocytosis
F. Wear sunglasses	B Orthostatic hypotension
G. Get up and dress early	G Sedation

EXERCISE 3.39 Exhibit-format:

The nurse reviews the patient data:

Vital signs (VS): Temperature: 98.2°F, respiratory rate (RR): 24 breaths per minute, heart rate (HR): 90 beats per minute (bpm): blood pressure (BP): 132/86 mmHg

Physical examination: Head symmetrical, dull affective responses, pupils equal and reactive to light and accommodation (PERLA), difficulty in fully extending arms and ataxic gait

The nurse suspects that these assessment findings are consistent with:

A. Parkinson's disease—NO; this is usually a gradual onset.
B. Extrapyramidal side effects (EPSE)—**YES.**
C. Transient ischemic attack (TIA)—NO; this is usually sudden and associated with high blood pressure.
D. Signs of overdose—NO; this usually manifests with decreased respirations.

EXERCISE 3.40 Select all that apply:

Which of the following is true about the atypical antipsychotics?

A. Cause fewer or no extrapyramidal side effects (EPSE)—**YES.**
B. Used to treat both positive and negative symptoms of schizophrenia—**YES.**
C. Exert both dopamine and serotonin receptor blocking action—**YES.**
D. Cause more EPSE—NO; they cause less.
E. Treat only positive symptoms of schizophrenia—NO; negative symptoms must also be treated.

EXERCISE 3.41 Select all that apply:

In teaching about the antipsychotics, the nurse would tell her to do the following:

A. Stop taking meds when you feel better—NO; do not stop taking prescribed medications.
B. Report adverse effects promptly—**YES.**
C. Do not drink alcohol—**YES.**
D. Do not take over-the-counter (OTC) meds causing drowsiness—**YES.**
E. Do not drive or use hazardous equipment or do activities needing alertness—**YES.**
F. Give medication 1 week to relieve symptoms—NO; long-term medication is needed.

EXERCISE 3.42 Fill in the blanks:

What two neurotransmitters in the body are targeted with atypical and typical antipsychotics?

1. **Serotonin**
2. **Dopamine**

EXERCISE 3.43 Matching:

Indicate whether the medication in Column A is a typical or atypical antipsychotic in Column B:

Column A	Column B
A. Chlorpromazine (Thorazine) B. Fluphenazine (Prolixin) C. Risperidone (Risperdal) D. Trifluoperazine (Stelazine) E. Olanzapine (Zyprexa) F. Haloperidol (Haldol) G. Aripiprazole (Abilify) H. Thioridazine (Loxapine) I. Clozapine (Clozaril) J. Thiothixene (Navane) K. Ziprasidone (Geodon)	**A, B, D, F, H, J** Typical antipsychotic **C, E, G, I, K** Atypical antipsychotic

EXERCISE 3.44 Matching:

Please match the effects in Column A with the medications in Column B:

Column A	Column B
A. Fixed false beliefs strongly held in spite of invalidating evidence B. Flat affect and apathy C. Reduction in the range and intensity of emotional expression D. Reduced ability, difficulty, or inability to initiate and persist in goal-directed behavior E. Marked decrease in reaction to the immediate surrounding environment F. Hallucinations and delusions G. Poverty of speech H. Distortions or exaggerations of perception in any of the senses I. Loss of feeling or an inability to experience pleasure	**A** Chlorpromazine (Thorazine) **H** Fluphenazine (Prolixin) **G** Risperidone (Risperidal) **C** Trifluoperazine (Stelazine) **D** Olanzapine (Zyprexa) **E** Haloperidol (Haldol) **F** Aripiprazole (Abilify) **B** Thoridazine (Loxapine) **I** Clozapine (Clozaril)

EXERCISE 3.45 Multiple-choice:

Angelique complains of itching and dermatitis after taking a medication for a psychiatric disorder; after 3 days, the nurse should:

A. Reassure the patient—NO; because it could be a serious reaction.

B. Offer the patient soothing lotions—NO; further assess the symptoms.

C. Contact the physician—**YES; antipsychotic and anticonvulsant agents have been associated with various dermatologic manifestations—including exanthems, pruritis, photosensitivity, angioedema, exfoliative dermatitis, cellulitis, Stevens–Johnson syndrome, and toxic epidermal necrolysis.**

D. Offer the patient a warm tub bath—NO; this is not the best option, although it may be temporarily soothing.

EXERCISE 3.46 Multiple-choice:

When Marina requires larger doses of a given medication to maintain its therapeutic effect, the nurse determines that she has developed:

A. Abuse—NO; this is use of illicit drugs or the abuse of prescription or over-the-counter drugs for purposes other than those for which they are indicated or in a manner or in quantities other than directed.

B. Tolerance—**YES; tolerance occurs when a person's reaction to a drug decreases so that larger doses are required to achieve the same effect. Drug tolerance can involve both *psychological drug tolerance and physiological factors*.**

C. Addiction—NO; this is a primary, chronic, neurobiological disease, with genetic, psychosocial, and environmental factors influencing its development and manifestations. It is characterized by behaviors that include one or more of the following: impaired control over drug use, compulsive use, continued use despite harm, and craving.

D. Allergies—NO; this is sensitivity (hypersensitivity) to a drug or other chemicals.

EXERCISE 3.47 Multiple-choice:

Which of the following atypical antipsychotic agents is associated with the most weight gain?

A. Ziprasidone (Geodon)—NO; ziprasidone and aripiprazole are associated with the least weight gain.

B. Aripiprazole (Abilify)—NO; ziprasidone and aripiprazole are associated with the least weight gain.

C. Olanzapine (Zyprexa)—**YES; olanzapine has been associated with the most weight gain.**

D. Quetiapine (Seroquel)—NO; a minimal amount of weight is gained with quetiapine and risperidone.

E. Risperidone (Risperdal)—NO; a minimal amount of weight is gained with quetiapine and risperidone.

EXERCISE 3.48 Select all that apply:

Schizophrenia spectrum includes:

A. Borderline personality—NO; borderline personality is not included in the schizophrenia spectrum.

B. Schizotypal personality—**YES; schizotypal personality is included in the schizophrenia spectrum.**

C. Schizophreniform disorder—**YES; schizophreniform disorder is included in the schizophrenia spectrum.**
D. Schizoaffective disorder—**YES; schizoaffective disorder is included in the schizophrenia spectrum.**
E. Psychosis not otherwise specified—NO; psychosis associated with substance use or medical conditions is not included in the schizophrenia spectrum.

EXERCISE 3.49 Select all that apply:

Which of the following is true about schizophrenia?

A. Initial symptoms most often occur in early adulthood—**YES; initial symptoms typically occur in late teens to early 30s.**
B. The patients usually do not need medication—NO; antipsychotic drugs that act on dopamine receptors are a common treatment.
C. It requires long-term treatment—**YES; most patients affected suffer frequent relapse that may require hospitalization, intensive treatment, or crisis management.**
D. Families require support and education—**YES; supportive psychotherapy or cognitive behavioral therapy may be helpful for the patient and family.**
E. Cause is clearly known—NO; the cause is unknown.

EXERCISE 3.50 Select all that apply:

What should the nurse do to provide culturally competent care for Marina?

A. Get a family member to translate—NO; a hospital translator should be contacted.
B. Insist Marina eat what other patients eat—NO; this is not a culturally competent action.
C. Contact a hospital-approved translator—**YES; a hospital translator is appropriate instead of using a family member or a friend.**
D. Meet Marina's request for dietary consult—**YES; this is being culturally sensitive to her requests.**
E. Ask Marina whether she would like to have clergy visit—**YES; this is a culturally competent action.**

EXERCISE 3.51 Select all that apply:

What should the nurse do?

A. Reassure Marina she will not tell—NO; do not swear to secrecy.
B. Tell Marina she cannot keep it a secret—**YES; never swear to secrecy.**
C. Notify the health team—**YES; it is important to involve the health team.**
D. Place Marina on one-to-one observation—**YES; one-to-one observation is a safety measure to implement when there is a risk of suicide.**
E. Ask Marina's roommate to watch her—NO; it is not appropriate to ask her roommate to watch her; a staff member needs to be assigned to observation.
F. Put Marina in a seclusion room—NO; placing her in seclusion is not an appropriate action to take.

EXERCISE 3.52 Fill in the blanks:

Anticholinergic: benztropine (Cogentin), trihexyphenidyl (Artane), biperiden (Akineton), and procyclidine (Kemadrin); Antihistamine: Diphenhydramine (Benadryl); Dopamine Agonist: amantadine (Symmetrel) are examples of anticholinergic, antihistamine, and dopamine agonists to treat extrapyramidal side effects (EPSE).

EXERCISE 3.53 Select all that apply:

What teaching should the nurse include for both Marina and her family caregiver?

A. Return for white blood cell (WBC) testing as prescribed—NO; this is not necessary.
B. Notify provider of any infection or fever—NO; manifestations of infection are not expected.
C. Take over-the-counter (OTC) medications as she wishes—NO; many OTC medications can cause serious drug–drug interactions.
D. Call 911 if Marina has command hallucinations to hurt herself or others—**YES; safety is a number-one priority.**
E. Do teach-back to evaluate what they understood—**YES; this will ensure they understand what has been taught.**
F. Have an interpreter present—**YES; have a hospital translator present as there is a language barrier.**

EXERCISE 3.54 Select all that apply:

Please select the top-10 signs of schizophrenia.

A. Delusions (believing things that are not true)—**YES.**
B. Hallucinations (seeing or hearing things that are not there)—**YES.**
C. Depression—NO.
D. Disorganized thinking—**YES.**
E. Agitation—**YES.**
F. Mania—NO.
G. Violence—NO.
H. Using drugs and alcohol—NO.
I. Low intellect—NO.
J. Disorganized speech (e.g., frequent derailment or incoherence)—**YES.**
K. Grossly disorganized or catatonic behavior—**YES.**
L. Lack of drive or initiative—**YES.**
M. Social withdrawal—**YES.**
N. Apathy—**YES.**
O. Emotional unresponsiveness—**YES.**

One of the most important kinds of impairment caused by schizophrenia involves the person's thought processes. The individual can lose much of the ability to rationally evaluate his or her surroundings and interactions with others. There can be hallucinations and delusions, which reflect distortions in the perception and interpretation of reality. The resulting behaviors may seem bizarre to the casual observer, even though they may be consistent with the abnormal perceptions and a belief according to the person who is suffering from schizophrenia.

EXERCISE 3.55 Multiple-choice:

Most drug metabolism occurs in the

A. Liver—**YES; most drug metabolism occurs in the liver, although some processes occur in the gut wall, lungs, and blood plasma.**

B. Stomach—NO; drugs may be absorbed here but not metabolized.

C. Brain—NO; drugs affect the brain but they are not metabolized there.

D. Gallbladder—NO; the gallbladder does not metabolize drugs.

EXERCISE 3.56 Multiple-choice:

If Marina is prescribed a neuroleptic drug to treat a psychiatric disorder, the nurse should explain to her and her family that neuroleptic drugs are the same as:

A. Antipsychotic medications—**YES; these are used to treat psychosis.**

B. Central nervous system depressants—NO; these are tranquilizers and sedatives.

C. Anticholinesterase inhibitors—NO; these break down acetylcholine (a chemical messenger in the brain) and can be used in conditions in which there is an apparent lack of this messenger transmission, such as in Alzheimer's disease.

D. Tranquilizers—NO; these are commonly prescribed as antianxiety drugs or anxiolytics.

EXERCISE 3.57 Multiple-choice:

A patient diagnosed with schizophrenia is being treated with traditional antipsychotic medications. The nurse should explain to the patient and the patient's family that one negative symptom that may worsen during drug therapy is:

A. Insomnia—NO; neither a positive nor a negative symptom.

B. Social withdrawal—**YES; this is a negative symptom.**

C. Hallucinations—NO; this is considered a positive symptom in mental health nursing.

D. Delusions—NO; this is considered a positive symptom in mental health nursing.

EXERCISE 3.58 Multiple-choice:

Marina has been taking clozapine (Clozaril) for 6 weeks and visits the clinic complaining of fever, sore throat, and mouth sores. The nurse contacts the patient's physician as these symptoms are indicative of:

A. Severe anemia—NO; this is a decrease in red blood cells or when the blood does not have enough hemoglobin; symptoms include tiredness, weakness, and pale color.

B. Bacterial infection—NO; this involves elevated numbers of circulating white blood cells (WBCs) in the bloodstream. Symptoms include an elevated body temperature, sweating, chills, confusion, and rapid breathing.

C. Viral infection—NO; this is an infection caused by the presence of a virus in the body. Symptoms include fever, diarrhea, and vomiting.

D. Agranulocytosis—**YES; this is a serious condition in which WBCs decrease in number or disappear altogether; early signs of agranulocytosis include mouth sores, sore throat, weakness, and fever.**

EXERCISE 3.59 Matching:

Match the symptoms in Column A to the disorder in Column B:

Column A	Column B
A. Subjective or inner restlessness resulting in difficulty sitting still, leg movement, and pacing; it produces intense anxiety and fidgeting	D Acute dystonia
B. Tremors, mask-like face, bradykinesia, loss of facial expression, flattening of vocal inflection, stiffness, cogwheel rigidity, and reduced social functioning	A Akathisia
C. Neuroleptic-induced delirium	B Parkinsonism
D. Acute spasms of the muscles of the jaw, face, eyes, trunk, and chest	C Neuroleptic malignant syndrome

EXERCISE 3.60 Multiple-choice:

The nurse is caring for José, who has been taking haloperidol (Haldol) for 3 days. To assess José for neuroleptic malignant syndrome (NMS), the nurse should assess the patient's:

A. Blood pressure—NO; this is not a symptom.

B. Serum sodium level—NO; this is not a symptom.

C. Temperature—**YES; NMS is a potentially fatal reaction to dopamine blockade caused by antipsychotic and other medications. Four cardinal symptoms of NMS are hyperthermia, muscle rigidity, mental status changes, and autonomic instability.**

D. Weight—NO; this is not a symptom.

EXERCISE 3.61 Multiple-choice:

Two medications that the nurse may give that are key in treating neuroleptic malignant syndrome (NMS) include:

A. Aspirin and lorazepam—NO; these are not used.

B. Calcium and lithium—NO; these are not used.

C. Bromocriptine (Parlodel) and dantrolene (Dantrium)—**YES; bromocriptine, a dopamine agonist, reverses the hypodopaminergic state that precipitates NMS. Dantrolene, a skeletal muscle relaxer, helps ameliorate the symptoms of muscle rigidity and the resulting muscle breakdown and heat generation.**

D. Lamictal (Lamotrigine) and olanzopine (Zyprexa)—NO; these are not used.

EXERCISE 3.62 Select all that apply:

Because neuroleptic malignant syndrome (NMS) is a life-threatening illness that may lead to rhabdomyolysis and renal failure, the nurse anticipates the following interventions:

A. Place patient on isolation precautions—NO; the patient does not need to be put on isolation.

B. Hold Haldol (or other antipsychotic) and call provider—**YES; speak with the provider before administering medication that causes NMS.**

C. Call 911 and prepare for transfer—NO; call the provider, not 911.

D. Admission to the intensive care unit (ICU)—**YES; NMS is a potentially fatal syndrome for which ICU care is recommended.**

E. Use cooling blanket, antipyretic, fluids, and hemodialysis at the medical hospital—**YES; these are common interventions taken with NMS.**

EXERCISE 3.63 Select all that apply:

In evaluating the intervention that was taken for meeting the Quality and Safety Education for Nurses (QSEN) standards, the nurse reviews:

A. Whether hospital procedure agrees with the literature best practices—**YES; evidence-based practice is a QSEN core competency.**

B. Whether staff like the interventions—NO; the effectiveness of the intervention is important, not the staff's like or dislike.

C. Whether staff collaborate as a team—**YES; teamwork/collaboration is a QSEN core competency.**

D. Whether staff could find the procedure—**YES; if the staff could not find the procedure, it might not meet the QSEN standard for quality improvement or informatics.**

E. Whether staff consider the patient response—**YES; patient-centered care is a QSEN core competency.**

EXERCISE 3.64 Select all that apply:

What are the risk factors that place José at risk for neuroleptic malignant syndrome (NMS)?

A. Young age—**YES.**

B. Hispanic ethnicity—NO; culture does not produce a risk factor.

C. Male gender—**YES.**

D. Presence of affective illness and agitation—**YES.**

EXERCISE 3.65 Select all that apply:

Which of the following statements are true of electroconvulsive therapy (ECT)?

A. Changes personality—**YES.**

B. Changes neurotransmitters—**YES.**

C. Causes a seizure—**YES.**

D. Uses muscle relaxant and general anesthesia—**YES.**

E. Always used before trying medication—NO; it is used when medications are not tolerated.

F. Is given in a series of treatments—**YES.**

EXERCISE 3.66 True/False:

A. Nurse can delegate pre- and post-electroconvulsive therapy (ECT) assessment to a mental health technician.

__X__ **False**

B. Patient may return to unit and sleep, then wake up confused.

__X__ **True**

C. Patient may complain of headache post-ECT.

__X__ **True**

D. Patient disorientation and short-term memory problem usually resolves within 24 hours.

__X__ **True**

E. Patient cannot refuse ECT.

__X__ **False**

F. Patient or guardian must sign an informed consent for ECT.

__X__ **True**

G. ECT cannot be done as an outpatient.

__X__ **False**

H. Nurse administers the voltage.

__X__ **False**

EXERCISE 3.67 Select all that apply:

The nurse would teach that Depakote:

A. Must be taken as directed—**YES.**
B. Is a neuroleptic—NO; it is not an antipsychotic medication.
C. Is an anticonvulsant used as a mood stabilizer—**YES.**
D. Can be stopped abruptly—NO; abruptly stopping this medication can cause status epilepticus.
E. Abrupt withdrawal can cause a seizure—**YES.**

EXERCISE 3.68 Select all that apply:

What should the nurse tell him about his plan to drink alcohol?

A. Alcohol use is fine.—NO; it is not safe to use alcohol while taking medications.
B. Alcohol use is not an effective way of coping.—**YES; alcohol should not be used to relax.**
C. Take his medication instead.—NO; the medication is not being used to replace alcohol.
D. Do not drink alcohol with medication.—**YES; alcohol should not be consumed while taking medication.**
E. Practice relaxation techniques or listen to music as good coping skills.—**YES; these are effective coping mechanisms.**

EXERCISE 3.69 Select all that apply:

The nurse addresses the following:

A. Family is highly valued—**YES.**

B. Religion, primarily Catholic, is important—**YES.**

C. Health is thought to be God's will—**YES.**

D. Religion is not important—NO; religion is an important aspect of the Hispanic culture.

E. Hispanics tend to be verbally expressive—NO; the Hispanic culture tends to be more quiet and respectful in unfamiliar conditions or around unfamiliar people; Hispanic people tend not to be assertive, respond with silence, and avoid direct eye contact.

EXERCISE 3.70 Select all that apply:

What interventions should the nurse make?

A. Forbid him from using the healer—NO; this is not a culturally competent action.

B. Tell him to listen to the healer—NO; this action is not in a nurse's scope of practice.

C. Explain the importance of taking medication—**YES; teaching is important to help patients understand and be compliant.**

D. Encourage family to support taking medication—**YES; family is very important in Hispanic culture.**

E. Discuss folk customs that complement Western medicine—**YES; this is a culturally competent action.**

EXERCISE 3.71 Multiple-choice:

The drug that is most successful in treating the side effect of akathisia is:

A. Carbamazepine (Tegretol)—NO; this is an anticonvulsant used to treat seizures and mania symptoms.

B. Diazepam (Valium)—NO; this is an antianxiety medication.

C. Lorazepam (Ativan)—NO; this is an antianxiety medication.

D. Propranolol (Inderal)—**YES; beta blockers, particularly lipophilic agents such as propranolol, have been suggested as the most effective antiakathitic.**

EXERCISE 3.72 Multiple-choice:

If José has been diagnosed with a manic disorder, the nurse anticipates that the physician will most likely prescribe:

A. Clonazepam (Klonopin)—NO; this is an anticonvulsant.

B. Lorazepam (Ativan)—NO; this is an antianxiety agent.

C. Imipramine (Tofranil)—NO; this is an antidepressant.

D. Lithium (Lithobid)—**YES; this is a mood stabilizer.**

EXERCISE 3.73 Multiple-choice:

When a patient is prescribed 300 mg of oral lithium three times a day, the nurse should instruct the patient to contact the physician if he or she experiences:

A. Metallic taste—**YES; metallic taste, diarrhea, ataxia and tremor (neurotoxicity), as well as nausea are early warning signs of lithium toxicity.**

B. Urinary frequency—NO; this is usually not a symptom.

C. Loose stools—NO; this is usually not a symptom.

D. Thirst—NO; this is usually not a symptom.

EXERCISE 3.74 Multiple-choice:

Lithium is:

A. An anticonvulsant—NO; it is not for seizures.

B. A salt—**YES; lithium is a salt used as a mood-altering drug.**

C. A nickel by-product—NO; it is not for seizures.

D. A thyroid-stimulating hormone—NO; it is not for seizures.

EXERCISE 3.75 Multiple-choice:

The nurse is caring for a hospitalized patient who has been diagnosed with mixed mania and is not responding to lithium therapy. The nurse anticipates that the physician will most likely prescribe:

A. Tricyclic antidepressants—NO; this would increase the mania.

B. Anticonvulsants—**YES; the simultaneous presence of both manic and depressive symptoms is referred to as a *mixed-manic state* or *dysphoric mania*. Mixed states are generally more responsive to anticonvulsants than more traditional antimanic agents like lithium.**

C. Sedatives—NO; this would increase the depressive state.

D. Stimulants—NO; this would increase the mania.

EXERCISE 3.76 True/False:

A. Lithium is contraindicated in pregnancy because of possible congenital defects.

__X__ **True**

B. Continuous gastrointestinal (GI) upset may be a sign of toxic reaction.

__X__ **True**

C. Lithium levels are not needed if the patient follows orders.

__X__ **False**

D. If sodium decreases, the lithium level decreases.

__X__ **False**

E. Full effect takes 2 to 3 weeks.

__X__ **True**

F. Long-term use may lead to hypothyroidism.

__X__ **True**

EXERCISE 3.77 Multiple-choice:

The nurse is caring for Tamara who has been hospitalized with mixed mania who is to receive lamotrigine (Lamictol) as a medication. The nurse should explain to the patient that the target symptom of this medication is:

A. Anxiety—NO; it is not an antianxiety medication.

B. Lethargy—NO; it has no effect on lethargic states.

C. Mood stability—**YES; lamotrigine is an antiepileptic medication, also called an *anticonvulsant*, which has been successful in controlling rapid cycling and mixed bipolar states.**

D. Sedation—NO; it is not used for sedative purposes.

EXERCISE 3.78 True/False:

A. Normal serum levels of divalproex sodium (Depakote) are 150 to 200 mcg/mL.

__X__ **True; this is a normal serum level.**

B. The therapeutic range for serum divalproex sodium (Depakote) is 50 to 120 mcg/mL.

__X__ **True; this is a normal dose.**

EXERCISE 3.79 Multiple-choice:

A patient with mixed mania is prescribed carbamazepine (Tegretol). The nurse should instruct the patient that toxic side effects can occur if he or she concurrently takes a medication such as:

A. Lithium—NO; lithium and carbamazepine are given concurrently to successfully treat manic episodes and rapid-cycling bipolar disorder.

B. Amoxicillin—NO; this is an antibiotic in the class of drugs called *penicillins*. It fights bacteria in your body.

C. Cimetidine—**YES; cimetidine has been shown to inhibit the elimination of carbamazepine after a single oral dose; therefore, patients can become toxic.**

D. Buspirone—NO; this is used to treat anxiety disorders or as short-term treatment of symptoms of anxiety.

EXERCISE 3.80 Multiple-choice:

A patient who has been taking the medication carbamazepine (Tegretol) tells the nurse that he has been continually nauseated. The nurse should explain to the patient that the nausea may be decreased if the medication is:

A. Decreased in dosage—NO; dosages should never be randomly adjusted.

B. Taken at bedtime—NO; this will not affect it.

C. Supplemented with zinc—NO; this will not affect it.

D. Taken with food—**YES; nausea usually goes away after several days to several weeks of being on the medication. To minimize these symptoms, carbamazepine should be taken with food.**

EXERCISE 3.81 True/False:

Electroconvulsive therapy (ECT) is a type of somatic treatment in which an electric current is applied to the chest area through electrodes placed on the chest. The current is sufficient to induce a grand mal seizure.

__X__ **False; ECT is a type of somatic treatment in which an electric current is applied to the brain through electrodes placed on the temples. The current is sufficient to induce a grand mal seizure.**

EXERCISE 3.82 Multiple-choice:

Electroconvulsive therapy (ECT) is thought to work by:

A. Decreasing dopamine levels—NO; it increases levels.
B. Increasing acetylcholine levels—NO; it does not increase these levels.
C. Stabilizing histamine and epinephrine levels—NO; this is not the action.
D. Increasing norepinephrine and serotonin levels—**YES; ECT is thought to produce biochemical changes in the brain by way of an increase in the levels of norepinephrine and serotonin, similar to the effects of antidepressant medications.**

EXERCISE 3.83 Matching:

Match the communication interventions between Columns A and B:

Column A	Column B
A. The nurse may enhance this by bringing attention to the progress of group members. It helps maintain the patients' faith in the therapeutic modality.	__A__ Instillation of hope
B. Prevents the patient from feeling unique or different.	__I__ Interpersonal learning
C. The act of giving, such as patients helping each other.	__C__ Altruism
D. Giving information in a planned and structured manner.	__D__ Imparting of information
E. Feedback and role playing are two methods used in group therapy to develop social skills.	__F__ Imitative behavior
F. Patients imitate healthy behavior of other group members and the leader, which demonstrates growth.	__G__ Universality
G. Correction of interpersonal distortions is the goal.	__E__ Development of socializing techniques
H. Relates to bonding in the group. The patient's role in the group influences self-esteem. Cohesive groups create positive patient results.	__B__ Catharsis
I. Expression of feelings; is effective when followed by insight and learning.	__J__ Existential factors
J. Emphasizes the present quality, content, subjective awareness, freedom of choice, and state of being. Examples are responsibility and recognition of mortality.	__H__ Group cohesiveness

EXERCISE 3.84 Select all that apply:

Advantages of a psychiatric advance directive include:

A. An advance directive empowers the patient to make his or her treatment preferences known.—**YES.**

B. An advance directive will improve communication between the patient and the physician.—**YES.**

C. It can prevent clashes with professionals over treatment and may prevent forced treatment.—**YES.**

D. Having an advance directive may shorten a patient's hospital stay.—**YES.**

EXERCISE 3.85 True/False:

A psychiatric advance directive can cover medical and surgical treatment.

__X__ False; the psychiatric advance directive will be an advance directive for mental health decision making only; it will not cover decisions about other medical or surgical treatments.

EXERCISE 3.86 Fill in the blanks:

Name two concerns noted in the changes Angelique intends to make after discharge from the hospital.

1. **Taking St. John's wort with herbs or supplements with antidepressants, such as Zoloft, may lead to increased side effects, including serotonin syndrome, mania, or severe increase in blood pressure.**
2. **Dietary changes that might reduce salt intake will affect lithium levels and cause lithium toxicity.**

EXERCISE 3.87 Multiple-choice:

Having a Spanish-speaking interpreter for the father during the family meeting demonstrates:

A. Marginalizing—NO; this actually includes him.

B. Cultural insensitivity—NO; this is culturally sensitive.

C. Support for the patient's recovery process—**YES; providing services that support family engagement contributes to Angelique's recovery process and displays respect and cultural competence.**

D. Assuming inferior cognition—NO; the language one speaks does not determine intelligence.

EXERCISE 3.88 True/False:

Good psychiatric nursing care involves treating all patients equally.

__X__ True; good psychiatric nursing adapts care to the patient's cultural needs and preferences.

EXERCISE 3.89 Select all that apply:

Patients' rights under the law include:

A. Right to treatment—**YES.**
B. Right to assent—NO; this is used to obtain consent for a child.
C. Right to refuse treatment—**YES.**
D. Right to informed consent—**YES.**
E. Rights surrounding involuntary commitment—**YES.**
F. Psychiatric advance directives—**YES.**
G. Rights regarding seclusion and restraint—**YES.**

EXERCISE 3.90 Multiple-choice:

What is the nurse's priority nursing diagnosis for Matthew?

A. Ineffective individual coping—NO; this is not a priority.
B. Alteration in thought process—**YES; having thoughts of killing himself is the priority.**
C. Alteration in self-concept—NO; this is not a priority.
D. Potential for violence (against self)—NO; this is important, but not the priority.

EXERCISE 3.91 Multiple-choice:

The nurse initiates a verbal contract with Matthew for which of the following?

A. Safety—**YES; it is important to verbally contract for safety.**
B. Admission—NO; a verbal contract is not needed for admission.
C. Monitoring—NO; a verbal contract is not needed for admission.
D. Drinking—NO; drinking is not permitted in the hospital.

EXERCISE 3.92 Multiple-choice:

The nurse recognizes that Matthew's symptoms may be consistent with which disorder?

A. Social anxiety disorder—NO; this is a mental health condition where social interactions cause irrational anxiety.
B. Posttraumatic stress disorder—**YES; this is a mental health condition triggered by experiencing or seeing a terrifying event.**
C. Dissociative identity disorder—NO; this is a mental health condition characterized by the presence of two or more distinct personalities.
D. Paranoid disorder—NO; this is a mental health condition characterized by a long-term pattern of distrust and suspicion in others.

EXERCISE 3.93 Select all that apply:

What other nursing diagnoses can the nurse record at this point?

A. Ineffective individual coping—**YES; he is not coping well because he has not gone to the VA for help.**
B. Ineffective family coping—**YES; he and his wife have been fighting.**
C. Alteration in sleep pattern—**YES; he is having nightmares.**
D. Anxiety—**YES; he gets anxious with loud noises.**
E. Alteration in self-concept—NO; he is not having issues with self-esteem or depending on others for help.
F. Alteration in thought process (suicidal ideation)—**YES; he is having thoughts of killing himself.**

EXERCISE 3.94 Select all that apply:

The nurse prepares a situation, background, assessment, recommendation (SBAR) report for the psychiatric inpatient unit nurse. What information is critical to convey in terms of safety and continuity?

A. Patient admission for depression not otherwise specified (NOS) with suicidal ideation—**YES.**
B. Patient has plan and weapon at home (gun)—**YES.**
C. Patient drinks heavily, last drink 1 day ago—**YES.**
D. Patient refuses to contract for safety—**YES.**
E. Patient is a computer technician—NO; does not relate to the patient's safety.
F. Maintain on one-to-one until further assessment—**YES.**

EXERCISE 3.95 True/False:

Which of the following statements are true or false in reference to suicidal/homicidal patients?

A. Ask patient directly about suicidal/homicidal thoughts
__X__ **True**
B. Ask the family whether the patient has suicidal/homicidal thoughts
__X__ **True**
C. Depressed patients are not high risk
__X__ **False**
D. Establish a safety contract with the patient
__X__ **True**
E. Assume that the patient is just seeking attention
__X__ **False**
F. Patient is thinking rationally
__X__ **False**
G. Remove access to weapons
__X__ **True**
H. Patient's right to bear arms is primary
__X__ **False**
I. Duty to inform potential victim of declared threat
__X__ **True**

EXERCISE 3.96 Select all that apply:

When the nurse goes to the medication-dispensing machine (Pyxis) for antianxiety medication, the drawer is empty. The nurse goes to another unit and takes lorazepam (Ativan) from the unit's supply. This system workaround works for the short term, but may cause a problem in the long term. Why?

A. Manager not informed—NO; pharmacy needs to be informed not the nurse manager.

B. Supply not replaced—**YES; supply needs to be replaced on this unit.**

C. Staff continues "time-saving" short cut—**YES; this does not help to replace the unit's supply.**

D. Identification of patient may be bypassed—**YES; that patient might not be listed on the other unit's Pyxis.**

E. Medication amount may be incorrect—**YES; it might not be resupplied because the medication count was wrong.**

F. Hospital does not want to know as long as patient is satisfied—NO; the hospital would want to know whether supplies are not being replenished.

EXERCISE 3.97 Select all that apply:

What issues about alcohol use would indicate that the nurse and Matthew are in the working phase of the nurse–patient relationship?

A. Patient denies he has a problem with alcohol.—NO; denying the problem would occur in the orientation phase.

B. Patient identifies problems in marriage related to alcohol use.—**YES.**

C. Patient discusses how alcohol impairs his work.—**YES.**

D. Patient claims arguments with boss are definitely harassment by the boss.—NO; denying the problem would occur during the orientation phase.

E. Patient feels remorse for being impatient with his children.—**YES.**

F. Patient says goodbye and states he will continue Alcoholics Anonymous (AA) meetings after discharge.—NO; this would be the termination phase.

EXERCISE 3.98 Multiple-choice:

One of the groups his wife will attend is Al Anon. Which statement by the wife demonstrates recovery and improvement in their relationship?

A. "When my husband comes home I will hide the bottles of alcohol."—NO; this is not a positive coping mechanism.

B. "If he doesn't go into work, I will call and say he is sick."—NO; this is promoting alteration in self-concept.

C. "I will continue to be both mother and father to the children."—NO; this is not a positive coping mechanism.

D. "I will take care of myself and let him manage his own responsibilities."—**YES.**

EXERCISE 3.99 Multiple-choice:

What is the best response by the nurse when Matthew tells the same story over and over again of how his buddies died?

A. Listen and be nonjudgmental—NO; the nurse should always listen and be nonjudgmental, but limitations have to be set.

B. Give suggestions for what he could do—NO; giving advice is not a therapeutic communication technique.

C. Set limits and terminate discussion—**YES; it is important to set boundaries for the conversation.**

D. Clarify and probe further—NO; exploring is a therapeutic communication technique but there must be limitations.

EXERCISE 3.100 Multiple-choice:

Which statement by Matthew best demonstrates that he is coping better with his survivor guilt?

A. "I wish I had died instead of my buddies."—NO.

B. "I don't know why they died, they were better than me."—NO.

C. "If I had fought harder my buddies would be here."—NO.

D. "I am still here; I can help others with their memories."—**YES.**

EXERCISE 3.101 Multiple-choice:

Which of the following conditions is the patient most likely experiencing?

A. Amphetamine intoxication—NO; these are not symptoms of amphetamine intoxication.

B. Alcohol withdrawal—NO; these are not symptoms of alcohol withdrawal.

C. Alcohol intoxication—**YES; these symptoms are indicative of alcohol intoxication.**

D. Alcoholic dementia—NO; this is a condition caused by long-term, excessive alcohol consumption.

EXERCISE 3.102 Select all that apply:

After Sarah is medically cleared, what disorder(s) is the crisis team focused on preventing?

A. Dissociative fugue—**YES; this is characterized by reversible amnesia for personal identity and can be caused by experiencing a traumatic event or substance abuse.**

B. Borderline personality disorder—NO; this is a disorder with unstable moods and behaviors. Impulsiveness and poor judgment in lifestyle choices can lead the individual to risky situations, but have not caused the trauma this patient experienced.

C. Acute stress disorder—**YES; this occurs within a month of a traumatic stressor.**

D. Depression—**YES; physical, emotional, and/or sexual abuse can increase the risk of depression.**

E. Delusional disorder—**YES; this is characterized by delusional thinking and can be caused by stress and/or substance abuse.**

F. Somatization disorder—NO; this is a mental disorder characterized by recurring complaints about somatic symptoms.

EXERCISE 3.103 Select all that apply:

Which of the following is true about rape?

A. It is never the victim's fault.—**YES; it is never the victim's fault.**

B. The victim probably provoked it.—NO; it is never the victim's fault.

C. Only women who lose control get raped.—NO; anyone can be the victim of rape.

D. "No" sometimes means "yes."—NO; when a victim says "no" it means "no."

E. If a person is drunk, he or she cannot consent.—**YES; alcohol intoxication impairs mental ability.**

F. It is an act of aggression and control.—**YES; rape is an act of power and control, not an act of sexual desire.**

EXERCISE 3.104 Multiple-choice:

Considering Sarah's chronic use of alcohol, what is the most important information that the nurse should obtain and report?

A. Type of alcoholic drink—NO; this is important to know, but is not the most important.

B. Time of last drink—**YES; this is the most important so that the nurse can anticipate when withdrawal might occur.**

C. Source of alcohol—NO; this is not the most important.

D. Drinking at home alone or in a bar—NO; this is important but not the most important.

EXERCISE 3.105 Multiple-choice:

Which of the following would be signs of alcohol withdrawal?

A. Slurred speech, ataxia, hypothermia—NO.

B. Decreased reflexes, hypotension, drowsiness—NO.

C. Bradycardia, sedation, decreased respiration—NO.

D. Mild tremors, tachycardia, hypertension—**YES.**

EXERCISE 3.106 Select all that apply:

The nurse has the responsibility to foster and document the following interventions for Sarah in order to adhere to The Joint Commission (TJC) and Centers for Medicare & Medicaid Core Measures for quality and safety, which is required for accreditation and reimbursement of hospitals.

A. Median time from emergency department (ED) arrival to ED departure—**YES.**

B. Admit decision time to ED transfer—**YES.**

C. Encourage and offer a smoking-cessation program; document acceptance or refusal—**YES.**

D. Screen and document alcohol intoxication; document treatment acceptance or refusal—**YES.**

E. Refuse admission to those who refuse screening and treatment for alcohol, drugs, tobacco use—NO; it is not right to refuse admission if a patient refuses screenings.

F. Report alcohol and drug use to police—NO; this is not an appropriate action to take.

EXERCISE 3.107 Select all that apply:

In the following list, which are the measures on which patients and families rate hospitals for quality?

A. Communication with doctors—**YES.**
B. Communication on social media—NO.
C. Communication with nurses—**YES.**
D. Responsiveness of hospital staff—**YES.**
E. Pain management—**YES.**
F. Medication communication—**YES.**
G. Pet therapy—NO.
H. Discharge information—**YES.**
I. Clean and quiet environment—**YES.**
J. Hotel accommodations—**YES.**

EXERCISE 3.108 Matching:

Sarah is in the process of being transferred to the inpatient psychiatric unit. The nurse, Kathy, is giving a situation, background, assessment, recommendation (SBAR) report to the psychiatric inpatient nurse, Marie. Based on the aforementioned progress note, Kathy gives a report to Marie. Match the information in Column A with the parts of SBAR in Column B:

Column A	Column B
A. Temperature: 98.6°F, pulse: 98 beats per minute (bpm), respiratory rate (RR): 28 breaths per minute, blood pressure (BP): 140/90 mmHg, anxious, hand tremors, 6 hours last drink	__B__ Situation
B. Sarah, 40 years old, alcohol withdrawal	__D__ Background
C. Needs medication for alcohol withdrawal	__A__ Assessment
D. Patient states "need drink," "usually needed in morning to calm nerves," has been drinking heavily for 12 years	__C__ Recommendation

EXERCISE 3.109 Select all that apply:

The nurse anticipates that the primary care provider (PCP) may order which of the following medications for withdrawal?

A. Sertraline (Zoloft)—NO.
B. Clonidine (Catapres)—**YES.**
C. Lithium carbonate (Lithobid)—NO.
D. Oxazepam (Serax)—**YES.**
E. Propanolol (Inderal)—**YES.**
F. Lorazepam (Ativan)—**YES.**

EXERCISE 3.110 Ordering:

What is the nurse's priority at this time in terms of Sarah's interdisciplinary care plan? Place the following nursing diagnoses in priority order from 1 to 6:

__1__ Ineffective individual coping
__2__ Ineffective parenting
__4__ Potential for violence (against self)
__3__ Ineffective grieving
__6__ Alteration in nutrition (less than requirements)
__5__ Risk for injury (seizure from withdrawal)

EXERCISE 3.111 Select all that apply:

The nurse implements nursing interventions for a suicidal patient. What does this include?

A. Establish a patient contract for safety—**YES; safety is a top concern.**
B. Place the patient in seclusion and restraints—NO; this is not an appropriate action.
C. Place the patient on one-to-one observation—**YES; this provides for safety.**
D. Allow the patient to go off unit—NO; this is not an appropriate action to take.
E. Give the patient knitting needles in group—NO; knitting needles are not a safe item.
F. Notify physician of suicide ideation—**YES; the physician needs to know the patient's condition.**

EXERCISE 3.112 Select all that apply:

Sarah has been dually diagnosed with major depression and substance use (alcohol). The medication group of first choice for depression is selective serotonin reuptake inhibitors (SSRIs). Why?

A. They have no adverse effects—NO.
B. They have side effects such as headache, nausea, drowsiness, insomnia, and sexual dysfunction—**YES.**
C. They are less expensive—**YES.**
D. They may take up to 5 weeks for full effect—**YES.**
E. Suicide risk increases in the first couple of weeks—**YES.**
F. They may be taken with alcohol—NO.

EXERCISE 3.113 Select all that apply:

Sarah is being discharged to a drug and alcohol rehabilitation program. What are the nurse's responsibilities?

A. Provide teaching about discharge plan—**YES; the patient needs to understand the discharge plan.**
B. Report patient dissatisfaction with discharge plan—NO; this is not important to report.
C. Give a situation, background, assessment, recommendation (SBAR) report to rehabilitation program—**YES; the rehab program needs to understand the patient's condition.**

D. Consult with social services for safety of children—**YES; the children's safety is very important.**
E. Tell the patient she may resume alcohol in future if she handles it better—NO; alcohol is not an effective coping mechanism.
F. Encourage continued participation in Alcoholics Anonymous (AA) and sexual trauma support group—**YES; support groups can provide positive coping.**

EXERCISE 3.114 Select all that apply:

What defense mechanism(s) is Sarah using?

A. Rationalization—**YES; she is justifying her behavior.**
B. Projection—**YES; she denies having a bad drinking problem, yet blames her drinking on the bar.**
C. Minimization—**YES; she said her drinking "wasn't that bad."**
D. Repression—NO; she is not excluding desires and impulses from her consciousness.
E. Denial—**YES; she is denying that her drinking problem was bad.**
F. Reaction formation—NO; she is not doing the opposite of what she wants.

Resources

American Psychiatric Association. (2013). *Diagnostic and statistical manual of mental disorders* (5th ed.). Arlington, VA: American Psychiatric Publishing.

AMN Healthcare Education Services. (2013). Core measures: The nurse's role. Retrieved from http://www.rn.com

Debono, D. S., Greenfield, D., Travaglia, J. F., Long, J. C., Black, D., Johnson, J., & Braithwaite, J. (2013). Nurses' workarounds in acute healthcare settings: A scoping review. *BMC Health Services Research, 13*, 175. Retrieved from http://www.ncbi.nlm.nih.gov/pubmed/23663305

ECRI Institute and Institute for Safe Medical Practices. (2005). Workarounds: A sign of opportunity knowing, *PA PSRS Patient Safety Advisory, 2*(4), 25–28.

Hansten, R. (2014). Follow the money: Nurses leading value based care. *Washington State Nurses Association Nursing Update.* Retrieved from https://www.wsna.org

HIMSS Media. (2013). Workarounds in health care a risky trend. *Med Tech Media.* New Gloucester, ME: Author.

Koppel, R., Wetterneck, T., & Karsh, B. T. (2008). Workarounds to barcode medication administration systems: Their occurrences, causes and threats to patient safety. *Journal of the American Medical Informatics Association, 15*(4), 408–423.

La Charity, L. A., Kumagal, C. K., & Bartz, B. (2010). *Prioritization, delegation and assignment* (2nd ed.). St. Louis, MO: Mosby.

National Council of State Boards of Nursing. (2013). *NCLEX-RN Program Reports.* Chicago, IL: Author.

National Council of State Boards of Nursing. (2014). *NCLEX-RN Plan.* Chicago, IL: Author.

Porter, M. E. (2009). A strategy for health care reform—Toward a value-based system. *New England Journal of Medicine, 361*, 109–112.

The Stellaris Core Measure Workgroup. (2014). Inpatient and outpatient quality measures (core measures) education program. *Stellaris Health*, 1–28.

Townsend, M. C. (2014). *Essentials of psychiatric mental health nursing: Concepts of care in evidence based practice* (6th ed.). Philadelphia, PA: F. A. Davis.

Tucker, A. L. (2009). Workarounds and resiliency on the front lines of healthcare. *Perspectives on Safety: Agency for Healthcare Research and Quality*. Retrieved from https://psnet.ahrq.gov/perspectives/perspective/78

Varcarolis, E. M. (2013). *Essentials of psychiatric mental health nursing: A communication approach to evidence based care* (2nd ed.). New York, NY: Elsevier.

Wood, D. (2013). The future of value-based nursing care. Retrieved from https://www.aacn.org/nursing-excellence/healthy-work-environments

CHAPTER 4

Women's Health Nursing

Mary Foster Cox and Ruth A. Wittmann-Price

Nurses dispense comfort, compassion, and caring without even a prescription.—Val Saintsbury

UNFOLDING CASE STUDY 1: Ava

Ava is a 16-year-old high school student who is involved with a 20-year-old man; she comes to the free clinic for birth control (BC). Ava is taught the basic differences among all methods of BC. The nurse explains that there are basically three types of BC: *mechanical, hormonal or chemical, and surgical.*

EXERCISE 4.1 Multiple-choice:

The nurse understands that when a 16-year-old reveals she is sexually active with a 20-year-old male, the implications are:

A. The nurse should counsel the teenager against continuing the relationship.
B. The nurse is obligated to tell the teenager's parents.
C. The teenager is emancipated as a result of being sexually active.
D. The nurse may be obligated to tell authorities.

The answer can be found on page 306

EXERCISE 4.2 Matching:

Classify each method listed by matching the type of birth control (BC) in Column A with the method in Column B (the methods in Column A may be used more than once):

Column A	Column B
A. Mechanical B. Hormonal/chemical C. Surgical	_____ Condom _____ Vaginal ring (NuvaRing) _____ Tubal ligation _____ Morning-after pill (emergency contraception) _____ Silicone tubal occlusion plug _____ BC pills _____ Intrauterine device _____ Male vasectomy _____ BC implants (Nexplanon/Implanon) _____ BC patch (Ortho Erva) _____ Diaphragm _____ Cervical cap (FemCap) _____ BC shot (Depo-Provera) _____ Abstinence _____ BC sponge (Today Sponge) _____ Female condom _____ Fertility awareness method (FAM) _____ Outercourse _____ Spermicide _____ Withdrawal

The answer can be found on page 306

EXERCISE 4.3 Fill in the blanks:

Which birth control (BC) method is most effective against sexually transmitted diseases (STDs)?

____

Which BC method may be ineffective with the antibiotic rifampin?

____

Which BC method can be effective for 5 or 10 years?

____

Which BC method may not be effective if the patient is more than 200 lb?

____

Which BC method is implanted under the skin?

____

Which BC method is administered intramuscularly (IM)?

____

The answer can be found on page 307

eRESOURCE

To supplement your understanding of BC, refer to the *Merck Manual*. [Pathway: www.merckmanuals.com/professional ➔ enter "Contraception" into the search field ➔ select "Overview of Contraception" ➔ click on "Comparison of Common Contraceptive Methods" and click again on the table to expand the view ➔ review content.]

Ava talks to the nurse about BC and openly expresses some of her ideas. The nurse uses therapeutic communication skills and listens to all Ava's concerns and provides information when needed.

eRESOURCE

To reinforce your understanding of therapeutic communication, refer to Nursing Planet. [Pathway: http://nursingplanet.com ➔ select "Mental Health Nursing" ➔ scroll down to the "Assessment and Evaluation" section and select "Therapeutic Communication" and review the content.]

EXERCISE 4.4 Multiple-choice:

The nurse understands that Ava needs additional information when she states:

A. "If I use the pills and I miss a day I may need emergency contraception."
B. "I can use the RU-486 pill as emergency contraception."
C. "If I become sick, I should tell my primary care provider (PCP) that I am on birth control (BC) before she prescribes antibiotics."
D. "If I skip my progesterone-only pill I should take it as soon as I remember."

The answer can be found on page 307

Ava chooses to use BC pills on a 4-week cycle. The nurse then does a Pap test to screen Ava for any cervical anomalies. The nurse also takes culture swabs to test Ava for any sexually transmitted diseases (STDs).

EXERCISE 4.5 Multiple-choice:

The nurse also tells Ava about Gardasil, the quadrivalent vaccine to prevent which sexually transmitted disease (STD)?

A. Hepatitis B (hep B)
B. Herpes type II
C. Herpes zoster
D. Human papillomavirus (HPV)

The answer can be found on page 308

Gardasil is Food and Drug Administration (FDA) approved and is given in three doses within 6 months.

EXERCISE 4.6 Multiple-choice:

The nurse explains that Gardasil is given to:

A. Both men and women to prevent cervical and penile human papillomavirus (HPV), which can cause cancer
B. Both men and women to prevent cervical cancer and penile dysfunction disease
C. Just women, to prevent cervical warts and vulva cancers
D. Just men, to prevent genital warts and penile and testicular cancer

The answer can be found on page 308

---

eRESOURCE

To reinforce your understanding of Gardasil, refer to Epocrates Online. [Pathway: http://online.epocrates.com ➔ under the "Drugs" tab, enter "Gardasil" in the search field ➔ select "Gardasil" ➔ review content, focusing on "Patient Education".]

Gynecological History

Ava had menarche at the age of 12 years and has regular menstrual cycles of 28 to 30 days. She has *dysmenorrhea* on the first day of menstruation, for which she takes ibuprofen 400 mg orally every 6 hours. Ava understands the concepts of the menstrual cycle and when her "fertile" time may be. The nurse reviews this with her just to make sure she understands how important it is to take BC regularly. The nurse reviews the hormones that affect the menstrual cycle to further Ava's understanding.

EXERCISE 4.7 Matching:

Match the hormones in Column A to the effects in Column B:

Column A	Column B
A. Luteinizing hormone (LH)	____ Under the influence of this hormone from the anterior pituitary gland, the ova matures during days 5 to 13.
B. Progesterone	____ The *corpus luteum* produces this hormone along with estrogen.
C. Follicle-stimulating hormone (FSH)	____ This hormone surges for 48 hours on day 12 to produce ovulation.

The answer can be found on page 308

Ava seems to understand the information provided to her at the clinic and makes an appointment to return in 6 months for a follow-up visit.

eRESOURCE

To supplement your understanding of dysmenorrhea, refer to the *Merck Manual.* [Pathway: www.merckmanuals.com/professional → enter "Dysmenorrhea" into the search field → select "Dysmenorrhea" → review content, focusing on "Treatment" and "General Measures."]

Ava's Next Clinic Appointment

Ava frantically calls the clinic during her senior year of high school and says that she has skipped her pills while away on a spring break trip and had unprotected sex. She comes to the office and is given emergency contraception or the morning-after pill. There are several types of emergency contraception available. Some types currently available are:

- Progestin-only pills, which are approved for unrestricted (over-the-counter) sale and have very few side effects. They are 88% effective in preventing pregnancy (FDA approved).
- Ulipristal acetate which is available by prescription (FDA approved).
- Progestin and estrogen pills are used many times in increased dosages. These have a 75% effective rate (not FDA approved).
- A fourth type of pill contains mifepristone and is sold only in specific countries, not in the United States. This is often called "the abortion pill" because it can terminate an established pregnancy (not FDA approved).

EXERCISE 4.8 Multiple-choice:

The nurse is counseling Ava and realizes that she needs further information when she states:

A. "I can't take emergency contraception because it has been 4 days since I had sex."
B. "I may have some slight side effects but they should not be severe."
C. "My next period should come about the same time it is supposed to."
D. "I know that emergency contraception is most likely not causing an abortion."

The answer can be found on page 308

EXERCISE 4.9 Select all that apply:

Possible side effects of high-dose progesterone pills include:

A. Nausea
B. Vomiting
C. Rash
D. Diarrhea
E. Bleeding

The answer can be found on page 309

EXERCISE 4.10 Multiple-choice:

The nurse tells Ava about another method of emergency contraception that is 99% effective but Ava does not consider it because in the past it has had some bad publicity concerning uterine infection rates. Therefore, Ava rejects the suggestion of using a(n):

A. Diaphragm
B. Vaginal ring
C. Intrauterine device
D. Female condom

The answer can be found on page 309

---

eRESOURCE

To reinforce your understanding of emergency contraception, refer to the *Merck Manual.* [Pathway: www.merckmanuals.com/professional ➔ enter "Emergency Contraception" into the search field ➔ select "Emergency Contraception" ➔ review content.]

Ava continues to have inconsistent BC use. She comes to the clinic after a missed period on August 19 and states that she thinks she is pregnant. Ava performed an at-home pregnancy test. Ava tells the nurse she feels tired and nauseous in the mornings. These are two presumptive signs of pregnancy.

EXERCISE 4.11 Multiple-choice:

At-home pregnancy tests detect which of the following hormones in the urine?

A. Progesterone
B. Estrogen
C. Prolactin
D. Human chorionic gonadotropin (hCG)

The answer can be found on page 309

The nurse reviews the presumptive and probable signs of pregnancy with Ava (Table 4.1).

TABLE 4.1 Presumptive and Probable Signs of Pregnancy

Presumptive Signs of Pregnancy	Probable Signs of Pregnancy
Fatigue (12 weeks)	Braxton–Hicks contractions (16–28 weeks)
Breast tenderness (3–4 weeks)	Positive pregnancy test (4–12 weeks)
Nausea and vomiting (4–14 weeks)	Abdominal enlargement (14 weeks)
Amenorrhea (4 weeks)	Ballottement (16–28 weeks)
Urinary frequency (6–12 weeks)	Goodell's sign (5 weeks)
Hyperpigmentation (16 weeks)	
Uterine enlargement (7–12 weeks)	
Breast enlargement (6 weeks)	

EXERCISE 4.12 Select all that apply:

Positive signs of pregnancy include the following:

A. Ultrasound
B. Chadwick's sign (6–8 weeks)
C. Hegar's sign (6–12 weeks)
D. Fetal movement felt by the mother
E. Fetal movement felt by the examiner

The answer can be found on page 309

EXERCISE 4.13 Matching:

Match the terms in Column A with the definitions in Column B:

Column A	Column B
A. Quickening	____ Reflex of the fetus moving away from the examiner's fingers
B. Braxton–Hicks contractions	____ Softening of the cervix
C. Ballottement	____ Maternal perception of feeling the baby move
D. Goodell's sign	____ Softening of the lower uterine segment
E. Chadwick's sign	____ False labor contractions
F. Hegar's sign	____ Increase vascularity and blueness to cervix

The answer can be found on page 310

After Ava's pregnancy is confirmed with an hCG-positive urine test, an ultrasound is ordered to visualize the fetal heart (FH).

eRESOURCE

To reinforce your understanding of the pregnancy diagnosis, refer to Medscape on your mobile device. [Pathway: Medscape → enter "Pregnancy" into the search field → select "Pregnancy Diagnosis" and review content, focusing on "History" and "Physical Examination," "Laboratory Evaluation," and "Ultrasonography."]

The FH can be seen beating. By the crown–rump length measurement, the fetus is at 7 weeks gestation. That would coincide with Ava's last menstrual period (LMP), which was July 1. The nurse compliments Ava for seeking help after her first missed period and not waiting. Now health care and education are able to begin early and often to ensure a good pregnancy outcome.

EXERCISE 4.14 Multiple-choice:

Using Naegel's rule, Ava's baby is due on:

A. March 8
B. May 8
C. April 1
D. April 8

The answer can be found on page 310

---

eRESOURCE

Use the American Congress of Obstetricians and Gynecologists (ACOG) mobile app to verify Ava's due date. To download the app, visit the following sites:

- Apple IOS: http://goo.gl/PkMA3W
- Android IOS: https://goo.gl/ONdbWq
  [Pathway: ACOG Mobile App ➔ select "EDD Calculator" ➔ select "EDD Based on LMP" ➔ enter "July 1" and review result.]

EXERCISE 4.15 Select all that apply:

During Ava's first prenatal visit, an assessment is performed and plans are being made. Select all the appropriate components of a first prenatal visit.

A. Blood drawn for type and Rh
B. Amniocentesis
C. Venereal Disease Research Laboratory (VDRL) test or rapid plasma reagin (RPR) test
D. Dietary history
E. Nonstress test (NST)

The answer can be found on page 310

Also, during the first prenatal visit, the nurse documents Ava's complete health status and does a physical assessment and weight check, records vital signs, and teaches Ava about caring for herself and organogenesis. Ava's blood type is O−. Her Venereal Disease Research Laboratory (VDRL) test or rapid plasma reagin (RPR) test is negative, and her Rubella titer is positive; therefore, she is negative for syphilis and she is immune to German measles (Rubella) and will not need the vaccine.

eRESOURCE

To supplement your understanding of routine prenatal care, refer to the *Merck Manual*. [Pathway: www.merckmanuals.com/professional ➔ enter "Prenatal Care" into the search field ➔ select "Evaluation of the Obstetric Patient" ➔ review content, including "Table 1: Components of Routine Prenatal Evaluation."]

EXERCISE 4.16 Multiple-choice:

It is clear Ava needs more information about immunizations when she states:

A. "I know I should receive an influenza vaccine this winter."
B. "I am glad I am immune to German measles, I would hate to have it again."
C. "I will get the rubella vaccine so my baby is protected against mumps."
D. "I understand that varicella is a live vaccine so I cannot receive it."

The answer can be found on page 310

---

eRESOURCE

To reinforce your understanding of recommended immunizations for pregnant women, refer to:

- ACOG app on your mobile device. [Pathway: ACOG Mobile App ➔ select "For Pregnancy" ➔ select "Influenza Inactivated" ➔ and review content. Repeat with "TD/Tdap" and review content.]
- *Merck Manual*. [Pathway: www.merckmanuals.com/professional ➔ enter "Prenatal Care" into the search field ➔ select "Evaluation of the Obstetric Patient" ➔ review content under "Immunizations."]

Social History

Ava lives with her mother and two younger brothers. Ava has a high school education and works full time in retail. She is a licensed driver and has health insurance. She is involved with the baby's father but has no plans, at this point in time, to move in with him or to get married. She states her mother is upset about the pregnancy but will be supportive. Ava's mother works full time. Ava's house has electricity, plumbing, and a refrigerator. She has her own room and plans to keep the baby in her room on the second floor.

EXERCISE 4.17 Select all that apply:

Safety issues that should be discussed with Ava include:

A. Fire safety
B. Proper refrigeration
C. Well-water sterilization
D. Infant sleeping safety
E. Safe childcare options

The answer can be found on page 311

Health History

Ava's health history is unremarkable. As a child the only surgeries she had are an adenoidectomy and a tonsillectomy. She is up to date on her immunizations. She had chicken pox as a child. The only referral that the nurse provides to Ava is to see a dentist, because she has not seen one in 2 years.

EXERCISE 4.18 Multiple-choice:

The nurse understands the importance of prenatal dental care because:

A. Pregnant women may drink too many soft drinks in an effort to decrease nausea.
B. Periodontal disease is associated with preterm labor.
C. Pregnant women often lose teeth because of the fetus's needs.
D. Tooth decay is accelerated during pregnancy.

The answer can be found on page 311

Family History

Ava's mother is 48 years old and in good health. Ava has two healthy younger brothers. Ava's father is not part of her life and she never interacts with him, but as far as she knows he is alive and in good health. Her grandparents on her mother's side are alive and well. Her grandfather takes medication for high cholesterol. She does not know her grandparents on her father's side but thinks one may have died.

Dietary History

Ava eats supper at home and her mom normally cooks a full meal. For lunch, she has fast food and she has only coffee for breakfast.

EXERCISE 4.19 Multiple-choice:

Ava's body mass index (BMI) is 22.9; therefore, she should gain:

A. 15 to 25 lb
B. 25 to 35 lb
C. 35 to 45 lb
D. 45 to 55 lb

The answer can be found on page 311

EXERCISE 4.20 Fill in the blanks:

The nurse makes the following recommendations for Ava's diet:

Protein intake should be ______________ g/d.
Iron intake/d should be 30 mg/d. Take supplement with __________ to increase absorption.

Have _________ servings of fruits and vegetables each day.
To prevent neural tube defects, take ______ mg of folic acid each day.

The answer can be found on page 311

Ava is given a prescription for prenatal vitamins and she is told not to have *any* alcohol because of the risk of fetal alcohol syndrome (FAS) and fetal alcohol effects (FAE). Ava does not smoke and denies using street drugs. She is told to check with the nurses at the clinic before consuming any herbal medications.

eRESOURCE

To supplement your understanding of FAS, refer to the *Merck Manual.* [Pathway: www.merckmanuals .com/professional ➔ enter "Fetal Alcohol Syndrome" into the search field ➔ select "Fetal Alcohol Syndrome" ➔ review content.]

EXERCISE 4.21 Matching:

Match the trimester(s) in Column A that the common complaints and discomfort are most likely to occur in to the discomfort described in Column B:

Column A	Column B
A. First trimester	____ Urinary frequency and nocturia
B. Second trimester	____ Backache
C. Third trimester	____ Increased vaginal discharge *(leukorrhea)*
	____ Nausea and vomiting
	____ Fatigue

The answer can be found on page 312

EXERCISE 4.22 Matching:

Match the common discomfort in Column A with the physiologic reason in Column B:

Column A	Column B
A. Urinary frequency	____ Change in center of gravity
B. Backache	____ Elevated human chorionic gonadotropin (hCG) levels
C. Leukorrhea	____ First trimester progesterone rise
D. Nausea and vomiting	____ Enlarged uterus
E. Fatigue	____ Elevated estrogen levels

The answer can be found on page 312

Physical Examination

A complete physical examination is performed on Ava; here are some of the findings:

Vital signs: Temperature: 98.2°F, heart rate (HR): 74 beats per minute (bpm), respiratory rate (RR): 18 breaths per minute, and blood pressure (BP): 104/62 mmHg
Weight and height: 125 lb at 5′2″
Her heart and lung sounds are normal.

Ava asks the nurse whether she will have to have genetic testing for her baby because she heard another mother speaking about a procedure that can "look at the baby's cells." The nurse asks Ava whether she is concerned about anything. Ava says that she is not concerned about anything specifically. The nurse discusses risk factors with Ava.

EXERCISE 4.23 Exhibit-format:

A complete physical examination is performed on Ava and here are some of the findings:

Vital signs: Temperature: 98.2°F, heart rate (HR): 74 beats per minute (bpm), respiration rate (RR): 18 breaths per minute, and blood pressure (BP): 104/62 mmHg

Weight and height: 125 lb at 5′2″

Her heart and lung sounds are normal

Understanding Ava's history, what risk factors does she have?

A. Advanced maternal age and poor family history
B. Poor family and social history
C. Mental health and physical risk factors
D. Emotional and economic risk factors

The answer can be found on page 312

EXERCISE 4.24 Multiple-choice:

The genetic test that Ava was referring to can be completed at 10 to 12 weeks gestation and can be performed transcervically or abdominally, guided by ultrasound. The test is:

A. Amniocentesis
B. Chorionic villi sampling
C. Biophysical profile
D. Level III ultrasound

The answer can be found on page 312

Before Ava leaves the clinic, two appointments are made for her:

- An appointment for a level II ultrasound for fetal nuchal translucency (FNT), which is done by ultrasonography (USG) at 10 to 14 weeks. The nape of the neck is measured and can indicate genetic disorders.
- Her next clinic appointment is made for 4 weeks hence.

Also before Ava leaves for the day, danger signs (manifestations that indicate complications) are reviewed.

EXERCISE 4.25 Matching:

Match the manifestation in Column A with the possible complication in Column B (complications can be used more than once):

Column A	Column B
A. Bright painless vaginal bleeding	___ Infection
B. Persistent vomiting	___ Placental abruption (separation of the placenta before fetus is delivered; condition is exacerbated by vasoconstriction such as in maternal hypertension, smoking, abdomenal trauma, and cocaine usage)
C. Fever (more than 101°F), chills	___ Premature rupture of membranes (PROM) or preterm premature rupture of membranes (pPROM)
D. Sudden gush of fluid from the vagina	___ Pregnancy-induced hypertension (PIH; elevated BP of 140/90 mmHg or above after 20 weeks in previously normotensive women—two occurrences 6 hours apart)
E. Abdominal pain	___ Placenta previa (implantation of the placenta in the lower uterine segment; it can be complete, covering all of the os; partial, covering part of os; or marginal—sometimes called *low lying*)
F. Dizziness, blurred, double vision	___ Hyperemesis gravidarum (persistent vomiting with 5% weight loss, dehydration, ketosis and acetonuria)
G. Bright painful vaginal bleeding	
H. Severe headache	
I. Edema of hands, face, legs, and feet	
J. Muscular irritability	
K. Maternal weight gain more than 2 lb in a week	

The answer can be found on page 313

eRESOURCE

To supplement your understanding of the risk factors associated with pregnancy, refer to the *Merck Manual*. [Pathway: www.merckmanuals.com/professional → enter "Risk Factors for Pregnancy" into the search field → select "Risk Factors for Complications During Pregnancy" → review content.]

Prenatal Visit 2: 15 Weeks, September 16

At the second prenatal visit, a quad screen is done on Ava to check four parameters in the maternal serum:

Alpha-fetoprotein (AFP): a protein that is produced by the fetus.
hCG: a hormone produced within the placenta.
Estriol: an estrogen produced by both the fetus and the placenta.
Inhibin-A: a protein produced by the placenta and ovaries.

EXERCISE 4.26 Multiple-choice:

The nurse realizes that Ava needs a better understanding of a quad screen when she states:

A. Elevated alpha-fetoprotein (AFP) may indicate neural tube defects or Down syndrome.
B. To maintain the pregnancy, human chorionic gonadotropin (hCG) is important in the first trimester.
C. Decreased AFP indicates fetal alcohol syndrome (FAS) or fetal alcohol effects (FAE).
D. The amount of hCG decreases in the second trimester.

The answer can be found on page 313

Ava is now officially in her second trimester and other fetal surveillance tests for fetal well-being are sometimes done at approximately the 15th week. These include amniocentesis, percutaneous umbilical blood sampling, and Doppler studies.

EXERCISE 4.27 Matching:

Match the fetal surveillance tests in Column A to the descriptions of the tests in Column B:

Column A	Column B
A. Amniocentesis	_____ This is done by ultrasound to visualize the velocity of blood flow and measures the amount of red blood cells (RBCs).
B. Percutaneous umbilical blood sampling	_____ This can be done after 16 weeks to sample fetal blood. One to 4 mL are collected near the cord insertion to look for hemolytic disease of the newborn. This is guided by ultrasound.
C. Doppler studies	_____ Amniotic fluid is removed to test cells for genetic makeup. This test is done at 16 to 18 weeks under ultrasound.

The answer can be found on page 314

Ava has gained 2 lb and is now 127 lb. She walks eight blocks to work every day for exercise. Ava's BP is 106/70 mmHg and her urine is negative for glucose and protein when tested by dipstick analysis. Ava complains of occasional leg cramps that wake her up at night. She has started to take her lunch to work and is now eating breakfast. Discomfort of the second trimester is discussed.

EXERCISE 4.28 Matching:

Match the discomfort in Column A to the appropriate nursing actions in Column B:

Column A	Column B
A. Heart burn and indigestion	___ Increase fiber
B. Flatus	___ Increase calcium and phosphorus
C. Constipation	___ Stay upright after meals
D. Hemorrhoids	___ Decrease gas-forming foods
E. Leg cramps	___ Use stool softeners

The answer can be found on page 314

Ava listens to the instructions for the second trimester and asks questions about her care.

EXERCISE 4.29 Multiple-choice:

Ava understands the teaching when she states:

A. "I know my heartburn is caused by human chorionic gonadotropin (hCG)."
B. "I think my heartburn has to do with eating fast."
C. "Estrogen increases heartburn."
D. "Progesterone increases heartburn."

The answer can be found on page 314

Ava leaves the clinic well informed and has supplemental reading material and, of course, numbers to call should she experience any issues or danger signs.

Prenatal Visit 3: 19 Weeks, October 11

The routine assessments are completed for Ava's third visit. A urine dipstick is done to monitor for any developing hypertension of pregnancy (protein) and pregnancy-onset diabetes (glucose). Ava is excited because she can finally "feel the baby." This feeling occurs at about 18 weeks in multiparous women (women with more than one pregnancy) and at about 20 weeks in nulliparous women (women with no gestations past 20 weeks) or primigravidas (first pregnancy).

EXERCISE 4.30 Multiple-choice:

The nurse explains to Ava that the maternal perception of feeling the baby move is called:

A. Lightening
B. Ballottement
C. Softening
D. Quickening

The answer can be found on page 314

Ava is interested in what manifestations of pregnancy are called; so the nurse teaches her some terminology and Ava writes down the words so that she can search them later on the Internet.

EXERCISE 4.31 Crossword:

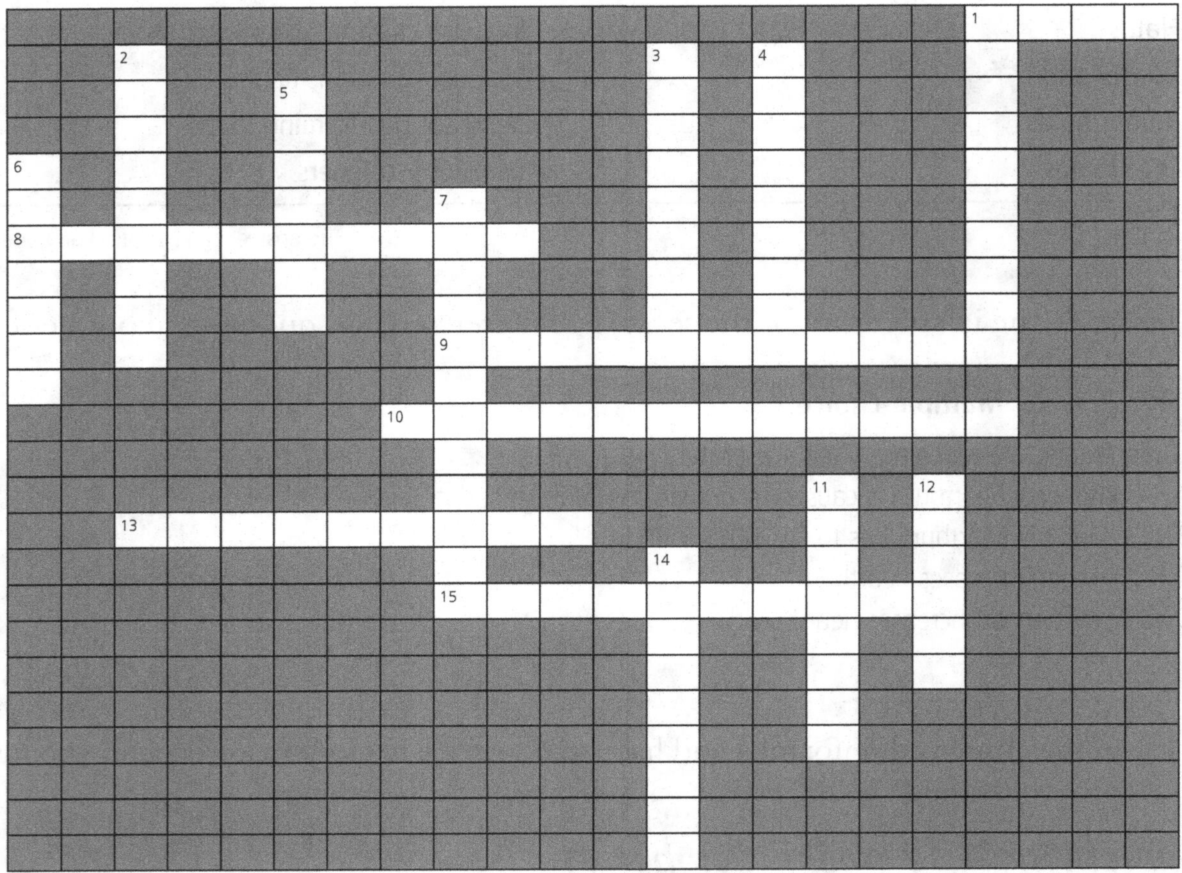

Across

1. Refers to the number of pregnancies that have reached viability
8. Time period between conception and labor
9. Onset of true labor to delivery of placenta
10. Woman pregnant for the first time
13. Process of producing and supplying milk
15. Placenta and membranes

Down

1. Period after delivery
2. Secretions from breast in the first few days after delivery
3. Two or more viable pregnancies
4. Woman who has never carried to viability
5. From birth to 28 days of life
6. Number of times a woman has been pregnant
7. Woman who has been pregnant two or more times
11. Another name for the postpartum period
12. Maternal discharge of blood, mucus, and tissue from uterus
14. Woman who has carried once to viability

Ava has gained an additional 3 lb and is 128 lb. Her blood pressure is 110/70 mmHg. Ava has no complaints and is excited because she is going to have an ultrasound, and she and her boyfriend would like to know the baby's gender. A transabdominal ultrasound or a level II ultrasound is recommended at 18 to 20 weeks for an anatomy check because congenital anomalies are best seen at this time. Pregnancy dating is done by biparietal diameter (BPD) and femur length.

The answer can be found on page 315

EXERCISE 4.32 Select all that apply:

Nursing care for a second-trimester transabdominal ultrasound includes the following interventions:

A. Fill bladder
B. Elevate head of bed
C. Place in stirrups
D. Tilt to the left side
E. Use gel conductor

The answer can be found on page 315

The baby is a *BOY!*

Prenatal Visit 4: 23 Weeks, November 9

Ava has now gained 5 lb since her last visit, for a total weight gain of 10 lb. Her blood pressure is 120/76 mmHg and her urine is negative for protein and glucose. She is registered for prenatal classes. Her mother will be going with her because she and the father of the baby are no longer together. She has a new boyfriend and is unsure whether she will give the baby the father's last name and ask him to sign paternity papers. Vaginal cultures are done on Ava since she reports being sexually active with her new boyfriend. The nurse also explains to Ava that the reason for measuring her belly with a tape measure is to assess fundal height and it is a good clinical method to estimate the growth of the baby.

EXERCISE 4.33 Multiple-choice:

The nurse explains to Ava that her fundal height at 23 weeks gestation should measure:

A. 22 to 24 in.
B. 22 to 24 cm
C. 24 to 26 in.
D. 24 to 26 cm

The answer can be found on page 315

Ava's culture is positive for chlamydia, and Ava is prescribed an antibiotic. She is encouraged to tell her new boyfriend so he can also get treatment. Ava comes in to pick up the prescription and the nurse reviews STDs and their implications to the baby.

EXERCISE 4.34 Fill in the blank:

If Ava is positive for chlamydia, what other sexually transmitted diseases (STDs) would you suspect that she might have?

The answer can be found on page 316

The nurse reviews some of the common STDs with Ava (Table 4.2).

eRESOURCE

To supplement your understanding of the risk factors associated with pregnancy, refer to the *Merck Manual.* [Pathway: www.merckmanuals.com/professional → enter "Risk Factors for Pregnancy" into the search field → select "Risk Factors for Complications During Pregnancy" → select "Sexually Transmitted Diseases (STDs)" and review content.]

Prenatal Visit 5: 27 Weeks, December 6

Ava has gained another 5 lb. Her blood pressure is 118/74 mmHg and her urine is negative for protein and glucose. The FH rate (FHR) is 138 bpm. Ava is given Rh immune globulin (RhoGAM®) intramuscular (IM), which is administered to all Rh-negative mothers at approximately 28 weeks gestation.

EXERCISE 4.35 Multiple-choice:

The nurse explains the reason for RhoGAM correctly when she states that Rh-negative mothers need RhoGAM to:

A. Change them to Rh positive temporarily
B. Produce antibodies against the fetal blood cells
C. Produce antigens against the RhoGAM
D. Change antibodies to antigens

The answer can be found on page 316

The nurse also explains that Ava should start doing a daily fetal movement count (DFMC). The nurse provides Ava with a chart on which to record her DFMC and explains DFMC is done each day by the mother. Ava is to record the number of kicks for 2 hours each day. Ava should feel at least 10 kicks during that time. A repeat hemoglobin (Hgb) and hematocrit (Hct) are drawn as well as another RPR. The repeat Hct it is slightly lower than the initial.

TABLE 4.2 Common STDs

Infectious Agents	Symptoms	Treatment	Effects in Pregnancy
Chlamydia trachomatis	Often asymptomatic. Can cause vaginal discharge, dysuria, or *pelvic inflammatory disease (PID)*	Antibiotics (eyrthromycin or azithroymcin)	Can be transmitted during birth and causes newborn conjunctivitis and/or chlamydia pneumonia in the newborn.
Gonorrhea (caused by gram-negative diplococcus) 30% of the time occurs as a coinfection with chlamydia	Most women show no symptoms or some vaginal discharge, pain and frequency on urination	Antibiotics (cephalosporins)	Newborn conjunctivitis
Herpes simplex virus (HSV)	Ulcerating blisters on the genitals or anal area; may be spread from the mouth; fatigue and fever are often experienced	The virus hides in nerve endings and reoccurs. There is no cure. It is treated with acyclovir to decrease the severity of outbreaks.	Can be spread through vaginal birth if there are open lesions; rarely is spread transplacentally. It has a high infant mortality and morbidity rate for those newborns who contract it during delivery.
Syphilis or *Treponema pallidum*	Early stages show painless sores, swollen glands, and skin rashes. Sores may be inside the vagina or anus and go unnoticed. Later stages show rashes, new sores, flu-like symptoms, swollen glands, and brain infection	Antibiotics (penicillin)	Congenital syphilis is transmitted by the placenta if the mother is not treated and 50% of fetuses will die before birth. Those born may have failure to gain weight, irritability, flat bridge of nose, rash, and pneumonia.

(*continued*)

TABLE 4.2 Common STDs (*continued*)

Infectious Agents	Symptoms	Treatment	Effects in Pregnancy
Hepatitis B Caused by a virus that invades the liver. This STI can be prevented by vaccine	Sudden flu-like illness with fatigue, nausea, vomiting, lack of appetite, and fever	No cure (preventative vaccine available)	Newborns are treated with hepatitis B vaccine in the nursery or at 1 month of age. If the mother is positive, baby is treated in the nursery with the vaccine and hepatitis B immune globulin.
AIDS Caused by the HIV virus, which invades the immune system	Flu-like symptoms may occur early or late. Skin and lung infections common in later years	There is no cure. Mothers are treated during pregnancy with zidovudine.	15% to 20% of infants born to untreated HIV-positive mothers will be infected. However, the risk of transmission can be dropped to as low as 1% with pre- and perinatal treatment. Mother should not breastfeed.
Human papillomavirus (HPV) Genital warts are associated with cancer	Soft, moist, pink growths on the penis, around the anus, and on or in the female genitals. May become stalked like a cauliflower.	There is no cure but there is a preventative vaccine. Topical agents are usually ordered and may decrease symptoms.	May be passed to infants.
Trichomoniasis Caused by the single-celled protozoan parasite *Trichomonas vaginalis*	Causes itching, burning, vaginal or vulva redness, and an unusual vaginal discharge	Antibiotics (Flagyl after the first trimester, clotrimazole suppositories during first trimester)	This is associated with premature delivery.

STDs, sexually transmitted diseases; STI, sexually transmitted infection.

EXERCISE 4.36 Exhibit-format:

Laboratory data: Hematocrit (Hct), 30.1; rapid plasma regain (RPR), negative

Vital signs: Temperature: 97.8°F, heart rate (HR): 68 beats per minute (bpm), respiratory rate (RR): 18 breaths per minute, blood pressure (BP): 110/72 mmHg

Fetal heart rate (FHR): 150 bpm

The nurse understands that Ava's slight drop in Hgb during the second trimester is caused by:

A. All patients get anemic during pregnancy, so it expected at this time.
B. There is an increase in fetal utilization of iron, so the baby is taking more.
C. Iron is poorly absorbed because of the gravid uterus pressing on the gastrointestinal (GI) tract.
D. The cellular content of blood increases at a lesser rate than the plasma.

The answer can be found on page 316

Also at 28 weeks gestation, the nurse schedules Ava for a glucose tolerance test (GTT).

EXERCISE 4.37 Multiple-choice:

The nurse understands that if Ava's repeat glucose tolerance test (GTT) is greater than 140 mg/dL she will be a candidate for:

A. Insulin therapy
B. Oral hypoglycemic medication
C. A 3-hour GTT
D. A fasting GTT

The answer can be found on page 316

In addition, before Ava leaves the clinic, the discomfort of the third trimester is reviewed with Ava.

eRESOURCE

To reinforce your understanding of GTT, refer to Medscape on your mobile device. [Pathway: Medscape ➔ enter "Glucose Tolerance Test" into the search field ➔ select "Glucose Tolerance Test" and review content.]

EXERCISE 4.38 Matching:

Match the common third-trimester discomfort in Column A with the description that matches in Column B:

Column A	Column B
A. Pica	_____ Caused by stretching and pressure from the gravid uterus
B. Backache	_____ Caused by uterus placing pressure on diaphragm
C. Round ligament pain	_____ Caused by pressure of gravid uterus on pelvic veins
D. Shortness of breath	_____ Caused by gravid uterus and softening of pelvic joints
E. Pedal edema	_____ Cravings of nonfood substances
F. Vulva and leg varicosities	_____ Impaired circulation caused by gravid uterus

The answer can be found on page 317

EXERCISE 4.39 Matching:

Match the third-trimester discomfort in Column A to the teaching that the nurse should provide in Column B:

Column A	Column B
A. Pica	___ Support hose
B. Backache	___ Flex legs onto abdomen
C. Round ligament pain	___ Check blood pressure, elevate feet
D. Shortness of breath	___ Proper nutrition
E. Pedal edema	___ Sit up straight and increase rest
F. Vulva and leg varicosities	___ Good posture and body mechanics

The answer can be found on page 317

Ava goes into spontaneous labor at 28 and 1/7 weeks gestation. She is contracting every 5 minutes and calls the clinic. Ava is told to go right to the emergency department (ED) at the hospital for assessment because of her gestational age (GA). When Ava arrives at the ED, she is admitted directly to the high-risk perinatal unit. She is given terbutaline (Brethine), a tocolytic agent to stop preterm labor. With three doses of terbutaline 0.25 mg subcutaneously (subq), her contractions stop.

EXERCISE 4.40 Calculation:

Order: Give terbutaline (Brethine) 0.25 mg subq, stat

On hand: Terbutaline 1 mg in 1 mL

How much do you give? ____________________

The answer can be found on page 317

Ava is also given betamethasone (Celestone) 12 mg IM now and again in 12 hours to help increase fetal lung maturity.

eRESOURCE

To reinforce your understanding of terbutaline, refer to Medscape on your mobile device. [Pathway: Medscape → enter "Terbutaline" into the search field → select "Terbutaline" and review content.]

EXERCISE 4.41 Calculation:

Order: Betamethasone 12 mg intramuscular (IM), stat

On hand: Betamethasone 50 mg/5 mL

How much do you give? ____________________

The answer can be found on page 317

Ava's contractions become intermittent and she is monitored on the high-risk perinatal unit for the next 2 days, and then discharged to home on modified bed rest.

UNFOLDING CASE STUDY 2: Jane

While Ava was on the perinatal unit, Jane was admitted into the next room. Jane's LMP was October 1, and it is January 15. This makes her 15 and 3/7 weeks gestation. Jane put off the first prenatal visit as this is her seventh child. Jane's case came through the ED because she has dark-brown vaginal discharge and she believes this time it is much more than in the past. Jane is hoping it is not twins again. On examination, the nurse assesses Jane's blood pressure and it is 154/92 mmHg. Jane denies a history of hypertension. Her past prenatal records are retrieved and verify that there was no gestational hypertension. Her uterus is large and measures 24 weeks gestation and the nurse cannot locate a FHR by Doppler. Jane also has very high hCG levels in her blood.

EXERCISE 4.42 Fill in the blanks:

Jane is pregnant for the seventh time. She has a 13-year-old girl who was delivered at 34 weeks gestational age (GA) but is doing well. She had a set of twins at 38 and 1/7 weeks who are now 10 years old. Jane has a 7-year-old and 5-year-old who were term babies. Jane had a miscarriage and then a preterm baby 3 years ago, who has mild cerebral palsy (CP).

Jane is a: G ____ P _____ T _____ A ______ L

The answer can be found on page 318

EXERCISE 4.43 Multiple-choice:

The nurse understands that the patient should most likely be prepared for which diagnostic procedure?

A. Ultrasound
B. Biophysical profile
C. Cesarean section
D. Amniocentesis

The answer can be found on page 318

The primary care provider (PCP) visualizes clear vesicles throughout the uterine cavity and makes the diagnosis of hydatidiform mole, a precancerous condition. No invasion into the uterus itself is visualized.

EXERCISE 4.44 Multiple-choice:

The most important education that the nurse can provide Jane after dilatation and curettage (D&C) of the hydatidiform mole is that she must:

A. Exercise regularly to get her abdominal tone back
B. Go to a support group for hydatidiform mole victims
C. Make sure she adheres to her birth control pills for at least a year
D. Get a second opinion about radiation therapy

The answer can be found on page 318

---

eRESOURCE

To reinforce your understanding of hydatidiform mole, refer to Medscape on your mobile device. [Pathway: Medscape ➔ enter "Hydatidiform Mole" into the search field ➔ select "Hydatidiform Mole" and review content.]

UNFOLDING CASE STUDY 3: Miracle

While in the high-risk perinatal unit, Ava shared a room with Miracle. Miracle is on complete bed rest at 36 weeks gestation for pregnancy-induced hypertension (PIH). She is a G1, 19-year-old patient whom Ava previously met in the clinic. Miracle has a blood pressure of 142/92 mmHg while resting on her left side. She has an intermittent frontal headache and 2+ edema of both ankles and calves. Miracle also has 2+ deep tendon reflexes (DTRs).

eRESOURCE

To reinforce your understanding of the clinical presentation and management of PIH, refer to Medscape on your mobile device. [Pathway: Medscape ➔ enter "Pregnancy and Hypertension" into the search field ➔ select "Pregnancy and Hypertension" and review content under "Gestational Hypertension," "Fetal Monitoring," and "Medical Therapy."]

EXERCISE 4.45 Multiple-choice:

The nurse caring for Miracle and Ava has a nursing student with her. The nurse assesses that the nursing student understands the patient's care when he states:

A. "Miracle's edema is slightly severe, I will continue strict input and output (I&O)."
B. "Miracle's edema is severe and pitting on palpation."
C. "Miracle's deep tendon reflexes (DTRs) are hypoactive."
D. "Miracle's DTRs are hyperactive."

The answer can be found on page 318

When Miracle arrived in the high-risk perinatal unit, she was given magnesium sulfate ($MgSO_4$) to prevent seizures by decreasing the neuromuscular transmissions at the junctions. The nurse has an order to hang a new bag of $MgSO_4$ and it is delivered from pharmacy premixed with 40 g in 500 mL. The order is to administer a continuous intravenous (IV) drip at 4 g/hr.

eRESOURCE

To reinforce your understanding of the prophylactic management of preeclampsia, refer to Medscape on your mobile device. [Pathway: Medscape ➔ enter "Preeclampsia" into the search field ➔ select "Preeclampsia" and review content under "Seizure Treatment and Prophylaxis With Magnesium Sulfate."]

EXERCISE 4.46 Calculation:

Order: Magnesium sulfate ($MgSO_4$) 4 g/hr

On hand: 40 g/500 mL

How much do you give? ____________________

The answer can be found on page 319

Later that day, the phlebotomist draws blood on Miracle for liver enzymes and clotting factors to rule out HELLP syndrome, which is hemolytic anemia, elevated liver enzyme, and low platelets.

EXERCISE 4.47 Multiple-choice:

A diagnostic finding in HELLP (hemolytic anemia, elevated liver enzyme, and low platelets) syndrome includes:

A. Decreased fibrinogen
B. Increased platelets
C. Decreased leukocytes
D. Increased fibrin-split products

The answer can be found on page 319

EXERCISE 4.48 Multiple-choice:

Miracle's labs show that her platelet count is $90,000/mm^3$. This would place her in which category?

A. Class I
B. Class II
C. Class III
D. Class IV

The answer can be found on page 319

EXERCISE 4.49 Multiple-choice:

The interprofessional group of health care providers has determined that Miracle is not in disseminated intravascular coagulation (DIC) because Miracle's laboratory results demonstrate:

A. A decrease in fibrin-split products
B. An increase in platelets
C. An increase in fibrin-split products
D. An increase in red blood cells (RBCs)

The answer can be found on page 319

eRESOURCE

To reinforce your understanding of the clinical presentation and management of DIC, refer to Medscape on your mobile device. [Pathway: Medscape ➔ enter "Disseminated Intravascular Coagulation" into the search field ➔ select "Disseminated Intravascular Coagulation" and review content under "Overview" and "Clinical Presentation."]

Miracle is also receiving daily nonstress tests (NSTs) because the baby has been diagnosed with intrauterine growth restriction (IUGR), which may indicate the infant will be small for gestational age (SGA). This is a consequence of vasoconstriction caused by the hypertension.

EXERCISE 4.50 Fill in the blank:

Small-for-gestational-age (SGA) babies' weights fall below the ___ percentile for weight when compared on the growth chart for their weeks of gestation.

The answer can be found on page 319

eRESOURCE

To reinforce your understanding of IUGR, refer to Medscape on your mobile device. [Pathway: Medscape ➔ enter "IUGR" into the search field ➔ select "Intrauterine Growth Restriction" and review content.]

Nonstress Test

This test is done after the 28th week by attaching the patient to the external fetal monitor (EFM) and assessing FHR in relation to movement. For a reactive test, there should be three movements with an acceleration of FHR 15 bpm for at least 15 second in 20 minutes.

EXERCISE 4.51 Select all that apply:

Nursing care for a patient having a nonstress test (NST) should include:

A. Tilting the patient to the side to prevent supine hypotension
B. Increasing the intravenous (IV) fluids to 250 mL/hr
C. Explaining the procedure to the patient and family
D. Keeping the room as quiet as possible
E. Placing a Foley catheter into the bladder

The answer can be found on page 320

If the NST was questionable, two other tests may be ordered:

Biophysical Profile

The biophysical profile (BPP) tests and scores five fetal wellness parameters as 0, 1, or 2. It scores the NST, amniotic fluid volume (AFV), fetal breathing movements, gross body movements, and fetal tone. A low score indicates fetal distress.

Contraction Stress Test

Exogenous oxytocin (IV oxytocin [Pitocin]) or (less often) nipple stimulation is used to stimulate uterine contractions (UCs). This evaluates placenta functioning and reserve. The goal is to stimulate three UCs of 40- to 60-second duration in 10 minutes and to evaluate the FHR. A negative result is a positive sign, meaning no fetal distress. A positive result indicates fetal distress.

EXERCISE 4.52 Select all that apply:

Miracle has been informed that because of its small-for-gestational-age (SGA) status, when the baby is born the newborn may need extra blood testing for:

A. Glucose
B. Polycythemia
C. Thyroid-stimulating hormone (TSH)
D. Phenylketonuria (PKU)
E. Bilirubin

The answer can be found on page 320

---

eRESOURCE

To supplement your understanding of SGA, refer to the *Merck Manual.* [Pathway: www.merckmanuals.com/professional ➔ enter "Small for Gestational" into the search field ➔ select "Small-for-Gestational-Age (SGA) Infant" ➔ review content.]

UNFOLDING CASE STUDY 4: Janelle

Janelle is another patient on the high-risk unit where Ava was admitted. Janelle is a 32-year-old G3, T0, P2, A0, L2. She is 14 weeks pregnant and 1 postoperative day from a cerclage for an incompetent cervix. Her previous babies were born at 24 and 32 weeks, respectively. She had a cerclage placed with the second pregnancy after the diagnosis of incompetent cervix.

EXERCISE 4.53 Select all that apply:

The following conditions place women at high risk for an incompetent cervix:

A. Diethylstilbestrol (DES) exposure while in utero
B. Cervical trauma
C. Congenitally shorter cervix
D. Large babies
E. Uterine anomalies
F. Overdistended bladder
G. Previous loop electrosurgical excision procedure (LEEP), cone, or other surgical procedures
H. Multiple gestations

The answer can be found on page 320

UNFOLDING CASE STUDY 1 (CONTINUED): Ava (At Home on Modified Bed Rest)

Ava was discharged from the hospital and is scheduled to return to the clinic every 2 weeks until 36 weeks, at which time she is seen every week (Table 4.3).

At 36 weeks gestational age Ava is cultured (vaginal and rectal) for group B *Streptococcus* (GBS), which is known to cause sepsis in otherwise healthy newborns. GBS is present in 10% to 30% of all women. It is colonized in the vagina, yet most women are usually asymptomatic. GBS has the potential to cause urinary tract infections (UTIs), which are one of the leading causes of preterm labor and neonatal septicemia.

EXERCISE 4.54 Multiple-choice:

Ava's group B streptococcal culture is positive, so the nurse would anticipate the following order once Ava shows signs of true labor:

A. Gentamycin every 2 hours until delivery
B. Ampicillin 4 hours before delivery
C. Pitocin 1 mU/min to start regular uterine contractions (UCs)
D. Terbutaline 0.25 subq to increase the time until delivery

The answer can be found on page 320

TABLE 4.3 Ava's Prenatal Record

Date	Week	Fundal Height (cms)	FHR	BP (mmHg)	Urine Pro/ Glucose	Tests	Comments
1–20	29	29	142 RLQ	106/72	N/N		C/O being tired—encouraged to rest during day
1–27	30	30.5	148 RLQ	108/70	N/N		Feeling Braxton–Hicks contractions
2–17	33	32.5	136 RLQ	110/70	N/N		Admitted for preterm labor
3–4	35	35	144 RLQ	112/76	N/N		Virtual tour of the L&D suite
3–11	36	36	140 RLQ	114/74	N/N	GBS culture	

BP, blood pressure; cm, centimeters; C/O, complains of; FHR, fetal heart rate; GBS, group B *Streptococcus*; L&D, labor and delivery; N/N, negative/negative; RLQ, right lower quadrant.

Ava calls the clinic at 36 and 5/7 weeks and states she is in labor. It is 3 a.m. and the answering service instructs her to go to the local ED. There she is evaluated and attached to the electronic fetal monitor (EFM).

EXERCISE 4.55 Matching:

Match the correct term describing uterine contractions (UCs) in Column A with the descriptions in Column B:

Column A	Column B
A. Intensity	____ The time in seconds in between contractions
B. Frequency	____ The firmness of the uterus, which can be demonstrated in three ways: By an external fetal monitor (EFM) as the uterus rises and falls with contractions but is not an exact pressure because of different abdominal thicknesses By an internal uterine pressure catheter (IUPC), which is inserted through the vagina into a pocket of fluid after rupture of membranes (ROM) By palpation: Mild is the consistency of the tip of your nose; moderate is the consistency of your chin; strong is the consistency of your forehead
C. Interval	____ From the onset of one contraction to the onset of the next contraction

The answer can be found on page 321

Ava is in labor.

EXERCISE 4.56 Fill in the blanks.

Fill in the blanks using these external fetal monitor strips:

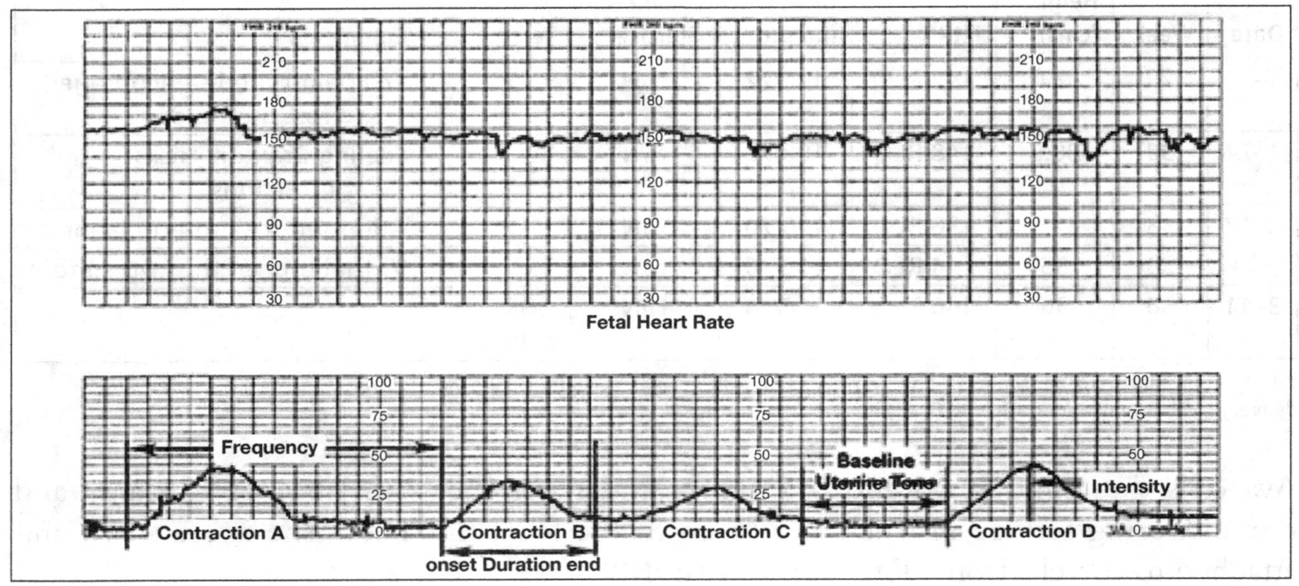

What is the frequency of Ava's contractions? ____________________
What is the duration of Ava's contractions? ____________________
What is the interval of Ava's contractions? ____________________
What is the intensity of Ava's contractions? ____________________

The answer can be found on page 321

Ava is admitted to the L&D suite.

UNFOLDING CASE STUDY 5: Mirabel

Mirabel comes into the ED approximately the same time as Ava. She is a 27-year-old G2, T0, P0, A1, L0. Mirabel states that she missed her period last month but was waiting to see whether it returned this month. Her primary complaint is pain in her left lower abdomen that radiates down her leg. On a pain scale of 0 to 10 she rates it a 6, and is visibly uncomfortable.

EXERCISE 4.57 Multiple-choice:

The nurse should anticipate that the primary care provider (PCP) will order:

A. A computerized axial tomography (CAT) scan and human chorionic gonadotropin (hCG) level
B. An MRI and ultrasound
C. An ultrasound and CAT scan
D. An hCG level and ultrasound

The answer can be found on page 322

These tests confirm that she is pregnant, but it is an unruptured ectopic pregnancy.

EXERCISE 4.58 Hot spot:

Place an X on the diagram the portion of the female anatomy where you believe the implantation is most likely to occur.

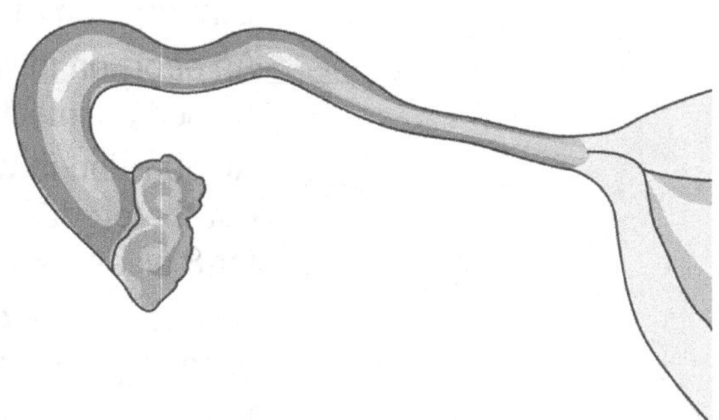

The answer can be found on page 322

Mirabel is given methotrexate, which is an antimetabolite drug that will stop rapidly dividing cells, such as an embryo, in order to save the fallopian tube. She is extremely lucky that the ectopic pregnancy did not rupture. Therefore, Mirabel has a better chance of becoming pregnant in the future.

eRESOURCE

To supplement your understanding of ectopic pregnancy, refer to the *Merck Manual.* [Pathway: www.merckmanuals.com/professional → enter "Ectopic Pregnancy" into the search field → select "Ectopic Pregnancy" → review content, particularly "Treatment and Management" and "Medication."]

UNFOLDING CASE STUDY 6: Sara

Sara comes to the ED while Ava is waiting to be taken to the L&D suite. Sara is pregnant and experiencing vaginal bleeding. She is in her first trimester. An ultrasound that was done 2 weeks ago dated the pregnancy at 9 weeks gestation, which is consistent with Sara's dates. Sara is G4, T1, P0, A2, L1. Since her son was born 6 years ago, she has experienced two spontaneous abortions. One was a complete abortion and the second one was an incomplete abortion, for which she had to be admitted to the hospital for a dilation and evacuation (D&E) at 7 weeks gestation. She is now under a threatened abortion and is placed on bed rest in the ED, after which she is transferred to the perinatal unit. During the next 2 hours of observation, the bleeding increases and an ultrasound shows no FHR. Sara is diagnosed with an inevitable abortion, which will be extremely difficult for her. She will need to be referred to the outpatient perinatal center for genetic studies because she is a habitual aborter.

EXERCISE 4.59 Matching:

Match the terms in Column A with the definitions in Column B:

Column A	Column B
A. Abortion	____ Bleeding and cramping that subside with continuation of the pregnancy
B. Therapeutic abortion	____ An abortion in which retained tissue has caused an infection
C. Induced abortion	____ An abortion in which the fetus died in utero, but the products of conception are retained for 8 weeks or longer
D. Spontaneous abortion	____ An abortion in which some of the products of conception are retained
E. Complete abortion	____ Termination of pregnancy before 20 to 24 weeks gestation; it differs from state to state
F. Incomplete abortion	____ Intentional termination of pregnancy by means of dilating the cervix and evacuating the uterus
G. Threatened abortion	____ An abortion in which the total products of conception are expelled
H. Inevitable abortion	____ A woman who has had three or more consecutive abortions
I. Infected abortion	____ A second- or third-trimester abortion
J. Partial-birth abortion	____ An abortion performed when the pregnancy endangers the mom or the fetus has a condition that is incompatible with life
K. Habitual aborter	____ An abortion that cannot be stopped
L. Missed abortion	____ Loss of a pregnancy before viability that has not been interfered with intentionally. Symptoms are cramping and bleeding. Most often caused by genetic disorders of the embryo, hormonal imbalances, infections, and abnormalities of the placenta.

The answer can be found on page 322

EXERCISE 4.60 Select all that apply:

Choose the appropriate nursing interventions for Sara.

A. Tell her she can get pregnant again
B. Tell her to adopt a child
C. Encourage her to verbalize about the loss
D. Give her a special memento, such as a silk rose, to remember the loss
E. Include her husband in the discussion

The answer can be found on page 323

eRESOURCE

To reinforce your understanding of therapeutic communication, refer to Nursing Planet. [Pathway: http://nursingplanet.com → select "Mental Health Nursing" → scroll down to the "Assessment and Evaluation" section and select "Therapeutic Communication" and review the content.]

UNFOLDING CASE STUDY 1 (CONTINUED): Ava

Ava is attached to the EFM. The FHR shows good variability or push and pull of the sympathetic and parasympathetic nervous system of the fetus. There are FHR accelerations with UCs and fetal movement. Therefore, the pattern is reassuring. Ava is allowed to walk around, off the monitor, for 40 minutes out of every hour and placed on the monitor for 20 minutes. The nurse evaluates the monitor for basic patterns every hour and uses the acronym *VEAL CHOP* (see Table 4.4).

TABLE 4.4 VEAL CHOP Mnemonic

V	Variable deceleration	C	Cord compression. The first nursing intervention is to reposition the patient.
E	Early deceleration	H	Head compression. Early decelerations occur as a mirror image of the uterine contractions (UCs) and are caused by the fetus moving down in the birth canal. The fetal head is compressed causing vagal stimulation that is recorded as a deceleration. There is a decrease in fetal heart rate at the beginning of the contraction and a return to baseline at the end of the contraction. These are usually benign and require no further intervention. Continue to monitor the patient. Vaginal examination should continue to determine whether the fetus is descending through the pelvis. If the fetus is not descending, the physician should be contacted.
A	Accelerations	O	These are OK and reassuring.
L	Late decelerations	P	Problem. Late decelerations begin after the onset of the contraction and are identified as a slow return to baseline after the UC. They inversely mirror the contraction but are late in onset and recovery. This is usually an ominous sign as it indicates uteroplacental insufficiency and poor perfusion. At the first sign of this pattern, the nurse should address oxygenation or fetal resuscitation: ■ Turn the patient to the left side; if that does not help try the right. ■ Provide oxygen by mask at 10 L ■ Turn up the plain IV to hydrate ■ Turn off the oxytocin (Pitocin) ■ Call the primary care provider

After 3 hours, Ava is 4-cm dilated and the PCP has decided that Ava will receive labor augmentation. Artificial rupture of membranes (AROM) is done with an amniohook to augment Ava's labor process.

EXERCISE 4.61 Multiple-choice:

The expert nurse understands that after artificial rupture of membranes (AROM), her first intervention will be:

A. Clean the patient's bed
B. Observe the fluid's color
C. Count the fetal heart rate (FHR)
D. Palpate the maternal pulse

The answer can be found on page 323

After the AROM, Ava's UCs become stronger and she receives butorphanol 1 mg.

EXERCISE 4.62 Multiple-choice:

The nurse understands that once a labor patient receives a narcotic, a priority intervention is:

A. Assist when out of bed (OOB)
B. Monitor the labor contractions, which may decrease in intensity
C. Provide oral hygiene to reduce dry mouth
D. Have naloxone (Narcan) available

The answer can be found on page 323

EXERCISE 4.63 Calculation:

Order: Give butorphanol 1 mg intravenous (IV) push, stat

On hand: Butorphanol 2 mg in 1 mL

How much do you give? ____________

The answer can be found on page 323

EXERCISE 4.64 Calculation:

Order: Have neonatal naloxone (Narcan) 0.1 mg/kg intramuscular (IM) on hand

On hand: Naloxone (Narcan) 0.4 mg /mL

How much would you give if you suspect a 7-lb baby? ____________

The answer can be found on page 323

Ava is now in bed and she is 5-cm dilated (Table 4.5). Ava is very uncomfortable and requests an epidural. The nurse increases her IV fluid rate, as ordered, to increase the vascular volume to offset the hypotensive effect of the epidural, which is produced by the vasodilation.

TABLE 4.5 Stages and Phases of Labor

First Stage (Dilating Stage)	Second Stage (Expulsion Stage)	Third Stage (Placental Stage)
Latent phase: 0–3 cm dilated, mild contractions q 5–10 min lasting 20–40 sec. The patient is usually social and calm. Active phase: 4–8 cm with moderate UC sq 2–5 min lasting 30–50 sec. Ava is introverted. Transition phase: 8–10 cm, strong contractions q 2–3 min lasting 45–90 sec. This is a difficult time and mother becomes irritable.	Full dilation to delivery of baby. Ava is relieved that she can start pushing.	Delivery of placenta. Ava is excited and talkative.

q, every; UCs, uterine contractions.

eRESOURCE

To reinforce your understanding of these medications, refer to Epocrates Online. [Pathway: http://online.epocrates.com ➔ under the "Drugs" tab, enter each medication name in the search field ➔ review "Adult Dosing," "Adverse Reactions," and "Safety/Monitoring."]

EXERCISE 4.65 Calculation:

Order: Increase Ringer's lactate (RL) to 500 mL bolus in 30 minutes.

On hand: 1,000-mL bag of RL on a pump that delivers mL/hr

What would the pump setting be for this bolus? ____________________

The answer can be found on page 323

Ava receives a continuous epidural infusion and the nurse checks her BP every minute for 5 minutes, then every 15 minutes for 1 hour to make sure it does not drop too low. A low blood pressure can severely affect placental perfusion of blood and therefore fetal oxygenation. The baby is continuously monitored and Ava rests in between UCs.

EXERCISE 4.66 Select all that apply:

Check all the appropriate nursing interventions for the first stage of the second phase of labor:

A. Catheterize or void every 4 hours
B. Change blue pads every 30 minutes
C. Allow her to order a regular full lunch
D. Turn lights on so she is alert
E. Take off the fetal monitor

The answer can be found on page 324

Ava's UCs slow down and oxytocin (Pitocin) stimulation or augmentation is given via IV.

EXERCISE 4.67 Calculation:

Calculate the correct dose if the primary care provider (PCP) orders a Pitocin intravenous (IV) to start at 2 mU/min.

On hand: 500-mL bag of Ringer's lactate (RL) with 30 units of Pitocin and a pump that delivers mL/hr

What is the correct pump setting? ______________________________

The answer can be found on page 324

Ava wakes up and is starting to feel the UCs again. She is short tempered with her mother and irritable with the nurse, but the nurse knows this is normal and reviews the stages and phases of labor with Ava's mother, so she understands Ava's behavior. The professional nurse notes early decelerations on the fetal monitor but the FHR remains at 130 to 140 in between contractions, which is the baseline.

eRESOURCE

To reinforce your understanding of the stages of labor, refer to Medscape on your mobile device. [Pathway: Medscape ➔ enter "Labor" into the search field ➔ select "Normal Labor and Delivery" and review content.]

EXERCISE 4.68 Fill in the blanks:

What is the normal fetal heart rate (FHR) range? The normal range is______ to _______ beats/min.

The answer can be found on page 324

The nurse has Ava checked internally and she is fully dilated (10 cm). The nurse repositions Ava so she can push. Ava pushes effectively for approximately an hour, and when rechecked the baby is + 3 station. The delivery table is brought into the room and the PCP is called. The baby is crowning and Ava feels the "ring of fire" sensation around her perineum. The PCP massages her perineum in an attempt to decreases perineal lacerations. The baby turns in external restitution and the nurse reviews the six cardinal processes of childbirth (Exhibit 4.1) with the graduate nurse who is being oriented and is observing the delivery. A right medial lateral (RML) episiotomy is made to prevent perineal tearing.

The baby is bigger than expected and the anterior shoulder gets caught under the symphysis pubis. An RML episiotomy is made. The PCP immediately puts on the call bell to alert the L&D team that there is shoulder dystocia. The McRobert's maneuver is performed. Ava's legs are flexed as far as possible to open the pelvic arch, and subrapubic pressure is applied to dislodge the fetal shoulder. The McRobert's maneuver is successful, anesthesia is not needed, and the baby is delivered.

EXHIBIT 4.1 Six Cardinal Processes of Labor

Engagement and descent. The presenting part moves through the false pelvis to the true pelvis and reaches the *ischial spines*.
Flexion. The fetal head is forced chin to chest so the *suboccipital bregmatic* presents.
Internal rotation. The fetus turns its head so the largest diameter is lined up with the widest part of the pelvis (anterior–posterior [AP] diameter of fetal head aligns with AP diameter of pelvis).
Extension. The fetal head passes under the *symphysis pubis*.
Restitution or external rotation. The fetal head turns 90° once outside the perineum to allow the shoulders to turn and pass through the wider diameter of the pelvis.
Expulsion. The anterior shoulder and then the posterior shoulder deliver under the symphysis pubis.

EXERCISE 4.69 Select all that apply:

The nurse understands that the baby is at high risk for:

A. Broken clavicle
B. Cephalhematoma
C. Caput succedaneum
D. Brachial plexus
E. Fractured humerus
F. Hydrocele

The answer can be found on page 324

EXERCISE 4.70 Multiple-choice:

The nurse understands that the proper interventions to expect at the delivery include:

A. Ritgen's maneuver, suction the infant's nose and then mouth
B. Suction the infant's nose, Ritgen's maneuver, and then suction the infant's mouth
C. Externally rotate the infant, Ritgen's maneuver, and suction the infant's mouth
D. Ritgen's maneuver, suction the infant's mouth and then nose

The answer can be found on page 324

UNFOLDING CASE STUDY 7: Baby Benjamin

The PCP places the baby on Ava's abdomen and cuts the cord.

EXERCISE 4.71 Fill in the blanks:

The umbilical cord should contain ___ vessels; there are two ________ and one _________.

The answer can be found on page 325

Ava's nurse remembers the important interventions for the baby after the delivery.

EXERCISE 4.72 Fill in the blanks:

One letter simply stands for a letter of the alphabet. See if you can break the code.

Y M N – A H W W D N O J O T Y M J C J G I

ONE— _ O N B _ _ _

W C Y – B G T

TWO— _ _ _

W D G N N – Z Y Q K W K Y M W D N D N J B

THREE— _ _ _ _ _ _ _ _ _ _ _ _ _ _ _ _ _ _

Z Y U G – Q H E W K Y M

FOUR— _ _ _ _ _ _ _

Z K X N – Q W K I H S J W N W Y O G N J W D N

FIVE— _

The answer can be found on page 325

EXERCISE 4.73 Matching:

Match the type of heat loss in Column A to the appropriate sentence in the neutral thermal environment (NTE) story in Column B:

Column A	Column B
A. Convection B. Evaporation C. Radiation D. Conduction	The delivery room nurse waits for the cord to be cut and carries the baby over to the bed, which is away from the windows to prevent __________, and away from the door, where people move quickly in and out to prevent __________ from air currents. The bed was warmed to prevent __________. The nurse vigorously dries the baby off to prevent cold stress from __________.

The answer can be found on page 325

Benjamin is 6 lb 4 ounces. He has central cyanosis and is hypotonic with poor reflexes. His respirations are gasping and he has a HR of 110 bpm. The nurse suctions him with the bulb syringe (mouth then nose) and provides him with free-flow or blow-by oxygen; the baby responds by crying.

EXERCISE 4.74 Fill in the blanks:

At 1 minute, the baby is responding to his extrauterine environment and is only acrocyanotic and slightly hyporeflexic with good reflexes. His respiratory rate is 70 breaths per minute and his HR is 170 bpm. The nurse assigns him an Apgar score of ______. At 5 minutes old, the baby is still acrocyanotic (which can be normal up to 24 hours) and has good reflexes and tone. His vital signs are 97.9°F axillary, HR 155 bpm, RR 60. His 5-minute Apgar score is _______.

The answer can be found on page 325

---

eRESOURCE

To verify your answer, consult MedCalc. [Pathway: www.medcalc.com ➔ select "Pediatrics" ➔ select "APGAR Score" and enter information into fields.]

EXERCISE 4.75 Select all that apply:

The delivery room nurse finishes the immediate care of the newborn; what interventions are normally completed in the delivery room?

A. Blood pressure measurement
B. Vital signs assessment
C. Identification bracelets and footprints completed
D. Vitamin K administered
E. Circumcision performed

The answer can be found on page 326

EXERCISE 4.76 Multiple-choice:

The nurse understands that the preferred site for an intramuscular (IM) injection of vitamin K for a newborn is the vastus lateralis because:

A. It is easily accessible
B. There is better blood flow in the legs
C. The dorsal gluteal is underdeveloped
D. Newborns have to sleep on their backs

The answer can be found on page 326

At 15 minutes, the placenta is delivered. The delivery nurse knows this is going to happen because of the four classic signs.

EXERCISE 4.77 Fill in the blanks:

Fill in the four classic signs of placental separation:

1. ____________________
2. ____________________
3. ____________________
4. ____________________

The answer can be found on page 326

If it is the shiny fetal side of the placenta that presents first, it is called *Schultz*; if it is the rough maternal side of the placenta that presents first, it is called *Duncan*. The fourth stage of labor is the recovery stage, which lasts 1 to 4 hours. Initially after delivery, the uterus contracts and is located between the symphysis pubis and the umbilicus. It then rises back up in the abdomen to the umbilicus and involutes 1 to 2 cm each day. It should be firm to the touch, and oxytocin (Pitocin) is often given after delivery to ensure the placenta contracts. Breastfeeding also helps it contract because the breastfeeding process releases indigenous oxytocin from the posterior pituitary gland. The lochia should be rubra and moderate in amount.

eRESOURCE

To verify your answer, consult Medscape on your mobile device. [Pathway: Medscape → enter "Labor" into the search field → select "Normal Labor and Delivery" and review content under "Intrapartum Management of Labor" focusing on the third stage of labor.]

UNFOLDING CASE STUDY 8: Paulette

Also on the L&D suite at this time is Paulette, who is a Class II cardiac patient in active labor. She had rheumatic heart disease when she was young and has had a valve replacement. Her pregnancy has gone well, but she was placed on modified bed rest during her third trimester to decrease the stress on her heart muscle.

EXERCISE 4.78 Select all that apply:

The nurse understands that manifestations of cardiac decompensation include:

A. Cough
B. Dyspnea
C. Edema
D. Heart murmur
E. Palpitations
F. Weight loss

The answer can be found on page 326

EXERCISE 4.79 Multiple-choice:

What kind of delivery would the nurse anticipate for Paulette in order to conserve cardiac output and maintain a more even thoracic pressure?

A. Cesarean
B. Natural vaginal birth
C. Low-forceps delivery
D. Midforceps delivery

The answer can be found on page 327

eRESOURCE

To supplement your understanding of the care required for a pregnant patient with cardiac disease; consult Medscape on your mobile device. [Pathway: Medscape ➔ enter "Pregnancy" into the search field ➔ select "Cardiovascular Disease and Pregnancy" and review content.]

eRESOURCE

To supplement your understanding of forceps delivery procedures, consult Medscape on your mobile device. [Pathway: Medscape ➔ select "Procedures" ➔ select "Obstetric and Gynecologic" ➔ select "Forceps Delivery Procedures" and review content.]

UNFOLDING CASE STUDY 9: Jacqueline

Right after Ava delivers, an emergency delivery is started and Ava can hear the commotion in the hall. Apparently, Jacqueline, the patient in the next room with hydramnios, had spontaneous rupture of membranes (SROM) and the baby's umbilical cord completely prolapsed.

EXERCISE 4.80 Multiple-choice:

The first nursing intervention for a prolapsed cord would be to:

A. Check the fetal heart rate (FHR)
B. Raise the patient's hips
C. Call the primary physician
D. Explain to the patient the baby will probably be born dead

The answer can be found on page 327

eRESOURCE

To learn more about your understanding of the management of an umbilical cord prolapse, refer to the *Merck Manual*. [Pathway: www.merckmanuals.com/professional → enter "Umbilical Cord Prolapse" into the search field → select "Umbilical Cord Prolapse" review content under "Overt Prolapse."]

UNFOLDING CASE STUDY 1 (CONTINUED): Ava

After Ava's delivery, postpartum assessments are completed by the nurse using the BUBBLE-HE (breasts, uterus, bladder, bowels, lochia, episiotomy, Homan's sign, edema/emotions) method:

EXERCISE 4.81 Fill in the blanks:

Use the following words to fill in the blanks in the BUBBLE-HE narrative in Table 4.6.

Ecchymosis
Taking hold
Rubra
Engorgement
Postpartum psychosis
Redness
Diuresis
Letting go
Deep vein thrombosis
Sulcus
Postpartum depression
Approximation
Hemorrhoids
Taking in
Edema
Serosa
Discharge
Afterbirth
Alba
Sims
Ambulation
Postpartum blues
Binding in

TABLE 4.6 Fill in for Exercise 4.81

B	Breasts	______ is the process of swelling of the breast tissue caused by an increase in blood and lymph supply as a precursor to lactation. This usually happens on postpartum days 3 to 5. On days 1 to 5, colostrum is secreted.
U	Uterus	Six to 12 hours after delivery, the fundus should be at the umbilicus. It then decreases 1 cm/d for approximately 10 days when it becomes a nonpalpable pelvic organ. Discomfort or cramping from involution is called _______pain. Afterbirth pains are increased in multiparous women, breastfeeders, and women with an overdistended uterus. Have the patient void before the examination.
B	Bladder	The bladder may be subjected to trauma that results in edema and diminished sensitivity to fluid pressure. This can lead to overdistention and incomplete emptying. Difficulty voiding may persist for the first 2 days. Hematuria reflects trauma or urinary tract infection. Acetone denotes dehydration after prolonged labor. _______ usually begins within 12 hours after delivery and eliminates excess body fluid.
B	Bowels	Bowel sounds (BS) should be assessed at each shift. Assess whether the patient is passing flatus. Use a high-fiber diet and increase fluid intake. Stool softeners (Colace) are usually ordered to decrease discomfort. Early______ should be encouraged.
L	Lochia	______ is the color of vaginal discharge for the first 3 to 4 days. It is a deep-red mixture of mucus, tissue debris, and blood. Lochia ______ starts from 3 to 10 days postpartum. It is pink to brown in color and contains leukocytes, decidual tissue, red blood cells, and serous fluid. Lochia ______ begins within 10 to 14 days and is creamy white or light brown in color and consists of leukocytes and decidua tissue. Lochia is described for quantity as scant, small, moderate, or large.
E	Episiotomy or incision if cesarean section	Episiotomy/laceration or cesarean incision repair should be assessed each shift. Use the REEDA acronym to assess and describe. If the patient had an episiotomy, laceration that was repaired, or a cesarean incision, that surgical site should be further assessed using the REEDA acronym. Fill in what the letters stand for: R: ______ E: ______ E: ______ D: ______ A: ______ Inspection of an episiotomy/laceration is best done in a lateral ______ position with a pen light. ______ are distended rectal veins and can be uncomfortable. Care measures include ice packs for the first 24 hours, peri bottle washing after each void, sitz baths, witch hazel pads (Tucks), and hydrocortisone cream. *Classifications of Perineal Lacerations*: First-degree laceration involves only skin and superficial structures above muscle.

(continued)

TABLE 4.6 Fill in for Exercise 4.81 (*continued*)

		Second-degree laceration extends through perineal muscles. Third-degree laceration extends through the anal sphincter muscle. Fourth-degree laceration continues through anterior rectal wall. *Classifications of Episiotomies*: Midline is made from the posterior vaginal vault toward the rectum. Right mediolateral is made from the vaginal vault to the right buttock. Left mediolateral is made on the left side. Mediolateral incisions increase room and decrease rectal tearing, but midline episiotomies heal easier. A ______tear is a tear through the vaginal wall. A cervical tear is an actual tear in the cervix of the uterus. This bleeds profusely.
H	Homan's	Positive Homan's sign may be present when there is a deep vein thrombosis of the leg. To elicit a Homan's sign, passive dorsiflexion of the ankle produces pain in the patient's leg. Postpartum is a state of hypercoagulability and moms are at 30% higher risk for _______.
E	Edema or emotional	*Pedal edema* should be assessed on postpartum patients as they have massive fluid shifts right after delivery. Pedal edema can indicate overhydration in labor, hypertension, or lack of normal diuresis. *Emotional assessment* must be made on each postpartum family. Initially, maternal touch of the newborn is by fingertip in an en face position that progresses to full hand touch. The mom should draw the infant close and usually strokes the baby. ______ is when the mother identifies specific features about the baby such as who he or she looks like. These are claiming behaviors. Verbal behavior is noticed because most mothers speak to infants in a high-pitched voice and progress from calling the baby "it" to "he" or "she," then they progress to using the baby's name. *Rubin (1984) describes three stages of maternal adjustment:* ______ (1–2 days). In this phase, the mother is passive and dependent as well as preoccupied with self. This is the time she reviews the birth experience. ______ (3–10 days). This is when she resumes control over her life and becomes concerned about self-care. During this time, she gains self-confidence as a mother. ______ (2–4 weeks). This is when she accomplishes maternal role attainment and makes relationship adjustments. *Emotional postpartum states:* ______are mood disorders that occur in most women usually within the first 4 weeks. They are hormonal in origin and are called *baby blues*. ______ should be assessed on every woman and is a true depressive state that affects daily function. ______ is a mental health illness characterized by delusions.

The answer can be found on page 327

UNFOLDING CASE STUDY 7 (CONTINUED): Baby Benjamin

Ava's baby boy, Benjamin, is tachypnic or has a resting respiratory rate (RRR) above 60 breaths per minute. Benjamin is also manifesting other common signs of respiratory distress.

EXERCISE 4.82 Multiple-choice:

The nurse understands that an infant may be manifesting signs of respiratory distress when the mother tells her:

A. "My baby is sleeping peacefully but his eyes look like they are moving under his lids."
B. "I can see that my baby stops breathing for about 10 seconds sometimes."
C. "My baby's breathing is very uneven, it is sometimes fast and at other times is slow."
D. "I love when my baby makes that squeaking sound every time he breaths."

The answer can be found on page 330

The newborn nursery nurse checks his pulse oximeter and it is 90% when placed on his left foot. The nurse calls the pediatrician, who calls for a neonatology consult, which is done by a neonatal nurse practitioner (NNP). The NNP transfers the baby to the neonatal intensive care unit (NICU) to be placed on an oxygen hood. A complete head-to-toe physical examination is done on Benjamin when he arrives in the NICU.

eRESOURCE

To learn more about the management of respiratory distress in neonates, refer to the *Merck Manual*. [Pathway: www.merckmanuals.com/professional → enter "Respiratory Distress Neonate" into the search field → select "Overview of Perinatal Respiratory Disorders" → review content under "Etiology," "Physiology," and "Evaluation."]

EXERCISE 4.83 Hot spot:

Place an X on the sagittal suture on the infant's head.

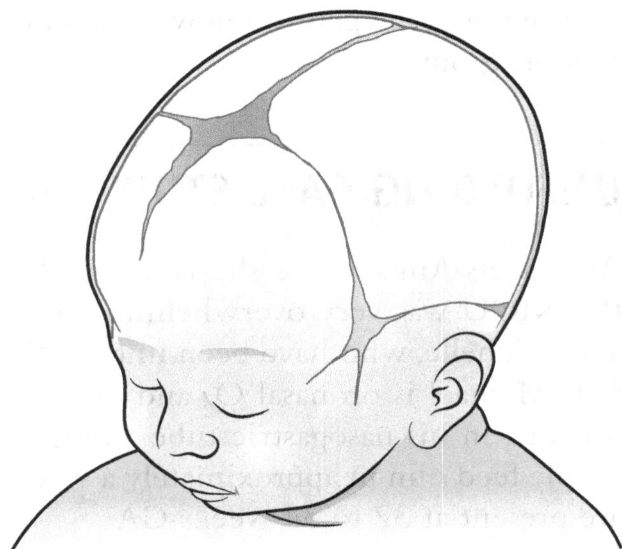

The answer can be found on page 330

EXERCISE 4.84 Matching:

Match the terms in Column A to the correct descriptions in Column B:

Column A	Column B
A. Universal newborn hearing screen (UNHS)	___ Folds on thigh
B. Epstein pearls	___ Edematous scrotum
C. Frenulum	___ Startle reflex
D. Crepitus	___ Hand-grasp object
E. Xiphoid	___ Ligament under tongue
F. Brachial	___ Palpation of bone over bone
G. Gluteal	___ Sebaceous cysts on hard palate
H. Ortolani	___ Toes spread when sole is stimulated
I. Hydrocele	___ Stops responding to repetitive stimuli
J. Pilonidal	___ End of sternum
K. Moro	___ Maneuver to check for hip dysplasia
L. Habituation	___ Used to rule out congenital deafness
M. Palmar grasp	___ Toes curl around an object
N. Plantar grasp	___ Indentation at the base of spine
O. Babinski reflex	___ Pulse found in arm

The answer can be found on page 331

Benjamin's vital signs are assessed every 3 to 4 hours during the first 24 hours to observe for signs of neonatal sepsis from vertical transmission (transmitted in the perinatal period). Ava is feeling well and goes over to the NICU to visit Benjamin frequently. While she is in the unit, she gets to know some of the other parents and they develop an informal support group.

UNFOLDING CASE STUDY 10: Michael and Michelle

Ava meets Anna while she is in the NICU. Anna is very familiar with the NICU; the NICU was very overwhelming to Ava at first. Anna has growing twins, Michael and Michelle, who have been in the NICU for 24 days. They were born at 28 weeks GA. Michael is on nasal O_2 and dressed in an open crib. He is tolerating premature formula in his nasogastric tube and growing appropriately. They are going to try to nipple feed him in approximately a week because the sucking and swallowing reflexes are present at 32 to 34 weeks GA.

EXERCISE 4.85 Calculation:

Yesterday Michael gained 15 g. How would you express that to Anna in ounces? ____ ounces

The answer can be found on page 331

eRESOURCE

To verify your answer, consult MedCalc. [Pathway: www.medcalc.com ➔ select "General" ➔ select "Weights and Measures" and enter information into weight conversion fields.]

Michelle is still in an incubator to maintain a neutral thermal environment (NTE) but she is breathing unassisted. Michelle was diagnosed with intraventricular hemorrhage (IVH) grade I, which is a bleeding into the ventricles of the brain; preterm babies have fragile vessels that are very susceptible to intracranial pressure changes. Michelle also had blood replacement for anemia as iron (Fe) is stored in the last months of pregnancy and she did not have that advantage. Michelle is also on caffeine to decrease her apnea and bradycardia episodes, which are common in preterm infants as a result of immature respiratory regulation.

EXERCISE 4.86 Multiple-choice:

The nurse understands that Michelle may need tactile stimulation in the following situation:

A. Her breathing is irregular and at a rate of 62 breaths per minute.
B. She is yawning excessively and turning away from her caregiver.
C. Her breathing stops periodically but resumes within 15 seconds with coughing.
D. She stops breathing for 20 seconds and does not cough or make sucking motions.

The answer can be found on page 331

eRESOURCE

To learn more about the care of the premature infant, refer to the *Merck Manual*. [Pathway: www.merckmanuals.com/professional ➔ enter "Premature" into the search field ➔ select "Premature Infant" review content, focusing on "Symptoms and Signs" and "Treatment."]

UNFOLDING CASE STUDY 11: William

The newborn in the open crib next to the twins is a postterm baby (more than 42 weeks GA) whose mother had only two prenatal visits at the clinic. William is 48 hours old and is becoming jaundiced as a result of polycythemia (venous Hct greater than 60%). He looks different from the preterm infants because he has dry, cracked, wrinkled skin and long, thin extremities. He is only 5 lb and 1 oz.

EXERCISE 4.87 Multiple-choice:

William is 42 weeks gestation and weighs 5 lb and 1 oz. This would most likely classify him as:

A. Small for gestational age (SGA)
B. Large for gestational age (LGA)
C. Average for gestational age (AGA)
D. Preterm

The answer can be found on page 332

eRESOURCE

To learn more about assessing GA, refer to the *Merck Manual.* [Pathway: www.merckmanuals.com/professional ➔ enter "Gestational Age" into the search field ➔ select "Gestational Age" and review content. You may also wish to review content under "Small-for-Gestational-Age (SGA) Infant" and "Large-for-Gestational-Age (LGA) Infant."]

There was meconium in the amniotic fluid when William was born and he was suctioned to prevent meconium aspiration syndrome (MAS), which can predispose a newborn to persistent pulmonary hypertension (PPN).

eRESOURCE

To learn more about MAS, refer to the *Merck Manual.* [Pathway: www.merckmanuals.com/professional ➔ enter "Meconium" into the search field ➔ select "Meconium Aspiration Syndrome" review content.]

PPN is serious and sometimes requires a risky procedure that is only done at well-equipped tertiary NICU centers. This procedure is called *extracorporeal membrane oxygenation* (ECMO) and is a mechanical heart/lung support.

eRESOURCE

To reinforce your understanding of the clinical presentation of PPN and its treatment, refer to Medscape on your mobile device. [Pathway: Medscape ➔ enter "Persistent Pulmonary Hypertension" into the search field ➔ select "Persistent Newborn Pulmonary Hypertension" and review content.]

William has been observed on a cardiorespiratory (CR) monitor and is being maintained without oxygen. Now at 48 hours old, William is displaying some irritability and hypertonicity. A drug screen that had been done on William's urine and meconium was positive for cocaine. Now he is being assessed every 3 hours for neonatal abstinence syndrome (NAS) using a scale that includes the following manifestations to assess the extent of his discomfort (Exhibit 4.2).

EXHIBIT 4.2 Neonatal Abstinence Syndrome (NAS) Manifestations

WITHDRAWAL Acronym for NAS
W = Wakefulness
I = Irritability
T = Temperature variation, tachycardia, tremors
H = Hyperactivity, high-pitched cry, hyperreflexia, hypertonus
D = Diarrhea, diaphoresis, disorganized suck
R = Respiratory distress, rub marks, rhinorrhea
A = Apneic attacks, autonomic dysfunction
W = Weight loss or failure to gain weight
A = Alkalosis (respiratory)
L = Lacrimation

EXERCISE 4.88 Select all that apply:

Which nursing interventions would be done for neonates experiencing neonatal abstinence syndrome (NAS)?

A. Hold in an upright position
B. Provide a pacifier
C. Obtain an order to medicate for moderate to severe withdrawal symptoms
D. Keep the lights on
E. Encourage parental participation
F. Undress under warmer
G. Provide a quiet environment
H. Provide good skin care to decrease diaper rash

The answer can be found on page 332

eRESOURCE

To learn more about prenatal drug exposure, refer to the *Merck Manual.* [Pathway: www.merckmanuals.com/professional → enter "Prenatal Drug Exposure" into the search field → select "Prenatal Drug Exposure" → review content, focusing on content under "Cocaine."]

UNFOLDING CASE STUDY 12: Mia

The newborn in the same room with Michael and Michelle is Mia, who is a preterm infant delivered 4 hours ago at 25 weeks GA. Mia has a patent ductus arteriosis (PDA) that cannot be addressed with indomethacin (Indocin) because she is on high-frequency ventilation. She was given surfactant in the delivery room via her endotracheal tube to decrease the respiratory distress.

eRESOURCE

To reinforce your understanding of the clinical presentation and management of PDA, refer to Medscape on your mobile device. [Pathway: Medscape ➔ enter "PDA" into the search field ➔ select "Patent Ductus Arteriosis (PDA)" and review content.]

One of the conditions that Mia is at risk of is retinopathy of prematurity (ROP) because of high concentrations of oxygen and its effect on the eyes.

EXERCISE 4.89 Multiple-choice:

The nurse understands that the best intervention to protect Mia from retinopathy of prematurity (ROP) is to:

A. Use eye covers while Mia is receiving oxygen
B. Keep the oxygen flow at a consistent level
C. Use as little oxygen as needed
D. Intermittently take Mia off oxygen for short periods

The answer can be found on page 332

ROP is a condition related directly to prolonged O_2 use that causes abnormal growth of blood vessels in the retina and can lead to blindness. This NICU unit has periodic eye checks for all the newborns who are born before 34 weeks, weigh under 1,500 g, or receive oxygen for an extended period of time. If ROP occurs, it can be treated with laser therapy.

eRESOURCE

To reinforce your understanding of ROP and related treatment, refer to the *Merck Manual.* [Pathway: www.merckmanuals.com/professional ➔ enter "ROP" into the search field ➔ select "Retinopathy of Prematurity" ➔ review content.]

UNFOLDING CASE STUDY 13: Dominic

Another patient in the NICU is Dominic. He is a growing preterm infant who had gastric surgery for necrotizing enterocolitis (NEC). He is now tolerating oral feedings of pumped breast milk and is gaining weight. NEC is a condition in which a section of the bowel becomes ischemic and often infected as a result of hypoxia in prematurity, although it can occur in term infants.

EXERCISE 4.90 Select all that apply:

To assess a newborn for necrotizing enterocolitis (NEC), the nurse should:

A. Measure the abdominal circumference
B. Check for aspirates
C. Take an x-ray before each feed
D. Check bowel sounds
E. Weigh every 2 hours

The answer can be found on page 332

EXERCISE 4.91 Select all that apply:

The nursing interventions for a newborn with suspected necrotizing enterocolitis (NEC) are:

A. Increase breast-milk feedings
B. Keep nothing orally (NPO) status
C. Suction vigorously
D. Call the primary care provider (PCP)
E. No longer check for aspirates

The answer can be found on page 333

eRESOURCE

To reinforce your understanding of the clinical presentation and management of NEC, refer to Medscape on your mobile device. [Pathway: Medscape → enter "Necrotizing Enterocolitis" into the search field → select "Necrotizing Enterocolitis" and review content, focusing on "Practice Essentials" and "Treatment and Management."]

UNFOLDING CASE STUDY 14: Chandelle

Chandelle is a 35-week GA newborn who is on isolation because she has *cytomegalovirus (CMV)*. When she was born, her physical examination showed that she was *microcephalic* (head circumference below the 10th percentile). CMV was cultured during the TORCH (toxoplasmosis; other infections, including treponema pallidum, varicella-zoster virus [VZV], and parvovirus B19; rubella virus; CMV; and herpes simplex virus [HSV]) studies that were done on chandelle. TORCH is a group of infections (Table 4.7) that can cross the placenta and harm the fetus, especially if exposure occurs during the first 12 weeks of pregnancy. During organogenesis, fetuses can cause developmental anomalies. Chandelle's mother is very attentive to her and is often in the NICU caring for her. She is knowledgeable about CMV, but often verbalizes that she is overwhelmed and depressed at the prospect of having a chronically ill child.

eRESOURCE

To reinforce your understanding of CMV, refer to Medscape on your mobile device. [Pathway: Medscape → enter "CMV" into the search field → select "CMV" and review content.]

EXERCISE 4.92 Multiple-choice:

An appropriate nursing intervention for a mother experiencing chronic sorrow is:

A. Tell her that it could be worse
B. Encourage her to look on the bright side
C. Distract her thoughts to something else
D. Encourage her to verbalize

The answer can be found on page 333

TABLE 4.7 TORCH Infections

T	*Toxoplasmosis* is an infection caused by a parasite, *Toxoplasma gondii*, which results from ingesting undercooked meat or contact with cat feces. Signs in the mom are fatigue, malaise, and muscle pain. It is diagnosed by IgM flourescent antibody testing. It is treated with 21 to 30 days of sulfadiazine. If contracted before 20 weeks, it can cause spontaneous abortion; preterm delivery; stillbirth; anomalies, including enlarged liver and spleen; or inflamed retinas, which may not appear until adolescence.
O	*Other* *Treponema pallidum* is the bacteria that causes syphilis (please refer to the STD section). *Varicella-zoster virus* (*VZV;* chickenpox) is a herpes virus transmitted via the respiratory tract or direct contact. The latent form is shingles. If the fetus is infected in the first trimester, it can cause limb hypoplasia, cutaneous scars, cataracts, microcephaly, and intrauterine growth restriction (IUGR). Neonatal varicella syndrome carries a 30% incidence of death even with varicella-zoster globulin (VZIG). *Parvovirus B19* (fifth disease). This virus can lead to hydrops fetalis if contracted in first 20 weeks. It has a distinctive facial rash.
R	*Rubella*. Droplet-transmitted virus to which 20% of adults are susceptible. Etiology— It crosses placental barrier; test mom for titre. Signs in mother are general malaise, and maculopapular rash. If the fetus is affected during the first trimester, it can cause deafness, cardiac malformation, cataracts, mental retardation, IUGR, microcephaly, spontaneous abortion, and can be contagious for months.
C	*Cytomegalovirus* (*CMV*)—Affects 3,000 infants per year and is the most prevalent of the TORCH infections. The mother is usually asymptomatic. CMV can cross the placenta and cause the fetus to be deaf, blind, have seizures, and causes dental deformities. Diagnosis is done by culturing the virus in urine and finding elevated IgM in the infant's blood.
H	*Herpes simplex virus* (see STI section).

IgM, immunoglobulin M; STD, sexually transmitted disease; STI, sexually transmitted infection.

eRESOURCE

To reinforce your understanding of therapeutic communication, refer to Nursing Planet. [Pathway: http://nursingplanet.com ➔ select "Mental Health Nursing" ➔ scroll down to the "Assessment and Evaluation" section and select "Therapeutic Communication" and review the content.

UNFOLDING CASE STUDY 15: Felix

Ironically, next to the preterm infants in the NICU is a 10 lb 4 oz boy named Felix. Felix is 40 weeks GA and his mom was a gestational diabetic whose diabetes was poorly controlled. Therefore, Felix is hypoglycemic. Felix is 48 hours old and is being weaned off a glucose IV. At birth, his blood glucose level at 30 minutes old was 24 mg/dL, and after gavaging 50 mL of formula, his glucose was 52 mg/dL at 1 hour. At 2 hours, it was down to 30 mg/dL and he was transferred to the NICU and an

IV of glucose was started. He has had 12 hours of normal glucose levels and is being weaned off the IV.

EXERCISE 4.93 Multiple-choice:

The nurse shows an understanding of the pathophysiology of neonatal hypoglycemia when she states:

A. "Infants of diabetic mothers have glucose levels that fluctuate from hyperglycemia to hypoglycemia in the first 24 hours."
B. "Infants of diabetic mothers need extra feedings because of hyperinsulinemia."
C. "Infants of diabetic mothers are hypersensitive to insulin infusions."
D. "Infants of diabetic mothers are always overweight."

The answer can be found on page 333

---

eRESOURCE

To reinforce your understanding of neonatal hypoglycemia and related treatment, refer to the *Merck Manual.* [Pathway: www.merckmanuals.com/professional ➔ enter "Neonatal Hypoglycemia" into the search field ➔ select "Neonatal Hypoglycemia" ➔ review content.]

EXERCISE 4.94 Select all that apply:

Felix is over the 90th percentile on the growth chart, which would classify him or place him at risk for the following manifestations or conditions:

A. Small for gestational age (SGA)
B. Broken clavicle
C. Brachial plexis injury
D. Average for gestational age (AGA)
E. Patent ductus arteriosis (PDA)

The answer can be found on page 333

---

eRESOURCE

To reinforce your understanding of neonatal hypoglycemia and related treatment, refer to the *Merck Manual.* [Pathway: www.merckmanuals.com/professional ➔ enter "Growth Parameters" into the search field ➔ select "Growth Parameters in Neonates" ➔ review content.]

UNFOLDING CASE STUDY 1 (CONTINUED): Ava

Ava has been pumping her breasts while Benjamin was in the NICU. After 48 hours, Benjamin's transitional tachypnea of the newborn (TTN) resolved, and he was readmitted to the newborn nursery for assessment and care, which will include Ava's discharge instructions. Ava also puts Benjamin to breast and he does fairly well, as you can see by his LATCH score (8; Exhibit 4.3).

EXHIBIT 4.3 LATCH Score

L = Latch—Benjamin latches by himself = 2
A = Audible suck—Benjamin has an audible suck 50% of the time = 1
T = Type of nipple—Ava's nipples are everted = 2
C = Comfort—at this point, Ava is comfortable with no soreness = 2
H = Hold—Ava needs help positioning belly to belly = 1

Infant-feeding principles are reviewed with Ava for discharge care.

EXERCISE 4.95 Select all that apply:

Correct information about bottle-feeding infants includes:

A. Mom should use heat packs to her breast
B. Recommended daily amount (RDA) of formula is 100 to 115 kcal/kg/d
C. There are 30 kcal in each ounce of newborn formula
D. Mothers lose 20 lb initially after delivery
E. Formula-fed infants should be at birth weight at approximately 10 days old

The answer can be found on page 334

EXERCISE 4.96 Select all that apply:

Correct information about breastfeeding infants includes:

A. Breastfeeding mothers should limit their fluid intake to avoid engorgement
B. Breastfeeding mothers should nurse every 4 hours
C. Warm showers help the milk flow
D. A supportive bra should be worn
E. Breastfeeding mothers should only nurse 20 minutes on each side

The answer can be found on page 334

EXERCISE 4.97 Matching:

Match the stage of milk in Column A with the description in Column B:

Column A	Column B
A. Colostrum	____ is produced in the beginning of the feeding
B. Transitional milk	____ is produced after letdown and is high in fat
C. Foremilk	____ is the first milk and it lasts 2 to 4 days; it is high in protein, vitamins, minerals, and immunoglobulin A (IgA)
D. Hind milk	____ starts at engorgement or 4 days to 2 weeks

The answer can be found on page 334

Benjamin's blood type is B+; so Ava receives RhoGAM. If the newborn's blood type is Rh^+ and the mother is Rh^-, this is given to prevent the mother's immune system from recognizing the Rh^+ antigens and building up permanent antibodies. The Rh immune globulin is a solution of gamma globulin, and is given via IM or IV within 72 hours after birth. It will attach to the anti-D antigens of the fetal blood that have passed into the maternal circulation, thereby preventing the maternal cells from building up antibodies.

EXERCISE 4.98 Fill in the blank:

The usual procedure for Rh^+ babies/Rh^- mothers is a 300-mcg dose of RhoGAM, and a _________ test, which detects fetal cells in the maternal blood. This is followed if a large feto–maternal transfusion is suspected. A larger dose can be given if needed.

The answer can be found on page 334

Ava's baby is B^+ and there is a positive Coombs test (which shows an antibody–antigen reaction has taken place). There is an ABO incompatibility reaction. ABO incompatibilities are never life threatening like Rh incompatibilities, but can cause neonatal jaundice. The antibody buildup in Ava caused hemolysis of the fetal cells.

eRESOURCE

To supplement your understanding of RhoGAM, refer to Epocrates Online. [Pathway: http://online.epocrates.com ➔ under the "Drugs" tab, enter "RhoGAM" in the search field ➔ select "RhoGAM" ➔ review "Adult Dosing," "Adverse Reactions," and "Safety/Monitoring."]

EXERCISE 4.99 Multiple-choice:

Hemolysis of fetal cells increases the likelihood of what neonatal condition?

A. Hypoglycemia
B. Hyperglycemia
C. Hyperbilirubinemia
D. Hypocalcemia

The answer can be found on page 334

A heel-stick total bilirubin test is drawn on Benjamin.

EXERCISE 4.100 Multiple-choice:

The nurse is careful to do the heel stick on the side of the heel in order to prevent:

A. Pain
B. Hemorrhage
C. Cellulites
D. Foot drop

The answer can be found on page 335

Jaundice should be assessed in the newborn. If it appears in the first 24 hours, it is considered to be pathological, and could indicate a blood dyscrasia. The blanch test differentiates jaundice from skin color. It is performed by applying pressure with the thumb to the infant's forehead, causing emptying of skin capillaries. When the pressure is released, the capillaries should fill with blood and return to a pink color. If the skin appears "yellow" before the capillaries fill, this is indicative of jaundice.

The total bilirubin test comes back 13.6 mg/dL at 48 hours with a weakly positive Coombs test. Bilirubin is a by-product of broken down red blood cells (RBCs), and is normally excreted by the liver. A newborn's liver is immature and sometimes cannot handle the bilirubin from the breakdown of fetal Hgb cells, which are more plentiful than adult Hgb and have a shorter life span. The unconjugated or indirect bilirubin circulates in the newborn's system and binds to a large albumin molecule, which makes it inaccessible to kidney excretion. Albumin-bound bilirubin is then conjugated (direct) by the liver enzyme glucuronyl transferase and excreted in bile (H_2O soluble) into the biliary tree and transported to the intestinal tract. The GI tract reduces it to urobilinogen using bacteria and excretes it in stool as yellow-brown pigment. If hyperbilirubinemia is not treated and becomes pathological, it can cross the blood–brain barrier and produce a condition called *kernicterus* or *bilirubin encephalopathy*, which can be fatal or lead to mental retardation.

EXERCISE 4.101 Multiple-choice:

The most important nursing intervention to decrease the incidence of newborn hyperbilirubinemia is:

A. Prevent cold stress
B. Early and frequent feeds
C. Placing the baby near the window of the nursery
D. Keeping the baby in the nursery at night

The answer can be found on page 335

Benjamin is placed on phototherapy, because light breaks down bilirubin or photooxidizes it in the skin. The by-products are water soluble and can be excreted in the bile.

EXERCISE 4.102 Select all that apply:

Select all the nursing interactions that are appropriate when caring for a newborn under phototherapy.

A. Cover the eyes and genitalia
B. Maintain a neutral thermal environment (NTE)
C. Early and frequent feeds
D. Dress the newborn to prevent cold stress
E. Check light-source strength with a light meter

The answer can be found on page 335

EXHIBIT 4.4 Nursing Interventions for a Newborn Circumcision Procedure

Make sure vitamin K is given
Informed consent
Have suction handy
Restrain
Antibiotic cream with surgical removal (not with a plastibell)
Check voiding and chart (before and after)
Gauze wrap
Keep clean and dry
Bleeding—apply pressure

eRESOURCE

To reinforce your understanding of the clinical presentation and management of jaundice, refer to Medscape on your mobile device. [Pathway: Medscape → enter "Jaundice" into the search field → select "Neonatal Jaundice" and review content.]

Ava signed the informed consent for her baby to have a circumcision. The nurse is aware of all the interventions that are needed for a circumcision (Exhibit 4.4).

eRESOURCE

To reinforce your understanding of the circumcision procedure and subsequent care, refer to Medscape on your mobile device. [Pathway: Medscape → enter "Circumcision" into the search field → select "Circumcision" and review content.]

In addition, before Ava is discharged with Benjamin, a newborn or metabolic screening is done to detect inborn errors of metabolism. A blood test is performed by heel stick after 24 hours of postoral intake. Four circles of blood are filled in on special absorbing paper and sent to the state lab. Hep B vaccine is also given to Benjamin before going home. The second dose will be given in 1 to 2 months, and the third within 6 months.

UNFOLDING CASE STUDY 16: Sophia

Also in the newborn nursery is a baby girl Sophia. Her mother was HIV positive.

EXERCISE 4.103 Fill in the blanks:

The nurse would be expected to give Sophia zidovudine (AZT) for ______________ weeks at 2 mg/kg every 12 hours. What route is used? ______________.

The answer can be found on page 335

EXERCISE 4.104 Calculation:

Sophia weighs 7 lb, 4 oz. How much Sophia zidovudine (AZT) do you give at each 12-hour dose? (The order reads 2 mg/kg every 12 hr.) ____________

The answer can be found on page 335

eRESOURCE

To reinforce your understanding of zidovudine, refer to Medscape on your mobile device. [Pathway: Medscape ➔ enter "Zidovudine" into the search field ➔ select "Zidovudine" and review content.]

Answers

EXERCISE 4.1 Multiple-choice:

The nurse understands that when a 16-year-old reveals she is sexually active with a 20-year-old male, the implications are:

A. The nurse should counsel the teenager against continuing the relationship.—NO; this is not the nurse's role and it will decrease the trust in the nurse–patient relationship.

B. The nurse is obligated to tell the teenager's parents.—NO; this is not the nurse's role and it will decrease the trust in the nurse–patient relationship.

C. The teenager is emancipated as a result of being sexually active.—NO; this may be true, but the circumstances are different because of the ages of the participants.

D. The nurse may be obligated to tell authorities.—**YES; this may qualify as statutory rape because the man is older than 18 years and Ava is not.**

EXERCISE 4.2 Matching:

Classify each method listed by matching the type of birth control (BC) in Column A with the method in Column B (the methods in Column A may be used more than once):

Column A	Column B
A. Mechanical	__A__ Condom
B. Hormonal/chemical	__B__ Vaginal ring (NuvaRing)
C. Surgical	__C__ Tubal ligation
	__B__ Morning-after pill (emergency contraception)
	__A__ Silicone tubal occlusion plug
	__B__ BC pills
	__A__ Intrauterine device
	__C__ Male vasectomy
	__B__ BC implants (Nexplanon/Implanon)
	__B__ BC patch (Ortho Erva)

(continued)

Column A	Column B
	A Diaphragm
	A Cervical Cap (FemCap)
	B BC shot (Depo-Provera)
	A Abstinence
	B BC sponge (Today Sponge)
	A Female condom
	A Fertility awareness method (FAMs)
	A Outercourse
	B Spermicide
	A Withdrawal

EXERCISE 4.3 Fill in the blanks:

Which birth control (BC) method is most effective against sexually transmitted diseases (STDs)?

Condom

Which BC method may be ineffective with the antibiotic rifampin?

BC pills

Which BC method can be effective for 5 or 10 years?

Intrauterine devices (IUDs)

Which BC method may not be effective if the patient is more than 200 lb?

BC patch

Which BC method is implanted under the skin?

BC implants (Nexplanon)

Which BC method is administered intramuscularly (IM)?

BC shot (Depo-Provera)

EXERCISE 4.4 Multiple-choice:

The nurse understands that Ava needs additional information when she states:

A. "If I use the pills and I miss a day I may need emergency contraception."—**YES; this is not true, after 1 day, Ava can catch up the next day**.

B. "I can use the RU-486 pill as emergency contraception."—NO; this is true but not the best method.

C. "If I become sick, I should tell my primary care provider (PCP) that I am on birth control (BC) before he or she prescribes antibiotics."—NO; this is true and a good idea.

D. "If I skip my progesterone-only pill I should take it as soon as I remember."—NO; this is true.

EXERCISE 4.5 Multiple-choice:

The nurse also tells Ava about Gardasil, the quadrivalent vaccine to prevent which sexually transmitted disease (STD)?

A. Hepatitis B (hep B)—NO; this is not the immunization for hep B.
B. Herpes type II—NO; this is not for herpes type II.
C. Herpes zoster—NO; this is not the immunization for herpes zoster or singles.
D. Human papillomavirus (HPV)—**YES**.

EXERCISE 4.6 Multiple-choice:

The nurse explains that Gardasil is given to:

A. Both men and women to prevent cervical and penile human papillomavirus (HPV), which can cause cancer—**YES; it is given to people of both genders to prevent cancer**.
B. Both men and women to prevent cervical cancer and penile dysfunction disease—NO; it is not for penile dysfunction.
C. Just women, to prevent cervical warts and vulva cancers—NO; it is not just for women.
D. Just men, to prevent genital warts and penile and testicular cancer—NO; it is not just for men.

EXERCISE 4.7 Matching:

Match the hormones in Column A to the effects in Column B:

Column A	Column B
A. Luteinizing hormone (LH)	C Under the influence of this hormone from the anterior pituitary gland, the ova matures during days 5 to 13.
B. Progesterone	B The *corpus luteum* produces this hormone along with estrogen.
C. Follicle-stimulating hormone (FSH)	A This hormone surges for 48 hours on day 12 to produce ovulation.

EXERCISE 4.8 Multiple-choice:

The nurse is counseling Ava and realizes that she needs further information when she states:

A. "I can't take emergency contraception because it has been 4 days since I had sex." —**YES; emergency contraception can be taken up to 5 days after unprotected sex.**
B. "I may have some slight side effects but they should not be severe."—NO; this is a true statement about treatment.
C. "My next period should come about the same time it is supposed to."—NO; this is a true statement.
D. "I know that emergency contraception is most likely not causing an abortion."—NO; this is a true statement because emergency contraception is thought to prevent sperm mobility before conception can occur.

EXERCISE 4.9 Select all that apply:

Possible side effects of high-dose progesterone pills include:

A. Nausea—**YES; nausea is a side effect of high-dose estrogen and progesterone 23% of the time.**
B. Vomiting—**YES; some women vomit with this treatment.**
C. Rash—NO; a rash is not usually a side effect.
D. Diarrhea—**YES; this is a possible side effect.**
E. Bleeding—**YES; 17% experience vaginal bleeding.**

EXERCISE 4.10 Multiple-choice:

The nurse tells Ava about another method of emergency contraception that is 99% effective but Ava does not consider it because in the past it has had some bad publicity concerning uterine infection rates. Therefore, Ava rejects the suggestion of using a(n):

A. Diaphragm—NO; this is not the method that was difficult in the past but is safe to use currently.
B. Vaginal ring—NO; this is not the method that was difficult in the past but is safe to use currently.
C. Intrauterine device—**YES; this is the one that is now safe**.
D. Female condom—NO; this is not the method that was difficult in the past but is safe to use currently.

EXERCISE 4.11 Multiple-choice:

At-home pregnancy tests detect which of the following hormones in the urine?

A. Progesterone—NO; progesterone is not detected.
B. Estrogen—NO; the test is not sensitive for estrogen, which is normally found in females.
C. Prolactin—NO; prolactin production should not be initiated yet.
D. Human chorionic gonadotropin (hCG)—**YES; hCG is the hormone found in urine**.

EXERCISE 4.12 Select all that apply:

Positive signs of pregnancy include the following:

A. Ultrasound—**YES; verification of embryo or fetus (4–6 weeks) or auscultation of fetal heart (FH) tones via Doppler (10–12 weeks). Doppler uses high-frequency sound waves to detect FH movement.**
B. Chadwick's sign—NO; this is a probable sign at 6 to 8 weeks.
C. Hegar's sign—NO; this is a probable sign at 6 to 12 weeks.
D. Fetal movement felt by the mother—NO; this is a possible sign (quickening) at 18 to 20 weeks.
E. Fetal movement felt by the examiner—**YES; this is a positive sign**.

EXERCISE 4.13 Matching:

Match the terms in Column A with the definitions in Column B:

Column A	Column B
A. Quickening	C Reflex of the fetus moving away from the examiner's fingers
B. Braxton–Hicks contractions	D Softening of the cervix
C. Ballottement	A Maternal perception of feeling the baby move
D. Goodell's sign	F Softening of the lower uterine segment
E. Chadwick's sign	B False labor contractions
F. Hegar's sign	E Increase vascularity and blueness to cervix

EXERCISE 4.14 Multiple-choice:

Using Naegel's rule, Ava's baby is due on:

A. March 8—NO; this is not correct if you count back 3 months, add 7 days, and increase the year by 1 if needed.
B. May 8—NO; this is not correct if you count back 3 months, add 7 days, and increase the year by 1 if needed.
C. April 1—NO; this is not correct if you count back 3 months, add 7 days, and increase the year by 1 if needed.
D. April 8—**YES; this is 10 lunar months, 9 calendar months, 40 weeks or 280 days from July 1**.

EXERCISE 4.15 Select all that apply:

During Ava's first prenatal visit, an assessment is performed and plans are being made. Select all the appropriate components of a first prenatal visit.

A. Blood drawn for type and Rh—**YES; this is needed to understand whether Ava will need RhoGAM at 28 weeks and possibly after delivery.**
B. Amniocentesis—NO; this is done at 18 to 20 weeks for genetic studies, or in the third trimester for lung maturity studies.
C. Venereal Disease Research Laboratory (VDRL) test or rapid plasma reagin (RPR) test—**YES; this is done to make sure that Ava does not have a sexually transmitted disease (STD).**
D. Dietary history—**YES; this is done to make sure that Ava's prenatal nutrition is adequate.**
E. Nonstress test (NST)—NO; this is done in the third trimester for fetal well-being.

EXERCISE 4.16 Multiple-choice:

It is clear Ava needs more information about immunizations when she states:

A. "I know I should receive an influenza vaccine this winter."—NO; this is correct.
B. "I am glad I am immune to German measles, I would hate to have it again."—NO; this is correct.
C. "I will get the rubella vaccine so my baby is protected against mumps."—**YES; rubella is a live virus and cannot be given to pregnant women.**
D. "I understand that varicella is a live vaccine so I cannot receive it."—NO; this is correct.

EXERCISE 4.17 Select all that apply:

Safety issues that should be discussed with Ava include:

A. Fire safety—**YES; she and the baby are on the second floor of the house.**

B. Proper refrigeration—**YES; proper care of food, and later, formula or breast milk are essential.**

C. Well-water sterilization—NO; the social history does not indicate that there is a well used for water.

D. Infant sleeping safety—NO; this will be done later in the pregnancy.

E. Safe childcare options—**YES; this is essential to start early because it is sometimes difficult to obtain childcare for infants.**

EXERCISE 4.18 Multiple-choice:

The nurse understands the importance of prenatal dental care because:

A. Pregnant women may drink too many soft drinks to decrease nausea.—NO; this is not necessarily true.

B. Periodontal disease is associated with preterm labor.—**YES; this is the reason.**

C. Pregnant women often lose teeth because of the fetus's needs.—NO; this is only true with poor nutrition.

D. Tooth decay is accelerated during pregnancy.—NO; this is only true with poor nutrition and poor dental care.

EXERCISE 4.19 Multiple-choice:

Ava's body mass index (BMI) is 22.9, therefore she should gain:

A. 15 to 25 lb—NO; this weight gain is for a woman who is overweight.

B. 25 to 35 lb—**YES; this is a normal weight gain.**

C. 35 to 45 lb—NO; this is for a woman who is underweight.

D. 45 to 55 lb—NO; this is too much weight.

EXERCISE 4.20 Fill in the blanks:

The nurse makes the following recommendations for Ava's diet:

Protein intake should be **60 to 80** g/d.

Iron intake/d should be 30 mg/d. Take supplement with **vitamin C** to increase absorption.

Have **five** servings of fruits and vegetables each day.

To prevent neural tube defects, take **0.4** mg of folic acid each day.

EXERCISE 4.21 Matching:

Match the trimester(s) in Column A that the common complaints and discomfort are most likely to occur in to the discomfort described in Column B:

Column A	Column B
A. First trimester	A Urinary frequency and noctoria
B. Second trimester	C Backache
C. Third trimester	C Increased vaginal discharge *(luekorrhea)*
	A Nausea and vomiting
	A Fatigue

EXERCISE 4.22 Matching:

Match the common discomfort in Column A with the physiologic reason in Column B:

Column A	Column B
A. Urinary frequency	B Change in center of gravity
B. Backache	D Elevated human chorionic gonadotropin (hCG) levels
C. Leukorrhea	E First-trimester progesterone rise
D. Nausea and vomiting	A Enlarged uterus
E. Fatigue	C Elevated estrogen levels

EXERCISE 4.23 Exhibit-format:

A complete physical examination is performed on Ava and here are some of the findings:

Vital signs: Temperature: 98.2°F, heart rate (HR): 74 beats per minute (bpm), respiratory rate (RR): 18 breaths per minute, and blood pressure (BP): 104/62 mmHg

Weight: 125 lb at 5′2″

Her heart and lung sounds are normal.

Understanding Ava's history, what risk factors does she have?

A. Advanced maternal age and poor family history—NO; she does not have advanced maternal age.
B. Poor family and social history—NO; her family is supportive.
C. Mental health and physical risk factors—NO; she does not display any physical or emotional risk factors.
D. Emotional and economic risk factors—**YES; she is not independent.**

EXERCISE 4.24 Multiple-choice:

The genetic test that Ava was referring to can be completed at 10 to 12 weeks gestation and can be performed transcervically or abdominally, guided by ultrasound. The test is:

A. Amniocenteses—NO; this is done between 15 and 18 weeks for genetic testing.
B. Chorionic villi sampling—**YES; this is the test that can take a sample of the villi for genetic testing of fetal cells.**
C. Biophysical profile—NO; this is a third-trimester test for fetal well-being.
D. Level III ultrasound—NO; this is usually done to detect congenital anomalies such as cardiac anomalies.

EXERCISE 4.25 Matching:

Match the manifestation in Column A with the possible complication in Column B (complications can be used more than once):

Column A	Column B
A. Bright painless vaginal bleeding	C Infection
B. Persistent vomiting	E, G Placenta abruption (separation of the placenta before fetus is delivered; condition is exacerbated by vasoconstriction, such as in maternal hypertension, smoking, abdomenal trauma, and cocaine usage)
C. Fever (more than 101°F), chills	D Premature rupture of membranes (PROM) or preterm premature rupture of membranes (pPROM)
D. Sudden gush of fluid from the vagina	E, F, H, I, J, K Pregnancy-induced hypertension (PIH; elevated BP of 140/90 mmHg or above after 20 weeks in previously normotensive women—two occurrences 6 hours apart)
E. Abdominal pain	A Placenta previa (implantation of the placenta in the lower uterine segment; it can be complete, covering all of the os; partial, covering part of os; or marginal—sometimes called *low lying*)
F. Dizziness, blurred, double vision	B Hyperemesis gravidarum (persistent vomiting with 5% weight loss, dehydration, ketosis and acetonuria)
G. Bright painful vaginal bleeding	
H. Severe headache	
I. Edema of hands, face, legs, and feet	
J. Muscular irritability	
K. Maternal weight gain more than 2 lb in a week	

EXERCISE 4.26 Multiple-choice:

The nurse realizes that Ava needs a better understanding of a quad screen when she states:

A. Elevated alpha-fetoprotein (AFP) may indicate neural tube defects or Down syndrome.—**YES; it would indicate a neural tube defect; a low AFP may indicate Down syndrome.**

B. To maintain the pregnancy, human chorionic gonadotropin (hCG) is important in the first trimester.—NO; this is correct.

C. Decreased AFP indicates fetal alcohol syndrome (FAS) or fetal alcohol effects (FAE).—NO; this is correct.

D. The amount of hCG decreases in the second trimester—NO; this is correct, because the placenta takes over producing hormones to maintain the pregnancy.

EXERCISE 4.27 Matching:

Match the fetal surveillance tests in Column A to the descriptions of the tests in Column B:

Column A	Column B
A. Amniocentesis B. Purtaneous umbilical blood sampling C. Doppler studies	C This is done by ultrasound to visualize the velocity of blood flow and measures the amount of red blood cells (RBCs). B This can be done after 16 weeks to sample fetal blood. One to 4 mL are collected near the cord insertion to look for hemolytic disease of the newborn. This is guided by ultrasound. A Amniotic fluid is removed to test cells for genetic makeup. This test is done at 16 to 18 weeks under ultrasound.

EXERCISE 4.28 Matching:

Match the discomfort in Column A to the appropriate nursing action in Column B:

Column A	Column B
A. Heart burn and indigestion	C Increase fiber
B. Flatus	E Increase calcium and phosphorus
C. Constipation	A Stay upright after meals
D. Hemorrhoids	B Decrease gas-forming foods
E. Leg cramps	D Use stool softeners

EXERCISE 4.29 Multiple-choice:

Ava understands the teaching when she states:

A. "I know my heartburn is caused by human chorionic gonadotropin (hCG)."—NO; heartburn is usually caused by a relaxed cardiac sphincter.
B. "I think my heartburn has to do with eating fast."—NO; heartburn is usually caused by a relaxed cardiac sphincter.
C. "Estrogen increases heartburn."—NO; the cardiac sphincter is relaxed because of progesterone.
D. "Progesterone increases heartburn."—**YES; the cardiac sphincter is relaxed because of progesterone.**

EXERCISE 4.30 Multiple-choice:

The nurse explains to Ava that the maternal perception of feeling the baby move is called:

A. Lightening—NO; this is the feeling that the baby moves down into the pelvis.
B. Ballottement—NO; this is the baby withdrawing from an internal examination.
C. Softening—NO; this is usually referred to as *cervical softening*.
D. Quickening—**YES.**

EXERCISE 4.31 Crossword:

																		1 P	A	R	A
		2 C										3 M		4 N				O			
		O			5 N							U		U				S			
		L			E							L		L				T			
6 G		O			O							T		L				P			
R		S			N			7 M				I		I				A			
8 A	N	T	E	P	A	R	T	U	M			P		P				R			
V		R			T			L				A		A				T			
I		U			E			T				R		R				U			
D		M						9 I	N	T	R	A	P	A	R	T	U	M			
A								G													
							10 P	R	I	M	I	G	R	A	V	I	D	A			
								A													
								V							11 P		12 L				
		13 L	A	C	T	A	T	I	O	N					U		O				
								D				14 P			E		C				
								15 A	F	T	E	R	B	I	R	T	H				
												I			P		I				
												M			E		A				
												I			R						
												P			A						
												A									
												R									
												A									

EXERCISE 4.32 Select all that apply:

Nursing care for a second-trimester transabdominal ultrasound includes the following interventions:

A. Fill bladder—NO; only needed in first trimester to lift the uterus out of the pelvic cavity.
B. Elevate head of bed—NO; this is not necessary for visualization.
C. Place in stirrups—NO; only needed for a transvaginal ultrasound.
D. Tilt to the left side—**YES; to prevent supine hypotension.**
E. Use gel conductor—**YES; needed to produce appropriate sound-wave picture.**

EXERCISE 4.33 Multiple-choice:

The nurse explains to Ava that her fundal height at 23 weeks gestation should measure:

A. 22 to 24 in.—NO; the measurement is taken in centimeters.
B. 22 to 24 cm—**YES; the fundus should grow 1 cm per week.**

C. 24 to 26 in.—NO; the measurement is taken in centimeters.
D. 24 to 26 cm—NO; this is for 24 to 26 weeks gestation.

EXERCISE 4.34 Fill in the blank:

If Ava is positive for chlamydia, what other sexually transmitted diseases (STDs) would you suspect that she might have?

Gonorrhea

EXERCISE 4.35 Multiple-choice:

The nurse explains the reason for RhoGAM correctly when she states that Rh-negative mothers need RhoGAM to:

A. Change them to Rh positive temporarily—NO; this is not the physiologic action of RhoGAM.
B. Produce antibodies against the fetal blood cells—NO; this is not the physiologic action of RhoGAM.
C. Produce antigens against the RhoGAM—**YES; this is the physiologic action of RhoGAM; the body produces antigens again.**
D. Change antibodies to antigens—NO; this is not the physiologic action of RhoGAM.

EXERCISE 4.36 Exhibit-format:

Laboratory data: Hematocrit (Hct), 30.1; rapid plasma regain (RPR), negative

Vital signs: Temperature: 97.8°F, heart rate (HR): 68 beats per minute (bpm), respiratory rate (RR): 18 breaths per minute, blood pressure (BP): 110/72 mmHg

Fetal heart rate (FHR): 150 bpm

The nurse understands that Ava's slight drop in Hgb during the second trimester is caused by:

A. All patients get anemic during pregnancy, so it expected at this time—NO; this is not true.
B. There is an increase in fetal utilization of iron, so the baby is taking more—NO; the fetus uses iron at a steady rate for its growth.
C. Iron is poorly absorbed because of the gravid uterus pressing on the GI tract—NO; this is also not true.
D. The cellular content of blood increases at a lesser rate than the plasma—**YES; there is blood volume expansion and the plasma portion increases more than the cellular.**

EXERCISE 4.37 Multiple-choice:

The nurse understands that if Ava's repeat glucose tolerance test (GTT) is greater than 140 mg/dL she will be a candidate for:

A. Insulin therapy—NO; this is not the next evidence-based-practice step.
B. Oral hypoglycemic medication—NO; this is not the next evidence-based-practice step.
C. A 3-hour GTT—**YES; this is the next step.**
D. A fasting GTT—NO; this was already completed, so there is no need to reassess.

EXERCISE 4.38 Matching:

Match the common third-trimester discomfort in Column A with the description that matches in Column B:

Column A	Column B
A. Pica	C Caused by stretching and pressure from the gravid uterus
B. Backache	D Caused by uterus placing pressure on diaphragm
C. Round ligament pain	F Caused by pressure of gravid uterus on pelvic veins
D. Shortness of breath	B Caused by gravid uterus and softening of pelvic joints
E. Pedal edema	A Cravings of nonfood substances
F. Vulva and leg varicosities	E Impaired circulation caused by gravid uterus

EXERCISE 4.39 Matching:

Match the third-trimester discomfort in Column A to the teaching that the nurse should provide in Column B:

Column A	Column B
A. Pica	F Support hose
B. Backache	C Flex legs onto abdomen
C. Round ligament pain	E Check blood pressure, elevate feet
D. Shortness of breath	A Proper nutrition
E. Pedal edema	D Sit up straight and increase rest
F. Vulva and leg varicosities	B Good posture and body mechanics

EXERCISE 4.40 Calculation:

Order: Give terbutaline (Brethine) 0.25 mg subq, stat

On hand: Terbutaline 1 mg in 1 mL

How much do you give?

0.25 mg

EXERCISE 4.41 Calculation:

Order: Betamethasone 12 mg intramuscular (IM), stat

On hand: Betamethasone 50 mg/5 mL

How much do you give?

1.2 mL

EXERCISE 4.42 Fill in the blanks:

Jane is pregnant for the seventh time. She has a 13-year-old girl who was delivered at 34 weeks gestational age (GA) but is doing well. She had a set of twins at 38 and 1/7 week who are now 10 years old. Jane has a 7-year-old and 5-year-old who were term babies. Jane had a miscarriage and then a preterm baby 3 years ago who has mild cerebral palsy (CP). Jane is a: G **7** P **2** T **3** A **1** L **6**

EXERCISE 4.43 Multiple-choice:

The nurse understands that the patient should most likely be prepared for which diagnostic procedure?

A. Ultrasound—**YES; this will assist the primary care provider (PCP) to know whether there is a live fetus in Jane's uterus.**
B. Biophysical profile—NO; this is done later on a live fetus to determine well-being.
C. Cesarean section—NO; this is done in an emergency for a viable infant.
D. Amniocentesis—NO; this is done on a live fetus for one of two reasons: (a) in the first trimester for genetic studies and (b) in the last trimester for fetal lung maturity studies.

EXERCISE 4.44 Multiple-choice:

The most important education that the nurse can provide Jane after dilatation and curettage (D&C) of the hydatidiform mole is that she must:

A. Exercise regularly to get her abdominal tone back—NO; this is important but not the priority.
B. Go to a support group for hydatidiform mole victims—NO; emotional support may be important but again it is not the priority.
C. Make sure she adheres to her birth control pills for at least a year—**YES; hydatidiform moles increase human chorionic gonadotropin (hCG) levels and a return to 0 indicates that the vesicles have been successfully removed in total. If Jane gets pregnant, the hCG levels from pregnancy will mask a proliferation because some tumors also produce hCG.**
D. Get a second opinion about radiation therapy—NO; this is usually not necessary because there was no uterine invasion seen.

EXERCISE 4.45 Multiple-choice:

The nurse caring for Miracle and Ava has a nursing student with her. The nurse assesses that the nursing student understands the patient's care when he states:

A. "Miracle's edema is slightly severe, I will continue strict input and output (I&O)."—**YES; this is correct and I&O should be continued.**
B. "Miracle's edema is severe and pitting on palpation."—NO; 3 or 4+ edema would be considered severe and pitting.
C. "Miracle's deep tendon reflexes (DTRs) are hypoactive."—NO; 2+ reflexes are normal.
D. "Miracle's DTRs are hyperactive."—NO; 2+ reflexes are normal.

EXERCISE 4.46 Calculation:

Order: Magnesium sulfate ($MgSO_4$) 4 g/hr

On hand: 40 g/500 mL

How much do you give?

50 mL/hr

EXERCISE 4.47 Multiple-choice:

A diagnostic finding in HELLP (hemolytic anemia, elevated liver enzyme, and low platelets) syndrome includes:

A. Decreased fibrinogen—NO; fibrinogen levels should be normal.
B. Increased platelets—NO; platelets are low.
C. Decreased leukocytes—NO; leukocytes are not affected.
D. Increased fibrin-split products—**YES; these are increased to try to assist the body to contain the hemorrhage.**

EXERCISE 4.48 Multiple-choice:

Miracle's labs show that her platelet count is 90,000/mm³. This would place her in which category?

A. Class I—NO; platelet count less than 50,000/mm³ and considered high risk.
B. Class II—**YES; platelet count of 50,000 to less than 100,000/mm³ is considered moderate risk.**
C. Class III—NO; platelet count of 100,000 to 150,000/mm³ is considered lower risk.
D. Class IV—NO; there is no class IV.

EXERCISE 4.49 Multiple-choice:

The interprofessional group of health care providers has determined that Miracle is not in disseminated intravascular coagulation (DIC) because Miracle's laboratory results demonstrate:

A. A decrease in fibrin-split products—NO; fibrin-split products are increased because they are trying to decrease bleeding.
B. An increase in platelets—NO; platelets are used excessively and are decreased.
C. An increase in fibrin-split products—**YES; fibrin-split products are increased to try to stop bleeding.**
D. An increase in RBCs—NO; these are not significantly affected.

EXERCISE 4.50 Fill in the blank:

Small-for-gestational-age (SGA) babies' weights fall below the **10th** percentile for weight when compared on the growth chart for their weeks of gestation.

EXERCISE 4.51 Select all that apply:

Nursing care for a patient having a nonstress test (NST) should include:

A. Tilting the patient to the side to prevent supine hypotension—**YES; this is an important point for all pregnant patients.**
B. Increasing the intravenous (IV) fluids to 250 mL/hr—NO; they do not necessarily need an IV.
C. Explaining the procedure to the patient and family—**YES; patient teaching is always a priority.**
D. Keep the room as quiet as possible—NO; there is no reason for the room to be quiet.
E. Place a Foley catheter into the bladder—NO; this is not necessary.

EXERCISE 4.52 Select all that apply:

Miracle has been informed that because of its small-for-gestational-age (SGA) status, when the baby is born the newborn may need extra blood testing for:

A. Glucose—**YES; SGA newborns do not have stored brown fat (5% of their body weight in term infants) for energy utilization.**
B. Polycythemia—**YES; SGA newborns produce more red blood cells (RBCs) in an attempt to increase their oxygen-carrying capacity.**
C. Thyroid-stimulating hormone (TSH)—NO; SGA newborns do not normally have thyroid difficulties.
D. Phenylketonuria (PKU)—NO; PKU is not a problem until a diet is established.
E. Bilirubin—**YES; SGA infants may have hyperbilirubinemia caused by polycythemia and excessive RBC breakdown.**

EXERCISE 4.53 Select all that apply:

A. Diethylstilbestrol (DES) exposure while in utero—**YES; studies show these women are prone to incompetent cervixes.**
B. Cervical trauma—**YES; trauma can disrupt the integrity of the cervix.**
C. Congenitally shorter cervix—**YES; shorter cervixes tend to be less stable during pregnancy.**
D. Large babies—NO; babies gain most of their weight in the last trimester and incompetent cervixes usually occur in the second trimester of pregnancy.
E. Uterine anomalies—**YES; anatomical anomalies can cause lack of cervical integrity.**
F. Overdistended bladder—NO; this would be anterior to the cervix.
G. Previous loop electrosurgical excision procedure (LEEP), cone, or other surgical procedures—**YES; surgery can also disrupt the integrity of the cervix.**
H. Multiple gestations—**YES; in this case there is more weight to carry in the second trimester.**

EXERCISE 4.54 Multiple-choice:

Ava's group B streptococcal culture is positive, so the nurse would anticipate the following order once Ava shows signs of true labor:

A. Gentamycin every 2 hours until delivery—NO; gentamycin would only be used if the patient was allergic to penicillin and this dose is excessive and dangerous.
B. Ampicillin 4 hours before delivery—**YES; this is the treatment of choice.**
C. Pitocin 1 mU/min to start regular uterine contractions (UCs)—NO; this is not related to GBS.
D. Terbutaline 0.25 subq to increase the time until delivery—NO; this is not done because it may increase the chances of other complications.

EXERCISE 4.55 Matching:

Match the correct term describing uterine contractions (UCs) in Column A with the descriptions in Column B:

Column A	Column B
A. Intensity	C The time in seconds in between contractions
B. Frequency	A The firmness of the uterus, which can be demonstrated in three ways: By an external fetal monitor (EFM) as the uterus rises and falls with contractions but is not an exact pressure because of different abdominal thicknesses. By an internal uterine pressure catheter (IUPC), which is inserted through the vagina into a pocket of fluid after rupture of membranes (ROM). By palpation: Mild is the consistency of the tip of your nose; moderate is the consistency of your chin; strong is the consistency of your forehead
C. Interval	B From the onset of one contraction to the onset of the next contraction

EXERCISE 4.56 Fill in the blanks.

Fill in the blanks using these external fetal monitor strips:

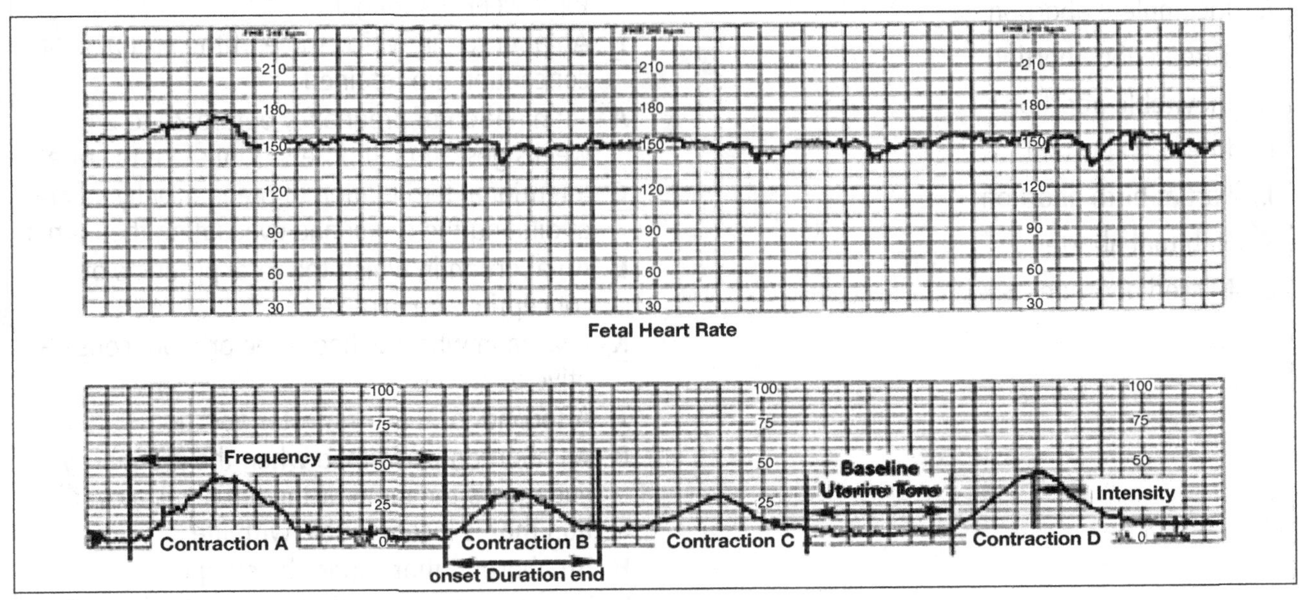

What is the frequency of Ava's contractions? **2 minutes**

What is the duration of Ava's contractions? **60 seconds**

What is the interval of Ava's contractions? **60 to 70 seconds**

What is the intensity of Ava's contractions? **Moderate**

EXERCISE 4.57 Multiple-choice:

The nurse should anticipate that the primary care provider (PCP) will order:

A. A computerized axial tomography (CAT) scan and human chorionic gonadotropin (hCG) level—NO; a CAT scan is not necessary.
B. An MRI and ultrasound—NO; an MRI is not necessary.
C. An ultrasound and CAT scan—NO; a CAT scan is not necessary.
D. An hCG level and ultrasound—**YES; both these tests are specific to possible pregnancy.**

EXERCISE 4.58 Hot spot:

Place an X on the diagram the portion of the female anatomy where you believe the implantation is most likely to occur.

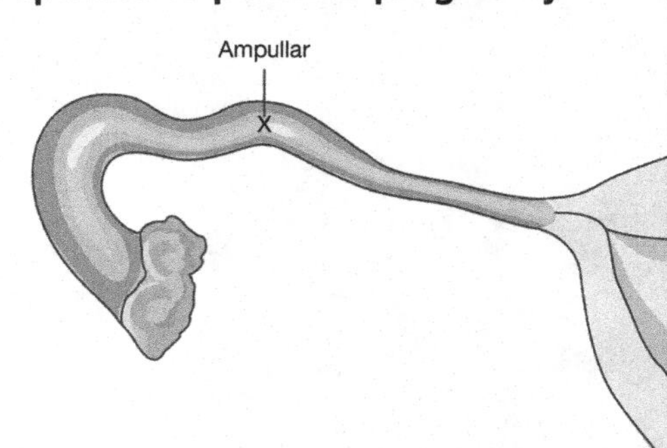

EXERCISE 4.59 Matching:

Match the term in Column A with the definition in Column B:

Column A	Column B
A. Abortion	G Bleeding and cramping that subside with continuation of the pregnancy
B. Therapeutic abortion	I An abortion in which retained tissue has caused an infection
C. Induced abortion	L An abortion in which the fetus died in utero, but the products of conception are retained for 8 weeks or longer
D. Spontaneous abortion	F An abortion in which some of the products of conception are retained
E. Complete abortion	A Termination of pregnancy before 20 to 24 weeks gestation; it differs from state to state
F. Incomplete abortion	C Intentional termination of pregnancy by means of dilating the cervix and evacuating the uterus
G. Threatened abortion	E An abortion in which the total products of conception are expelled
H. Inevitable abortion	K A woman who has had three or more consecutive abortions
I. Infected abortion	J A second- or third-trimester abortion
J. Partial-birth abortion	B An abortion performed when the pregnancy endangers the mom or the fetus has a condition that is incompatible with life
K. Habitual aborter	H An abortion that cannot be stopped
L. Missed abortion	D Loss of a pregnancy before viability that has not been interfered with intentionally. Symptoms are cramping and bleeding. Most often caused by genetic disorders of the embryo, hormonal imbalances, infections, and abnormalities of the placenta

EXERCISE 4.60 Select all that apply:

Choose the appropriate nursing interventions for Sara.

A. Tell her she can get pregnant again—NO; this is inappropriate while a person is grieving a loss.
B. Tell her to adopt a child—NO; this is also inappropriate while a person is grieving a loss.
C. Encourage her to verbalize about the loss—**YES; she should be encouraged to verbalize.**
D. Give her a special memento, such as a silk rose, to remember the loss—**YES; providing mementos lets the patient know that you understand it is difficult.**
E. Include her husband in the discussion—**YES; her husband is also grieving and should be encouraged to verbalize.**

EXERCISE 4.61 Multiple-choice:

The expert nurse understands that after artificial rupture of membranes (AROM), her first intervention will be:

A. Clean the patient's bed—NO; this is not the first priority for safe care.
B. Observe the fluid's color—NO; this is important but not the first priority.
C. Count the fetal heart rate (FHR)—**YES; this is most important.**
D. Palpate the maternal pulse—NO; this is important but not the first priority.

EXERCISE 4.62 Multiple-choice:

The nurse understands that once a labor patient receives a narcotic, a priority intervention is:

A. Assist when out of bed (OOB)—NO; they should not be ambulating.
B. Monitor the labor contractions, which may decrease in intensity—NO; this is not a safety priority.
C. Provide oral hygiene to reduce dry mouth—NO; this is not a safety priority.
D. Have naloxone (Narcan) available—**YES; the infant may need to be resuscitated if born within a short time of the narcotic administration.**

EXERCISE 4.63 Calculation:

Order: Give butorphanol 1 mg intravenous (IV) push, stat

On hand: Butorphanol 2 mg in 1 mL

How much do you give?

0.5 mL

EXERCISE 4.64 Calculation:

Order: Have neonatal naloxone (Narcan) 0.1 mg /kg intramuscular (IM) on hand

On hand: Naloxone (Narcan) 0.4 mg /mL

How much would you give if you suspect a 7-lb baby?

0.3 mg

EXERCISE 4.65 Calculation:

Order: Increase Ringer's lactate (RL) to 500 mL bolus in 30 minutes.

On hand: 1,000-mL bag of RL on a pump that runs mL/hr

What would the pump setting be for this bolus?

1,000 mL/hr

EXERCISE 4.66 Select all that apply:

Check all the appropriate nursing interventions for the first stage of the second phase of labor:

A. Catheterize or void every 4 hours—NO; labor patients should void or be catheterized every 2 hours.
B. Change blue pads every 30 minutes—**YES; this will decrease ascending bacterial contamination.**
C. Allow her to order a regular full lunch—NO; she will most likely throw it up when she is in transition.
D. Turn lights on so she is alert—NO; decrease environmental stimuli so she can concentrate on getting through each uterine contraction.
E. Take off the fetal monitor—NO; after an epidural patient should be monitored continuously.

EXERCISE 4.67 Calculation:

Calculate the correct dose if the primary care provider (PCP) orders a Pitocin intravenous (IV) to start at 2 mU/min.

On hand: 500-mL bag of Ringer's lactate (RL) with 30 units of Pitocin and a pump that delivers mL/hr

What is the correct pump setting?

30 U = 30,000 mU/500 mL or 60 mU/mL

2 mU/min × 60 min = 120 = 2 mL/hr

EXERCISE 4.68 Fill in the blanks:

What is the normal fetal heart rate (FHR) range? **The normal range is <u>110</u> to <u>160</u> beats/min.**

EXERCISE 4.69 Select all that apply:

The nurse understands that the baby is at high risk for:

A. Broken clavicle—**YES; this is the most commonly broken bone on a newborn.**
B. Cephalhematoma—**YES; this is a collection of blood under the periosteum; it produces a visible bump on one side of the newborn's head but because it is under the periosteum, it does not cross the suture line.**
C. Caput succedaneum—NO; caputs are normal edema of the crowning part of the head.
D. Brachial plexus—**YES; these are nerves that run from the neck into the arm that can be injured. The classic sign is that the infant does not flex that extremity.**
E. Fractured humerus—**YES; this bone can also be broken in a traumatic delivery.**
F. Hydrocele—NO; there should be no genital injury in a vertex-presenting delivery.

EXERCISE 4.70 Multiple-choice:

The nurse understands that the proper interventions to expect at the delivery include:

A. Ritgen's maneuver, suction the infant's nose and then mouth—NO; the mouth is suctioned first.
B. Suction the infant's nose, Ritgen's maneuver, and then suction the infant's mouth—NO; first the infant needs to be delivered using the Ritgen's maneuver.

C. Externally rotate the infant, Ritgen's maneuver, and suction the infant's mouth—NO; the Ritgen's maneuver is first.

D. Ritgen's maneuver, suction the infant's mouth and then nose—**YES; this is the expected order of the interventions.**

EXERCISE 4.71 Fill in the blank:

The umbilical cord should contain **three** vessels; there are two **arteries** and one **vein**.

EXERCISE 4.72 Fill in the blanks:

One letter simply stands for a letter of the alphabet. See if you can break the code.

ONE—**put the baby on a warm bed**
TWO—**dry**
THREE—**position the head**
FOUR—**suction**
FIVE—**stimulate to breathe**

EXERCISE 4.73 Matching:

Match the type of heat loss in Column A with the appropriate sentence in the neutral thermal environment (NTE) story in Column B:

Column A	Column B
A. Convection B. Evaporation C. Radiation D. Conduction	The delivery room nurse waits for the cord to be cut and carries the baby over to the bed, which is away from the windows to prevent **C,** and away from the door, where people move quickly in and out to prevent **A** from air currents. The bed was warmed to prevent **D.** The nurse vigorously dries the baby off to prevent cold stress from **B.**

EXERCISE 4.74 Fill in the blanks:

At 1 minute, the baby is responding to his extrauterine environment and is only acrocyanotic and slightly hyporeflexic with good reflexes. His respiratory rate is 70 breaths per minute and his HR is 170 bpm. The nurse assigns him an Apgar score of **8.** At 5 minutes old, the baby is still acrocyanotic (which can be normal up to 24 hours) and has good reflexes and tone. His vital signs are 97.9°F axillary, HR 155 bpm, RR 60. His 5-minute Apgar score is **9.**

EXERCISE 4.75 Select all that apply:

The delivery room nurse finishes the immediate care of the newborn; what interventions are normally completed in the delivery room?

A. Blood pressure measurement—NO; blood pressures on infants are usually not routine but are completed if a murmur is heard.
B. Vital signs assessment—**YES; vital signs are done frequently to make sure the infant is adjusting well and staying warm.**
C. Identification bracelets and footprints completed—**YES; infants cannot be removed from the delivery room without identification.**
D. Vitamin K administered—NO; most times this is done in the newborn nursery, but some places may do it in the delivery room.
E. Circumcision performed—NO; this is done later, once the infant is stabilized.

EXERCISE 4.76 Multiple-choice:

The nurse understands that the preferred site for an intramuscular (IM) injection of vitamin K for a newborn is the vastus lateralis because:

A. It is easily accessible—NO; this is not the reason, although it is accessible.
B. There is better blood flow in the legs—NO; this is not true; it is an IM not an intravenous (IV) injection.
C. The dorsal gluteal is underdeveloped—**YES; this muscle is not developed until the child is walking for a time, usually about 2 years old.**
D. Newborns have to sleep on their backs—NO; this is true but would not interfere with a dorsal gluteal injection.

EXERCISE 4.77 Fill in the blanks:

Fill in the four classic signs of placental separation:

1. **The uterus rises in the abdominal cavity.**
2. **The uterus becomes globular in shape.**
3. **There is a gush of blood (normal: 250–300 mL).**
4. **The cord spontaneously lengthens.**

EXERCISE 4.78 Select all that apply:

The nurse understands that manifestations of cardiac decompensation include:

A. Cough—**YES; congestive heart failure increases the fluid around the lungs.**
B. Dyspnea—**YES; the increased fluid makes breathing more difficult.**
C. Edema—**YES; veinous return is slower and fluid leaks into the extravascular spaces.**
D. Heart murmur—**YES; often there is a heart murmur especially if a valve is involved.**
E. Palpitations—**YES; often the HR is increased to compensate for poor circulation.**
F. Weight loss—NO; the edema usually promotes weight gain.

EXERCISE 4.79 Multiple-choice:

What kind of delivery would the nurse anticipate for Paulette in order to conserve cardiac output and maintain a more even thoracic pressure?

A. Cesarean—NO; anesthesia may put more stress on the heart and circulatory system.
B. Natural vaginal birth—NO; prolonged pushing will increase thoracic pressure.
C. Low-forceps delivery—**YES; this will accomplish delivery with less pushing.**
D. Mid forceps delivery—NO; this can injure the fetus.

EXERCISE 4.80 Multiple-choice:

The first nursing intervention for a prolapsed cord would be to:

A. Check the fetal heart rate (FHR)—NO; this can be done after the patient's hips are raised.
B. Raise the patient's hips—**YES; this keeps the presenting part from compressing the cord.**
C. Call the primary physician—NO; this can be done after the patient's hips are raised.
D. Explain to the patient the baby will probably be born dead—NO; this may be necessary but attempts to save the fetus must be made.

EXERCISE 4.81 Fill in the blanks:

Use the following words to fill in the blanks in the BUBBLE-HE narrative in Table 4.6.

Ecchymosis
Taking hold
Rubra
Engorgement
Postpartum psychosis
Redness
Diuresis
Letting go
Deep vein thrombosis
Sulcus
Postpartum depression
Approximation
Hemorrhoids
Taking in
Edema
Serosa
Discharge
Afterbirth
Alba
Sims
Ambulation
Postpartum blues
Binding in

TABLE 4.6 Answers to Exercise 4.81

<table>
<tr><td>B</td><td>Breasts</td><td>Engorgement is the process of swelling of the breast tissue caused by an increase in blood and lymph supply as a precursor to lactation. This usually happens on postpartum days 3 to 5. On days 1 to 5, colostrum is secreted.</td></tr>
<tr><td>U</td><td>Uterus</td><td>Six to 12 hours after delivery, the fundus should be at the umbilicus. It then decreases 1 cm/d for approximately 10 days when it becomes a nonpalpable pelvic organ. Discomfort or cramping from involution is called "afterbirth" pain. Afterbirth pains are increased in multiparous women, breastfeeders, and women with an overdistended uterus. Have the patient void before the examination.</td></tr>
<tr><td>B</td><td>Bladder</td><td>The bladder may be subjected to trauma that results in edema and diminished sensitivity to fluid pressure. This can lead to overdistention and incomplete emptying. Difficulty voiding may persist for the first 2 days. Hematuria reflects trauma or urinary tract infection. Acetone denotes dehydration after prolonged labor. Diuresis usually begins within 12 hours after delivery and eliminates excess body fluid.</td></tr>
<tr><td>B</td><td>Bowels</td><td>Bowel sounds (BS) should be assessed at each shift. Assess whether the patient is passing flatus. Use a high-fiber diet and increase fluid intake. Stool softeners (Colace) are usually ordered to decrease discomfort. Early ambulation should be encouraged.</td></tr>
<tr><td>L</td><td>Lochia</td><td>Rubra is the color of vaginal discharge for the first 3 to 4 days. It is a deep-red mixture of mucus, tissue debris, and blood. Lochia serosa starts within 3 to 10 days postpartum. It is pink to brown in color and contains leukocytes, decidual tissue, red blood cells, and serous fluid. Lochia alba begins within 10 to 14 days and is creamy white or light brown in color and consists of leukocytes and decidua tissue. Lochia is described for quantity as scant, small, moderate, or large.</td></tr>
<tr><td>E</td><td>Episiotomy or incision if cesarean section</td><td>Episiotomy/laceration or cesarean incision repair should be assessed each shift. Use the REEDA acronym to assess and describe. If the patient had an episiotomy, laceration that was repaired, or a cesarean incision, that surgical site should be further assessed using the REEDA acronym.

Fill in what the letters stand for:
<table>
<tr><td>R</td><td>Redness</td></tr>
<tr><td>E</td><td>Edema</td></tr>
<tr><td>E</td><td>Ecchymosis (bruising)</td></tr>
<tr><td>D</td><td>Discharge</td></tr>
<tr><td>A</td><td>Approximation</td></tr>
</table>
Inspection of an episiotomy/laceration is best done in a lateral (T) Sims position with a pen light.</td></tr>
</table>

(continued)

TABLE 4.6 Answers to Exercise 4.81 (*continued*)

		Hemorrhoids are distended rectal veins and can be uncomfortable. Care measures include ice packs for the first 24 hours, peri bottle washing after each void, sitz baths, witch hazel pads (Tucks), and hydrocortisone cream. *Classifications of Perineal Lacerations* First-degree laceration involves only skin and superficial structures above muscle. Second-degree laceration extends through perineal muscles. Third-degree laceration extends through the anal sphincter muscle. Fourth-degree laceration continues through anterior rectal wall. *Classifications of Episiotomies* Midline is made from the posterior vaginal vault toward the rectum. Right mediolateral is made from the vaginal vault to the right buttock Left mediolateral is made on the left side. Mediolateral incisions increase room and decrease rectal tearing, but midline episiotomies heal easier. A Sulcus tear is a tear through the vaginal wall. A cervical tear is an actual tear in the cervix of the uterus. This bleeds profusely.
H	Homan's	Positive Homan's sign may be present when there is a deep vein thrombosis of the leg. To elicit a Homan's sign, passive dorsiflexion of the ankle produces pain in the patient's leg. Postpartum is a state of hypercoagulability and moms are a 30% higher risk for deep vein thrombosis.
E	Edema or emotional	*Pedal edema* should be assessed on postpartum patients as they have massive fluid shifts right after delivery. Pedal edema can indicate overhydration in labor, hypertension, or lack of normal diuresis. *Emotional assessment* must be made on each postpartum family. Initially, maternal touch of the newborn is by fingertip in an en face position that progresses to full hand touch. The mom should draw the infant close and usually strokes the baby. Binding-in is when the mother identifies specific features about the baby such as who he or she looks like. These are claiming behaviors. Verbal behavior is noticed because most mothers speak to infants in a high-pitched voice and progress from calling the baby "it" to "he" or "she," then they progress to using the baby's name. *Rubin (1984) describes three stages of maternal adjustment.* Taking in (1–2 days). In this phase, the mother is passive and dependent as well as preoccupied with self. This is the time she reviews the birth experience. Taking hold (3–10 days). This is when she resumes control over her life and becomes concerned about self-care. During this time, she gains self-confidence as a mother. Letting go (2–4 weeks). This is when she accomplishes maternal role attainment and makes relationship adjustments. *Emotional postpartum states* Postpartum "blues" are mood disorders that occur to most women usually within the first 4 weeks. They are hormonal in origin and are called *baby blues*. Postpartum "depression" should be assessed on every woman and is a true depressive state that affects daily function. Postpartum "psychosis" is a mental health illness characterized by delusions.

EXERCISE 4.82 Multiple-choice:

The nurse understands that an infant may be manifesting signs of respiratory distress when the mother tells her:

A. "My baby is sleeping peacefully but his eyes look like they are moving under his lids."—NO; the mother is describing rapid eye movement (REM) sleep, which is normal.

B. "I can see that my baby stops breathing for about 10 seconds sometimes."—NO; irregular or periodic breathing is normal for a newborn as long as the apnea does not last longer than 15 seconds.

C. "My baby's breathing is very uneven, it is sometimes fast and at other times is slow."—NO; irregular or periodic breathing is normal for a newborn.

D. "I love when my baby makes that squeaking sound every time he breaths."—**YES; the squeaking sound is grunting and is one of the first signs of respiratory distress and is usually accompanied by nasal flaring.**

EXERCISE 4.83: Hot spot:

Place an X on the sagittal suture on the infant's head.

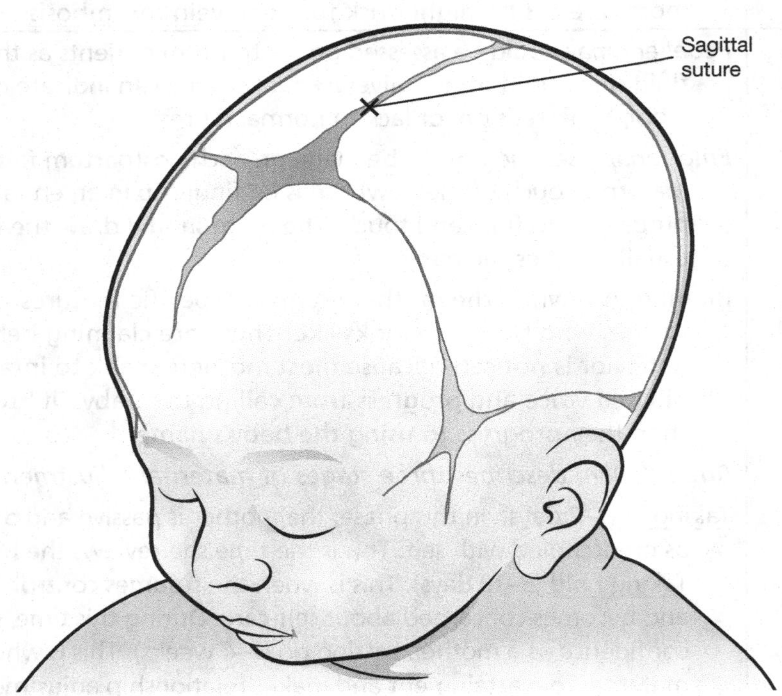

EXERCISE 4.84 Matching:

Match the terms in Column A to the correct descriptions in Column B:

Column A	Column B
A. Universal newborn hearing screen (UNHS)	**G** Folds on thigh
B. Epstein pearls	**I** Edematous scrotum
C. Frenulum	**K** Startle reflex
D. Crepitus	**M** Hand-grasp object
E. Xiphoid	**C** Ligament under tongue
F. Brachial	**D** Palpation of bone over bone
G. Gluteal	**B** Sebaceous cysts on hard palate
H. Ortolani	**O** Toes spread when sole is stimulated
I. Hydrocele	**L** Stops responding to repetitive stimuli
J. Pilonidal	**E** End of sternum
K. Moro	**H** Maneuver to check for hip dysplasia
L. Habituation	**A** Used to rule out congenital deafness
M. Palmar grasp	**N** Toes curl around an object
N. Plantar grasp	**J** Indentation at the base of spine
O. Babinski reflex	**F** Pulse found in arm

EXERCISE 4.85 Calculation:

Yesterday Michael gained 15 g. How would you express that to Anna in ounces?

0.5 ounces

EXERCISE 4.86 Multiple-choice:

The nurse understands that Michelle may need tactile stimulation in the following situation:

A. Her breathing is irregular and at a rate of 62 breaths per minute.—NO; this is normal and Michelle should not be stimulated to breath faster.

B. She is yawning excessively and turning away from her caregiver.—NO; this indicates that she is overstimulated.

C. Her breathing stops periodically but resumes within 15 seconds with coughing.—NO; this is a normal span of apnea and is self-limiting because Michelle resumes normal breathing without intervention.

D. She stops breathing for 20 seconds and does not cough or make sucking motions.—**YES; 20 seconds is prolonged apnea and Michelle is not self-limiting it because she is not moving.**

EXERCISE 4.87 Multiple-choice:

William is 42 weeks gestation and weighs 5 lb, 1 oz. This would most likely classify him as:

A. Small for gestational age (SGA)—**YES; William is SGA.**
B. Large for gestational age (LGA)—NO; LGA newborns are over the 90th percentile on the growth chart.
C. Average for gestational age (AGA)—NO; AGA is between the 10th and 90th percentiles on the growth chart.
D. Preterm—NO; preterm newborns are born before the completion of the 37th week GA.

EXERCISE 4.88 Select all that apply:

Which nursing interventions would be done for neonates experiencing neonatal abstinence syndrome (NAS)?

A. Hold in an upright position—**YES; studies show they like to be held upright.**
B. Provide a pacifier—**YES; this is for nonnutritive sucking and comfort.**
C. Obtain an order to medicate for moderate to severe withdrawal symptoms—**YES; they are in actual pain from the withdrawal symptoms.**
D. Keep the lights on—NO; too much stimulation.
E. Encourage parental participation—**YES; they need to know how to care for the baby when they take him or her home.**
F. Undress under warmer—NO; they like to be swaddled.
G. Provide a quiet environment—**YES; this decreases stimulation.**
H. Provide good skin care to decrease diaper rash—**YES; they have loose stools while they metabolize the drug.**

EXERCISE 4.89 Multiple-choice:

The nurse understands that the best intervention to protect Mia from retinopathy of prematurity (ROP) is to:

A. Use eye covers while Mia is receiving oxygen—NO; this is done for bili-lights, not oxygen.
B. Keep the oxygen flow at a consistent level—NO; this is not the best intervention to decrease the risk of ROP.
C. Use as little oxygen as needed—**YES; oxygen is the causative agent, so reducing it is the best intervention.**
D. Intermittently take Mia off oxygen for short periods—NO; this will compromise her oxygenation.

EXERCISE 4.90 Select all that apply:

To assess a newborn for necrotizing enterocolitis (NEC), the nurse should:

A. Measure the abdominal circumference—**YES; increased abdominal circumference is a symptom of NEC.**
B. Check for aspirates—**YES; increased aspirates is also a sign of NEC.**
C. Take an x-ray before each feed—NO; only if NEC is suspected would you call the primary care provider, and he or she may order an abdominal x-ray.
D. Check bowel sounds—**YES; always check before each feed.**
E. Weigh every 2 hours—NO; this will not assist the assessment.

EXERCISE 4.91 Select all that apply:

The nursing interventions for a newborn with suspected necrotizing enterocolitis (NEC) are:

A. Increase breast-milk feedings—NO; feedings are held.
B. Keep nothing orally (NPO) status—**YES; this will provide time for a diagnosis and treatment.**
C. Suction vigorously—NO; this increases stress on a possibly compromised newborn.
D. Call the primary care provider (PCP)—**YES; report your findings.**
E. No longer check for aspirates—NO; always check for aspirates; they need to be reported if excessive.

EXERCISE 4.92 Multiple-choice:

An appropriate nursing intervention for a mother experiencing chronic sorrow is:

A. Tell her that it could be worse—NO; this is not helpful; it only minimizes her feelings.
B. Encourage her to look on the bright side—NO; this is not helpful; it minimizes her feelings.
C. Distract her thoughts to something else—NO; this tries to decrease the importance of a very serious concern.
D. Encourage her to verbalize—**YES; this will help her reflect on the situation and work toward understanding.**

EXERCISE 4.93 Multiple-choice:

The nurse shows understanding of pathophysiology of neonatal hypoglycemia when she states:

A. "Infants of diabetic mothers have glucose levels that fluctuate from hyperglycemia to hypoglycemia in the first 24 hours."—NO; they are hypoglycemic.
B. "Infants of diabetic mothers need extra feedings because of hyperinsulinemia."—**YES; they put out extra insulin because of excessive glucose in utero.**
C. "Infants of diabetic mothers are hypersensitive to insulin infusions."—NO; they usually need insulin to cope with the glucose.
D. "Infants of diabetic mothers are always overweight."—NO; some are small if the mother has vascular disease resulting from advanced diabetes.

EXERCISE 4.94 Select all that apply:

Felix is over the 90th percentile on the growth chart, which would classify him or place him at risk for the following manifestations or conditions:

A. Small for gestational age (SGA)—NO; he is large for gestational age (LGA).
B. Broken clavicle—**YES; LGA infants are at risk.**
C. Brachial plexis injury—**YES; LGA infants are at risk because of pressure on the arm during delivery.**
D. Average for gestational age (AGA)—NO; he is LGA.
E. Patent ductus arteriosis (PDA)—NO; preterm infants are at risk.

EXERCISE 4.95 Select all that apply:

Correct information about bottle-feeding infants includes:

A. Mom should use heat packs to her breast—NO; bottle-feeding moms should use ice to dry up their breast milk.
B. Recommended daily amount (RDA) of formula is 100 to 115 kcal/kg/d—**YES; this is approximately 140 to 150 mL/kg/d.**
C. There are 30 kcal in each ounce of newborn formula—NO; there are 20 kcal/oz.
D. Mothers lose 20 lb initially after delivery—NO; moms lose 10 to 12 lb.
E. Formula-fed infants should be at birth weight at approximately 10 days old—**YES; this is a normal weight gain.**

EXERCISE 4.96 Select all that apply:

Correct information about breastfeeding infants includes:

A. Breastfeeding mothers should limit their fluid intake to avoid engorgement.—NO; increased fluid is needed for milk production.
B. Breastfeeding mothers should nurse every 4 hours.—NO; nursing mothers should feed at least every 3 hours or on demand.
C. Warm showers help the milk flow.—**YES; this is true.**
D. A supportive bra should be worn.—**YES; this is true.**
E. Breastfeeding mothers should only nurse 20 minutes on each side.—NO; the mother will regulate the time to the needs of the infant.

EXERCISE 4.97 Matching:

Match the stages of milk in Column A with the descriptions in Column B:

Column A	Column B
A. Colostrum	__C__ is produced in the beginning of the feeding
B. Transitional milk	__D__ is produced after letdown and is high in fat
C. Foremilk	__A__ is the first milk and it lasts 2 to 4 days; it is high in protein, vitamins, minerals, and immunoglobulin A (IgA)
D. Hind milk	__B__ starts at engorgement or 4 days to 2 weeks

EXERCISE 4.98 Fill in the blank:

The usual procedure for Rh+ babies/Rh– mothers is a 300-mcg dose of RhoGAM, and a **Kleihauer–Betke** test, which detects fetal cells in the maternal blood. This is followed if a large feto–maternal transfusion is suspected. A larger dose can be given if needed.

EXERCISE 4.99 Multiple-choice:

Hemolysis of fetal cells increases the likelihood of which neonatal condition?

A. Hypoglycemia—NO; hypoglycemia is caused by decreased glucose intake or increased insulin production.

B. Hyperglycemia—NO; hyperglycemia in newborns is usually caused by distress and brown fat breakdown.
C. Hyperbilirubinemia—**YES; antibodies cause hemolysis of red blood cells and bilirubin is a by-product that accumulates in the skin and organs.**
D. Hypocalcemia—NO; hypocalcemia is related to hypoglycemia.

EXERCISE 4.100 Multiple-choice:

The nurse is careful to do the heel stick on the side of the heel in order to prevent:

A. Pain—NO; this is not the primary reason.
B. Hemorrhage—NO; this is not the primary reason.
C. Cellulites—NO; this is not the primary reason.
D. Foot drop—**YES; nerve damage can occur if the infant's heel is stuck directly in the back of the heel.**

EXERCISE 4.101 Multiple-choice:

The most important nursing intervention to decrease the incidence of newborn hyperbilirubinemia is:

A. Prevent cold stress—NO; although this is always important, it is not directly related to hyperbilirubinemia.
B. Early and frequent feeds—**YES; this will assist the gasrointestinal tract to reduce and excrete the bilirubin.**
C. Placing the baby near the window of the nursery—NO; studies show this is not helpful, although it is still a practice that is followed.
D. Keeping the baby in the nursery at night—NO; this is just a hospital routine.

EXERCISE 4.102 Select all that apply:

Select all the nursing interactions that are appropriate when caring for a newborn under phototherapy.

A. Cover the eyes and genitalia—**YES; this is to protect them from the light rays.**
B. Maintain an neutral thermal environment (NTE)—**YES; this is to decrease cold stress.**
C. Early and frequent feeds—**YES; this helps the gastroinstestinal tract excrete the bilirubin.**
D. Dress the newborn to prevent cold stress—NO; this prevents the lights from reaching the newborn's skin.
E. Check light-source strength with a light meter—**YES; the light output should be checked at each shift.**

EXERCISE 4.103 Fill in the blanks:

The nurse would be expected to give Sophia zidovudine (AZT) for **6** weeks at 2 mg/kg every 12 hours. What route is used? **PO** (by mouth).

EXERCISE 4.104 Calculation:

Sophia weighs 7 lb, 4 oz. How much Sophia zidovudine (AZT) do you give at each 12-hour dose? (The order reads 2 mg/kg every 12 hr.)

7 lb, 4 oz = 3.3 kg

2 mg × 3.3 kg = 6.6 mg every 12 hours

Resources

Amendolia, B., Fisher, K., Wittmann-Price, R. A., Bloch, J. R., Gardner, M., Badit, M., & Aghai, Z. H. (2014). Feeding tolerance in preterm infants on noninvasive respiratory support. *Journal of Perinatal Neonatal Nursing, 28*(4), 300–304.

Cornelius, F. H., & Wittmann-Price, R. A. (2013). *Community nursing test success: An unfolding case study review.* New York, NY: Springer Publishing.

Gittings, K. K., Brogdon, R., Cornelius, F. H., & Wittmann-Price, R. A. (2013). *Medical-surgical nursing test success: An unfolding case study review.* New York, NY: Springer Publishing.

Rubin, R. (1984). *Maternal identity and maternal experience.* New York, NY: Springer Publishing.

Scaffidi, R. M., Posmontier, B., Bloch, B. R., & Wittmann-Price, R. A. (2014). The relationship between personal knowledge and decision self-efficacy in choosing trial of labor after cesarean. *Journal of Midwifery & Women's Health, 59*(3), 246–253.

Scholtz, S. P., Martin, V. A., & Cornelius, F. H. (2015). *Pediatric nursing test success: An unfolding case study review.* New York, NY: Springer Publishing.

Wittmann-Price, R. A., & Cornelius, F. H. (2013). *Fundamentals of nursing test success: An unfolding case study review.* New York, NY: Springer Publishing.

Wittmann-Price, R. A., Reap Thompson, B., Sutton, S., & Eskew, S. (2013). *Nursing concept care maps for safe patient care.* Philadelphia, PA: F. A. Davis.

Wittmann-Price, R. A., & Cornelius, F. H. (2011). *Maternal-child nursing test success: An unfolding case study review.* New York, NY: Springer Publishing.

Wittmann-Price, R. A., & Reap Thompson, B. (Eds.) (2010). *NCLEX-RN® EXCEL: Test success through unfolding case study review.* New York, NY: Springer Publishing.

CHAPTER 5

Pediatric Nursing

Maryann Godshall

Be the change you want to see in the world.—Gandhi

UNFOLDING CASE STUDY 1: Justin

Justin is 2 weeks old and has a temperature of 101.2°F. He has not been eating well for the past 2 days and is lethargic. He is also irritable. His mother says that "all he wants to do is sleep." She takes him to visit the pediatrician, who determines that he should be admitted to the hospital. They arrive on the inpatient pediatric unit and are taken to the treatment room.

History

There is no significant medical history. After a normal vaginal delivery at term, Justin's birth weight was 8 lb, 13 oz. He has no known allergies.

Assessment

- Respiratory: His lung sounds are clear and equal, his respiratory rate (RR) is 54 with no signs of respiratory distress.
- Cardiovascular (CV): His heart rate (HR) is 168 beats per minute (bpm) and regular. No murmur is auscultated.
- Gastrointestinal (GI): His abdomen is soft and nondistended, active bowel sounds.
- Genitourinary (GU): Circumcised male. He has wet only one diaper in the last 24 hours.
- Skin: No rashes, jaundice, or petechiae noted.
- Vital signs (VS): His temperature on admission is 100.8°F axillary.

RAPID RESPONSE TIPS

Normal respiratory rate by pediatric age

Newborn—30 to 60 breaths per minute

2 years—30 breaths per minute

4 years—25 breaths per minute

10 years—20 breaths per minute

RAPID RESPONSE TIPS

Normal heart rate by pediatric age

Age	Awake	Sleeping
Newborn	100–180 bpm	80–160 bpm
1 year	80–150 bpm	70–120 bpm
2–10 years	70–110 bpm	60–100 bpm

EXERCISE 5.1 Multiple-choice:

Which of the following assessments is a priority nursing concern?

A. Heart rate (HR) of 168 beats per minute (bpm)
B. Respiratory rate of 54 breaths per minute
C. Irritability
D. One wet diaper in 24 hours

The answer can be found on page 381

The physician orders a complete blood count (CBC) as well as an electrolyte profile and blood cultures; the physician also does a lumbar puncture. The physician orders an intravenous (IV) line started and IV antibiotics to be given immediately. The lab studies come back and Justin's white blood cell (WBC) count is 3.8/mm^3 (normal WBC count is approximately 4.5–11.0/mm^3).

EXERCISE 5.2 Multiple-choice:

Justin's lab studies are: White blood cell (WBC) count: 3.8/mm^3; vital signs (VS): Temperature: 97.6°F, heart rate (HR): 134 beats per minute (bpm), respiratory rate (RR): 26 breaths per minute

The nurse would suspect:

A. Leukemia
B. HIV
C. Overwhelmed immune system
D. This is normal for a 2-week-old infant

The answer can be found on page 381

The IV line is started and ampicillin (Omnipen, Polycillin, and Principen) and cefotaxime (Claforan) are ordered. The doses are as follows:

Ampicillin: 160 mg IV every 6 hours

Cefotaxime: 200 mg IV every 8 hours

RAPID RESPONSE TIPS

Converting a weight to kilograms

Divide the weight by 2.2 to get kilograms (kg).

If Justin weighs 8 lb, 6 oz, how many kilograms is that?

8 lb and 6 oz = 134 oz; divide by 16 oz = 8.375 lbs and divide by 2.2 = 3.8 kg

All pediatric medications are weight based. It is important to know the weight of the patient in kilograms before attempting to calculate a therapeutic dosage for that patient.

RAPID RESPONSE TIPS

Calculating the therapeutic range for medications

Medication ordered: ampicillin (Omnipen)

Dose given: 160 mg IV every 6 hours

Patient's weight is 3.6 kg

1. First confirm the therapeutic dose range for the medication given in a pediatric drug reference. The range for ampicillin (Omnipen) for a 2-week-old infant is IV/IM 100 to 200 mg/kg/day divided into four doses (drug is administered every 6 hours).
2. Calculate the therapeutic range for the infant's weight:

   3.6 kg × 100 = 360 mg/kg/d

   3.6 kg × 200 = 720 mg/kg/d

   Therapeutic range is 360 to 720 mg/kg/d
3. A nurse needs to know the therapeutic range per *dose* (divide by 4, because a dose is given every 6 hours × 4 = 24 hours in a day):

   360 mg/kg/day divided by 4 = 90 mg/dose

   720 mg/kg/day divided by 4 = 180 mg/dose

   Therapeutic range is 90 to 180 mg/dose
4. Then check to see whether the ordered dose of 160 mg IV every 6 hours falls within the therapeutic range of 90 to 180 mg/dose; it does. So *this is a good therapeutic dose for this patient.*

EXERCISE 5.3 Calculation:

Calculate the therapeutic range for Justin, whose weight is 3.6 kg using the information in the preceding Rapid Response Tip.

The order stated:

Ampicillin: 160 mg intravenous (IV) every 6 hours

Cefotaxime: 200 mg IV every 8 hours

- The medication ordered is Cefotaxime
- Dose ordered: 200 mg IV every 8 hours

What is the therapeutic dose range for Cefotaxime for Justin?

Is the dose therapeutic?

Would you give Justin this dose of medication?

The answer can be found on page 381

---

eRESOURCE

To verify your answer, consult MedCalc. [Pathway: www.medcalc.com → select "Pediatrics" → select "Pediatric Dosing Calculator" and enter information into fields.]

EXERCISE 5.4 Multiple-choice:

What is the priority for calculating the therapeutic dose for pediatric patients based on body weight?

A. To check that the physician's medication order is correct
B. To check that the pharmacy sent the correct medication
C. To provide adequate treatment to the patient
D. To provide safe patient medication administration

The answer can be found on page 382

In conducting an admission assessment, the nurse asks the mother whether Justin has had any childhood immunizations yet. She replies "yes," but forgets which ones.

EXERCISE 5.5 Multiple-choice:

Justin, at 2 weeks of age, would have had which typical childhood immunizations?

A. Diphtheria, tetanus toxoids, and pertussis (DTP)
B. Measles, mumps, and rubella (MMR)
C. Hepatitis B vaccine
D. Varicella vaccine

The answer can be found on page 382

---

eRESOURCE

Consult the Centers for Disease Control (CDC) Recommended Immunization Schedules:

- Online: [Pathway: www.cdc.gov ➔ enter "Immunization schedule" into the search field ➔ select "Childhood & Adolescent Immunization Schedule" and review content.]
- Mobile App: [Pathway: CDC Vaccine Schedule ➔ select "Child (Birth-6 Years)" ➔ review content] (obtain mobile apps from CDC: http://goo.gl/I7ikb2)

EXERCISE 5.6 Matching:

In assessing growth and development, match the stages of development in Column A that Justin would be in according to the developmental and cognitive theorists listed in Column B:

Column A	Column B
A. Sensorimotor	____ Erickson
B. Trust versus mistrust	____ Freud
C. Oral	____ Piaget

The answer can be found on page 382

UNFOLDING CASE STUDY 2: Sasha

Sasha, a 6-month-old female infant, is having difficulty breathing and is brought to the hospital as an emergency admission from the pediatric clinic. According to her mother, she has been sick for about 2 days with a runny nose.

History

Normal 34-week vaginal delivery, birth weight: 5 lb, 11 ounces (2.32 kg). Sasha was in the neonatal intensive care unit (NICU) for 2 weeks with respiratory distress. She received continuous positive airway pressure (CPAP) for 2 days and then oxygen by nasal cannula for 5 days. She has a heart murmur and has been examined by a cardiologist. It is a patent ductus arteriosus (PDA), which is common for a preterm infant. Her childhood immunizations are up to date. Sasha had otitis media at 4 months of age, which was treated with amoxicillin.

Assessment

EXERCISE 5.7 Multiple-choice:

What is a priority for the nurse to assess?

A. Respirations
B. Cardiac sounds
C. Bowel sounds
D. Skin turgor

The answer can be found on page 382

EXERCISE 5.8 Fill in the blanks:

As part of the respiratory assessment, what should the nurse observe?

____

____

____

____

The answer can be found on page 382

In conducting a respiratory assessment, it is very important to take a minute before approaching the child to observe her or his respiratory effort. Does the child look relaxed, is the child breathing easily, or is the child "working" harder than normal to breathe? Remember, as the nurse approaches the child, he or she may begin to cry, causing him or her to breathe at a faster rate. Approach the child slowly, while addressing the child in a soft voice. Also, speak with the parents, if present, to help establish a trusting relationship.

RAPID RESPONSE TIPS

Signs and symptoms of respiratory distress syndrome

Restlessness
Retractions
Poor oral feeding and intake
Elevated temperature
Tachycardia initially (bradycardia is an ominous sign; increased heart rate)
Tachypnea (increased respiratory rate)
Duskiness or cyanosis
Periorbital or perioral cyanosis
Pale, mottled skin
Nasal flaring

eRESOURCE

To reinforce your understanding of the clinical presentation of a respiratory distress syndrome (RDS), refer to Medscape on your mobile device. [Pathway: Medscape → enter "RDS" into the search field → select "RDS" and review content under "Clinical Presentation."]

RAPID RESPONSE TIPS

Auscultation of lung sounds

When the nurse listens to lung sounds, he or she has to listen for the quality and characteristics of breath sounds in order to identify any abnormal lung sounds. Auscultate the entire chest, comparing sounds between the sides. Also listen to the lateral lung fields. Listen to an entire inspiratory and expiratory phase for each area before moving to the next one. Normal breath sounds are vesicular and low pitched. Bronchovesicular and bronchial or tracheal breath sounds should be heard at the correct position. Absent or diminished breath sounds usually indicate a partial or total obstruction to airflow. Listen for intensity, pitch, and rhythm. Also listen for adventitious breath sounds. Assess the lungs of an infant or young child when he or she is sleeping or quiet.

Sasha's temperature is 101.8°F rectally. Her RR is 68 breaths per minute. Her HR is 152 bpm at rest. Sasha is exhibiting nasal flaring and grunting on expiration. Retractions are present. She looks very pale and tired. The parents state that she "has had a cold" for the past few days. An IV line is ordered as well as a nasal aspirate/swab for respiratory syncytial virus (RSV). The primary nursing goal is to maintain a patent airway.

EXERCISE 5.9 Fill in the blank:

What are retractions and why do they occur?

____

The answer can be found on page 383

EXERCISE 5.10 Fill in the blanks:

The severity of retractions is noted as ___________, ___________, and ___________.

The answer can be found on page 383

EXERCISE 5.11 Hot spot:

Please draw a line to the area where retraction would be assessed and label each line using the supplied terms:

Supraclavicular
Suprasternal
Intercostal
Substernal
Subcostal

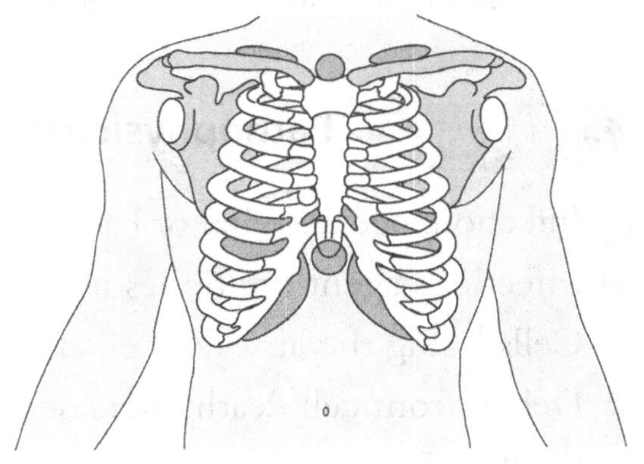

The answer can be found on page 383

EXERCISE 5.12 Fill in the blanks:

Name two priority nursing diagnoses for Sasha:

1. ________________________________
2. ________________________________

The answer can be found on page 383

Sasha's RSV specimen comes back positive. Her pulse oximetry reading is 90% on room air. Sasha is placed on 1 L of oxygen via nasal cannula. Her pulse oximetry reading is now 98%. Her lung sounds demonstrate expiratory wheezing bilaterally. Her retractions and nasal flaring disappear with the oxygen. She stops grunting. She is placed on the pediatric unit.

EXERCISE 5.13 Select all that apply:

Which of the following should the nurse implement for a child hospitalized with respiratory syncytial virus (RSV)?

A. Antipyretics to reduce the fever
B. Oxygen therapy
C. Intravenous (IV) and/or oral rehydration
D. IV administration of antibiotics
E. Frequent monitoring and suctioning of the nasal airway
F. Monitoring on a cardiac/respiratory monitor
G. Routine intubation to protect the airway
H. Monitoring by continuous pulse oximetry

The answer can be found on page 383

eRESOURCE

To reinforce your understanding of the treatment of RDS, refer to Medscape on your mobile device. [Pathway: Medscape ➔ enter "RDS" into the search field ➔ select "RDS" and review content under "Treatment and Management."]

RAPID RESPONSE TIPS **Pathophysiology of bronchiolitis or respiratory syncytial virus**

- Infectious agent—viral or bacterial—penetrates the mucosal cells lining the bronchioles.
- Infectious agent multiplies in mucosal cells.
- Cells lining the airway swell and produce mucus.
- Debris from cell death, increased mucus, and swollen cells compromises the size of the airway.
- As the diameter of the airway is reduced, air exchange becomes more difficult, resulting in respiratory distress and wheezing.

UNFOLDING CASE STUDY 3: Jenifer

Jenifer, a 4-week-old infant, is brought to the emergency department (ED) by her parents. Her mother says, "When I held her, I felt her heartbeat racing against my chest. Is that normal?" They also say that they think she is breathing faster than normal.

History

The parents report that Jenifer was born at 39 weeks gestational age (GA) by spontaneous vaginal delivery. Her Apgar scores were 9 and 10 at 1 and 5 minutes, respectively. Jenifer was discharged home on the second day of life and had a normal 2-week checkup, at which time she received her hepatitis B vaccine. She had been eating well until yesterday. Now she is not taking her full bottle. She has no fever, cough, vomiting, or diarrhea. She has not been around anyone who was sick.

Assessment

Upon initial assessment, Jenifer's skin is pale but pink. She is looking around and has an appropriate neurological examination. Her anterior fontanel is open and flat. Her lung fields are clear to auscultation bilaterally. Her oxygen saturation is 96% on room air and her abdomen is soft and nondistended, with active bowel sounds. She has voided six wet diapers in the past day. She had a soft stool just this morning. Her HR is fast and her rhythm is normal, without a murmur. The nurse places Jenifer on a cardiac respiratory monitor and observes the following:

EXERCISE 5.14 Exhibit-format:

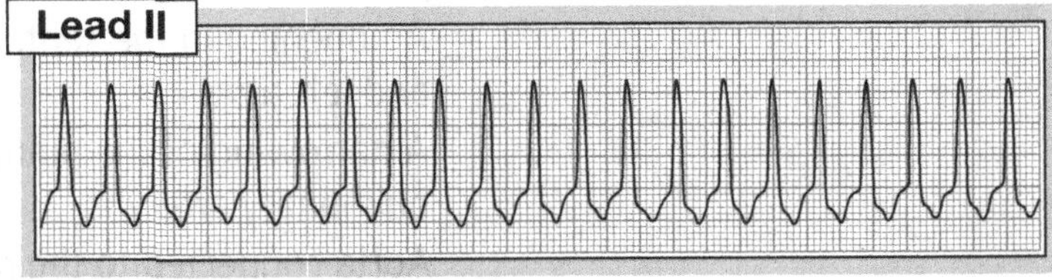

HR = 210

Using this electrocardiogram (EKG) monitor strip the nurse would suspect:

A. Normal sinus rhythm
B. Tachycardia
C. Supraventricular tachycardia
D. Congestive heart failure

The answer can be found on page 384

eRESOURCE

To reinforce your understanding of EKG interpretation, view the following resources:

- *Intro EKG Interpretation Part 1:* http://youtu.be/ex1k_MPF-w4
- *Intro EKG Interpretation Part 2:* http://youtu.be/ecTM2O940mg

EXERCISE 5.15 Fill in the blank:

What would be the most appropriate, nonhematological diagnostic test to perform at this time?

____

The answer can be found on page 384

Jenifer is transferred to the pediatric unit for further workup. An echocardiogram is done to determine if she has a congenital heart defect.

EXERCISE 5.16 Matching:

Match the structural defects in Column A with the correct descriptions in Column B:

Column A	Column B
A. Ventricular septal defect (VSD)	___A narrowing at, above, or below the aortic valve
B. Atrial septal defect (ASD)	___A narrowing of the lumen of the aorta usually at or near the ductus arteriosus
C. Patent ductus arteriosus (PDA)	___A hole in the septum between the right and left ventricles
D. Aortic stenosis (AS)	___ Complete closure of the tricuspid valve
E. Pulmonary stenosis (PS)	___ Consists of four anomalies: pulmonary stenosis (PS), ventricular septal defect (VSD), overriding aorta, and right ventricular hypertrophy
F. Tricuspid atresia (TA)	___ Normal fetal circulatory opening between the pulmonary artery and the aorta that fails to close
G. Coarctation of the aorta (CoA)	___ An opening in the septum between the right and left atria
H. Transposition of the great vessels (arteries; TGA)	___A narrowing of the pulmonary valve or pulmonary artery
I. Tetralogy of Fallot (TOF)	___Aorta connected to the right ventricle instead of the left; pulmonary artery connected to the left ventricle instead of the right

The answer can be found on page 384

Jenifer's history is negative for other cardiac events, but she is noted to have some edema. The nurses on this pediatric unit assess many children with cardiac disease and are well versed on the medications used.

eRESOURCE

To supplement your understanding of congenital heart defects, refer to the *Merck Manual.* [Pathway: www.merckmanuals.com/professional ➔ enter "Congenital Heart Defects" into the search field ➔ select "Overview of Congenital Cardiovascular Anomalies" ➔ review content.]

EXERCISE 5.17 Matching:

Match the common cardiac medications listed in Column A with the uses for pediatric patients in Column B:

Column A	Column B
A. Digoxin (Lanoxin)	___A potent loop diuretic that rids the body of excess fluid. Used to treat congestive heart failure (CHF).
B. Furosemide (Lasix)	___A medication that is given to convert supraventricular tachycardia (SVT) back to normal sinus rhythm (NSR).
C. Captopril (Capoten)	___A diuretic that is potassium sparing.
D. Adenosine (Adenocard)	___An angiotensin converting enzyme (ACE) inhibitor that causes vasoconstriction, which reduces afterload.
E. Spironolactone (Aldactone)	___A medication that improves cardiac contractility.

The answer can be found on page 385

The treatment for supraventricular tachycardia would be to first attempt a vagal maneuver (ice to the face, have the patient bear down if possible). If that does not work, adenosine would be administered. The half-life of adenosine is less than 10 seconds. It is, therefore, vital that the medication be given by a physician via rapid push followed by a rapid saline flush. Note that adenosine stops the heart to allow time to "break the irregular rhythm"; it is hoped that the heart will restart with a regular rhythm.

eRESOURCE

To supplement your understanding of the clinical presentation and treatment of supraventricular tachycardia, refer to the *Merck Manual.* [Pathway: www.merckmanuals.com/professional ➔ enter "SVT" into the search field ➔ select "Reentrant Supraventricular Tachycardias" ➔ review content.]

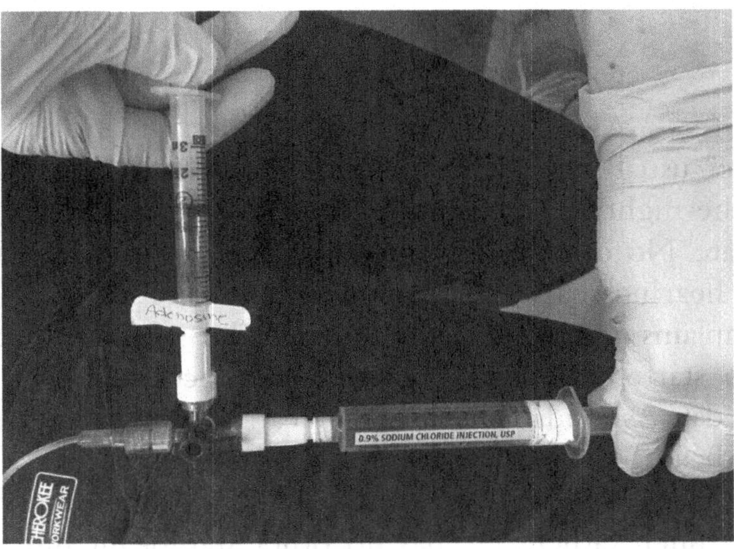

FIGURE 5.1 Administering adenosine.

The following strip is on the monitor during the adenosine administration.

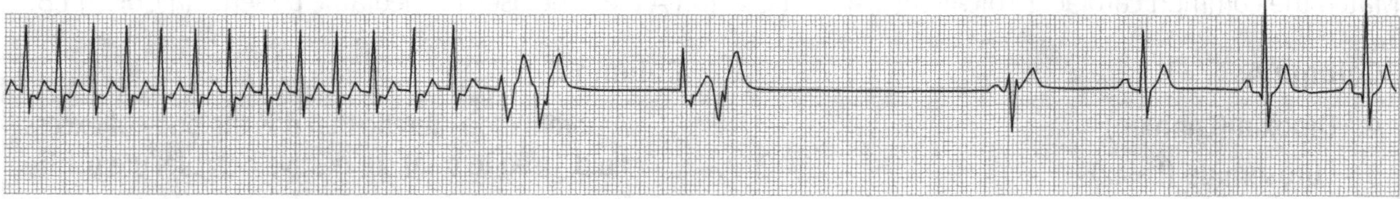

eRESOURCE

To reinforce your understanding of the clinical presentation and treatment of supraventricular tachycardia, refer to the Life in the Fastlane web resource. [Pathway: http://lifeinthefastlane.com ➔ select "ECG Library" tab ➔ enter "SVT" into the search field ➔ select "Supraventricular Tachycardia (SVT)" ➔ review content.]

The adenosine dose can be doubled for a total of three doses. If the supraventricular tachycardia (SVT) rhythm does not convert with medications, the patient may need to be cardioverted.

eRESOURCE

To reinforce your understanding of the cardioversion procedure, refer to Medscape on your mobile device. [Pathway: Medscape ➔ enter "Cardioversion" into the search field ➔ select "Synchronized Electrical Cardioversion" and review content.]

UNFOLDING CASE STUDY 4: Ashonda

Ashonda, a 2-year-old, is presented to the pediatric clinic with a 2-day history of vomiting and diarrhea.

History

Ashonda was in her usual state of health until about 2 days ago, when she woke up in the middle of the night and began vomiting. She had pizza for dinner, which the entire family also ate. No other family members became ill. She attends day care and the mother recalls hearing that other children there were also sick about a week earlier. Ashonda complains that "her belly hurts." The mother reports that last evening Ashonda also started having diarrhea, which occurred five or six times over the course of the day. Ashonda is refusing to eat. Her mother has given her Gatorade (a clear liquid), but she vomits immediately after she drinks it. She has had a fever of 99°F to 100.5°F (axillary) over the past day. The mother states that Ashonda hasn't voided very much either. She has no other significant history and she has no allergies.

Assessment

Ashonda is awake but lethargic in her mother's arms. She appears pale and is crying (tears are present). Her lung sounds are clear. Her RR is 28 breaths per minute and HR is 110 bpm and regular without a murmur. Abdomen is soft, mildly tender, nondistended, and bowel sounds are noted. Her temperature is now 101.2°F rectally. Her cheeks are slightly flushed. Ashonda has been vomiting and has had diarrhea for 24 hours.

EXERCISE 5.18 Fill in the blank:

What is a nursing priority with this patient?

____

The answer can be found on page 385

EXERCISE 5.19 Multiple-choice:

The nurse may suspect which diagnosis for Ashonda?

A. Appendicitis
B. Intussusception
C. Viral gastroenteritis
D. Intestinal obstruction

The answer can be found on page 385

EXERCISE 5.20 Multiple-choice:

What is the most likely cause of the viral gastroenteritis?

A. *Salmonella*
B. *Escherichia coli*
C. *Clostridium difficile*
D. Rotavirus

The answer can be found on page 385

eRESOURCE

To reinforce your understanding of viral gastroenteritis, refer to Medscape on your mobile device. [Pathway: Medscape ➔ enter "Gastroenteritis" into the search field ➔ select "Viral Gastroenteritis" and review "Overview" and "Clinical Presentation."]

Because of the vomiting and diarrhea and suspected diagnosis of viral gastroenteritis, it is decided that the patient should be placed in isolation.

EXERCISE 5.21 Multiple-choice:

What type of isolation precautions does the nurse expect Ashonda will require related to potential transmission of illness?

A. Contact isolation
B. Droplet isolation
C. Airborne isolation
D. Standard precautions

The answer can be found on page 385

EXERCISE 5.22 Select all that apply:

Which of the following are reasons for Ashonda being placed in the type of isolation that was chosen?

A. The risk of transmission via the fecal–oral route.
B. Rotavirus lives on hands for hours and contact surfaces are not cleaned for days.
C. Rotavirus can be transmitted through droplets in the air.
D. The transmission of the virus can be prevented by wearing gloves and good handwashing.
E. Families should be told why the patient is in isolation, so they can comply with isolation precautions too.
F. Standard precautions are good enough to prevent transmission.

The answer can be found on page 386

EXERCISE 5.23 Multiple-choice:

What is the most appropriate treatment for a mildly dehydrated patient with viral gastroenteritis?

A. Keep on nothing orally (NPO) status
B. Send the child home and tell the parents to give her apple juice as tolerated
C. Try oral rehydration therapy with Pedialyte; if ineffective, administer intravenous (IV) fluids
D. IV fluids followed by peritoneal lavage

The answer can be found on page 386

eRESOURCE

To reinforce your understanding of isolation precautions, refer to MedlinePlus. [Pathway: www.nlm.nih.gov/medlineplus ➔ enter "Isolation Precautions" into the search field ➔ select "Isolation Precautions" and review content.]

EXERCISE 5.24 Multiple-choice:

Which of the following assessments would be indicative of dehydration?

A. Dry mucous membranes
B. Increased skin turgor
C. Decreased thirst
D. Dilute urine

The answer can be found on page 386

Other signs that would point to dehydration would be dry, pale skin, a rapid pulse or HR (the body is trying to compensate for low vascular volume by circulating the low volume it has more rapidly), sunken fontanels (in an infant), and diminished urinary output.

EXERCISE 5.25 Multiple-choice:

What would be the *most appropriate* nursing diagnosis for moderate dehydration?

A. Anxiety
B. Fluid volume deficit
C. Acute pain
D. Alteration in cardiac output

The answer can be found on page 387

TABLE 5.1 Rapid Response Terms: Stages of Dehydration

Mild dehydration	■ In mild dehydration there is up to a 5% weight loss ■ Patients appears restless if they cannot verbalize that they are thirsty ■ Mucous membranes are still moist ■ Still urinating ■ Younger than a year, their anterior fontanel is flat and normal to palpation
Moderate dehydration	■ Greater weight loss; can be as high as 9% ■ Irritability and lethargy can be seen ■ Pulse is rapid, respiratory rate increases, capillary refill is delayed, and blood pressure is decreased ■ Mucous membranes are dry ■ Urine output is below 1 mL/kg/hr ■ Young child may display sunken fontanels
Severe dehydration	■ Weight loss greater than 10% ■ Lethargy ■ Low blood pressure ■ Pulse is rapid and capillary refill is greater than 4 seconds ■ Extremities are cool ■ Low blood pressure ■ In young children the fontanels are sunken and respiratory rate is rapid

EXERCISE 5.26 Matching:

Match the correct description in Column A with the appropriate disorder in Column B:

Column A	Column B
A. Cleft lip/palate	___ Protrusion of abdominal contents through the abdominal wall at the umbilical area
B. Pyloric stenosis	___ Aganglionic segments of the bowel cause the formation of a megacolon
C. Tracheoesophageal (TE) fistula	___ Twisting of the bowel upon itself, causing obstruction
D. Gastroesophageal (GE) reflux	___ Bowel inflammation with a "cobblestone-like" appearance
E. Crohn's disease	___ Necrosis of the mucosa of the intestine
F. Omphalocele	___ Inflammation of continuous segments of the bowel; bloody stools
G. Gastroschisis	___ Constricting band ("vestigial structure") of the bowel
H. Diaphragmatic hernia	___ "Telescoping" of the bowel
I. Hirschsprung's disease	___ Failure of the normal rotation of viscera
J. Malrotation	___ Failure of fusion of the maxillary and median nasal process
K. Intussusception	___ Abnormal connection between the trachea and esophagus
L. Ulcerative colitis	___ Characterized by projectile vomiting
M. Meckel's diverticulum	___ Diagnosed with a pH probe study
N. Necrotizing enterocolitis	___ Abdominal wall defect in which abdominal contents are not contained in a peritoneal membrane
O. Volvulus	___ Protrusion of abdominal contents into the chest cavity

The answer can be found on page 387

After 2 days of rehydration, Ashonda is discharged; she will require follow-up in the pediatric clinic in 48 hours to make sure she is maintaining fluids.

eRESOURCE

To reinforce your understanding of dehydration, refer to Medscape on your mobile device. [Pathway: Medscape ➔ enter "Dehydration" into the search field ➔ select "Dehydration" and review content.]

UNFOLDING CASE STUDY 5: Stevie

Stevie is a 5-year-old who has been potty rained without any "accidents" since age 4 years. He has begun to have accidents both at night and during the day. His parents are very concerned and Stevie is embarrassed. Stevie's parents have been trying to help the situation by not letting Stevie drink anything after 7 p.m. This has not been helpful. Stevie is still having enuresis.

EXERCISE 5.27 Select all that apply:

Which of the following could be possible causes of Stevie's enuresis?

A. Glomerulonephritis
B. Urinary tract infection (UTI)
C. New onset of diabetes mellitus
D. Epispadias
E. Exstrophy of the bladder
F. Hypospadias

The answer can be found on page 387

History

Stevie's parents bring him to the pediatric clinic. Stevie was born at term; it was a normal vaginal delivery without complications; no GU defects were noted. He has no known medical allergies. He has no prior hospitalizations. He has been on medicine for frequent ear infections and has bilateral myringotomy tubes. His mother also states that he had several urinary tract infections (UTIs) in the past.

Assessment

On admission, Stevie appears nervous and embarrassed. He is alert but avoiding eye contact with the pediatric nurse practitioner (PNP) during the examination and when asked questions. Breath sounds are clear and equal bilaterally. HR is regular at 76 bpm; his abdomen is soft and nondistended, with active bowel sounds. His parents state that he says he has to go to the bathroom, but by the time he gets there he has already voided in his clothes. When the PNP asks whether it hurts when he urinates, he does not reply. He has a temperature of 101.8°F tympanic. Because of the history of frequent UTIs in the past, the physician orders a urine specimen to be collected by urinary catheterization.

EXERCISE 5.28 Multiple-choice:

What symptoms would the nurse expect for a urinary tract infection (UTI)?

A. Dysuria, thirst, light-colored urine, ammonia smell in the urine
B. Dysuria; left-sided flank pain; and dark, foul-smelling urine
C. Oliguria, lower abdominal pain, yellow urine, ammonia smell in the urine, and epigastric pain
D. Polyuria, lower abdominal pain, yellow urine, ammonia smell in the urine

The answer can be found on page 388

eRESOURCE

To supplement your understanding of the clinical presentation and treatment of supraventricular tachycardia, refer to the *Merck Manual.* [Pathway: www.merckmanuals.com/professional ➔ enter "UTI" into the search field ➔ select "Urinary Tract Infection (UTI) in Children" ➔ review content.]

Stevie's urinalysis reveals WBCs. The urine culture shows 20,000 colonies of *E. coli*. The physician orders antibiotics and a voiding cystourethrogram (VCUG).

EXERCISE 5.29 Select all that apply:

The mother asks what a voiding cystourethrogram (VCUG) is and why it is being ordered. Which of the following statements are correct?

A. It is an x-ray of the child's bladder and lower urinary tract.
B. A tube or catheter will be inserted into the child's penis.
C. It is a tube or catheter that will be inserted up into your child's kidneys.
D. It has radioactive dye that will be instilled into the child's penis through a tube.
E. The child may cry through the entire procedure.
F. The test checks for urinary reflux.
G. The test checks whether the child has diabetes mellitus.
H. The test will tell whether the child has a urinary tract infection (UTI).

The answer can be found on page 388

UNFOLDING CASE STUDY 6: Marianne and Hashama

Marianne is a 7-year-old with a 4-day history of abdominal pain and weight gain of 10 lb in 1 week. Marianne's mother noticed that her urine is very dark and foamy. After a brief assessment by the PNP, Marianne is admitted to the pediatric inpatient unit at the hospital.

History

Marianne was born at term via a normal vaginal delivery. Her birth weight was 7 lb, 3 ounces. She has no allergies. She has no significant medical history other than that she has had two UTIs, both of which were treated with trimethoprim/sulfamethoxazole (Bactrim). She has just recovered from strep throat, which began 2 weeks ago. She likes to play video games and watch television.

Assessment

Marianne is alert but appears tired. Her lung sounds have fine crackles in the bases bilaterally. HR is normal at 110 bpm. Her RR is 28 breaths per minute. Her blood pressure is 155/92 mmHg. Her temperature is 101°F. She has periorbital edema and pedal edema +2. Her skin is pale, pink, and taut.

EXERCISE 5.30 Multiple-choice:

Because Marianne has suspected glomerulonephritis, the nurse would expect to see that she had a recent ____________ infection.

A. Urinary tract
B. Streptococcal
C. Blood
D. Ear

The answer can be found on page 388

Exercise 5.31 Multiple-choice:

For Marianne, which of the following nursing diagnoses should receive priority?

A. Excess fluid volume
B. Risk for infection
C. Knowledge deficit
D. Activity intolerance

The answer can be found on page 389

---

eRESOURCE

To reinforce your understanding of glomerulonephritis, refer to Medscape on your mobile device. [Pathway: Medscape ➔ enter "Glomerulonephritis" into the search field ➔ select "Poststreptoccal Glomerulonephritis" and review content.]

Hashama is a 7-year-old girl who was also admitted to the pediatric inpatient unit and placed in the same room as Marianne. Over the past few weeks, Hashama has become edematous. Her mother noticed that her clothes were fitting tighter and that she was gaining weight. Hashama also told her mother that "it hurts to wear my shoes." Hashama's mother reports that her child has been "just lying around the house." The mother also noticed that Hashama's urine is very dark and foamy. When Hashama has gym class, she gets winded easily.

History

Hashama was a normal-term vaginal delivery with a birth weight of 8 lb, 4 ounces. She has no known allergies. She had "a cold" for the past 2 weeks. She was never hospitalized. Family history indicates Hashama's mother has hypertension and her father had asthma as a child, which he later grew out of.

Assessment

Hashama's skin is pale and taut. Her lungs are clear. Her respiratory rate is 28 breaths per minute. Her heart is slightly tachycardic at 90 bpm. No murmur is noted. Her abdomen is soft but slightly distended, with positive bowel sounds. She has pitting edema of the feet as well as generalized edema about the hands and face; periorbital edema is noted. She appears tired. Temperature is 99.2°F orally.

EXERCISE 5.32 Multiple-choice:

What classic symptoms would the nurse expect Hashama to have if she has nephrotic syndrome?

A. Hypotension, hypernatremia, hyperproteinuria
B. Hypernatremia, hypoalbuminemia, hypertension
C. Hematuria, hypotension, tachycardia
D. Hyperalbuminemia, hypolipidemia, hypotension

The answer can be found on page 389

EXERCISE 5.33 Multiple-choice:

A child with nephrotic syndrome has a platelet count of 750,000 mm³. Which of the following signs and symptoms should the nurse monitor?

A. Thrombosis
B. Bruising and petechiae
C. Pulmonary edema
D. Infection

The answer can be found on page 389

The physician orders a urinalysis for Hashama, which shows massive proteinuria negative for blood and a trace of glucose; the specific gravity is 1.025. The mother asks why the urine is dark and foamy. The best response would be to tell her that this is caused by albumin and protein in the urine.

EXERCISE 5.34 Select all that apply:

Which of the following would be appropriate nursing measures for Hashama?

A. Strictly monitor input and output (I&O)
B. Maintain a diet low in sodium
C. Weigh the patient every day
D. Maintain a diet low in protein

The answer can be found on page 389

Hashama is transferred from the general pediatric unit to the pediatric intensive care unit (PICU).

eRESOURCE

To reinforce your understanding of nephrotic syndrome, refer to Medscape on your mobile device. [Pathway: Medscape ➔ enter "Nephrotic" into the search field ➔ select "Nephrotic Syndrome" and review content.]

UNFOLDING CASE STUDY 7: Sam

Sam, age 4 years, is a patient in the PICU. He has been in the PICU for 2 weeks. He had an unknown illness complicated by severe diarrhea. Sam is in renal failure because his kidneys are unable to maintain electrolyte and fluid balance. Nursing assessment of the GI tract finds no genetic anomalies.

EXERCISE 5.35 Matching:

Match the best description of the urinary defect listed in Column A with the definition in Column B:

Column A	Column B
A. Hypospadias	____ Congenital defect in which the bladder protrudes through the abdominal wall
B. Epispadias	____ Accumulation of urine in the renal pelvis
C. Exstrophy of the bladder	____ Urethral meatus located on the ventral surface of the penile shaft
D. Chordee	____ Narrowing or stenosis of preputial opening of foreskin
E. Hydronephrosis	____ Fluid in the scrotum
F. Hydrocele	____ Ventral curvature of the penis
G. Cryptorchidism	____ Urethral meatus located on the dorsal surface of the penile shaft
H. Phimosis	____ Undescended testes

The answer can be found on page 390

EXERCISE 5.36 Multiple-choice:

Which of the following is the most common cause of acute renal failure in children?

A. Pyelonephritis
B. Uremic syndrome
C. Urinary tract obstruction
D. Severe dehydration

The answer can be found on page 390

EXERCISE 5.37 Multiple-choice:

Which of the following is the primary clinical manifestation of acute renal failure?

A. Oliguria
B. Hematuria
C. Proteinuria
D. Bacteriuria

The answer can be found on page 390

Sam's laboratory studies indicate a hemoglobin of 7 g/dL, platelets are 50,000 μL. His blood urea nitrogen (BUN) is 32 mg/dL and creatinine is 1.5 mg/dL. His potassium level is 6.5 mEq/L. Hemolytic uremic syndrome (HUS) is suspected. The physicians tell the parents that Sam may need hemodialysis or plasmapheresis. His parents are very upset and tell the nurse they feel guilty for not getting him to the pediatrician sooner.

EXERCISE 5.38 Multiple-choice:

What is the best intervention to help the parents in coping with this illness?

A. Suggest to the parents that they get some rest so they will feel better
B. Tell the parents not to worry, it was not their fault
C. Call the nursing supervisor to talk with the parents
D. Be supportive of the parents and allow them to verbalize their feelings

The answer can be found on page 390

---

eRESOURCE

To further reinforce your understanding of acute renal failure, refer to Medscape on your mobile device. [Pathway: Medscape → enter "Acute Renal" into the search field → select "Acute Renal Failure Complications" and review content focusing on "Emergency Department Care," "Inpatient Care," and "Transfer Considerations."]

UNFOLDING CASE STUDY 8: Jeffrey

Jeffrey, who is 15 months old, was brought to the ED by his parents after having a generalized seizure. His parents state that he was well until the previous day, when he developed a runny nose and cough. They report that he was "not himself" and put him to bed at 8 p.m. At 1 a.m. they heard him crying; then, when they went into his room, he was silent and they saw him make rhythmic jerking movements with both his legs and arms for about 3 minutes. After he stopped jerking, he fell asleep. They gathered him up, put him in the car, and rushed him to the ED. They did not think to call 911. When asked whether he had a fever, his mother said that "he felt warm, but we don't have a thermometer."

History

Jeffrey was a full-term infant who had a spontaneous vaginal delivery. He had Apgar scores of 9 and 9 at 1 and 5 minutes, respectively. He was discharged to home at 2 days of age. There is no family history of seizures. He lives at home with his parents and attends day care. He is taking no medications other than daily vitamins. He has no known allergies.

Assessment

Jeffrey has a seizure again in the ED and is a direct admission to the PICU. On initial assessment, his skin appears flushed and is hot to the touch. His temperature is 102.5°F rectally. He is sleeping on the stretcher. His lungs are clear and a yellow mucous discharge from his nose is noted. Oxygen saturation is 99% on room air. HR is regular at 112 bpm without a murmur. His abdomen is soft, with positive bowel sounds. He has normal reflexes. Ear, nose, and throat are normal. As the nurse conducts her examination, Jeffrey wakes up and moves over, close to his mother. It is suspected that Jeffrey had a febrile seizure.

EXERCISE 5.39 Multiple-choice:

Which of the following statements is true about febrile seizures?

A. Febrile seizures are usually associated only with bacterial infections.
B. There is a genetic link to febrile seizures.
C. Febrile seizures are not associated with any long-term complications.
D. A febrile seizure usually indicates that the child will develop epilepsy later on.

The answer can be found on page 391

EXERCISE 5.40 Multiple-choice:

What is the most common age for seizures to occur in children?

A. Birth through 1 month of age
B. 1 month to 6 months of age
C. 6 months through 5 years of age
D. 5 years to 8 years of age

The answer can be found on page 391

Jeffrey is discharged from the PICU because he does not need cardiac or respiratory support, but he is admitted to the pediatric unit for further observation.

EXERCISE 5.41 Multiple-choice:

The nurse prepares the room for Jeffrey, what items would be a priority?

A. Working suction and oxygen
B. A drink to maintain hydration
C. Tongue blade and rail pads
D. Albuterol and an intravenous (IV) setup

The answer can be found on page 391

Jeffrey and his family get settled in his room. Jeffrey is placed on a cardiac–respiratory monitor as well as a pulse oximeter to measure his oxygen saturation. About 2 hours later, Jeffrey's parents ring the call bell. The nurse responds to find Jeffrey having another seizure. He is jerking both his arms and legs rhythmically.

EXERCISE 5.42 Multiple-choice:

What is the nursing priority for this patient?

A. Place a tongue depressor in his mouth to prevent him from swallowing his tongue
B. Maintain a patent airway
C. Start an intravenous (IV) line to give medications
D. Leave the room to get help and call the primary care provider

The answer can be found on page 391

During the seizure, the nurse reassures Jeffrey's parents that he will be all right. The nurse speaks to Jeffrey to reassure him and notices on the monitor that his HR has increased to 122 bpm and his pulse oximeter dropped to 89% during the seizure.

EXERCISE 5.43 True/False:

During a seizure, the nurse would expect Jeffrey's heart rate to increase and his oxygen saturation to drop.

_____ True
_____ False

The answer can be found on page 392

EXERCISE 5.44 Fill in the blank:

What is the name of the condition in which a seizure lasts longer than 30 minutes or a series of seizures that last longer than 30 minutes in which consciousness is not regained between episodes? __________

The answer can be found on page 392

---

eRESOURCE

To further reinforce your understanding of febrile seizures, refer to Medscape on your mobile device. [Pathway: Medscape → enter "Febrile Seizures" into the search field → select "Pediatric Febrile Seizures" and review content.]

EXERCISE 5.45 Multiple-choice:

Which of the following medications used for seizures has the side effect of gingival hyperplasia?

A. Phenobarbital (Luminal)
B. Valproic acid (Depakote)
C. Carbamazapine (Tegretol)
D. Phenytoin (Dilantin)

The answer can be found on page 392

EXERCISE 5.46 Fill in the blank:

What is the name of a medication similar to phenytoin (Dilantin) that can be given more quickly intravenously and is compatible with dextrose-containing intravenous (IV) solutions?__________

The answer can be found on page 392

---

eRESOURCE

To reinforce your understanding of specific medications used in the treatment of seizures, refer to Epocrates Online. [Pathway: http://online.epocrates.com → under the "Drugs" tab, select the "Drugs" tab → in the "Classes" column, select "Neurologic" → under that subclass, select "Seizure Disorders" and review the drugs listed, focusing on "Adverse Reactions" and "Safety/Monitoring."]

EXERCISE 5.47 Matching:

Match the seizure types in Column A with the correct descriptions in Column B:

Column A	Column B
A. Tonic–clonic	___ A brief loss of consciousness that looks like daydreaming
B. Absence seizure	___ Most severe and difficult to control
C. Febrile seizure	___ Strong rhythmic jerking of the body
D. Complex partial seizure	___ A phase of the seizure during which the person may sleep
E. Lennox–Gastaut seizure	___ May be caused by a sudden dramatic change in body temperature
F. Akinetic seizure	___ Usually starts in the focal area and then spreads to the other hemisphere, with some impairment or loss of consciousness
G. Aura	___ Phase of a seizure during which a feeling or smell is recognized before a seizure begins
H. Postictal phase	___ Person may "freeze into place"

The answer can be found on page 393

The next day Jeffrey starts showing signs of an upper respiratory infection (URI). He complains of a very bad headache. He also says it hurts his eyes to look in the light. On initial examination, he is seen lying on his side in the fetal position, lethargic, and somewhat unresponsive. The nurse turns him on his back and notes that he has nuchal rigidity (resistance to neck flexion). He also has positive Kernig's and Brudzinski's signs. The nurse suspects possible meningitis. The nurse obtains the lab orders for a CBC and electrolytes.

RAPID RESPONSE TIPS

Assessing for meningeal inflammation

Assessment Technique	Normal	Abnormal
Brudzinski's sign: Flex the client's neck while observing the reaction of the hips and knees	Hips and knees remain relaxed and motionless	Hips and knees become flexed
Kernig's sign: Flex the client's leg at the hip and knee; while the hip remains flexed, try to straighten the knee	No pain	Pain and increased resistance to extending the knee

EXERCISE 5.48 Fill in the blank:

What other test would the nurse expect the physician to perform to confirm the diagnosis of meningitis?

____

The answer can be found on page 393

EXERCISE 5.49 Select all that apply:

Which of the following nursing interventions are appropriate for Jeffrey?

A. Maintain Jeffrey on droplet or respiratory isolation
B. Perform neurological checks frequently
C. Administer antibiotics as ordered
D. Monitor the skin for petechiae or purpura
E. Keep the room bright and sunny to avoid depression

The answer can be found on page 393

EXERCISE 5.50 Select all that apply:

Which of the following vaccines protect infants from bacterial meningitis?

A. IPV (inactivated polio vaccine)
B. PCV (pneumococcal vaccine)

C. DTP (diphtheria, tetanus, and pertussis vaccine)
D. HiB (*Haemophilus influenzae* type B vaccine)
E. Measles, mumps, and rubella (MMR) vaccine

The answer can be found on page 393

eRESOURCE

To supplement your understanding of the clinical presentation associated with meningitis as well as preventative measures, refer to the *Merck Manual.* [Pathway: www.merckmanuals.com/professional ➔ enter "Meningitis" into the search field ➔ select "Acute Bacterial Meningitis" ➔ review "Pathophysiology," "Signs & Symptoms," and "Prevention."]

EXERCISE 5.51 Fill in the blank:

What is the name of the neurological disorder that can result when children are given aspirin? This disorder is a life-threatening condition that affects the liver and the brain. A high ammonia level, elevated liver enzymes, poor clotting ability, and hypoglycemia are definitive laboratory studies for this condition.

____

The answer can be found on page 394

UNFOLDING CASE STUDY 9: Rashad

Rashad, who is a 2-month-old infant with hydrocephalus caused by a Chiari II malformation, was discharged from the NICU 1 week ago after insertion of a ventriculoperitoneal shunt (VP). He is one of triplets born at 24 weeks gestation. His mother noticed that he seems very weak. His siblings are holding their heads up and he is content to just lie there. His mother says, "he feels like a rag doll when I hold him" as compared with his siblings. He usually eats and sleeps fairly well. Rashad is noted to be irritable and his mother states, "he is crying all the time like he is in pain." He has a fever. His head circumference has increased 5 cm in 1 week. His anterior fontanel is full and bulging. He is being evaluated in the children's ED.

EXERCISE 5.52 Select all that apply:

Which of the following assessments are *most* concerning in evaluating for a neurological problem related to a potential ventriculoperitoneal (VP) shunt malfunction?

A. He is one of a set of triplets.
B. He has a fever.
C. He "feels like a rag doll when I hold him."
D. His head circumference has increased 5 cm in 1 week.
E. His anterior fontanel is full and bulging.
F. He is "irritable and crying like he is in pain."

The answer can be found on page 394

eRESOURCE

To reinforce your understanding of the clinical presentation of a Chiari II malformation, refer to Medscape on your mobile device. [Pathway: Medscape ➔ enter "Chiari" into the search field ➔ select "Chiari Malformation" and review content.]

UNFOLDING CASE STUDY 10: Matthew

Matthew is a premature infant born at 32 weeks with a myelomenigocele. He is admitted to the NICU.

EXERCISE 5.53 Multiple-choice:

Look at the following illustration. Which of the following statements about Matthew's myelomenigocele is accurate?

A. He has a normal spinal cord and vertebrae that are not covered.
B. He has a normal spinal cord and vertebrae but a tuft of hair is noted at the base of his spine.
C. He has protrusion of a sac through his vertebrae that contains the meninges and cerebrospinal fluid.
D. He has protrusion of a sac through his vertebrae that contains the meninges, cerebrospinal fluid, and spinal cord or nerve root.

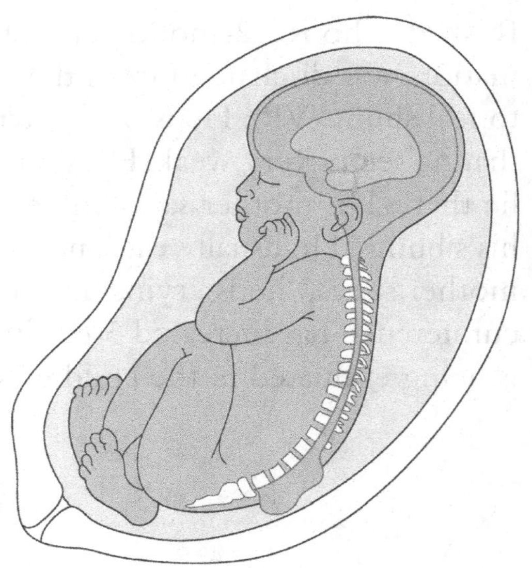

The answer can be found on page 395

EXERCISE 5.54 True/False:

Children with a myelomeningocele often have bowel and bladder incontinence problems.

_____ True

_____ False

The answer can be found on page 395

EXERCISE 5.55 True/False:

Matthew, who has spina bifida and needs to be intermittently catheterized for urine, should be taught, when he is older, to catheterize himself using a clean latex catheter.

_____ True

_____ False

The answer can be found on page 395

Matthew's parents verbalize to the nurse that they feel guilty for having given Matthew spina bifida. The mother also states, "This is all my fault, he was born too early."

EXERCISE 5.56 Multiple-choice:

What should the nurse caring for Matthew say to the parents?

A. "Don't worry; you didn't cause this problem."
B. "I can understand your feelings; spina bifida is hereditary and he gets the gene from the mother."
C. "You should have taken your folic acid when you were pregnant with Matthew."
D. "Tell me why you feel guilty for causing Mathew's spina bifida."

The answer can be found on page 395

---

eRESOURCE

To reinforce your understanding of the clinical presentation of spina bifida, refer to:

- Medscape on your mobile device: [Pathway: Medscape → enter "Spina Bifida" into the search field → select "Spina Bifida" and review content.]
- *Merck Manual*: [Pathway: www.merckmanuals.com/professional → enter "Spina Bifida" into the search field → select "Spina Bifida" and review content.]

EXERCISE 5.57 Multiple-choice:

Which type of medications would the nurse expect Matthew to be placed on to help with his reflux?

A. Rantidine (Zantac)
B. Caffeine citrate
C. Odanstron (Zofran)
D. Bismuth subsalicylate (Pepto-Bismol)

The answer can be found on page 396

eRESOURCE

To reinforce your understanding of the management of reflux in the pediatric population, refer to Medscape on your mobile device. [Pathway: Medscape ➔ enter "Reflux" into the search field ➔ select "Pediatric Gastroesophageal Reflux" and review content, focusing on "Treatment & Management" and "Medications."]

After 2 more weeks, Matthew is discharged to home. After being home 3 months, his vomiting becomes worse. It has become more forceful with every feeding. In fact, being the first-born male, Matthew is at risk for developing hypertrophic pyloric stenosis. His pediatrician has tried Matthew on several different formulas. He is diagnosed with having hypertrophic pyloric stenosis and is brought back to the hospital.

EXERCISE 5.58 Select all that apply:

Which of the following are symptoms of hypertrophic pyloric stenosis?

A. Projectile vomiting
B. Dry mucous membranes
C. Currant jelly stools
D. Constant crying and hunger
E. Walnut-shaped mass in his abdomen

The answer can be found on page 396

Matthew is admitted to the inpatient pediatric unit and has a pylorotomy to correct his hypertrophic pyloric stenosis. He begins to eat and goes home the next day.

Matthew follows up with his pediatrician a few weeks later. He is due for a complete examination. The pediatrician does a full examination and looks at his developmental state.

EXERCISE 5.59 Multiple-choice:

What is the most common test or tool pediatricians use to determine whether an infant is meeting his or her developmental goals?

A. An IQ test
B. Denver Developmental Screening Test II
C. Brainstem auditory evoked response (BAER) test
D. Battelle Developmental Inventory

The answer can be found on page 396

---

eRESOURCE

To supplement your understanding of normal growth and development for Mathew, consult the *Merck Manual.* [Pathway: www.merckmanuals.com/professional ➔ enter "Development" into the search field ➔ select "Childhood Development" and review content.]

Matthew's mother is concerned he may develop cerebral palsy since he was born prematurely at 32 weeks gestation. To reassure the mother, the nurse identifies reasons why Matthew will not have cerebral palsy.

EXERCISE 5.60 Multiple-choice:

Which of the following is *not* a cause of cerebral palsy?

A. Anoxia during delivery
B. Being born prematurely at 32 weeks
C. Cerebral infections
D. Early hospitalizations

The answer can be found on page 397

EXERCISE 5.61 Multiple-choice:

Which of the following types of cerebral palsy has the most severe symptoms, including both motor problems and speech problems related to involuntary facial movements?

A. Mixed type
B. Athetoid/dyskinetic
C. Ataxic
D. Spastic

The answer can be found on page 397

---

eRESOURCE

To reinforce your understanding of cerebral palsy, refer to Medscape on your mobile device. [Pathway: Medscape ➔ enter "Cerebral Palsy" into the search field ➔ select "Cerebral Palsy" and review content.]

UNFOLDING CASE STUDY 11: Natalie

Natalie, age 12 years, presents to her pediatrician for an annual checkup. Natalie's physical examination is normal except that she is diagnosed with scoliosis. She has a 40% lateral "S" curvature. She says that from time to time her back hurts. She finds it difficult to be in a crouched position when she plays softball. The pediatrician refers her to an orthopedic specialist, who orders an x-ray. The x-ray confirms a 42% "S" curvature. She is scheduled for surgical fusion with Harrington rods.

EXERCISE 5.62 Multiple-choice:

A 42% curvature is considered:

A. Mild scoliosis
B. Moderate scoliosis
C. Severe scoliosis
D. Total scoliosis

The answer can be found on page 397

Natalie is admitted to the PICU postoperatively. She is having a great deal of pain and is placed on a patient-controlled analgesia (PCA) pump, which is infusing morphine.

EXERCISE 5.63 Multiple-choice:

Which of the following nursing interventions is *most* important in caring for Natalie?

A. Making sure her Foley catheter is patent
B. Monitoring her respirations
C. Monitoring the pulses in her feet
D. Making sure Natalie does not become constipated

The answer can be found on page 397

EXERCISE 5.64 Select all that apply:

When setting up the patient-controlled analgesia (PCA) pump, which of the following nursing procedures must be followed to ensure safety and accuracy?

A. Two RNs must verify the medication.
B. An RN and a medical assistant need to verify the dosage settings on the pump.
C. The pump must be locked.
D. The pump tubing should be free of kinks and twists.
E. A pharmacist must verify the correct medication is in the pump.

The answer can be found on page 398

Natalie is still having considerable pain. She states her pain is 10 out of 10 (using the 0–10 scale). She is crying, hyperventilating, and becoming diaphoretic. Her mother is at her bedside and is very upset.

EXERCISE 5.65 Select all that apply:

Which of the following assessments and interventions would be an accurate interpretation of Natalie's pain-management scenario?

A. Wait to see whether the pain is relieved because it has only been 6 hours since surgery
B. Check the patient-controlled analgesia (PCA) pump and infusion set to be sure that it is working properly
C. Ask the mother to push the PCA control button for the patient in case she forgets
D. Call the primary care provider to report her pain is not being controlled
E. Tell her mother to talk with her and get her to calm down

The answer can be found on page 398

eRESOURCE

To complement your understanding of pain assessment, refer to Medscape on your mobile device. [Pathway: Medscape → enter "Pain" into the search field → select "Pain Assessment" and review content.]

UNFOLDING CASE STUDY 12: Pedro

Pedro, age 4 years, was involved in a four-wheeler bicycle accident. He was riding on the back of a four-wheeler with his father when his father ran into a tree. Pedro was thrown from the four-wheeler; he was not wearing a helmet. He was brought to the ED with a Glasgow Coma Scale score of 15. He is awake and crying. His HR is 120 bpm, RR is 36 breaths per minute, BP is 113/56 mmHg, and his temperature is 97.7°F rectally. His oxygen saturation is 98% on room air. On further assessment, a deformity to his left upper leg is noted. An x-ray is ordered; it shows a fractured left femur. He is admitted to the pediatric floor. His orders include placing him in 5 lb of Buck's traction.

EXERCISE 5.66 Multiple-choice:

Buck's traction is a type of:

A. Skin traction
B. Skeletal traction
C. Manual traction
D. Plaster traction

The answer can be found on page 398

The nurse walks into Pedro's room and notices that the 5-lb weight is resting on the floor just below his bed. Pedro is playing cars in bed with the television on and seems comfortable.

EXERCISE 5.67 Multiple-choice:

The appropriate intervention for the nurse to perform for Pedro in Buck's traction is to:

A. Do nothing, Pedro is comfortable. Play cars with him to gain his trust.
B. Add another 5-lb weight to the traction, so that it works properly.
C. Remove the weight, reposition the boot, then replace the weight making sure it is not sitting on the floor.
D. Pull Pedro up in bed to get the weight off the floor.

The answer can be found on page 399

EXERCISE 5.68 Multiple-choice:

The nurse is caring for a 7-year-old boy in Buck's traction for a fractured left femur. What would be included in a neurovascular assessment of the affected leg?

A. Pain level, temperature in the affected extremity, color, and a Doppler scan of the pedal pulse of the left leg
B. Vital signs (VS), bilateral lung sounds, pain level, and pulse oximetry done on the toes of both legs
C. Sensation, movement, capillary refill, and pulse of affected extremity and VS of the right leg
D. Color, sensation, movement, capillary refill, and pulse of affected extremity of the left leg

The answer can be found on page 399

EXERCISE 5.69 Choose all that apply:

Which of the following nursing actions would be appropriate for Pedro while in Buck's traction?

A. Maintain straight body alignment
B. Do frequent neurovascular checks to the lower extremities
C. Make sure the patient's buttocks are off the bed
D. Do pin care every 8 hours
E. Make sure the weights are free hanging and off the floor
F. Notify the physician if Pedro experiences any pain from muscle spasm

The answer can be found on page 400

---

eRESOURCE

To reinforce your understanding of the clinical presentation and management of a fracture of the femur, refer to Medscape on your mobile device. [Pathway: Medscape → enter "Femur" into the search field → select "Femur Fracture" and review content. Repeat and select "Femur Injuries and Fracture" → review content.]

A few hours later Pedro wakes, screaming out in pain. His mother says that she noticed his leg "jump." He had been given a therapeutic dose of acetaminophen (Tylenol) with codeine an hour earlier.

EXERCISE 5.70 Multiple-choice:

Pedro's as-needed orders are as follows. Of these, which medication should the nurse administer?

A. Tylenol (acetaminophen) with codeine one teaspoon every 4 hours
B. Morphine 2 mg intravenous (IV) every 2 hours for pain
C. Valium (diazepam) 5 mg IV every 6 hours
D. Demerol (meperidine) 3 mg IV every 4 hours

The answer can be found on page 400

Pedro was taken to the operating room the next morning and had a rod placed in his femur. He recovered well from anesthesia. The next day (48 hours after the accident), his mother indicates that he just "doesn't seem himself." He started complaining of a headache, not watching television or playing with his toys. He also seems to be sleeping more. When he wakes up, he cries and then falls back to sleep. Within the past hour he has vomited. While Pedro was wearing a helmet, the nurse is suspecting a closed head injury.

EXERCISE 5.71 Select all that apply:

A nurse assessing Pedro for a suspected closed, mild head injury would expect to see which of the following clinical manifestations?

A. Vomiting
B. Delayed pupillary response
C. Drowsiness and increased sleeping
D. Report of a headache
E. Confusion

The answer can be found on page 400

Pedro is taken for a CT scan of his head, which reveals a very small parietal hematoma. He is kept for observation for a few days and then is discharged to home.

eRESOURCE

To reinforce your understanding of closed head injury, refer to Medscape on your mobile device. [Pathway: Medscape → enter "Closed Head Injury" into the search field → select "Closed Head Injury" and review content.]

UNFOLDING CASE STUDY 13: Tyla

Tyla, age 12 years, is admitted with the diagnosis of sickle cell crisis. She is experiencing severe pain in her knees. Her mother reports that Tyla has not been herself lately. On entering Tyla's room, she found her lying in a fetal position and moaning.

EXERCISE 5.72 Multiple-choice:

Which of the following is the *most* common type of anemia in children?

A. Pernicious anemia
B. Iron-deficiency anemia
C. Sickle cell anemia
D. Aplastic anemia

The answer can be found on page 401

EXERCISE 5.73 Ordering:

The nurse is admitting Tyla to the emergency department (ED). Place the interventions in order of priority:

___ Obtain a throat culture
___ Start an intravenous (IV) of D5/0.9% normal saline
___ Administer nasal oxygen
___ Administer analgesics IV

The answer can be found on page 401

EXERCISE 5.74 Select all that apply:

Which of the following are conditions that can predispose to sickling of red blood cells, or sickling crisis?

A. Infection
B. Hypertension
C. Hypoxia
D. Emotional stress
E. Dehydration

The answer can be found on page 401

The nurse notices that Tyla's parents seem to be crying and withdrawn when they come to visit Tyla. They are tired after being at work all day and they are not sleeping at night because they are upset. The nurse talks with them and offers them support.

EXERCISE 5.75 Multiple-choice:

The nurse is talking with Tyla's parents about sickle cell anemia. The nurse explores the feelings of the parents and finds that both parents are admitting to feeling guilty a lot of the time. Which of the following causes will the nurse most likely find as the greatest contributor and/or cause of this guilt?

A. Both parents are working and cannot spend as much time with their child as they would like.
B. The parents are not able to help their child more and fear that the child is suffering a great amount of the time.
C. Both parents are carrying at least one recessive gene for sickle cell anemia.
D. The child wants more and more things that cost a lot and the parents cannot buy them because they do not have enough money.

The answer can be found on page 401

eRESOURCE

To supplement your understanding of sickle cell disease, consult the *Merck Manual.* [Pathway: www.merckmanuals.com/professional ➔ enter "Sickle Cell" into the search field ➔ select "Sickle Cell Disease" and review content.]

Tyla gets a roommate whose name is Jin. Jin is 7 years old and is admitted to the pediatric unit with suspected hemophilia. Her parents noticed that she has a lot of bruises. She is not noted to fall a lot but does feel week. She prefers to play with her stuffed animals and dolls instead of playing outside.

EXERCISE 5.76 Multiple-choice:

What is the most common type of hemophilia?

A. Hemophilia A
B. Hemophilia B
C. Hemophilia C
D. Hemophilia D

The answer can be found on page 402

EXERCISE 5.77 Multiple-choice:

In the most common type or classic form of hemophilia, which factor is deficient?

A. Factor VIII
B. Factor VII
C. Factor IX
D. vWF (von Willebrand factor)

The answer can be found on page 402

eRESOURCE

To supplement your understanding of hemophilia, consult the *Merck Manual.* [Pathway: www.merckmanuals.com/professional ➔ enter "Hemophilia" into the search field ➔ select "Hemophilia" and review content.]

When Tyla and Jin feel a little better, they go to the play room and meet a new friend whose name is Keoni.

Keoni, age 6 years, was noted by his mother's friend to be very pale. When she mentioned this to his mother, Keoni's mother replied that he does look a little pale. His mother reports that he seems to always feel warm, "like he has a fever." She is worried about him and brings him to the pediatrician's office. Keoni is not eating well and just seems to lie around and watch cartoons all the time. The mother senses that "something just isn't right." On examination, the pediatrician notes that Keoni's liver is enlarged. The primary care provider then orders some blood work.

EXERCISE 5.78 Multiple-choice:

Which of the following laboratory values could indicate that a child has leukemia?

A. White blood cells (WBCs): 32,000/mm^3
B. Platelets: 300,000/mm^3
C. Hemoglobin: 15 g/dL
D. Blood pH: 7.35

The answer can be found on page 402

EXERCISE 5.79 Multiple-choice:

The pediatric nurse understands that the most common cancer found in children is:

A. Non-Hodgkin's lymphoma
B. Acute lymphocytic leukemia
C. Chronic lymphocytic leukemia
D. Ewing's sarcoma

The answer can be found on page 402

EXERCISE 5.80 Select all that apply:

The nurse knows which of the following symptoms are early clinical manifestations of leukemia?

A. Anorexia
B. Hematuria
C. Petechiae

D. Unsteady gait and falling
E. Ulcerations in the mouth

The answer can be found on page 403

EXERCISE 5.81 Select all that apply:

Keoni develops thrombocytopenia after receiving chemotherapy. Which of the following should the nurse do?

A. Monitor for signs of bleeding
B. Obtain all temperatures by the rectal route
C. Administer all routine immunizations
D. Avoid unnecessary venipunctures
E. Limit the number of visitors

The answer can be found on page 403

Keoni's mother comes out of the room to get the nurse and runs into her neighbor. Keoni's mother asks whether she came to visit Keoni and the neighbor says she is actually here because of her daughter Amber. Amber was admitted 2 days ago.

eRESOURCE

To supplement your understanding of leukemia, consult the *Merck Manual.* [Pathway: www.merckmanuals.com/professional ➔ enter "Leukemia" into the search field ➔ select "Overview of Leukemia" and review content.]

UNFOLDING CASE STUDY 14: Amber and Andy

Amber is 18 months old. Her mother noticed a lump in her abdomen while giving her a bath and was concerned; she brought Amber to the pediatrician to be checked. Amber is eating and sleeping normally. She also seems happy and is playing with her toys. When the pediatrician examined Amber, she palpates a firm lobulated mass just to the right of midline on Amber's abdomen. She ordered a CT scan of the abdomen, and the report shows that Amber has a Wilms tumor (nephroblastoma). Amber is admitted to the pediatric unit. Amber's mother shares with Keoni's mother how scared she is about what is going to happen to Amber.

EXERCISE 5.82 Multiple-choice:

That evening, the nurse caring for Amber notices a group of medical students standing outside Amber's room reviewing her chart. When the nurse approaches and asks them what they are doing, they respond "we heard this child has a Wilms tumor and we want to palpate her abdomen to see the size of the tumor." What is the result of abdominal palpation of a Wilms tumor?

A. Palpation will be painful.
B. The lymph nodes may swell.
C. Only physicians can feel the tumor.
D. The tumor may spread if palpation is done.

The answer can be found on page 403

Amber is started on chemotherapy and monitored on the pediatric unit.

eRESOURCE

To supplement your understanding of the clinical presentation and treatment of Wilms tumor, consult the *Merck Manual.* [Pathway: www.merckmanuals.com/professional ➔ enter "Wilms" into the search field ➔ select "Wilms Tumor" and review content, focusing on "Symptoms and Signs" and "Treatment."]

EXERCISE 5.83 Multiple-choice:

As a result of chemotherapy's side effects of nausea and vomiting, the pediatric nurse administered which medication?

A. Ondansetron (Zofran)
B. Prochloroperazine (Compazine)
C. Doxorubicin (Myocet)
D. Neupogen (granulocyte-colony stimulating factor [G-CSF])

The answer can be found on page 404

eRESOURCE

To supplement your understanding of chemotherapy, consult the *Merck Manual.* [Pathway: www .merckmanuals.com/professional ➔ enter "Cancer Therapy" into the search field ➔ select "Modalities of Cancer Therapy" and review content, focusing on "Chemotherapy."]

The nurse begins teaching Amber's mother about Wilms tumor.

EXERCISE 5.84 Select all that apply

Which of the following statements should the nurse include in her teaching?

A. "Your child will need chemotherapy for about 12 months."
B. "Wilms tumors are caused by an inherited genetic trait."
C. "Surgery is usually done within 48 hours of diagnosis."
D. "Touching or palpating the tumor could spread it, so don't rub it."
E. "Further treatment will begin immediately after surgery."

The answer can be found on page 404

EXERCISE 5.85 Multiple-choice:

Amber has her surgery and is being cared for postoperatively. The nurse receives a report that Amber is NPO (nothing by mouth). Which of the following assessments is an indication to continue Amber's NPO status?

A. Her abdominal girth is 1 cm larger than yesterday.
B. Amber is crying and has pain at the surgical site.
C. Amber is passing flatus every 30 minutes.
D. There are absent bowel sounds.

The answer can be found on page 404

Amber slowly recovers and her mother asks whether her brother could come in to visit her. The nurse says, "of course." Amber's brother Andy comes in and the nurse notices fluid-filled pimples on his skin. The skin around the pimples is swollen and red. These pimples popped over the past few days and are now crusty and yellow. They seem to be itchy. Andy keeps scratching them. Andy and his family live in a middle-class neighborhood, where Andy has lots of playmates. The primary care provider walks in the room and diagnoses Andy with impetigo. The nurse tells the mother Andy is going to need to go home.

EXERCISE 5.86 Multiple-choice:

Which of the following is an important nursing consideration in caring for a child with impetigo?

A. Apply topical corticosteroids to decrease inflammation.
B. Carefully remove dressings so as not to dislodge undermined skin, crusts, and debris. Keep lesions covered for several days before changing.
C. Carefully wash hands and maintain cleanliness in caring for an infected child and apply antibiotic cream as ordered.
D. Examine child under a Wood's lamp for possible spread of lesions.

The answer can be found on page 405

---

eRESOURCE

To reinforce your understanding of the clinical presentation of impetigo, refer to Medscape on your mobile device. [Pathway: Medscape ➔ enter "Impetigo" into the search field ➔ select "Impetigo" and review content.]

EXERCISE 5.87 Multiple-choice:

Therapeutic management of a child with a ringworm infection (tinea capitis) would include which of the following?

A. Administer oral griseofulvin (antifungal)
B. Administer topical or oral antibiotics
C. Apply topical sulfonamides
D. Apply Burow's solution compresses to affected areas

The answer can be found on page 405

---

eRESOURCE

To reinforce your understanding of the clinical presentation of ringworm, refer to Medscape on your mobile device. [Pathway: Medscape ➔ enter "Tinea Capitis" into the search field ➔ select "Tinia Capitis" and review content.]

EXERCISE 5.88 Multiple-choice:

Which of the following is usually the only symptom of pediculosis capitis (head lice)?

A. Itching
B. Vesicles
C. Scalp rash
D. Localized inflammatory response

The answer can be found on page 405

eRESOURCE

To reinforce your understanding of the clinical presentation of head lice, refer to Medscape on your mobile device. [Pathway: Medscape ➔ enter "Lice" into the search field ➔ select "Pediculosis Capitus (Head Lice)" and review content.]

EXERCISE 5.89 Multiple-choice:

Which skin disorder is characterized by linear, thread-like, grayish burrows on the skin?

A. Impetigo
B. Ringworm
C. Pinworm
D. Scabies

The answer can be found on page 405

EXERCISE 5.90 Select all that apply:

The nurse is discussing the management of atopic dermatitis (eczema) with a parent. Which of the following teaching points should be included?

A. Dress infant warmly in woollen clothes to prevent chilling
B. Keep fingernails and toenails short and clean to prevent transfer of bacteria
C. Give bubble baths instead of washing lesions with soap
D. Launder clothes in mild detergent

The answer can be found on page 406

UNFOLDING CASE STUDY 15: Emma

Emma is 14 months old and just learning to walk by herself. She is with her family on a camping trip, and they have set up a campfire. Emma's dad started the fire while her mother prepared dinner in the camper. Emma's father sat her on a blanket a safe distance away from the fire. He walked over to the tree line to get some more wood for later when he heard a scream. Emma had gotten up, toddled over to the fire, and fallen hands first into the fire.

EXERCISE 5.91 Multiple-choice:

Which of the following treatments would be best to use for Emma's burns initially?

A. Quickly place ice on them to cool the burns
B. Place butter or Crisco on the wounds, because they had some in the camper
C. Soak Emma's hands in cold water from the lake to cool the burns
D. Use tepid water to cool the burns

The answer can be found on page 406

Emma is taken to the hospital. The skin on her hands is blistered in various areas and she is having some pain.

EXERCISE 5.92 Multiple-choice:

Considering the blisters on Emma's hands, what type of burn would this be?

A. Superficial thickness: first degree
B. Epidermal thickness: second degree
C. Partial thickness: second degree
D. Full thickness: third degree

The answer can be found on page 406

EXERCISE 5.93 Multiple-choice:

If Emma was not experiencing any pain from her burn injury, what type of burn would it be?

A. Superficial thickness: first degree
B. Epidermal thickness: second degree
C. Partial thickness: second degree
D. Full thickness: third degree

The answer can be found on page 406

RAPID RESPONSE TIPS **Burns**

Classification	Involvement
Superficial: first degree	The epidermis is injured and there is pain, swelling, and erythema.
Partial thickness: second degree	Both the epidermis and dermis are injured and the injury presents as a fluid-filled vesicle. The patient has severe pain because of nerve damage.
Full thickness: third degree	All layers of skin are injured; the injury sometimes extends deeper into the muscle, tendons, and bones. There is less or no pain because of severe nerve damage. Many times the healed skin is waxy and leathery.

Emma is admitted to the inpatient pediatric unit for her burns. Preventing infection is a very important goal of her burn injury.

EXERCISE 5.94 Multiple-choice:

Which of the following actions is important for Emma's nurse to take?

A. Implement contact isolation
B. Implement droplet isolation
C. Restrict her visitors to immediate family only
D. Place Emma on neutropenic precautions

The answer can be found on page 407

eRESOURCE

To supplement your understanding of the management of thermal burns, consult the *Merck Manual.* [Pathway: www.merckmanuals.com/professional ➔ enter "Burns" into the search field ➔ select "Burns" and review content.]

Answers

EXERCISE 5.1 Multiple-choice:

Which of the following assessments is a priority nursing concern?

A. Heart rate (HR) of 168 beats per minute (bpm)—NO; an infant's HR may be increased to 180 with crying.
B. Respiratory rate of 54 breaths per minute—NO; this is within the normal limits of 30 to 60 breaths per minute for an infant.
C. Irritability—NO; irritability is an infant's way of showing that he or she needs something or that something is wrong or painful.
D. One wet diaper in 24 hours—**YES; he should be wetting six to eight diapers a day; therefore, this could be a sign of dehydration.**

EXERCISE 5.2 Multiple-choice:

Justin's lab studies are: White blood cell (WBC) count: 3.8/mm^3; vital signs (VS): Temperature: 97.6°F, heart rate (HR): 134 beats per minute (bpm), respiratory rate (RR): 26 breaths per minute

The nurse would suspect:

A. Leukemia—NO; leukemia is signaled by a high WBC count.
B. HIV—NO; the test for HIV was not done.
C. Overwhelmed immune system—**YES; the baby's immune system might be overwhelmed and unable to produce enough WBCs to fight the infection. This is why the WBC count is low.**
D. This is normal for a 2-week-old infant—NO; this is a below-normal WBC count.

EXERCISE 5.3 Calculation:

Calculate the therapeutic range for Justin, whose weight is 3.6 kg using the information in the preceding Rapid Response Tip.

The order stated:

Ampicillin: 160 mg intravenous (IV) every 6 hours

Cefotaxime: 200 mg IV every 8 hours

- The medication ordered is Cefotaxime
- Dose ordered: 200 mg IV every 8 hours

What is the therapeutic dose range for Cefotaxime for Justin?

The therapeutic range is 360 to 720 mg/kg/day.

Is the dose therapeutic?

YES, I would give this dose to Justin.

The dose is ordered every 8 hours so divide the above therapeutic range by 3 (8 hours x 3 + 24 hours/day)

360 ÷ 3 = 120 mg/dose

720 ÷ 3 = 240 mg/dose

Per dose the therapeutic range is 120 to 240 mg/dose

The ordered dose is 200 mg.

YES, it is within the therapeutic range.

Would you give Justin this dose of medication?

YES I would give this dose to Justin.

EXERCISE 5.4 Multiple-choice:

What is the priority for calculating the therapeutic dose for pediatric patients based on body weight?

A. To check that the physician's medication order is correct—NO; this is just one aspect of double checking medications.
B. To check that the pharmacy sent the correct medication—NO; this is just one aspect of double checking medications.
C. To provide adequate treatment to the patient—NO; treatment should be evidence based and appropriate, which is more than adequate.
D. To provide safe patient medication administration—**YES; it is important to check therapeutic dose ranges to ensure safe medication administration to all pediatric patients. A double-check system is helpful in preventing medication errors. The nurse is the last line of defense for pediatric patients and must protect them from adverse events.**

EXERCISE 5.5 Multiple-choice:

Justin, at 2 weeks of age, would have had which typical childhood immunizations?

A. Diphtheria, tetanus toxoids, and pertussis (DTP)—NO; DTP is first given at 2 months of age.
B. Measles, mumps, and rubella (MMR)—NO; MMR is not given until 12 months of age.
C. Hepatitis B vaccine—**YES; hepatitis B vaccine is typically given at birth or at 2 weeks of age.**
D. Varicella vaccine—NO; varicella vaccine is not given until 12 months of age.

EXERCISE 5.6 Matching:

In assessing growth and development, match the stages of development in Column A that Justin would be in according to the developmental and cognitive theorists listed in Column B:

Column A	Column B	
A. Sensorimotor	B	Erickson
B. Trust versus mistrust	C	Freud
C. Oral	A	Piaget

EXERCISE 5.7 Multiple-choice:

What is a priority for the nurse to assess?

A. Respirations—**YES; A for airway is first, followed by B for breathing.**
B. Cardiac sounds—NO; airway and breathing are the priority, then C, circulation.
C. Bowel sounds—NO; not a priority in this case.
D. Skin turgor—NO; dehydration signs are important but are not the priority.

EXERCISE 5.8 Fill in the blanks:

As part of the respiratory assessment, what should the nurse observe?

Rate

Depth

Rhythm

Effort

EXERCISE 5.9 Fill in the blank:

What are retractions and why do they occur?

The chest wall is flexible in infants and young children because the chest muscles are immature and the ribs are cartilaginous. With respiratory distress, the negative pressure created by the downward movement of the diaphragm to draw in air is increased and the chest wall is pulled inward, causing retractions. As respiratory distress progresses, accessory muscles are used and retractions may be noted in the supraclavicular and suprasternal area (Ball, Bindler, & Cowen, 2015).

EXERCISE 5.10 Fill in the blanks:

The severity of retractions is noted as **mild**, **moderate**, and **severe**.

EXERCISE 5.11 Hot spot:

Please draw a line to the area where retraction would be assessed and label each line using the supplied terms:

Supraclavicular

Suprasternal

Intercostal

Substernal

Subcostal

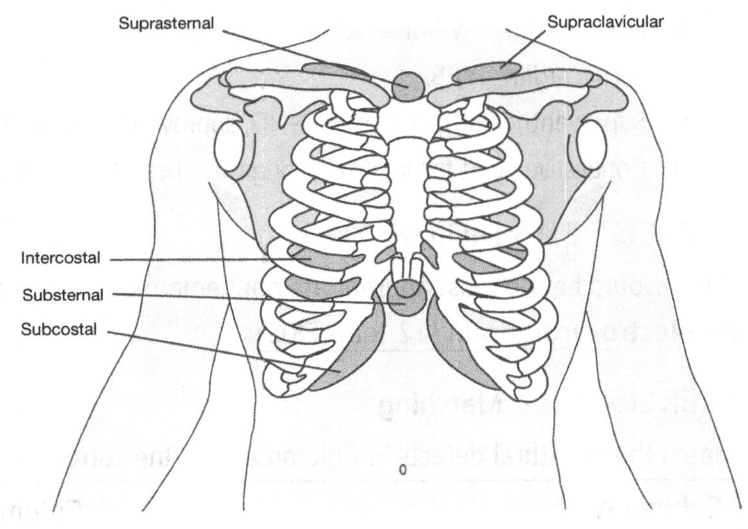

EXERCISE 5.12 Fill in the blanks:

Name two priority nursing diagnoses for Sasha.

The three possible answers are:

1. **Impaired gas exchange**
2. **Ineffective breathing pattern**
3. **Ineffective airway clearance**

EXERCISE 5.13 Select all that apply:

Which of the following should the nurse implement for a child hospitalized with respiratory syncytial virus (RSV)?

A. Antipyretics to reduce the fever—**YES.**

B. Oxygen therapy—**YES.**

C. Intravenous (IV) and/or oral rehydration—**YES.**

D. IV administration of antibiotics—NO; antibiotics will not work on viruses.

E. Frequent monitoring and suctioning of the nasal airway—**YES.**

F. Monitoring on a cardiac/respiratory monitor—**YES.**

G. Routine intubation to protect the airway—NO; this is not necessarily needed if other means of oxygenation are adequate.
H. Monitoring by continuous pulse oximetry—**YES.**

EXERCISE 5.14 Exhibit-format:

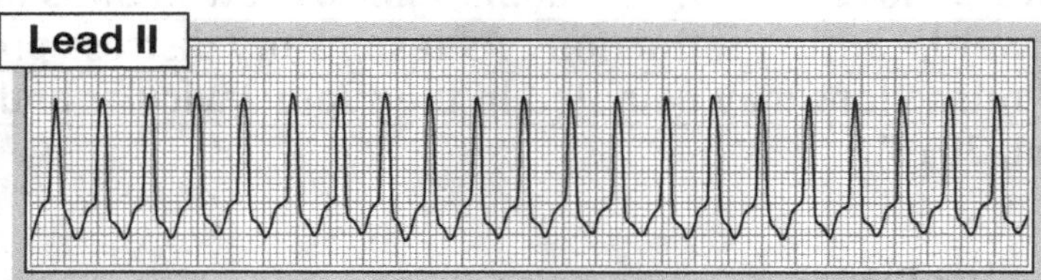

HR = 210

Using this electrocardiogram (EKG) monitor strip the nurse would suspect:

A. Normal sinus rhythm—NO, this is tachycardia.
B. Tachycardia—**YES.**
C. Supraventricular tachycardia—NO, supraventricular tachycardia is over 220 bpm for infants.
D. Congestive heart failure—NO, congestive heart failure may produce bradycardia and other symptoms.

EXERCISE 5.15 Fill in the blank:

What would be the most appropriate nonhematological test to perform at this time?

An electrocardiogram (12-lead EKG)

EXERCISE 5.16 Matching:

Match the structural defects in Column A with the correct descriptions in Column B:

Column A	Column B
A. Ventricular septal defect (VSD)	**D** A narrowing at, above, or below the aortic valve
B. Atrial septal defect (ASD)	**G** A narrowing of the lumen of the aorta usually at or near the ductus arteriosus
C. Patent ductus arteriosus (PDA)	**A** A hole in the septum between the right and left ventricles
D. Aortic stenosis (AS)	**F** Complete closure of the tricuspid valve
E. Pulmonary stenosis (PS)	**I** Consists of four anomalies: pulmonary stenosis (PS), ventricular septal defect (VSD), overriding aorta, and right ventricular hypertrophy
F. Tricuspid atresia (TA)	**C** Normal fetal circulatory opening between the pulmonary artery and the aorta that fails to close
G. Coarctation of the aorta (CoA)	**B** An opening in the septum between the right and left atria
H. Transposition of the great vessels (arteries; TGA)	**E** A narrowing of the pulmonary valve or pulmonary artery
I. Tetralogy of Fallot (TOF)	**H** Aorta connected to the right ventricle instead of the left; pulmonary artery connected to the left ventricle instead of the right

EXERCISE 5.17 Matching:

Match the common cardiac medications listed in Column A with the uses for pediatric patients in Column B:

Column A	Column B
A. Digoxin (Lanoxin)	**B** A potent loop diuretic that rids the body of excess fluid. Used to treat congestive heart failure (CHF).
B. Furosemide (Lasix)	**D** A medication that is given to convert supraventricular tachycardia (SVT) back to normal sinus rhythm (NSR).
C. Captopril (Capoten)	**E** A diuretic that is potassium sparing.
D. Adenosine (Adenocard)	**C** An angiotensin converting enzyme (ACE) inhibitor that causes vasoconstriction, which reduces afterload.
E. Spironolactone (Aldactone)	**A** A medication that improves cardiac contractility.

EXERCISE 5.18 Fill in the blank:

What is a nursing priority with this patient?

Hydration status would be the priority.

EXERCISE 5.19 Multiple-choice:

The nurse may suspect which diagnosis for Ashonda?

A. Appendicitis—NO; this would be indicated by severe abdominal pain.

B. Intussusception—NO; this is usually a colon obstruction.

C. Viral gastroenteritis—**YES; this is an infectious process, therefore, running a temperature is the key symptom.**

D. Intestinal obstruction—NO; Ashonda is passing stool.

EXERCISE 5.20 Multiple-choice:

What is the most likely cause of the viral gastroenteritis?

A. *Salmonella*—NO; *Salmonella* is a bacterial infection.

B. *Escherichia coli*—NO; *E. coli* frequently causes more severe symptoms, with a watery stool.

C. *Clostridium difficile*—NO; Ashonda has no history of antibiotics, so *C. difficile* is unlikely.

D. Rotavirus—**YES; the most common cause of viral gastroenteritis is rotavirus.**

EXERCISE 5.21 Multiple-choice:

What type of isolation precautions do you expect Ashonda will require related to potential transmission of illness?

A. Contact isolation—**YES; suspected rotavirus is spread through contact, via the fecal–oral route, and because it lives on hands for hours and contact surfaces not cleaned for days, contact isolation should be instituted.**

B. Droplet isolation—NO.

C. Airborne isolation—NO.

D. Standard precautions—NO.

EXERCISE 5.22 Select all that apply:

Which of the following are reasons for Ashonda being placed in the type of isolation that was chosen?

A. The risk of transmission via the fecal–oral route.—**YES; the fecal–oral route is the route of transmission for suspected viral gastrointestinal illnesses like rotavirus.**

B. Rotavirus lives on hands for hours and contact surfaces are not cleaned for days.—**YES; this is true. The virus can live on the hands if not washed, and on contact surfaces for days if not cleaned and wiped down with appropriate antiviral cleaning products.**

C. Rotavirus can be transmitted through droplets in the air.—NO; this is not true. Rotavirus is spread through contact with the virus, not through coughing or droplets in the air.

D. The transmission of the virus can be prevented by wearing gloves and good handwashing.—**YES; this is true and how to prevent the spread of the virus.**

E. Families should be told why the patient is in isolation, so they can comply with isolation precautions too.—**YES; this is true. The family needs to know so as to help prevent the transmission of the virus to themselves and other patients. In fact, encourage family members to use gloves when changing diapers.**

F. Standard precautions are good enough to prevent transmission.—NO; although standard precautions are good, rotavirus needs contact isolation. The nurse should wear a protective gown in addition to gloves to avoid transmitting the virus to other patients. Also, a designated stethoscope and equipment should be kept in the room and not carried or used between patients.

EXERCISE 5.23 Multiple-choice:

What is the most appropriate treatment for a mildly dehydrated patient with viral gastroenteritis?

A. Keep on nothing orally (NPO) status—NO; this would increase the dehydration.

B. Send the child home and tell the parents to give her apple juice as tolerated—NO; Ashley has been unable to tolerate fluids at home.

C. Try oral rehydration therapy with Pedialyte; if ineffective, administer intravenous (IV) fluids—**YES; Ashley has already not tolerated Gatorade at home, so this is the next logical step to rehydration.**

D. IV fluids followed by peritoneal lavage—NO; lavaging would dehydrate Ashley further.

EXERCISE 5.24 Multiple-choice:

Which of the following assessments would be indicative of dehydration?

A. Dry mucous membranes—**YES; dry mucous membranes would be indicative of dehydration. It is also important to note that if the child is crying, whether she is crying tears. If she is not, this is another sign of dehydration.**

B. Increased skin turgor—NO; skin turgor would be decreased in dehydration.

C. Decreased thirst—NO; thirst would be increased in dehydration.

D. Dilute urine—NO; the urine would appear more dark and concentrated in dehydration.

EXERCISE 5.25 Multiple-choice:

What would be the *most appropriate* nursing diagnosis for moderate dehydration?

A. Anxiety—NO; a child may be anxious but fluid volume would be a greater concern.
B. Fluid volume deficit—**YES; fluid volume deficit would be the most appropriate choice for a child who is dehydrated.**
C. Acute pain—NO; a child should not have acute pain because of dehydration.
D. Alteration in cardiac output—NO; alteration in cardiac output would be a very late problem with severe dehydration.

EXERCISE 5.26 Matching:

Match the correct description in Column A with the appropriate disorder in Column B:

Column A	Column B
A. Cleft lip/palate	**F** Protrusion of abdominal contents through the abdominal wall at the umbilical area
B. Pyloric stenosis	**I** Aganglionic segments of the bowel cause the formation of a megacolon
C. Tracheoesophageal (TE) fistula	**O** Twisting of the bowel upon itself, causing obstruction
D. Gastroesophageal (GE) reflux	**E** Bowel inflammation with a "cobblestone-like" appearance
E. Crohn's disease	**N** Necrosis of the mucosa of the intestine
F. Omphalocele	**L** Inflammation of continuous segments of the bowel; bloody stools
G. Gastroschisis	**M** Constricting band ("vestigial structure") of the bowel
H. Diaphragmatic hernia	**K** "Telescoping" of the bowel
I. Hirschsprung's disease	**J** Failure of the normal rotation of viscera
J. Malrotation	**A** Failure of fusion of the maxillary and median nasal process
K. Intussusception	**C** Abnormal connection between the trachea and esophagus
L. Ulcerative colitis	**B** Characterized by projectile vomiting
M. Meckel's diverticulum	**D** Diagnosed with a pH probe study
N. Necrotizing enterocolitis	**G** Abdominal wall defect in which abdominal contents are not contained in a peritoneal membrane
O. Volvulus	**H** Protrusion of abdominal contents into the chest cavity

EXERCISE 5.27 Select all that apply:

Which of the following could be possible causes of Stevie's enuresis?

A. Glomerulonephritis—NO; this does not cause enuresis.
B. Urinary tract infection (UTI)—**YES; enuresis is a symptom.**

C. New onset of diabetes mellitus—**YES; enuresis is a symptom.**
D. Epispadias—NO; this is a structural defect from birth.
E. Exstrophy of the bladder—NO; this is a structural defect from birth.
F. Hypospadias—NO; this is a structural defect from birth.

EXERCISE 5.28 Multiple-choice question:

What symptoms would the nurse expect for a urinary tract infection (UTI)?

A. Dysuria, thirst, light-colored urine, ammonia smell in the urine—NO; urine that has a light color and smells like ammonia is normal.
B. Dysuria, left-sided flank pain, and dark, foul-smelling urine—**YES; the nurse would expect painful urination with left-sided flank pain as well as a foul odor and dark color to the urine.**
C. Oliguria, lower abdominal pain, yellow urine, ammonia smell in the urine, and epigastric pain—NO; oliguria and epigrastric pain are symptoms of renal failure.
D. Polyuria, lower abdominal pain, yellow urine, ammonia smell in the urine—NO; frequent urination and urine that smells sweet would be indicative of diabetes mellitus.

EXERCISE 5.29 Select all that apply:

The mother asks what a voiding cystourethrogram (VCUG) is and why it is being ordered. Which of the following statements are correct?

A. It is an x-ray of the child's bladder and lower urinary tract.—**YES.**
B. A tube or catheter will be inserted into the child's penis.—**YES.**
C. It is a tube or catheter that will be inserted up into your child's kidneys.—NO; the catheter extends into the child's bladder, not into the kidneys.
D. It has radioactive dye that will be instilled into the child's penis through a tube.—**YES.**
E. The child may cry through the entire procedure.—NO; the child will not necessarily cry for the entire procedure if prepared and supported through the procedure.
F. The test checks for urinary reflux.—**YES.**
G. The test checks whether the child has diabetes mellitus.—NO; this procedure does not check for diabetes mellitus.
H. The test will tell whether the child has a urinary tract infection (UTI).—NO; this procedure does not check for a UTI; it will check why he is getting recurrent UTIs.

EXERCISE 5.30 Multiple-choice:

Because Marianne has suspected glomerulonephritis, the nurse would expect to see that she had a recent ____________ infection.

A. Urinary tract—NO; a urinary tract infection (UTI) is not typically the problem because there is inflammation of the glomeruli or small blood vessels in the kidney.
B. Streptococcal.—**YES; most often a recent streptococcal infection precedes acute glomerulonephritis.**
C. Blood—NO; blood infections do not usually precede glomerulonephritis.
D. Ear—NO; ear infections do not usually precede glomerulonephritis.

EXERCISE 5.31 Multiple-choice:

For Marianne, which of the following nursing diagnoses should receive priority?

A. Excess fluid volume—**YES; Marianne has gained 10 lb or 4.54 kg in the past week, meaning that she has gained 4.5 L of fluid in 1 week. This is an indication that the kidneys may not be functioning efficiently.**

B. Risk for infection—NO; there is no indication of an infection.

C. Knowledge deficit—NO; neither Marianne nor her mother has denied understanding.

D. Activity intolerance—NO; Marianne has not complained about being unable to function.

EXERCISE 5.32 Multiple-choice:

What classic symptoms would the nurse expect Hashama to have if she has nephrotic syndrome?

A. Hypotension, hypernatremia, hyperproteinuria—NO; hypertension is present, not hypotension.

B. Hypernatremia, hypoalbuminemia, hypertension—**YES; a child with nephrotic syndrome retains fluid and has increased permeability at the basement membrane. She is losing albumin in the urine, which leads to hypoalbuminemia. The renal tubules are unable to reabsorb all the filtered proteins. Immunoglobulins are lost, resulting in altered immunity. Edema occurs as a result of decreased intravascular oncotic pressure, secondary to urinary protein losses. She will be hemoconcentrated, which results in hypernatremia. The liver is stimulated and responds by increasing synthesis of lipoprotein (cholesterol) and hyperlipidemia results. Hypertension is a result of sodium and water retention.**

C. Hematuria, hypotension, tachycardia—NO; hypertension is present, not hypotension.

D. Hyperalbuminemia, hypolipidemia, hypotension—NO; hypertension is present, not hypotension.

EXERCISE 5.33 Multiple-choice:

A child with nephrotic syndrome has a platelet count of 750,000 mm^3. Which of the following signs and symptoms should the nurse monitor?

A. Thrombosis—**YES; a high platelet count can cause hypercoagulation, which could lead to thrombus formation. A normal thrombocyte or platelet count is 150,000 to 450,000 mm^3. The loss of antithrombin III and reduced levels of factors IX, XI, and XII because of urinary loss may lead to hypercoagulability and hyperlipidemia, which will increase the platelet count. This condition will place a child at risk for thrombus formation.**

B. Bruising and petechiae—NO; this would be a low platelet count.

C. Pulmonary edema—NO; this is unrelated.

D. Infection—NO; this is unrelated.

EXERCISE 5.34 Select all that apply:

Which of the following would be appropriate nursing measures for Hashama?

A. Strictly monitor input and output (I&O)—**YES.**

B. Maintain a diet low in sodium—**YES.**

C. Weigh the patient every day—**YES.**

D. Maintain a diet low in protein—NO; the diet should be high in protein, as protein is lost in the urine.

EXERCISE 5.35 Matching:

Place the best description of the urinary defect listed in Column A with the definition in Column B:

Column A	Column B
A. Hypospadias	C Congenital defect in which the bladder protrudes through the abdominal wall
B. Epispadias	E Accumulation of urine in the renal pelvis
C. Exstrophy of the bladder	A Urethral meatus located on the ventral surface of the penile shaft
D. Chordee	H Narrowing or stenosis of preputial opening of foreskin
E. Hydronephrosis	F Fluid in the scrotum
F. Hydrocele	D Ventral curvature of the penis
G. Cryptorchidism	B Urethral meatus located on the dorsal surface of the penile shaft
H. Phimosis	G Undescended testes

EXERCISE 5.36 Multiple-choice:

Which of the following is the most common cause of acute renal failure in children?

A. Pyelonephritis—NO; this is not the most common cause.

B. Uremic syndrome—**YES; hemolytic uremic syndrome (HUS) is the most frequent cause of intrarenal or intrinsic renal failure. The most common form of the disease is associated with *E. coli.***

C. Urinary tract obstruction—NO; this is not the most common cause.

D. Severe dehydration—NO; this is not the most common cause.

EXERCISE 5.37 Multiple-choice:

Which of the following is the primary clinical manifestation of acute renal failure?

A. Oliguria—**YES; oliguria is a clinical manifestation of renal failure. A child should have a urine output of 1.0 mL/kg/hr.**

B. Hematuria—NO; there is usually no bleeding into the urine.

C. Proteinuria—NO; there is usually no protein in the urine.

D. Bacteriuria—NO; there are usually no bacteria in the urine.

EXERCISE 5.38 Multiple-choice:

What is the best intervention to help the parents in coping with this illness?

A. Suggest to the parents that they get some rest so they will feel better—NO; suggesting to the parents to get rest is good, but they really need to work through their feelings of guilt.

B. Tell the parents not to worry, it was not their fault—NO; telling the parents not to worry will not relieve their feelings of guilt.

C. Call the nursing supervisor to talk with the parents—NO; calling the nursing supervisor is not appropriate because this is your responsibility and within your nursing scope of practice.

D. Be supportive of the parents and allow them to verbalize their feelings—**YES; the best thing to do is to be supportive of the parents and allow them to verbalize their feelings of guilt.**

EXERCISE 5.39 Multiple-choice:

Which of the following statements is true about febrile seizures?

A. Febrile seizures are usually associated only with bacterial infections.—NO; febrile seizures are not associated only with bacterial infections, they can be related to viral infections as well.

B. There is a genetic link to febrile seizures.—NO; there is no genetic link to a febrile seizure.

C. Febrile seizures are not associated with any long-term complications.—**YES; a febrile seizure usually has no long-term consequences.**

D. A febrile seizure usually indicates that the child will develop epilepsy later on.—NO; febrile seizures do not indicate that a child will later develop epilepsy.

EXERCISE 5.40 Multiple-choice:

What is the most common age for seizures to occur in children?

A. Birth through 1 month of age—NO; this is not the typical age.

B. 1 month to 6 months of age—NO; this is not the typical age.

C. 6 months through 5 years of age—**YES; febrile seizures most often occur from 6 months to 5 years of age. They peak from 14 to 28 months of age.**

D. 5 years to 8 years of age—NO; this is not the typical age.

EXERCISE 5.41 Multiple-choice:

As the nurse prepares the room for Jeffrey, what items are a priority?

A. Working suction and oxygen—**YES; it is necessary to have working suction to clear the airway and oxygen available if needed.**

B. A drink to maintain hydration—NO; this is not a priority.

C. Tongue blade and rail pads—NO; tongue blades and extra pads are no longer used.

D. Albuterol and an intravenous (IV) setup—NO; there is no need for albuterol, a bronchodilator, at this time.

EXERCISE 5.42 Multiple-choice:

What is the nursing priority for this patient?

A. Place a tongue depressor in his mouth to prevent him from swallowing his tongue—NO; this can damage the teeth.

B. Maintain a patent airway—**YES; the nursing priority for Jeffrey is to stay with him and maintain a patent airway.**

C. Start an intravenous (IV) line to give medications—NO; these are interventions that need orders from the primary care practitioner.
D. Leave the room to get help and call the primary care provider—NO; the nurse should never leave a patient who is having a seizure.

EXERCISE 5.43 True/False:

During a seizure, the nurse would expect Jeffrey's heart rate to increase and his oxygen saturation to drop.

__X__ True; this is normal during a seizure. Because Jeffrey's oxygen saturation dropped to 89%, the nurse should give him some blow-by oxygen until the seizure is over.

EXERCISE 5.44 Fill in the blank:

What is the name of the condition in which a seizure lasts longer than 30 minutes or a series of seizures that last longer than 30 minutes in which consciousness is not regained between episodes?

Status epilepticus. **However, the Epilepsy Foundation recommends parents and the public to call for help for any seizure lasting more than 5 minutes that does not show signs of stopping.**

EXERCISE 5.45 Multiple-choice:

Which of the following medications used for seizures has the side effect of gingival hyperplasia?

A. Phenobarbital (Luminal)—NO; this is not a side effect.
B. Valproic acid (Depakote)—NO; this is not a side effect.
C. Carbamazapine (Tegretol)—NO; this is not a side effect.
D. Phenytoin (Dilantin)—**YES; this is the medication that causes the gums in the mouth to enlarge and decreases some teenager's compliance. It cannot be given fast via the intravenous (IV) route. (The normal dose is 0.5 mg/kg/min for neonates; 1 to 3 mg/kg/min for infants, children, and adults.) If given by rapid IV administration, it can cause profound bradycardia, hypotension, arrhythmias, and cardiovascular collapse. It is also very irritating to the veins. Finally, it is compatible only in normal saline solution. It must be given with saline. If given with IV fluids containing dextrose, it will immediately precipitate out into a white powder inside the tubing and veins. Phenytoin can also cause venous irritation, pain, and thrombophlebitis.**

EXERCISE 5.46 Fill in the blank:

What is the name of a medication similar to phenytoin (Dilantin) that can be given more quickly intravenously and is compatible with dextrose-containing intravenous (IV) solutions?

Fosphenytoin (Cerebyx). **Fosphenytoin can be given at a rate of 150 phenytoin equivalents (PEs)/minute. This medication breaks down inside the body into phenytoin (Dilantin). Blood levels for both phenytoin and fosphenytoin must be measured to be sure it is therapeutic. A normal blood level of Dilantin is 10 to 20 µg/mL. Note that fosphenytoin is ordered in PEs and *not* milligrams! It should be used for all children, because it is less caustic to the veins.**

EXERCISE 5.47 Matching:

Match the seizure types in Column A with the correct descriptions in Column B:

Column A	Column B
A. Tonic–clonic	B A brief loss of consciousness that looks like daydreaming
B. Absence seizure	E Most severe and difficult to control
C. Febrile seizure	A Strong rhythmic jerking of the body
D. Complex partial seizure	H A phase of the seizure during which the person may sleep
E. Lennox–Gastaut seizure	C May be caused by a sudden dramatic change in body temperature
F. Akinetic seizure	D Usually starts in the focal area and then spreads to the other hemisphere, with some impairment or loss of consciousness
G. Aura	G Phase of a seizure during which a feeling or smell is recognized before a seizure begins
H. Postictal phase	F Person may "freeze into place"

EXERCISE 5.48 Fill in the blank:

What other test would the nurse expect the physician to perform to confirm the diagnosis of meningitis?
Lumbar puncture (LP). **An LP will be performed to obtain a small amount of spinal fluid to evaluate for white blood cells (WBCs), protein, and glucose. Cerebrospinal fluid with greater than 10,000 WBCs and a high protein count with low glucose is indicative of meningitis.**

EXERCISE 5.49 Select all that apply:

Which of the following nursing interventions are appropriate for Jeffrey?

A. Maintain Jeffrey on droplet or respiratory isolation—**YES; it is important to maintain isolation precautions until he has been treated for at least 24 hours with intravenous (IV) antibiotics.**
B. Perform neurological checks frequently—**YES; neurological checks should be performed frequently.**
C. Administer antibiotics as ordered—**YES; to fight the infection.**
D. Monitor the skin for petechiae or purpura—**YES; the skin should be monitored in the event that Jeffrey has meningococcal meningitis.**
E. Keep the room bright and sunny to avoid depression—NO; the room should be kept dark and quiet for comfort. In the initial case presentation, it is noted that Jeffrey has photophobia. Keeping the room bright and sunny will aggravate his photophobia and worsen the headache. He will not become depressed. Rest and comfort are best for Jeffrey.

EXERCISE 5.50 Select all that apply:

Which of the following vaccines protect infants from bacterial meningitis?

A. IPV (inactivated polio vaccine)—NO.
B. PCV (pneumococcal vaccine)—**YES; both the PCV and the HiB protect infants from bacterial meningitis).**

C. DTP (diphtheria, tetanus, and pertussis vaccine)—NO.

D. HiB (*Haemophilus influenzae* type B vaccine)—**YES; both the PCV and the HiB protect infants from bacterial meningitis. For older children and particularly college-bound students, it is important to also obtain the vaccine for meningococcal meningitis (MPSV4, or Menomune, or MCV4, or Menactra). As of May 2005, the American Academy of Pediatrics recommends that this vaccine be given to children at the age of 11 or 12. Many schools are requiring this prior to entering high school or by the age of 15.**

E. Measles, mumps, and rubella (MMR) vaccine—NO.

EXERCISE 5.51 Fill in the blank:

What is the name of the neurological disorder that can result when children are given aspirin?

***Reye's syndrome*. This is a life-threatening condition that affects the liver and the brain. A high ammonia level, elevated liver enzymes, poor clotting ability, and hypoglycemia are definitive laboratory studies for this condition.**

EXERCISE 5.52 Select all that apply:

Which of the following assessments are most concerning in evaluating for a neurological problem related to a potential ventriculoperitoneal (VP) shunt malfunction?

A. He is one of a set of triplets.—NO; just being premature should have no effect on a VP shunt malfunction.

B. He has a fever.—NO; a fever is a sign of infection, not that a shunt has malfunctioned unless it has been a prolonged time and the patient now has meningitis.

C. He "feels like a rag doll when I hold him."—NO; this statement needs more clarification. The mother seems to be referring to lack of tone and could be a result of motor delay related to prematurity. Further clarification is especially so because the mother states he is crying now and appears to be in pain.

D. His head circumference has increased 5 cm in 1 week.—**YES; this is *most* concerning. The fact that his head circumference has increased 5 cm in 1 week shows that the cerebral spinal fluid is not properly draining with the shunt and indicates a potential shunt malfunction.**

E. His anterior fontanel is full and bulging.—**YES; very concerning, his bulging fontanel is a sign that the cerebral spinal fluid has nowhere to go and is not draining. It also indicates increasing intracranial pressure.**

F. He is "irritable and crying like he is in pain."—**YES; the child is irritable because of the increasing intracranial pressure and the cerebral spinal fluid is not draining and has nowhere to go. This will cause a tremendous headache. Infants cannot verbalize pain, so when they cry, it is an indication that they might be in pain. The last three signs definitely indicate a potential shunt malfunction and increasing intracranial pressure. This is a medical emergency and needs to be addressed promptly.**

EXERCISE 5.53 Multiple-choice:

Look at the following illustration. Which of the following statements about Matthew's myelomenigocele is accurate?

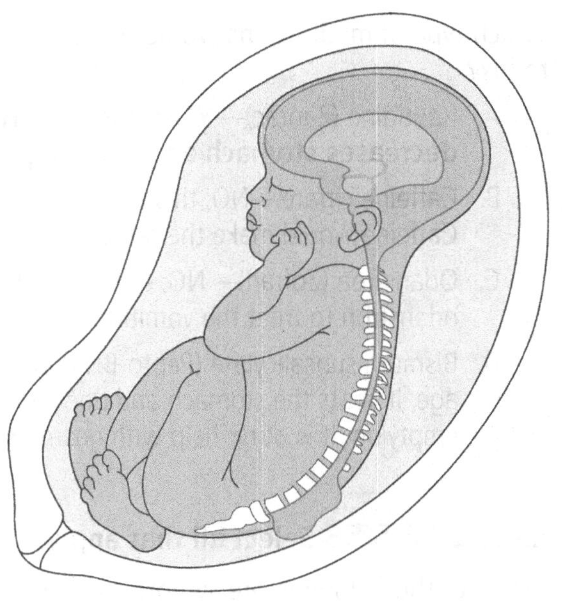

A. He has a normal spinal cord and vertebrae that are not covered.—NO; look at the illustration.

B. He has a normal spinal cord and vertebrae but a tuft of hair is noted at the base of his spine.—NO; look at the illustration.

C. He has protrusion of a sac through his vertebrae that contains the meninges and cerebrospinal fluid.—NO; look at the illustration.

D. He has protrusion of a sac through his vertebrae that contains the meninges, cerebrospinal fluid, and spinal cord or nerve root.—**YES; this is what happens in this case.**

EXERCISE 5.54 True/False:

Children with myelomeningocele often have bowel and bladder incontinence problems.

_X_ True; caused by decreased innervation in the sacral area of the cord, which is responsible for bowel and bladder function.

EXERCISE 5.55 True/False:

Matthew, who has spina bifida and needs to be intermittently catheterized for urine, should be taught, when he is older, to catheterize himself using a clean latex catheter.

_X_ False; a child with spina bifida should use a nonlatex catheter owing to potential latex allergy. The child should be considered latex sensitive for every hospital admission. He or she should always be treated with materials that are latex free and maintained in a latex-free environment using a high-efficiency particulate arrestance (HEPA) filter.

EXERCISE 5.56 Multiple-choice:

What should the nurse caring for Matthew say to the parents?

A. "Don't worry; you didn't cause this problem."—NO; telling them not to worry will not help them.

B. "I can understand your feelings, spina bifida is hereditary and he gets the gene from the mother."—NO; although there are risk factors that predispose a child for spina bifida, such as low maternal level of folic acid at the time of conception, a family history of spina bifida, a mother who had a previous pregnancy with a neural tube defect, a mother of European, Caucasian, or Hispanic descent or if she took certain medications during the pregnancy, there is no actual gene identified that has a marker for spina bifida at this time.

C. "You should have taken your folic acid when you were pregnant with Matthew."—NO; telling the mother she should have taken her folic acid will only add to her feelings of guilt.

D. "Tell me why you feel guilty for causing Mathew's spina bifida."—**YES; exploring the mother's feelings by asking her to tell you more allows her to openly verbalize her feelings.**

EXERCISE 5.57 Multiple-choice:

Which type of medications would the nurse expect Matthew to be placed on to help with his reflux?

A. Rantidine (Zantac)—**YES; this is an H2 blocker and would be appropriate for Matthew. It decreases stomach acid and helps ease the side effects of reflux.**

B. Caffeine citrate—NO; this is a xanthine stimulant and is used in babies to treat apnea of prematurity. Caffeine would make the reflux worse, so is not the choice of medication to be given.

C. Odanstron (Zofran)—NO; even though Matthew is vomiting, the nurse would not routinely give odanstron to treat the vomiting. The source of the vomiting needs to be identified.

D. Bismuth subsalicylate (Pepto-Bismol)—NO; this would not be an appropriate choice for a baby of this age. It coats the stomach and does not decrease stomach acid production or enhance gastric emptying. It is of no help with gastroesophageal reflux.

EXERCISE 5.58 Select all that apply:

Which of the following are symptoms of hypertrophic pyloric stenosis?

A. Projectile vomiting—**YES; projectile vomiting is a symptom of pyloric stenosis. An infant who has a pyloric stricture has thickening of the pyloric sphincter, which results in projectile vomiting.**

B. Dry mucous membranes—**YES; dry mucous membranes are a symptom of pyloric stenosis because the infant is unable to consume adequate food and fluid and becomes dehydrated.**

C. Currant jelly stools—NO; currant jelly stools are a symptom of a patient with an intussusception. They have bloody mucousy stools and pass a currant-like substance, which is from the sloughing of the gastric mucousa.

D. Constant crying and hunger—**YES; constant crying and hunger are symptoms of pyloric stenosis. Children are unable to consume enough food and become very irritable from the lack of food and from pain caused by the refluxing of stomach acid into the esophagus.**

E. Walnut-shaped mass in his abdomen—**YES; a walnut-shaped mass in the abdomen in the lower right quadrant is palpable and sometimes visible on the abdomen of an infant with pyloric stenosis.**

EXERCISE 5.59 Multiple-choice:

What is the most common test or tool pediatricians use to determine whether an infant is meeting his or her developmental goals?

A. An IQ test—NO; this is not appropriate for this age.

B. Denver Developmental Screening Test II—**YES; the Denver developmental II test is the most commonly used developmental screening tool.**

C. Brainstem auditory evoked response (BAER) test—NO; this is not appropriate for this age.

D. Battelle Developmental Inventory—NO; this is not appropriate for this age.

EXERCISE 5.60 Multiple-choice:

Which of the following is *not a cause* of cerebral palsy?

A. Anoxia during delivery—NO; anoxia does indeed cause cerebral palsy.

B. Being born prematurely at 32 weeks—NO; being a baby of a multiple birth or being premature may predispose an infant to cerebral palsy, but is not likely if there were no other complications at 32 weeks. The infant will need to be followed for normal growth and development patterns.

C. Cerebral infections—NO; cerebral infection does indeed cause cerebral palsy.

D. Early hospitalizations—**YES; early hospitalization alone is not a reason for the development of cerebral palsy. It may impede maternal/infant bonding but is not a cause of cerebral palsy.**

EXERCISE 5.61 Multiple-choice:

Which of the following types of cerebral palsy has the most severe symptoms, including both motor problems and speech problems related to involuntary facial movements?

A. Mixed type—**YES; the mixed type of cerebral palsy has both spastic and athetoid components, which include speech and involuntary movements that are uncontrollable by the patient.**

B. Athetoid/dyskinetic—NO; this is not the mixed type.

C. Ataxic—NO; this is not the mixed type.

D. Spastic—NO; this is not the mixed type.

EXERCISE 5.62 Multiple-choice:

A 42% curvature is considered:

A. Mild scoliosis—NO; mild scoliosis is curvature of 10% to 20%.

B. Moderate scoliosis—NO; moderate scoliosis is curvature of 20% to 40% and is treated with bracing, using a Boston or Milwaukee brace.

C. Severe scoliosis—**YES; severe scoliosis is a curvature greater than 40% and is usually treated with surgery.**

D. Total scoliosis—NO; this is not a term used.

EXERCISE 5.63 Multiple-choice:

Which of the following nursing interventions is *most* important in caring for Natalie?

A. Making sure her Foley catheter is patent—NO; airway and breathing are most important.

B. Monitoring her respirations—**YES; monitoring Natalie for respiratory depression while on the morphine patient-controlled analgesia (PCA) pump is the most important intervention.**

C. Monitoring the pulses in her feet—NO; airway and breathing are most important.

D. Making sure Natalie does not become constipated—NO; airway and breathing are most important.

EXERCISE 5.64 Select all that apply:

When setting up the patient-controlled analgesia (PCA) pump, which of the following nursing procedures must be followed to ensure safety and accuracy?

A. Two RNs must verify the medication.—**YES; two licensed individuals like RNs must not only verify the medication, they must witness and document any discard any time a new bag is changed, and verify the settings are correct as ordered on the pump.**

B. An RN and a medical assistant need to verify the dosage settings on the pump.—NO; it has to be two trained and registered health care workers who are competent in the operation of the pump.

C. The pump must be locked.—**YES; whenever a narcotic is used, the pump should have a lock and the lock must be utilized on the pump. Many PCA pumps will not operate if the pump is not in a locked position.**

D. The pump tubing should be free of kinks and twists.—**YES; be sure the tubing is free of kinks or twists. They could occlude the adequate flow of medication to the patient.**

E. A pharmacist must verify the correct medication is in the pump.—NO; a pharmacist is not mandated to verify the correct medication in the pump but could, in some institutions, verify the medication on hanging it. However, pharmacists are not usually validated on how to set up the pump. Verify at the institution who are the acceptable licensed individuals as per the administrative policy.

EXERCISE 5.65 Select all that apply:

Which of the following assessments and interventions would be an accurate interpretation of Natalie's pain-management scenario?

A. Wait to see whether the pain is relieved because it has only been 6 hours since surgery.—NO; it has already been 6 hours and her pain is not being controlled.

B. Check the patient-controlled analgesia (PCA) pump and infusion set to be sure that it is working properly.—**YES; do check that the pump is functioning correctly and no tubing is kinked.**

C. Ask the mother to push the PCA control button for the patient in case she forgets.—NO; the family should never push the button for the patient. The patient is to determine when he or she needs pain relief.

D. Call the primary care provider to report her pain is not being controlled.—**YES; notify the primary care provider that her pain control is not working for her.**

E. Tell her mother to talk with her and get her to calm down.—NO; the nurse should not direct the mother to get the daughter to calm down. The problem of inadequate pain control needs to be addressed with the attending physician.

EXERCISE 5.66 Multiple-choice:

Buck's traction is a type of:

A. Skin traction—**YES; Buck's traction is a type of skin traction. Skin traction is applied to the skin surface with adhesive materials or straps.**

B. Skeletal traction—NO; skeletal traction is pulled directly into the bone and involves pins, wires, or tongs. Skeletal traction must be placed surgically.

C. Manual traction—NO; manual traction is a type of external traction in which someone's hands exert a pulling force.

D. Plaster traction—NO; plaster traction is a type of skeletal traction except that it utilizes pins or wires in a cast to maintain a continuous pulling force.

EXERCISE 5.67 Multiple-choice:

The appropriate intervention for the nurse to perform for Pedro in Buck's traction is to:

A. Do nothing, Pedro is comfortable. Play cars with him to gain his trust.—NO; if the weight is on the floor there is no traction being applied to the leg. The traction must be fixed.

B. Add another 5-lb weight to the traction, so that it works properly.—NO; adding additional weight will not fix the malaligned traction. Also a physician's order is needed to add more weight to traction.

C. Remove the weight, reposition the boot, then replace the weight making sure it is not sitting on the floor.—**YES; first remove the weight, reposition the boot on the patient's lower leg to be sure it did not slide down, make sure the patient has not slid down in the bed and move him to a good position, then gently replace the 5-lb weight, making sure it is not sitting on the floor. The weight should be free hanging and not touching the bed either.**

D. Pull Pedro up in bed to get the weights off the floor.—NO; do not just pull Pedro up in bed; it will cause undue pain by pulling him to lift the weights up off the floor. Also, the boots need to be checked to verify they are positioned correctly on his lower legs. The safer way to do this is provided in answer C.

EXERCISE 5.68 Multiple-choice:

The nurse is caring for a 7-year-old boy in Buck's traction for a fractured femur. What would be included in a neurovascular assessment of the affected leg?

A. Pain level, temperature in the affected extremity, color, and a Doppler scan of the pedal pulse of the left leg—NO; pain level is important but not really most important in a neurovascular check. The temperature in the affected left extremity, especially if it is cool, could be an indicator of perfusion to the foot. Color is an indicator of blood flow to the foot. Doppler scan of the pedal pulse if one is unable to be palpated would be part of a good neurovascular assessment.

B. Vital signs (VS), bilateral lung sounds, pain level, and pulse oximetry done on the toes of both legs—NO; although VS are important, they are not always a strong indicator of the lack of perfusion to the affected left lower leg. Lung sounds obviously are not a concern in this situation. Pain level is important and could be a good indicator that something is wrong. Pulse oximetry done on any of the toes of the affected leg could indicate blood flow to the foot. If there is decreased perfusion to the foot, the pulse oximeter may not pick this up. Moreover, although it is important to check both legs and feet and for comparison, a definite priority should be given to the left affected leg.

C. Sensation, movement, capillary refill, and pulse of affected extremity and VS of the right leg—NO; these are all important as stated, but it is more important to do the assessment on the affected left leg, not the right leg, unless done for comparison.

D. Color, sensation, movement, capillary refill, and pulse of affected extremity of the left leg—**YES; of all the choices this one is the best. Color is a great indicator of blood flow. If pink, there is adequate blood flow, and if pale or blue, it is indicative of poor to bad blood flow. Sensation is important in that if a patient cannot feel his or her foot, poor blood flow may be indicated. The ability to move the extremity is important to a neurovascular assessment. If one can at least wiggle his or her toes, that indicates good perfusion and muscle and nerve innervation to the foot. Capillary refill and pulse of affected extremity are crucial to determining adequate blood flow to the foot and toes. Capillary refill should be 1 to 2 seconds. If it is prolonged, inadequate blood flow to the foot is definite. This is especially so of the left affected leg.**

Exercise 5.69 Choose all that apply:

Which of the following nursing actions would be appropriate for Pedro while in Buck's traction?

A. Maintain straight body alignment—**YES; make sure Pedro's body is in straight alignment.**

B. Do frequent neurovascular checks to the lower extremities—**YES; do this to be sure there is adequate circulation.**

C. Make sure the patient's buttocks are off the bed—NO; the patient's buttocks should not be off the bed. That is done with Bryant's traction, in which the legs are pulled upward at a 90° angle and the buttocks are slightly lifted off the bed.

D. Do pin care every 8 hours—NO; there are no pins in Buck's traction. Buck's traction is external and does not involve any pins into the bone. That is done with skeletal traction.

E. Make sure the weights are free hanging and off the floor—**YES; do make sure that the weights are free hanging and off the floor.**

F. Notify the physician if Pedro experiences any pain from muscle spasm—**YES; and obtain an order for a muscle relaxant. Muscle spasm can be very painful with a femur fracture.**

Exercise 5.70 Multiple-choice question:

Pedro's as-needed orders are as follows. Of these, which medication would the nurse administer?

A. Tylenol (acetaminophen) with codeine one teaspoon every 4 hours—NO; a dose of Tylenol with codeine was just given, so he cannot have that for another 3 hours.

B. Morphine 2 mg intravenous (IV) every 2 hours for pain—NO; the mother's description of "leg jumping" is evidence of muscle spasm and not pain, so the morphine would not be as effective.

C. Valium (diazepam) 5 mg IV every 6 hours—**YES; the child is most likely having muscle spasm associated with a fractured femur. Valium would be the drug of choice for that.**

D. Demerol (meperidine) 3 mg IV every 4 hours—NO; Demerol is not routinely used in children of this age because it breaks down into a toxic metabolite of normeperidine. For this reason, morphine is the narcotic of choice for children.

Exercise 5.71 Select all that apply:

A nurse assessing Pedro for a suspected closed, mild head injury would expect to see which of the following clinical manifestations?

A. Vomiting—**YES; vomiting is a clinical sign of a minor head injury.**

B. Delayed pupillary response—NO; delayed pupillary response would be a manifestation of a major head injury usually with associated increased intracranial pressure (ICP).

C. Drowsiness and increased sleeping—**YES; drowsiness and increased sleeping are an indication of an evolving head injury. Any alteration in consciousness or a child not playing are important signs.**

D. Report of a headache—**YES; report of a headache should be handled with great concern in any child after an accident even if he or she was wearing a helmet.**

E. Confusion—**YES; confusion or forgetfulness are also signs of a suspected mild closed head injury or a concussion.**

Exercise 5.72 Multiple-choice:

Which of the following is the *most* common type of anemia in children?

A. Pernicious anemia—NO; iron deficiency is more common.

B. Iron-deficiency anemia—**YES; iron-deficiency anemia is the most common type of anemia in children.**

C. Sickle cell anemia—NO; iron deficiency is more common.

D. Aplastic anemia—NO; iron deficiency is more common.

Exercise 5.73 Ordering:

The nurse is admitting Tyla to the emergency department (ED). Place the interventions in order of priority:

__4__ Obtain a throat culture. This is fourth, a broad-spectrum antibiotic will be ordered until the result of the culture is available. The culture should be obtained after the analgesic is administered.

__2__ Start an intravenous (IV) of D5/0.9% normal saline. This is second because it improves hydration.

__1__ Administer nasal oxygen. This is done first because it improves oxygenation and may prevent more sickling.

__3__ Administer analgesics IV. This is third because it is IV and must be administered after the IV is started.

Exercise 5.74 Select all that apply:

Which of the following are conditions that can predispose to sickling of red blood cells, or sickling crisis?

A. Infection—**YES; infection can precipitate a sickling crisis.**

B. Hypertension—NO; hypertension will not cause a sickling crisis.

C. Hypoxia—**YES; hypoxia can also precipitate a sickling crisis.**

D. Emotional stress—**YES; emotional stress can also precipitate a sickling crisis.**

E. Dehydration—**YES; dehydration can also precipitate a sickling crisis.**

Exercise 5.75 Multiple-choice:

The nurse is talking with Tyla's parents about sickle cell anemia. The nurse explores the feelings of the parents and finds that both parents are admitting to feeling guilty a lot of the time. Which of the following causes will the nurse most likely find as the greatest contributor and/or cause of this guilt?

A. Both parents are working and cannot spend as much time with their child as they would like.—NO; although both parents are working and cannot spend as much time with the child as they would like, this is not the main source of their feelings of guilt.

B. The parents are not able to help their child more and fear that the child is suffering a great amount of the time.—NO; the parents do have concerns about their child being in pain, but this is not the source of their guilt feelings.

C. Both parents are carrying at least one recessive gene for sickle cell anemia.—**YES; sickle cell anemia is an autosomal recessive condition; both parents must carry at least one recessive gene for sickle cell anemia to occur. The parents share they are feeling guilty because "it is my fault she has sickle cell, we gave this to her in our genes." The nurse assures them that although this is true, they had no way of knowing that they carried the gene. She supports them, allows them to verbalize their feelings of guilt, but reassures them that they cannot blame themselves for their child acquiring sickle cell anemia.**

D. The child wants more and more things that cost a lot and the parents cannot buy them because they do not have enough money.—NO; this is not the real reason for the parent's guilt. Not being able to buy her more things is not of importance.

Exercise 5.76 Multiple-choice:

What is the most common type of hemophilia?

A. Hemophilia A—**YES; hemophilia A is typically what we refer to as *hemophilia*, and it typically occurs in males.**

B. Hemophilia B—NO; only 15% of people with hemophilia have this form of hemophilia, which is also known as Christmas disease.

C. Hemophilia C—NO; hemophilia C has milder symptoms and occurs in both sexes.

D. Hemophilia D—NO; there is no hemophilia D.

Exercise 5.77 Multiple-choice:

In the most common type or classic form of hemophilia, which factor is deficient?

A. Factor VIII—**YES; in the most common type of hemophilia, type A, factor VIII is deficient.**

B. Factor VII—NO; in hemophilia C, factor XI is deficient.

C. Factor IX—NO; in hemophilia B, factor IX is deficient.

D. vWF (von Willebrand factor)—NO; vWF is needed for platelet adhesion.

Exercise 5.78 Multiple-choice:

Which of the following laboratory values could indicate that a child has leukemia?

A. White blood cells (WBCs): 32,000/mm^3—**YES; a normal WBC count is approximately 4.5/mm^3 to 11.0/mm^3. In leukemia, a high WBC count is diagnostic of the disease. This is usually confirmed with a blood smear. Leukemia occurs when the stem cells in the bone marrow produce immature WBCs that cannot function normally. These cells proliferate rapidly by cloning instead of mitosis, causing the bone marrow to fill with abnormal WBCs. These abnormal cells then spill out into the circulatory system, where they take the place of normally functioning WBCs.**

B. Platelets: 300,000/mm^3—NO; this does not indicate leukemia.

C. Hemoglobin: 15 g/dL—NO; this does not indicate leukemia.

D. Blood pH: 7.35—NO; this does not indicate leukemia.

Exercise 5.79 Multiple-choice:

The pediatric nurse understands that the most common cancer found in children is:

A. Non-Hodgkin's lymphoma—NO; this is not a common cancer in children.

B. Acute lymphocytic leukemia—**YES; the most common form of cancer found in children is acute lymphocytic leukemia (ALL). ALL accounts for 25% of all childhood cancers and 75% of leukemias in children.**

C. Chronic lymphocytic leukemia—NO; this is not a common cancer in children.

D. Ewing's sarcoma—NO; this is not a common cancer in children.

Exercise 5.80 Select all that apply:

The nurse knows which of the following symptoms are early clinical manifestations of leukemia?

A. Anorexia—**YES; anorexia and decreased appetite are early signs of leukemia.**

B. Hematuria—NO; hematuria is a late clinical manifestation of leukemia.

C. Petechiae—**YES; petechiae, or small red dots that do not fade with pressure, are small capillaries that have ruptured under the skin and are a sign of leukemia.**

D. Unsteady gait and falling—**YES; having an unsteady gait and falling are very common; this is frequently what parents notice and is an early sign of leukemia.**

E. Ulcerations in the mouth—NO; ulcerations in the mouth are usually a later sign of leukemia and usually occur after chemotherapy begins.

Exercise 5.81 Select all that apply:

Keoni develops thrombocytopenia after receiving chemotherapy. Which of the following should the nurse do?

A. Monitor for signs of bleeding—**YES; the child who has thrombocytopenia is at risk for bleeding and hemorrhage. Monitoring for signs of bleeding is a very important assessment.**

B. Obtain all temperatures by the rectal route—NO; temperatures should *not* be taken by the rectal route. The anal sphinchter is vascular and taking the temperature by this route could cause tissue injury and lead to bleeding and is *not* advised for oncology patients.

C. Administer all routine immunizations—NO; the child who has thrombocytopenia is at risk for bleeding and therefore all venipunctures, including routine immunizations, should be avoided.

D. Avoid unnecessary venipunctures—**YES; avoid unnecessary venipunctures because of the increased risk for bleeding resulting from the thrombocytopenia.**

E. Limit the number of visitors—NO; limiting the number of visitors protects the child from infection, so, if the child was neutropenic, it would be wise to limit the number of visitors, but visitors will have no impact on thrombocytopenia.

Exercise 5.82 Multiple-choice:

That evening, the nurse caring for Amber notices a group of medical students standing outside Amber's room reviewing her chart. When the nurse approaches and asks them what they are doing, they respond "we heard this child has a Wilms tumor and we want to palpate her abdomen to see the size of the tumor." What is the result of abdominal palpation of a Wilms tumor?

A. Palpation will be painful—NO; although this may be true, it is not the most urgent reason.

B. The lymph nodes may swell—NO; although this is not unusual.

C. Only physicians can feel the tumor—NO; this is not true.

D. The tumor may spread if palpation is done—**YES; for a child with a Wilms tumor or, if any mass is felt while palpating a child's abdomen, the nurse should stop palpating and immediately notify the physician. When the mass is palpated, a piece of the tumor might break off, allowing the cancerous cells to spread to other parts of the body**.

Exercise 5.83 Multiple-choice:

As a result of chemotherapy's side effects of nausea and vomiting, the pediatric nurse administered which medication?

A. Ondansetron (Zofran)—**YES; ondansetron is typically used to manage the side effects of nausea and vomiting in the pediatric population.**

B. Prochloroperazine (Compazine)—NO; compazine should not be used in children, especially at the age of 18 months. It can cause dystonic reactions in children.

C. Doxorubicin (Myocet)—NO; doxorubicin is a chemotherapy agent.

D. Neupogen (granulocyte-colony stimulating factor [G-CSF])—NO; neupogen is a colony-stimulating factor that stimulates the production of white blood cells.

Exercise 5.84 Select all that apply:

Which of the following statements should the nurse include in her teaching?

A. "Your child will need chemotherapy for about 12 months."—NO; chemotherapy depends on the stage of the tumor. The nurse should not give a time frame for chemotherapy. The nurse does not have enough information.

B. "Wilms tumors are caused by an inherited genetic trait."—NO; only about 2% of Wilms tumors have a familial origin; however, research continues as an absent tumor suppressor gene has been identified in children with Wilms tumor. Although Wilms tumors are sometimes caused by an inherited genetic trait, at this time there is no conclusive proof that familial origin is widespread.

C. "Surgery is usually done within 48 hours of diagnosis."—**YES; prompt removal of the tumor is best practice and best prognosis in the treatment of a Wilms tumor. Therefore, this should be included in the teaching to the parents/caregivers.**

D. "Touching or palpating the tumor could spread it, so don't rub it."—**YES; touching or rubbing the tumor could cause the encapsulated tumor to rupture and spread and therefore should be included in the teaching.**

E. "Further treatment will begin immediately after surgery."—**YES; further treatment will begin immediately after surgery. This will include chemotherapy and/or radiation.**

Exercise 5.85 Multiple-choice:

Amber has her surgery and is being cared for postoperatively. The nurse receives a report that Amber is NPO (nothing by mouth). Which of the following assessments is an indication to continue Amber's NPO status?

A. Her abdominal girth is 1 cm larger than yesterday.—NO; her abdominal girth increasing could be a result of edema. It is not a good indication of NPO status.

B. Amber is crying and has pain at the surgical site.—NO; Amber's crying and pain at the surgical site are not reasons to continue with NPO status. She may be hungry and postop surgical pain is common.

C. Amber is passing flatus every 30 minutes.—NO; Amber passing flatus is not an indication to continue NPO status. In fact, it indicates that gastrointestinal (GI) motility is returning to normal and the diet should be advanced.

D. There are absent bowel sounds.—**YES, if there are absent bowel sounds it means GI motility has not returned and is a reason to maintain NPO status.**

Exercise 5.86 Multiple-choice:

Which of the following is an important nursing consideration in caring for a child with impetigo?

A. Apply topical corticosteroids to decrease inflammation.—NO; it is an infection.

B. Carefully remove dressings so as not to dislodge undermined skin, crusts, and debris. Keep lesions covered for several days before changing.—NO; it requires treatment with antibiotics.

C. Carefully wash hands and maintain cleanliness in caring for an infected child and apply antibiotic cream as ordered.—**YES; treatment for impetigo is removal of crusts with warm water and application of a topical antimicrobial ointment for 5 to 7 days. Impetigo is highly infectious and spreads very easily. Carefully washing hands is paramount.**

D. Examine child under a Wood's lamp for possible spread of lesions.—NO; this is for parasites.

Exercise 5.87 Multiple-choice:

Therapeutic management of a child with a ringworm infection (tinea capitis) would include which of the following?

A. Administer oral griseofulvin (antifungal)—**YES; ringworm is a fungal infection that affects the skin, hair, or nails. The treatment of choice is griseofulvin, an antifungal.**

B. Administer topical or oral antibiotics—NO; fungal infections are not treated with antibiotics, bacterial infections are.

C. Apply topical sulfonamides—NO; fungal infections are not treated with sulfonamides, bacterial infections are.

D. Apply Burow's solution compresses to affected areas—NO; fungal infections are not treated with antibiotics and astringents, bacterial infections are.

Exercise 5.88 Multiple-choice:

Which of the following is usually the only symptom of pediculosis capitis (head lice)?

A. Itching—**YES; the classic sign of head lice is intense itching.**

B. Vesicles—NO; there are no vesicles.

C. Scalp rash—NO; there can be skin breakdown from the itching.

D. Localized inflammatory response—NO; there is only the itching.

Exercise 5.89 Multiple-choice:

Which skin disorder is characterized by linear, thread-like, grayish burrows on the skin?

A. Impetigo—NO; this is a rash.

B. Ringworm—NO; this is a circular lesion.

C. Pinworm—NO; this is a parasite.

D. Scabies—**YES; scabies is characterized by linear, thread-like, grayish burrows made by the female mite, which burrows into the outer layer of the epidermis (stratum corneum) to lay her eggs, leaving a trail of debris and feces. The larvae hatch in approximately 2 to 4 days and proceed toward the surface of the skin. This cycle is repeated every 7 to 14 days.**

Exercise 5.90 Select all that apply:

The nurse is discussing the management of atopic dermatitis (eczema) with a parent. Which of the following teaching points should be included?

A. Dress infant warmly in woollen clothes to prevent chilling—NO; woollen clothes irritate the skin.

B. Keep fingernails and toenails short and clean to prevent transfer of bacteria—**YES; this will help to avoid infection of the involved skin.**

C. Give bubble baths instead of washing lesions with soap—NO; bubble bath and harsh soaps should be avoided.

D. Launder clothes in mild detergent—**YES; atopic dermatitis is not a bacterial condition. It is an allergic or hypersensitivity response in a person who has a genetic predisposition.**

Exercise 5.91 Multiple-choice:

Which of the following treatments would be best to use for Emma's burns initially?

A. Quickly place ice on them to cool the burns—NO; ice water will cause vasoconstriction.

B. Place butter or Crisco on the wounds, because they had some in the camper.—NO; butter or Crisco should never be placed on a burn because it creates an insulated barrier that allows the burn to continue to evolve.

C. Soak Emma's hands in cold water from the lake to cool the burns—NO; lake water contains bacteria.

D. Use tepid water to cool the burns—**YES; tepid water is not very cold.**

Exercise 5.92 Multiple-choice:

Considering the blisters on Emma's hands, what type of burn would this be?

A. Superficial thickness: first-degree—NO; this is not associated with blistering.

B. Epidermal thickness: second-degree—NO; epidermal is not a category.

C. Partial thickness: second-degree—**YES; blistering is a sign of second-degree partial-thickness burns.**

D. Full thickness: third-degree—NO; this is a more severe burn.

Exercise 5.93 Multiple-choice:

If Emma was not experiencing any pain from her burn injury, what type of burn would it be?

A. Superficial thickness: first-degree—NO; this is painful.

B. Epidermal thickness: second-degree—NO; epidermal is not a category.

C. Partial thickness: second-degree—NO; this is painful.

D. Full thickness: third-degree—**YES; third-degree burns typically do not have pain associated with them because the nerve endings have been destroyed.**

Exercise 5.94 Multiple-choice:

Which of the following actions is important for Emma's nurse to take?

A. Implement contact isolation—**YES; contact precautions are recommended to decrease the risk of acquiring an infection when working with burn patients.**

B. Implement droplet isolation—NO; no need for droplet isolation. This type of isolation is usually initiated for someone with a respiratory illness.

C. Restrict her visitors to immediate family only—NO; no need to restrict her visitors to immediate family only as long as the nurse follows contact isolation precautions and keeps her burn wounds covered.

D. Place Emma on neutropenic precautions—NO; Emma is not neutropenic, so there is no need to place her on this type of isolation.

Resources

Ball, J. W., Bindler, R. C., & Cowen, K. (2015). *Principles of pediatric nursing: Caring for children* (6th ed.). Upper Saddle River, NJ: Pearson.

Centers for Disease Control and Prevention. (2015). 2015 Recommended immunizations for children from birth through 6 years old. Retrieved from http://www.cdc.gov/vaccines/schedules

Godshall, M. (2009). Caring for the child with cancer. In S. L. Ward & S. M. Hisley (Eds.), *Maternal child nursing care* (pp. 1104–1132). Philadelphia, PA: F. A. Davis.

CHAPTER 6

Pharmacology

Brian J. Fasolka

Nurses are I. V. leaguers.—Author unknown

UNFOLDING CASE STUDY 1: Robert

Robert, age 47 years, presents to a walk-in clinic with a complaint of a throbbing frontal headache that has lasted for 10 days. Robert initially denies having any past medical or surgical history. Robert's vital signs upon initial assessment are: blood pressure (BP): 224/112 mmHg, heart rate (HR): 84 beats per minute (bpm), respiratory rate (RR): 16 breaths per minute, oral temperature: 98.7°F (37°C). On further questioning by the nurse, Robert reports taking medication for hypertension in the past. He was asymptomatic but was diagnosed by his health care provider. He cannot recall the name of the medication, but reports he stopped taking it over 1 year ago because he "felt fine."

Although Robert is unable to recall the name of the antihypertensive medication he was prescribed, it likely belonged to one of the classes indicated in Exercise 6.1.

EXERCISE 6.1 Matching:

Match the antihypertensive classes in Column A with the mechanisms in Column B:

Column A	Column B
Antihypertensive Class	**Mechanism by Which It Decreases Blood Pressure (BP)**
A. Diuretics	_____ Decreases sympathetic stimulation from the central nervous system (CNS), resulting in decreased heart rate, decreased vasoconstriction, and decreased vascular resistance within the kidneys.

(continued)

Column A	Column B
Antihypertensive Class	**Mechanism by Which It Decreases blood pressure (BP)**
B. Beta blockers	____ Causes vasodilation by blocking the receptor sites of alpha-1 adrenergic receptors.
C. Calcium channel blockers	____ Blocks the receptor sites of angiotensin II, thus preventing the vasoconstricting effects. Prevents the release of aldosterone, which causes increased sodium and water reabsorption.
D. Angiotensin-converting enzyme inhibitors (ACE inhibitors)	____ Decreases heart rate, resulting in decreased cardiac output.
E. Angiotensin II receptor antagonists	____ Causes direct relaxation to arterioles, resulting in decreased peripheral resistance.
F. Centrally acting alpha-2 stimulators	____ Inhibits the conversion of angiotensin I to angiotensin II, thereby preventing the vasoconstrictive actions of angiotensin II. Prevents the release of aldosterone, which causes increased sodium and water reabsorption.
G. Peripherally acting alpha-1 blockers	____ Decreases reabsorption of water in the kidneys, resulting in decreased circulating volume and decreased peripheral resistance.
H. Alpha-1 beta blockers	____ Decreases heart rate, resulting in decreased cardiac output, and causes dilation of peripheral vessels resulting in decreased vascular resistance.
I. Direct vasodilators	____ Decreases the mechanical contraction of the heart by inhibiting the movement of calcium across cell membranes. Also dilates coronary vessels and peripheral arteries.

The answer can be found on page 452

eRESOURCE

To supplement your understanding of drugs used to treat hypertension, refer to the *Merck Manual*. [Pathway: www.merckmanuals.com/professional ➔ enter "Hypertension" into the search field ➔ select "Drugs for Hypertension" ➔ review content.]

The health care provider at the clinic determines that Robert requires treatment in an emergency department (ED). Robert is transferred via ambulance to the nearest ED. On arrival, Robert continues to report a headache of moderate severity.

EXERCISE 6.2 List:

The health care provider prescribes labetalol 10 mg intravenous (IV) push as a stat, one-time prescription. After preparing the medication using the aseptic technique, the nurse enters Robert's room and prepares to administer the medication. On entering the room, the nurse pauses to check the "six rights" of medication administration. List these rights, which the nurse must check before medication administration.

1. ______________________________
2. ______________________________
3. ______________________________
4. ______________________________
5. ______________________________
6. ______________________________

The answer can be found on page 453

EXERCISE 6.3 Multiple-choice:

After identifying the six rights, the nurse notes Robert's blood pressure (BP), heart rate (HR), and cardiac rhythm. Robert's BP is 218/108 mmHg, and his cardiac rhythm is sinus bradycardia at a rate of 50 beats per minute (bpm). What action should the nurse take?

A. Administer the medication as prescribed
B. Ask the physician to change the prescription to PO (oral) labetalol
C. Obtain a 12-lead electrocardiogram (EKG) before administering the medication
D. Hold the medication and request a different antihypertensive medication

The answer can be found on page 454

The health care provider prescribes hydralazine 10 mg IV push × 1, stat.

eRESOURCE

To reinforce your understanding of hydralazine, refer to Epocrates Online. [Pathway: http://online.epocrates.com → under the "Drugs" tab, enter "Hydralazine" in the search field → select "Heparin" → review "Adult Dosing," "Adverse Reactions," and "Safety/Monitoring."]

EXERCISE 6.4 Select all that apply:

The nurse understands that labetalol was discontinued for this patient because of the adverse effects of:

A. Agranulocytosis
B. Heart block
C. Bradycardia
D. Hypotension

The answer can be found on page 454

EXERCISE 6.5 Calculation:

Hydralazine is available in a concentration of 20 mg/mL. How many milliliters of medication must be withdrawn from the vial to administer 10 mg?

The answer can be found on page 454

Per hospital policy in the ED, IV hydralazine is administered undiluted over 1 minute as a slow IV push. Place in correct order the steps of administering this medication.

EXERCISE 6.6 Ordering:

In what order should the following be done? Place a number next to each.

_____ Administer the medication over a 1-minute period
_____ Clean the hub of the intravenous (IV) port using an alcohol pad
_____ Flush the IV with 3 mL of normal saline to assess its patency
_____ Identify the patient per hospital policy
_____ Flush the IV with 3 mL of normal saline to clear site of medication

The answer can be found on page 454

One hour has passed since Robert received the IV hydralazine. He now reports a severe pounding headache and blurred vision. His BP is 244/122 mmHg and heart rate is 90 bpm, normal sinus rhythm. Robert is diagnosed with hypertensive emergency.

EXERCISE 6.7 Multiple-choice:

Which of the following medications would the nurse anticipate administering to Robert next?

A. PO hydrochlorothiazide
B. Intravenous (IV) sodium nitroprusside infusion
C. PO clonodine
D. IV metoprolol

The answer can be found on page 455

The following prescriptions are received.

Furosemide 20 mg IV push × 1 dose, stat.

Continuous nitroprusside IV infusion 0.5 mcg/kg/min, titrated to mean arterial pressure (MAP) of 130 mmHg over 1 hour.

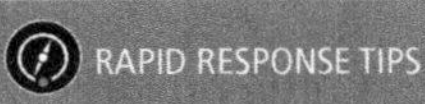

Mean arterial pressure (MAP)

MAP is measured directly with an arterial line; however, to calculate the MAP, the formula is MAP = (systolic BP + 2 × diastolic BP)/3.

The MAP should be 60 or above in order to adequately perfuse the coronary arteries, brain, and kidneys.

Adapted from Lewis, Dirksen, Heitkemper, and Bucher (2014).

EXERCISE 6.8 Multiple-choice:

Furosemide is prescribed in combination with the vasodilator in order to:

A. Decrease cardiac workload by decreasing afterload
B. Increase potassium excretion by the kidneys to prevent hyperkalemia
C. Decrease systolic blood pressure (BP) by decreasing preload
D. Prevent sodium and water retention caused by sodium nitroprusside

The answer can be found on page 455

EXERCISE 6.9 Multiple-choice:

The nurse understands that the intravenous (IV) sodium nitroprusside solution must be protected from light with an opaque sleeve to:

A. Prevent the medication from being degraded by light
B. Decrease replication of any bacterial contaminants
C. Increase the vasodilatory properties of the medication
D. Prevent the solution from developing crystallized precipitates

The answer can be found on page 455

EXERCISE 6.10 Multiple-choice:

Ten minutes after the sodium nitroprusside infusion is initiated, Robert's blood pressure (BP) is 240/120 mmHg and the mean arterial pressure (MAP) is 160 mmHg. Which action by the nurse is most appropriate?

A. Notify the health care provider of the BP
B. Stop the sodium nitroprusside infusion and request a change in medication
C. Increase the sodium nitroprusside infusion to 1 mcg/kg/min
D. Continue the infusion at the same rate allowing more time for medication to work

The answer can be found on page 455

EXERCISE 6.11 Multiple-choice:

In managing Robert's care at this time, which task can the nurse delegate to an experienced unlicensed assistive personnel (UAP)?

A. Measure the blood pressure (BP)
B. Assess pain level on 0 to 10 scale
C. Empty the urinal and document output
D. Silence the alarm on the volumetric pump

The answer can be found on page 456

Fifteen minutes later, Robert's MAP is 150 and he reports that his headache is beginning to improve. Laboratory studies reveal that Robert has a serum glucose of 620 mg/dL. Robert is diagnosed with new-onset type 2 diabetes mellitus.

eRESOURCE

To supplement your understanding of the treatment of type 2 diabetes mellitus, refer to the *Merck Manual.* [Pathway: www.merckmanuals.com/professional ➔ enter "Diabetes" into the search field ➔ select " Diabetes Mellitus (DM)" ➔ review " General Characteristics of Types 1 and 2 Diabetes Mellitus" and "Treatment."]

A continuous insulin infusion is prescribed at 4 units/hr.

EXERCISE 6.12 Multiple-choice:

The hospital's standard concentration is 100 units of insulin in 100 mL of 0.9% normal saline (NS) (1 unit/mL concentration). What type of insulin would the nurse add to the bag of normal saline (NS)?

A. Neutral protamine Hagedorn (NPH) insulin
B. Insulin glargine
C. Mixed NPH/regular insulin 70/30
D. Regular insulin

The answer can be found on page 456

EXERCISE 6.13 Multiple-choice:

Which of the following measures should the nurse implement in order to ensure patient safety when using a continuous insulin infusion?

A. Check capillary blood glucose every 8 hours
B. Administer the insulin as a piggyback to 0.9% normal saline
C. Infuse the insulin using an intravenous (IV) volumetric pump
D. Have the unlicensed assistive personnel (UAP) perform a double check of the infusion rate

The answer can be found on page 456

---

eRESOURCE

To supplement your understanding of the treatment of type 2 diabetes mellitus, refer to the *Merck Manual.* [Pathway: www.merckmanuals.com/professional ➔ enter "Diabetes" into the search field ➔ select " Diabetes Mellitus (DM)" ➔ review "Onset, Peak, and Duration of Action of Human Insulin Preparations" and "Complications of Treatment."]

Robert is transferred from the ED to the medical intensive care unit (MICU), where he is admitted for the diagnoses of:

1. Hypertensive emergency
2. New-onset type 2 diabetes mellitus

EXERCISE 6.14 Fill in the blank:

Robert's initial medication prescriptions include famotidine 20 mg intravenous (IV) every 12 hours. The nurse reviews the medication prescriptions with Robert before administration. Robert asks, "Why am I taking that heartburn medicine? I don't have any heartburn and I never had stomach problems." How should the nurse respond to Robert's question? ______________________________

The answer can be found on page 457

After he has been in the MICU for 2 days, Robert's hypertension and hyperglycemia improve. The sodium nitroprusside infusion and insulin infusion are discontinued. Robert is transferred to a medical–surgical unit. His BP is now under control with lisinopril 10 mg daily and hydrochlorothiazide 25 mg daily. His blood sugar is managed with insulin glargine at bedtime, 10 units administered subcutaneously (subq), and subq insulin determined on a sliding scale before meals and before bedtime using insulin aspart.

eRESOURCE

To reinforce your understanding of these medications, refer to Epocrates Online. [Pathway: http://online.epocrates.com → under the "Drugs" tab, enter "Insulin Aspart" in the search field → select "Heparin" → review in particular "Adult Dosing," "Adverse Reactions," and "Safety/Monitoring." Repeat with "Insulin Glargine" and "Lisinopril."]

In addition, Robert now reports five episodes of foul-smelling, liquid diarrhea over the past 12 hours. Stool cultures are sent to the microbiology lab for culture and sensitivity analysis.

EXERCISE 6.15 Multiple-choice:

In preparation for discharge, what teaching should the nurse include regarding the use of hydrochlorothiazide?

A. Decrease intake of foods high in potassium
B. Take this medication upon waking in the morning
C. Expect to gain weight while taking this medication
D. Report impaired hearing to health care provider immediately

The answer can be found on page 455

Robert asks why the insulin glargine is given only once daily.

EXERCISE 6.16 Fill in the blank:

Based on the pharmacokinetics of insulin glargine, how should the nurse respond to Robert's question?

The answer can be found on page 457

eRESOURCE

To reinforce your understanding of insulin glargine so that you can respond to Robert's question, refer to Medscape on your mobile device. [Pathway: Medscape ➔ enter "Insulin" into the search field ➔ select "Insulin Glargine" and review content.]

The insulin aspart sliding scale in Table 6.1 is prescribed for Robert.

EXERCISE 6.17 Fill in the blank:

At 11:30 a.m., Robert's finger-stick blood glucose is 257 mg/dL. Based on the information in Table 6.1, what action should the nurse take?

TABLE 6.1 Insulin Aspart Sliding Scale

Capillary Glucose Level	Dose of Subq Insulin Aspart
< 70 mg/dL	Initiate hypoglycemia protocol; contact health care provider
70–125 mg/dL	0 units
126–150 mg/dL	2 units
151–175 mg/dL	3 units
176–200 mg/dL	4 units
201–225 mg/dL	5 units
226–250 mg/dL	6 units
251–275 mg/dL	7 units
276–300 mg/dL	8 units
301–325 mg/dL	9 units
326–350 mg/dL	10 units
> 350 mg/dL	10 units; contact health care provider

subq, administered subcutaneously.

The answer can be found on page 457

EXERCISE 6.18 Fill in the blanks:

Based on the pharmacokinetics of insulin aspart, the nurse should expect to note a decrease in capillary glucose within what period of time after administering subcutaneous insulin aspart? ____________

During what period after administration of subcutaneous insulin aspart is Robert most likely to experience a hypoglycemic event? ____________

The answer can be found on page 457

EXERCISE 6.19 Multiple-choice:

Ninety minutes after the subcutaneous insulin aspart is administered, Robert rings his call light. The nurse enters the room and observes that Robert is awake and oriented but anxious and diaphoretic. Robert reports a headache and feelings of fatigue. His capillary blood glucose is 51 mg/dL. What action should the nurse take *first*?

A. Contact the health care provider
B. Prepare intravenous (IV) dextrose 50%
C. Have the patient drink orange juice
D. Ensure the patency of the peripheral IV

The answer can be found on page 458

---

eRESOURCE

To reinforce your understanding of insulin aspart, refer to Medscape on your mobile device. [Pathway: Medscape → enter "Insulin" into the search field → select "Insulin Aspart" and review content.]

EXERCISE 6.20 Multiple-choice:

Before Robert can finish drinking the orange juice he becomes confused, tachycardic, and increasingly diaphoretic. Robert then becomes unresponsive to verbal and painful stimuli. Robert has a patent airway and has an respiratory rate (RR) of 12 breaths per minute. The nurse understands that the best intervention for this patient is to:

A. Call a Code Blue (cardiac arrest/emergency response)
B. Place oral glucose under the patient's tongue
C. Administer intravenous (IV) glucagon
D. Administer IV dextrose 50%

The answer can be found on page 458

Shortly after receiving treatment, Robert is awake and oriented to person, place, and time. Robert's capillary blood glucose is now 135 mg/dL and he is given his lunch tray to prevent a recurrence of hypoglycemia. The health care provider is notified about the hypoglycemic event, and the doses of the insulin aspart on the sliding scale are decreased by the health care provider.

The following day the health care team is collaborating to switch Robert from insulin to an oral hypoglycemic medication in preparation for discharge.

EXERCISE 6.21 Matching:

Match the classes of oral hypoglycemic agents for type 2 diabetes mellitus in Column A with the actions and prototypes in Column B:

Column A	Column B
A. Meglitinides	_____ Increases insulin secretion by pancreas. Prototype: glipizide
B. Thiazolidinediones	_____ Increases insulin secretion by pancreas. Prototype: repaglinide
C. Alpha-glucosidase inhibitors	_____ [Inhibitors]. Inhibits the digestion and absorption of carbohydrates. Prototype: acarbose
D. Biguanides	_____ Increases muscle utilization of glucose, decreases glucose production by liver. Prototype: metformin
E. Sulfonylureas	_____ Decreases cellular resistance to insulin. Prototype: rosiglitazone

The answer can be found on page 458

Robert is prescribed the combination medication glipizide/metformin 2.5 mg/250 mg once daily with meal.

eRESOURCE

To reinforce your understanding of glipizide/metformin, refer to Medscape on your mobile device. [Pathway: Medscape → enter "Glipizide" into the search field → select "Glipizide/Metformin(Rx)" and review content.]

EXERCISE 6.22 Multiple-choice:

The nurse provides education about the glipizide/metformin tablet. Which statement, if made by Robert, indicates correct understanding of the education?

A. "I will need to temporarily stop this medication if I need a radiological study with intravenous (IV) dyes."
B. "Excessive thirst may indicate that my blood sugar has dropped too low."
C. "I will need to have my complete blood count (CBC) tested regularly while taking this."
D. "If I forget to take a dose one day, I should double my dose the following day."

The answer can be found on page 459

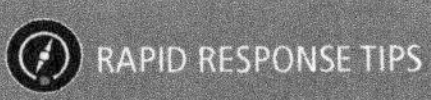

Inhaled medication for type 1 and type 2 diabetes mellitus

Exubera inhaler delivers regular insulin that acts in 30 minutes and lasts 6.5 hours. Patients with type 1 diabetes mellitus usually need a long-acting insulin daily; patients with type 2 diabetes mellitus usually need an oral hypoglycemic in addition to Exubera.

The following day a lipid profile, also drawn during Robert's hospital admission, reveals elevated low-density lipoproteins (LDL). Robert is prescribed rosuvastatin 10 mg at bedtime. Robert asks what benefit taking this medication will have.

EXERCISE 6.23 Select all that apply:

Which of the following are therapeutic uses for rosuvastatin?

A. Decreases low-density lipoproteins (LDLs).

B. Increases high-density lipoprotein

C. Decreases risk of a heart attack or stroke

D. Helps to maintain blood glucose within normal limits

The answer can be found on page 459

In providing patient teaching about use of rosuvastatin, the nurse identifies the known adverse effects of the medication for Robert.

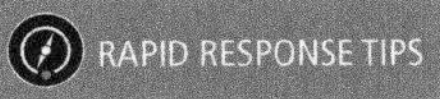

Side effects of statins

Hepatotoxicity

Myositis can progress to rhabdomyolysis

EXERCISE 6.24 Multiple-choice:

The following are known adverse effects of rosuvastatin. Which of these should the patient be instructed to report to the health care provider immediately if noted?

A. Flatus

B. Abdominal cramps

C. Muscle tenderness

D. Diarrhea

The answer can be found on page 459

eRESOURCE

To reinforce your understanding of rosuvastatin, refer to Medscape on your mobile device. [Pathway: Medscape → enter "Rosuvastatin" into the search field → select "Rosuvastatin (Rx)" and review content.]

Robert continues to have foul-smelling, watery diarrhea. The culture and sensitivity analysis is positive for *Clostridium difficile*. Robert is prescribed metronidazole 500 mg three times a day for 7 days by the health care provider.

EXERCISE 6.25 Multiple-choice:

The nurse is providing medication education about metronidazole. Which statement from Robert indicates a need for additional teaching?

A. "I can continue to eat yogurt each morning."
B. "I am able to continue taking acetaminophen for headaches."
C. "I can still have a few beers with my friends on Friday."
D. "I can eat cooked or raw fruits and vegetables while taking this."

The answer can be found on page 459

---

eRESOURCE

To reinforce your understanding of metronidazole, refer to Medscape on your mobile device. [Pathway: Medscape → enter "Metronidazole" into the search field → select "Metronidazole (Rx)" and review content.]

Follow-up care is arranged for Robert at the hospital's medical clinic. Robert is given prescriptions for all his medications and case management arranges for him to receive low-cost medications through a local health agency. Robert indicates that he understands all of his discharge instructions and is discharged from the hospital. Six months later, he returns to the ED reporting nausea, vomiting, fatigue, and shortness of breath for the past month. He also reports a decreased urine output over the past 2 months and a minimal amount of urine produced over the week. Robert states that he stopped taking his antihypertension and oral hypoglycemic medications about 5 months earlier. His vital signs are as follows: BP: 180/102 mmHg, HR: 110 (irregular) bpm, RR: 24 breaths per minute, temperature: 97.9°F (36.6°C; oral), pulse oximetry: 92% on room air. On physical examination, he has bilateral basilar fine crackles. His skin is pale, dry, and scaly. His cardiac rhythm is sinus tachycardia with about six premature ventricular contractions (PVCs) per minute and peaked T waves.

Laboratory studies reveal the following (Table 6.2):

TABLE 6.2 Laboratory Results

Hemoglobin: 8.2 g/dL
Glucose: 190 mg/dL
Potassium: 7.0 mEq/L
Sodium: 127 mEq/L
Phosphorus: 6.1 mg/dL
Calcium: 3.2 mEq/L
Creatinine: 8.5mg/dL
Blood urea nitrogen (BUN): 56 mg/dL
Glomerular filtration rate: 13 mL/min/1.72 m^2
pH: 7.28
$PaCO_2$: 30 mmHg
PaO_2: 60 mmHg
Bicarbonate: 17 mEq/L

Robert is diagnosed with end-stage renal disease (ESRD). The health care provider informs Robert that he will require hemodialysis.

EXERCISE 6.26 Fill in the blanks:

Describe why each of the following medications may be given in the treatment of hyperkalemia.

Intravenous (IV) regular insulin and IV dextrose 50%

____

IV calcium gluconate

____

IV sodium bicarbonate

____

PO or retention enema of sodium polystyrene sulfonate

____

The answer can be found on page 460

The health care provider prescribes sodium bicarbonate 50 mEq IV and sodium polystyrene sulfonate 15 g PO. The following day a temporary hemodialysis access device is placed in Robert's left internal jugular vein, and he has his first hemodialysis treatment. It is determined that Robert is an appropriate candidate for kidney transplantation, so he is placed on the regional kidney transplant list. He is prescribed alprazolam 0.25 mg three times daily as needed for severe anxiety. Six days later, Robert remains on the step-down telemetry unit. He is informed that a donor kidney has been matched. Robert is immediately prepped for surgery and taken to the operating room a short time later. On arriving in the surgical intensive care unit (SICU) from the operating room, new medication prescriptions for Robert include:

- Tacrolimus, 0.1 mg/kg/d IV, given as a continuous infusion over 24 hours
- Mycophenolate mofetil, 1 g IV twice a day
- Methylprednisolone, 125 mg IV every 6 hours
- Morphine, 4 mg IV every 2 hours as needed for pain

EXERCISE 6.27 Multiple-choice:

After noting the change in Robert's medication prescriptions, which of the following is the priority nursing diagnosis for Robert?

A. Activity intolerance
B. Chronic pain
C. Risk for infection
D. Risk for unstable glucose level

The answer can be found on page 460

EXERCISE 6.28 Calculation:

Robert weighs 75 kg; calculate the hourly dosage of tacrolimus given this prescription (Tacrolimus, 0.1 mg/kg/d IV, given as a continuous infusion over 24 hours; round to the nearest hundredth of a milligram).

The answer can be found on page 460

eRESOURCE

To verify your answer, consult MedCalc. [Pathway: www.medcalc.com ➔ select "Fluids/Electrolytes" ➔ select "IV Rate" and enter information into fields.]

Robert is drowsy, but reports moderate pain at the incision site on the right lower quadrant of his abdomen.

EXERCISE 6.29 Select all that apply:

What would the nurse check before administering the prescribed morphine?

A. Temperature
B. Respiratory rate (RR)
C. Blood pressure (BP)
D. Pulse

The answer can be found on page 460

It is determined that the morphine can be administered as prescribed.

EXERCISE 6.30 Multiple-choice:

Ten minutes after administering the intravenous (IV) morphine, the nurse returns to Robert's room in response to an alarm from the heart rate (HR) monitor. The nurse finds that Robert has an HR of 58 beats per minute (bpm), prolonged apnea, and constricted pupils. What is the priority nursing intervention?

A. Check pulse oximeter
B. Listen to breath sounds
C. Provide supplemental oxygen
D. Administer naloxone

The answer can be found on page 461

After the intervention, Robert is fully awake and oriented, has an RR of 12 breaths per minute, heart rate of 66 bpm, and pulse oximetry of 99% on room air.

EXERCISE 6.31 Select all that apply:

Nurses administer naloxone to patients to reverse the effects of opioids. After administration, what symptoms of naloxone would the nurse report immediately?

A. Dilated pupils
B. Rhinorrhea
C. Abdominal aches
D. Perspiration

The answer can be found on page 461

eRESOURCE

To reinforce your understanding of naloxone, refer to Epocrates Online. [Pathway: http://online.epocrates.com ➔ under the "Drugs" tab, enter "Naloxone" in the search field ➔ select "Naloxone" ➔ review "Contraindications/Cautions," "Adverse Reactions," and "Safety/Monitoring."]

EXERCISE 6.32 Fill in the blank:

What effects will naloxone have on Robert's incisional pain at this time? ______________________

The answer can be found on page 461

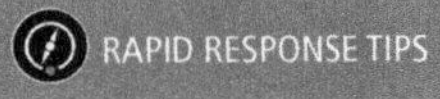

Morphine

Assess level of consciousness, BP, pulse, and RR before and periodically after administration. Watch for RR below 12 breaths per minute per minute.

Three days after the transplantation, Robert is being prepared for discharge. To prevent organ rejection, Robert has been placed on tacrolimus PO, mycophenolate mofetil PO, and prednisone PO. For pain management at home, Robert is prescribed oxycodone/acetaminophen.

EXERCISE 6.33 Select all that apply:

Which statement(s) made by Robert indicate that medication discharge teaching has been successful?

A. "I should avoid contact with anyone who is ill to the best of my ability."
B. "My blood count will need to be monitored regularly."
C. "My serum tacrolimus level will need to be monitored."
D. "I should take an oxycodone/acetaminophen before driving to my follow-up appointment."
E. "I should notify the health care provider if my blood pressure is elevated."
F. "I will immediately stop taking the prednisone if I develop nausea."

The answer can be found on page 461

Robert is discharged from the hospital and during the next 6 months he makes very positive lifestyle changes to improve his health. Robert maintains his regimen of medications to keep his blood glucose well controlled, BP normotensive, lipids within normal limits, and renal allograft functioning. Robert joins a gym and begins an exercise regimen in collaboration with his health care provider and a personal trainer. Robert presents to the ED for lower back pain, which he has experienced for the past 24 hours. He notes that the pain started while he was doing sit-ups, and it has not improved with acetaminophen. The health care provider diagnoses Robert with an acute lumbosacral muscle strain. He writes a prescription for cyclobenzaprine 10 mg every 8 hours as needed and asks the nurse to discharge Robert.

EXERCISE 6.34 Multiple-choice:

Which statement, if made by Robert, indicates the need for further teaching about cyclobenzaprine?

A. "I should chew gum if I develop dry mouth."
B. "I will return to the ED if I cannot urinate."
C. "I should not take this medication before going to sleep."
D. "This medication relaxes the muscle spasm."

The answer can be found on page 462

---

eRESOURCE

To reinforce your understanding of the patient teaching warranted for cyclobenzaprine, refer to Epocrates Online. [Pathway: http://online.epocrates.com → under the "Drugs" tab, enter "Cyclobenzaprine" in the search field → select "Cyclobenzaprine" → review "Patient Education," "Adverse Reactions," and "Safety/Monitoring."]

EXERCISE 6.35 Fill in the blank:

Robert asks the nurse whether he can take over-the-counter nonsteroidal antiinflammatory drugs (NSAIDs), such as ibuprofen or naproxen, to treat the back pain. How should the nurse respond to this question?

The answer can be found on page 462

---

eRESOURCE

For your answer, refer to Epocrates Online. [Pathway: http://online.epocrates.com → select the "Interaction Check" tab → enter all medications Robert is currently taking → review results.]

Robert is discharged and his lower back pain improves after 3 days of resting and taking cyclobenzaprine.

UNFOLDING CASE STUDY 2: Wanda

Wanda, age 56 years, is assessed by the ED triage nurse. Wanda reports a sudden onset of left shoulder pain, left-sided jaw pain, shortness of breath, and tingling in her left hand that started 30 minutes before arrival. She rates her pain as 10/10. She has a family history of coronary artery disease (CAD). She states that her medical history includes hypertension, for which she takes hydrochlorothiazide, and migraine headaches. Her skin is pale and diaphoretic; she appears anxious. Her vital signs are BP: 146/86 mmHg, HR: 110 bpm, RR: 24 breaths per minute, pulse oximetry: 96% on room air. Her temperature is 98.1°F (36.7°C) oral. Wanda is taken to a treatment room and a 12-lead EKG is completed. The EKG reveals ST-segment elevation consistent with an anterior wall myocardial infarction (MI). On the nurse's arrival in the room, the UAP is placing Wanda on supplemental oxygen and on the cardiac monitor.

EXERCISE 6.36 Fill in the blanks:

Review the following medication prescriptions that are initially written for Wanda. Describe the pharmacological rationale for each of these medications for a patient having a myocardial infarction.

Clopidogrel 300 mg orally, one dose now

Nitroglycerin 0.4 mg sublingual every 5 minutes, three times now

---

Metoprolol 5 mg intravenous (IV) push, one dose now

The answer can be found on page 462

---

eRESOURCE

To check your answer, refer to Medscape on your mobile device. [Pathway: Medscape ➔ enter "Clopidogrel" into the search field ➔ select "Clopidogrel" and review content. Repeat with "Nitroglycerin" and "Metoprolol."]

EXERCISE 6.37 Select all that apply:

Sublingual nitroglycerin has an onset of 1 to 3 minutes. Before and after each dose of sublingual nitroglycerin, the nurse should assess which of the following?

A. Blood pressure (BP)
B. Pupil size
C. Deep tendon reflexes (DTR)
D. Heart rate (HR)
E. Location, severity of pain
F. Temperature

The answer can be found on page 463

eRESOURCE

To reinforce your understanding of heparin, refer to Epocrates Online. [Pathway: http://online.epocrates.com ➔ under the "Drugs" tab, enter "Nitroglycerin" in the search field ➔ select "Nitroglycerin" ➔ review "Safety/Monitoring."]

After the third dose of sublingual nitroglycerin, Wanda reports that her pain has decreased to 4/10. Wanda's BP is now 118/64 mmHg and her HR is 88 bpm, sinus rhythm. The cardiologist is at her bedside to discuss percutaneous coronary intervention (PCI). The cardiologist prescribes a 5,000-unit bolus of IV heparin followed by a non-weight-based heparin infusion at 1,000 units/hr.

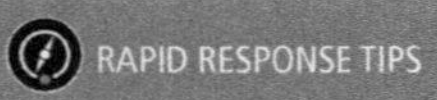

Heparin

Protamine sulfate is the antidote for heparin overdose.

The cardiologist also prescribes an IV nitroglycerin infusion at 15 mcg/min. Wanda's family questions why nitroglycerin is going to be administered via IV after she has already received three doses sublingually. They are concerned that she may experience an overdose of nitroglycerin. Her family also would like to know how the IV nitroglycerin differs from that which she received sublingually.

EXERCISE 6.38 Fill in the blanks:

Explain the rationale for administering intravenous (IV) nitroglycerin.

How would you respond to the family's concerns about a potential overdose of nitroglycerin?

Briefly summarize the difference in pharmacokinetics between IV and sublingual nitroglycerin.

The answer can be found on page 463

You know that heparin administration must be done carefully because of all the IV medication errors that occur in the United States, most occur with heparin and insulin.

EXERCISE 6.39 Calculation:

After administering the intravenous (IV) heparin bolus, the nurse prepares the continuous IV heparin infusion. The concentration of heparin is 25,000 units/250 mL 0.9% normal saline (NS). At what rate would the volumetric pump be set to administer 1,000 units/hr?

The answer can be found on page 463

EXERCISE 6.40 Calculation:

The nitroglycerin is set to infuse at 9 mL/hr. The concentration is 25 mg of nitroglycerin in 250 mL 0.9% normal saline (NS). Calculate the micrograms per hour.

The answer can be found on page 463

eRESOURCE

To verify your answers, consult MedCalc. [Pathway: www.medcalc.com ➔ select "Fluids/Electrolytes" ➔ select "IV Rate" and enter information into fields.]

EXERCISE 6.41 Multiple-choice:

Ten minutes after the nitroglycerin infusion is initiated, Wanda reports a headache of moderate severity. Her blood pressure (BP) is 105/68 mmHg, heart rate (HR) is 80 beats per minute (bpm), sinus rhythm. What action should the nurse take?

A. Immediately notify the cardiologist
B. Decrease the infusion in 5 mcg/min increments until headache improves
C. Turn off the nitroglycerin infusion
D. Reassure Wanda that a headache is an expected adverse effect

The answer can be found on page 463

EXERCISE 6.42 Multiple-choice:

Shortly after being reassured, Wanda complains of feeling dizzy and light-headed. Her blood pressure (BP) is 70/30 mmHg, heart rate (HR) is 88 beats per minute (bpm), sinus rhythm. Which of the following actions would be the initial priority?

A. Place the patient in a supine position
B. Administer a bolus of intravenous (IV) normal saline
C. Stop the nitroglycerin infusion
D. Notify the physician

The answer can be found on page 464

eRESOURCE

To review the adverse effects of nitroglycerine infusion, refer to Medscape on your mobile device. [Pathway: Medscape ➔ enter "Nitroglycerin" into the search field ➔ select "Nitroglycerine Infusion (Rx)" and review "Adverse Effects."]

The infusion of nitroglycerin is stopped and 5 minutes later Wanda's BP is 94/45 mmHg; HR is 90 bpm, sinus rhythm; with multiple unifocal PVCs. Wanda reports increased shortness of breath and palpitations. Wanda appears increasingly anxious when her cardiac rhythm converts to ventricular tachycardia (VT) with a palpable pulse.

EXERCISE 6.43 Fill in the blank:

What class of medication would the nurse expect to be prescribed for Wanda?

____

The answer can be found on page 464

EXERCISE 6.44 Calculation:

An amiodarone bolus of 150 mg intravenous (IV) × 1 dose is now prescribed, followed by an amiodarone infusion of 1 mg/hr × 6 hours. The initial amiodarone bolus of 150 mg is prepared in a 100-mL bag of 0.9% normal saline solution (NSS) and should be infused over 10 minutes. At what rate (mL/hr) should the bolus infuse?

The answer can be found on page 464

eRESOURCE

To verify your answers, consult MedCalc. [Pathway: www.medcalc.com ➔ select "Fluids/Electrolytes" ➔ select "IV Rate" and enter information into fields.]

EXERCISE 6.45 Multiple-choice:

The nurse continues to monitor Wanda while she receives the amiodarone infusion. Which assessment finding should be reported to the health care provider immediately?

A. Normal sinus rhythm with 4 premature ventricular contractions (PVCs) per minute
B. Generalized weakness and slight tremor to both hands
C. Nausea and one episode of vomiting with tan-colored emesis
D. Cough with white sputum and crackles in both lung fields

The answer can be found on page 464

Wanda is then transferred from the ED to the cardiac catheterization suite for PCI. From there, Wanda is taken to the coronary care unit (CCU). She is on a continuous infusion of abciximab and remains on an IV heparin infusion.

eRESOURCE

To reinforce your understanding of these medications, refer to Epocrates Online. [Pathway: http://online.epocrates.com → under the "Drugs" tab, enter "Heparin" in the search field → select "Heparin" → review "Adult Dosing," "Adverse Reactions," and "Safety/Monitoring." Repeat with "Abciximab."]

EXERCISE 6.46 Multiple-choice:

Which of the following would be a priority nursing assessment for Wanda?

A. Deep tendon reflexes (DTR)
B. Monitor urine specific gravity
C. Assess percutaneous coronary intervention (PCI) insertion site
D. Strict intake and output measurement

The answer can be found on page 465

Twelve hours after arriving at the CCU, Wanda develops right-sided weakness, slurred speech, and a right-sided facial droop. The health care team suspects that Wanda has experienced a stroke as a complication from the PCI. A CT scan of the head is performed and shows no cerebral hemorrhage. Neurology arrives at the CCU to evaluate Wanda's condition. It is determined that Wanda is a not a candidate for intravenous (IV) thrombolytic treatment with a tissue plasminogen activator (tPA).

EXERCISE 6.47 Fill in the blank:

Why has Wanda been excluded as a candidate for intravenous (IV) thrombolytic treatment?

The answer can be found on page 465

EXERCISE 6.48 Multiple-choice:

Wanda starts having a tonic–clonic seizure. What medication should the nurse prepare to administer first?

A. Phenytoin
B. Carbamazepine
C. Lorazepam
D. Hydromorphone

The answer can be found on page 465

The nurse administers 2 mg of lorazepam through the IV. Wanda continues with tonic–clonic seizure activity. A second dose of IV lorazapem is prescribed and administered by the nurse. The seizure stops after the administration of the second dose of lorazepam. A loading dose of phenytoin 1 g IV is prescribed to prevent further seizures.

EXERCISE 6.49 Select all that apply:

The nurse recognizes that intravenous (IV) phenytoin must be given slowly (no faster than 50 mg/min), as more rapid administration can cause what serious complications?

A. Cardiac dysrythmias
B. Coma
C. Cough
D. Mania
E. Hypotension

The answer can be found on page 465

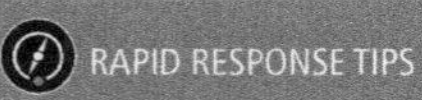

Phenytoin (Dilantin)

Phenytoin (Dilantin) is not mixed with other medications. It cannot infuse into an IV tubing at the same time as another medication.

EXERCISE 6.50 Fill in the blank:

What is the rationale for not mixing phenytoin with other medications?

The answer can be found on page 465

EXERCISE 6.51 Fill in the blank:

What action can the nurse take to reduce venous irritation when administering intravenous (IV) phenytoin?

The answer can be found on page 465

eRESOURCE

To reinforce your understanding of phenytoin, refer to Epocrates Online. [Pathway: http://online.epocrates.com → under the "Drugs" tab, enter "Phenytoin" in the search field → select "Phenytoin" → review content.]

After the seizure has resolved Wanda is somnolent. Her Glasgow Coma Scale (GCS) score is 7. Her respirations are rapid and shallow and the nurse notes a significant amount of secretions from Wanda's mouth. The health care team determines that Wanda requires intubation and mechanical ventilation. The health care provider prescribes etomidate 10 mg IV push, stat, followed by succinylcholine 100 mg IV push, stat.

EXERCISE 6.52 Fill in the blanks:

What is the rationale for giving etomidate to Wanda?

What type of medication should always be given in combination with neuromuscular blockers, such as succinylcholine (Anectine)?

What laboratory value should be monitored carefully with use of succinylcholine?

The answer can be found on page 466

eRESOURCE

To reinforce your understanding of etomidate, refer to Epocrates Online. [Pathway: http://online.epocrates.com → under the "Drugs" tab, enter "Etomidate" in the search field → select "Etomidate" → review content under "Adult Dosing."]

eRESOURCE

To reinforce your understanding of succinylcholine, refer to Epocrates Online. [Pathway: http://online.epocrates.com → under the "Drugs" tab, enter "Succinylcholine" in the search field → select "Succinylcholine" → review content under "Adult Dosing" focusing on "Neuromuscular Blockade Induction" and "Neuromuscular Blockade Maintenance."]

TABLE 6.3 Wanda's Vital Sign Results

Vital Sign Assessed	Finding
Heart rate (HR)	120, sinus tachycardia
Respiratory rate (RR)	12, assist control on ventilator
Blood pressure (BP)	88/70 mmHg
Pulse oximetry	93% on FiO_2 60

eRESOURCE

To reinforce your understanding of succinylcholine, refer to Epocrates Online. [Pathway: http://online.epocrates.com → under the "Drugs" tab, enter "Succinylcholine" in the search field → select "Succinylcholine" → review content under "Safety/Monitoring."]

The following day, Wanda's nurse notes the following vital signs found in Table 6.3.

The nurse notes jugular venous distention, auscultates crackles over bilateral basilar lung fields, and notes urine output of 20 mL over the past 2 hours. The nurse immediately calls the health care provider to Wanda's bedside. The health care provider determines that Wanda is in cardiogenic shock.

eRESOURCE

To review lung sounds, go to Practical Clinical Skills. [Pathway: http://www.practicalclinicalskills.com/mobile/ or http://goo.gl/KjzYuC → select "Lung Sounds" → review lung sounds.]

The health care provider prescribes dopamine IV 5 mcg/kg/min.

EXERCISE 6.53 Exhibit-format:

The nurse sets up the infusion and a second nurse independently confirms the medication. Wanda has two peripheral intravenous (IV) sites and a triple-lumen subclavian central venous line.

A. Which IV access site would be the ***best*** to use for IV administration of dopamine?

B. Which IV access site would ***not be appropriate*** for IV administration of dopamine?

Explain your rationale:

IV site A: Right subclavian triple-lumen central venous line

IV site B: Distal left-hand 22-gauge peripheral IV

IV site C: Right antecubital 18-gauge peripheral IV

The answer can be found on page 466

eRESOURCE

To reinforce your understanding of the rationale for IV administration of dopamine, refer to Epocrates Online. [Pathway: http://online.epocrates.com ➔ under the "Drugs" tab, enter "Dopamine" in the search field ➔ select "Dopamine" ➔ review content under "Black Box Warnings."]

EXERCISE 6.54 Fill in the blank:

Five minutes after the dopamine infusion is initiated, Wanda's vital signs and physical assessment are unchanged. What action should the nurse anticipate taking?

The answer can be found on page 466

Five minutes later, Wanda's BP is 100/68 mmHg and her heart rate remains at 120 bpm, sinus tachycardia.

EXERCISE 6.55 Select the correct response:

As dopamine in higher doses (such as 5–10 mcg/kg/min) stimulates beta-1 adrenergic receptors, the nurse would anticipate a(n) (*increase/decrease*) in heart rate as an expected effect.

The answer can be found on page 466

Three days later, Wanda's hypotension improves. The dopamine infusion is discontinued. Wanda is weaned from the ventilator. The neurological symptoms from the stroke appear to have improved, although Wanda still has weakness of the right upper extremity. Wanda has developed a stage 2 pressure ulcer on her sacrum during hospitalization in the intensive care unit (ICU). Wanda is now assisted with repositioning in bed every 2 hours and the wound care RN applies a dressing to the ulcer. Wanda is transferred to a medical–surgical unit.

eRESOURCE

To reinforce your understanding of the management of pressure ulcers, refer to Medscape on your mobile device. [Pathway: Medscape ➔ enter "Pressure Ulcer" into the search field ➔ select "Pressure Ulcers and Wound Care" and review content.]

While in the ICU, Wanda had subsequent tonic–clonic seizures. Carbamazepine was added to her medication profile. A therapeutic level was achieved with carbamazepine extended-release tablets 400 mg twice daily.

eRESOURCE

To reinforce your understanding of therapeutic levels for carbamazepine, refer to Epocrates Online. [Pathway: http://online.epocrates.com → under the "Drugs" tab, enter "Carbamazepine" in the search field → select "Carbamazepine" → review content under "Safety/Monitoring."]

EXERCISE 6.56 Fill in the blank:

The nurse notices a nursing student crushing the carbamazepine (Tegretol XR) extended-release tablet in applesauce. What action, if any, should the nurse take?

___

The answer can be found on page 467

EXERCISE 6.57 Fill in the blank:

The nurse must carefully monitor the complete blood count (CBC) when a patient is on carbamazepine. Explain why.

___

The answer can be found on page 467

eRESOURCE

To reinforce your understanding of the rationale for monitoring patients taking carbamazepine, refer to Epocrates Online. [Pathway: http://online.epocrates.com → under the "Drugs" tab, enter "Carbamazepine" in the search field → select "Carbamazepine" → review content under "Adverse Reactions" and also review "Safety/Monitoring."]

The sacral wound develops a bacterial infection. Empiric antibiotic therapy is initiated with vancomycin and cefepime. The health care provider prescribes cefepime 2 g IV every 12 hours and vancomycin 1 g IV every 12 hours.

EXERCISE 6.58 Multiple-choice:

Before administering vancomycin, the nurse should be sure to assess which of the following laboratory values?

A. Hemoglobin and hematocrit
B. Prothrombin time (PT) and international normalized ratio (INR)
C. Albumin and glucose
D. Serum creatinine and blood urea nitrogen (BUN)

The answer can be found on page 467

eRESOURCE

To reinforce your understanding of what labs should be checked before administering vancomycin, refer to Epocrates Online. [Pathway: http://online.epocrates.com ➔ under the "Drugs" tab, enter "Vancomycin" in the search field ➔ select "Vancomycin" ➔ review "Monitoring Parameters" under "Safety/Monitoring."]

Vancomycin 1 g is prepared in 250 mL of NSS by the pharmacy.

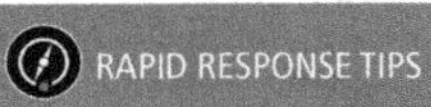

Vancomycin

Vancomycin is infused over a period of *no less than 60 minutes.*

EXERCISE 6.59 Multiple-choice:

Wanda is also receiving intravenous (IV) furosemide when vancomycin is added to her medication profile. Which of the following symptoms should the nurse advise Wanda to report immediately?

A. Urinary urgency
B. Tinnitus
C. Diarrhea
D. Chills

The answer can be found on page 467

EXERCISE 6.60 Select all that apply:

Too rapid administration of intravenous (IV) vancomycin may place the patient at increased risk for an adverse reaction such as:

A. Nausea and vomiting
B. Red man syndrome
C. Superinfection
D. Phlebitis

The answer can be found on page 467

Approximately 5 minutes after beginning the vancomycin infusion, the UAP tells the nurse that Wanda has developed a rash over her face, neck, and chest and her BP is 76/46 mmHg. The nurse immediately enters the room and finds that Wanda is not in respiratory distress but complains of feeling dizzy, hot, and anxious.

EXERCISE 6.61 Multiple-choice:

Which action should be taken by the nurse *first*?

A. Administer a 500-mL bolus of normal saline intravenous (IV)
B. Give 50 mg of diphenhydramine IV push
C. Page the health care provider to the unit, stat
D. Discontinue the vancomycin infusion

The answer can be found on page 468

The health care provider prescribes 50 mg IV diphenhydramine.

EXERCISE 6.62 Fill in the blank:

What most common central nervous system (CNS) adverse effect of diphenhydramine should the nurse explain to Wanda when she is administering this medication?

____

The answer can be found on page 468

---

eRESOURCE

To reinforce your understanding of what patient education should be provided, refer to Epocrates Online. [Pathway: http://online.epocrates.com ➔ under the "Drugs" tab, enter "Diphenhydramine" in the search field ➔ select "Diphenhydramine" ➔ review "Patient Education."]

Wanda's BP improves to 110/66 mmHg. The rash and other symptoms improve shortly after the administration of IV normal saline and diphenhydramine. With subsequent doses, Wanda is able to receive vancomycin without symptoms of red man syndrome when the medication is delivered over a 3-hour period.

EXERCISE 6.63 Fill in the blank:

Before administering cefepime, the nurse should be certain that Wanda does not have a history of serious allergic reactions to cephalosporins and what other class of anti-infectives?

____

The answer can be found on page 468

---

eRESOURCE

To reinforce your understanding of what allergies should be checked before administering cefepime, refer to Epocrates Online. [Pathway: http://online.epocrates.com ➔ under the "Drugs" tab, enter "Cefepime" in the search field ➔ select "Cefepime" ➔ select "Patient Education" and review information under "What Is the Most Important Information I Should Know About Cefepime?" and "What Should I Discuss With My Health Care Provider Before Using Cefepime?"]

Two days later, the nurse hears Wanda's telemetry alarm for a high heart rate. The nurse notes that Wanda's heart rate is irregular and varies from 110 to 130 bpm. She also notes the absence of p waves and determines that Wanda's heart rhythm is atrial fibrillation. She enters Wanda's room and finds her awake, alert, and oriented to person, place, and time. Wanda is not in any respiratory distress but reports palpitations. Wanda's BP is 122/76 mmHg.

Wanda remains on a continuous infusion of IV heparin. Her activated partial thromboplastin time (aPTT) is 60 seconds; therefore, she does not require additional anticoagulation therapy for new-onset atrial fibrillation.

EXERCISE 6.64 Fill in the blank:

Wanda has now been on intravenous (IV) heparin therapy for 7 days. In addition to monitoring the activated partial thromboplastin time (aPTT), the nurse should very carefully monitor which other hematological laboratory value?

The answer can be found on page 468

eRESOURCE

To reinforce your understanding of what other lab values should be monitored, refer to Epocrates Online. [Pathway: http://online.epocrates.com → under the "Drugs" tab, enter "Heparin" in the search field → select "Heparin" → select "Safety/Monitoring" and review content.]

The health care provider prescribes IV diltiazem for ventricular rate control. The diltiazem is prescribed as a bolus dose followed by a continuous infusion.

Wanda now weighs 154 lb. She is given IV diltiazem (Cardizem) 0.25 mg/kg as a loading dose followed by a continuous infusion at 10 mg/hr.

EXERCISE 6.65 Calculation:

If diltiazem is available in vials of 25 mg/5 mL, how many milliliters of diltiazem must the nurse give via intravenous (IV) push?

The answer can be found on page 468

EXERCISE 6.66 Calculation:

The diltiazem infusion is prepared as 125 mg in 250 mL of normal saline solution (NSS). At what rate should the diltiazem be infused?

The answer can be found on page 469

EXERCISE 6.67 List:

What three cardiac assessments must be done periodically while Wanda is on the diltiazem infusion?

1. ______
2. ______
3. ______

The answer can be found on page 469

eRESOURCE

To reinforce your understanding of diltiazem, refer to Epocrates Online. [Pathway: http://online.epocrates.com → under the "Drugs" tab, enter "Diltiazem" in the search field → select "Diltiazem" → select "Safety/Monitoring" and review content.]

The following day the health care team decides to discontinue the diltiazem infusion and to place Wanda on PO digoxin. A digitalizing dose of 500 mcg is prescribed at 6:00 p.m. followed by 250 mcg at midnight and 250 mcg at 6:00 a.m. the next morning.

EXERCISE 6.68 Fill in the blank:

Before administering digoxin, the nurse listens to the apical heart rate for 1 minute. If the apical heart rate is less than 60, what action should the nurse take?

______

The answer can be found on page 469

Wanda receives the digitalizing dose over a 12-hour period and then is placed on digoxin 125 mcg PO daily.

EXERCISE 6.69 Fill in the blanks:

As Wanda remains on a loop diuretic, what laboratory value must be carefully monitored to prevent a serious complication from digoxin therapy?

______

What is the therapeutic serum range for digoxin?

______

The answer can be found on page 469

eRESOURCE

To reinforce your understanding of digoxin, refer to Epocrates Online. [Pathway: http://online.epocrates.com → under the "Drugs" tab, enter "Digoxin" in the search field → select "Digoxin" → select "Safety/Monitoring" and review content.]

eRESOURCE

To check your answer, refer to Medscape on your mobile device. [Pathway: Medscape ➔ enter "Digoxin" into the search field ➔ select "Digoxin Level" and review content under "Reference Range" and "Collection and Panels."]

In preparation for discharge, the nurse must educate Wanda about signs and symptoms of digoxin toxicity.

EXERCISE 6.70 List:

Name five signs/symptoms of digoxin toxicity:

1. ______________________________
2. ______________________________
3. ______________________________
4. ______________________________
5. ______________________________

The answer can be found on page 469

eRESOURCE

To check your answer, refer to Medscape on your mobile device. [Pathway: Medscape ➔ enter "Digoxin" into the search field ➔ select "Digoxin Level" and review content under "Interpretation."]

In severe cases of digoxin toxicity, the antidote to digoxin may be administered.

EXERCISE 6.71 Fill in the blank:

What is the antidote to digoxin?

____

The answer can be found on page 470

In preparation for discharge, warfarin is added to Wanda's medication profile.

EXERCISE 6.72 Fill in the blank:

Explain why Wanda is able to receive both warfarin and heparin concurrently.

____

The answer can be found on page 470

Wafarin prevents coagulation by blocking the synthesis of vitamin K. Consumption of foods rich in vitamin K will cause a patient to have a subtherapeutic INR.

EXERCISE 6.73 List:

In order to provide medication teaching to Wanda, list four or more foods rich in vitamin K:

1. ______
2. ______
3. ______
4. ______
5. ______
6. ______
7. ______
8. ______

The answer can be found on page 470

Three days later, Wanda is discharged home with daily visits from a home-care registered nurse. Nine months later, Wanda presents to her primary health care provider for severe epigastric pain that worsens with eating food. Since her previous hospitalization, Wanda's heart rhythm has converted back to normal sinus rhythm and digoxin and warfarin have been discontinued. Furosemide and carbamazepine have also been discontinued. Wanda is presently taking aspirin (ASA), hydrochlorothiazide, lisinopril, and clopidogrel. Based on Wanda's symptoms, the health care provider makes a preliminary diagnosis of peptic ulcer disease. Generally, a combination of medication agents are used for the treatment of peptic ulcer disease.

EXERCISE 6.74 Matching:

Match the drug classes in Column A with the functions in Column B:

Column A	Column B
A. Proton pump inhibitors (PPIs)	______ Inhibits parietal cells from secreting gastric acid. Prototype: famotidine
B. Histamine 2 (H2) receptor blockers	______ Neutralizes gastric contents. Prototype: magnesium hydroxide/aluminum hydroxide
C. Gastrointestinal protectants	______ Prevents hydrogen ions from being transported into the gastric lumen. Prototype: pantoprazole
D. Antacids	______ Forms a paste when exposed to gastric acid which then covers the surface of peptic ulcers. Prototype: sucralfate

The answer can be found on page 470

Wanda is prescribed pantoprozale 40 mg PO daily and magnesium hydroxide/aluminum hydroxide 30 mL PO three times a day after meals. Four days later, Wanda calls her health care provider and reports three to four episodes of nonbloody diarrhea.

EXERCISE 6.75 Fill in the blank:

What might be the cause of Wanda's diarrhea?

The answer can be found on page 471

The health care provider prescribes loperamide for symptomatic treatment of the diarrhea. Wanda states that the epigastric pain is improving, but she is still experiencing some discomfort.

One week later, Wanda receives a phone call from her health care provider stating that the diagnostic study performed revealed the presence of *Helicobacter pylori* (*H. pylori*). The health care provider prescribes doxycycline and bismuth subsalicylate. The office nurse provides medication teaching to Wanda over the phone.

EXERCISE 6.76 Fill in the blank:

Which of the medications prescribed for Wanda should not be taken within 1 to 3 hours of doxycycline, and why?

The answer can be found on page 471

EXERCISE 6.77 Fill in the blank:

What change in the appearance of her stools should Wanda be instructed to expect while taking bismuth subsalicylate?

The answer can be found on page 471

---

eRESOURCE

To review the patient teaching required for these new medications, refer to Epocrates Online. [Pathway: http://online.epocrates.com → under the "Drugs" tab, enter "Doxycycline" in the search field → select "Doxycycline" → select "Patient Education" and review content. Repeat this for "Bismuth Subsalicylate."]

On completing treatment for *H. pylori*, Wanda's epigastric pain improves without any further complications.

UNFOLDING CASE STUDY 3: Joyce

Joyce, age 21 years, presents to the college health center for a dry, nonproductive cough, nasal drainage, malaise, low-grade fever, and wheezing for the past 2 days. Her vital signs on arrival to the clinic are: BP: 116/76 mmHg, HR: 98 bpm, RR: 24 breaths per minute, temperature: 99.6°F (37.5°C) orally; pulse oximetry saturation: 93% on room air. She reports a past medical history of asthma and seasonal allergies. She states she presently takes loratidine daily and uses an albuterol hydrofluoroalkane (HFA) metered-dose inhaler, as needed. On physical examination, Joyce is moderately dyspneic and has wheezes auscultated throughout all lung fields. The health care provider prescribes albuterol 2.5 mg mixed with ipratropium 0.5 mg administered via nebulizer, stat.

EXERCISE 6.78 Fill in the blanks:

What is the rationale for administering albuterol and ipratropium to Joyce?

____

Describe the basic mechanism by which albuterol and ipratropium will improve Joyce's symptoms.

____

The answer can be found on page 471

eRESOURCE

To review how medications can manage asthma, refer to Medscape on your mobile device. [Pathway: Medscape ➔ enter "Asthma" into the search field ➔ select "Asthma" and review content under "Medications."]

Joyce reports improvement after completing the nebulizer treatment. On physical examination, the nurse notes that the wheezing is improving. The health care provider writes a prescription to repeat the albuterol and ipratropium nebulizer treatment. On completing the second nebulizer treatment in the health clinic, Joyce reports feeling tremulous and like her heart is racing. Her apical heart rate is 110 bpm, capillary refill is less than 2 seconds, and her skin is warm and dry to the touch.

EXERCISE 6.79 Multiple-choice:

What action should the nurse take?

A. Immediately notify the health care provider of this potential complication
B. Position the patient in a modified Trendelenburg position
C. Place the patient on telemetry and prepare to administer a beta-2 receptor antagonist
D. Reassure the patient that this is an expected adverse effect from albuterol

The answer can be found on page 471

Joyce is diagnosed with exacerbation of asthma and bronchitis in the health center. The health care provider prescribes prednisone 60 mg PO now and writes a prescription for a tapering dose of prednisone for Joyce to take over 10 days. Joyce is also given erythromycin stearate 500 mg four times a day for 10 days to treat the bronchitis.

EXERCISE 6.80 Multiple-choice:

What instructions should the nurse include for Joyce when providing discharge teaching about erythromycin stearate?

A. "Discontinue the medication and notify the health care provider if you have multiple loose stools."
B. "Take the medication on an empty stomach with a glass of water."
C. "Discontinue the medication once presenting symptoms have completely improved to reduce side effects."
D. "Vaginal itching is common while taking this medication, but it is expected and not a concern."

The answer can be found on page 472

eRESOURCE

To review the patient teaching required for these new medications, refer to Epocrates Online. [Pathway: http://online.epocrates.com ➔ under the "Drugs" tab, enter "Erythromycin" in the search field ➔ select "Erythromycin Stearate" ➔ select "Patient Education" and review content.]

Joyce asks about the types of medications that are available to suppress her cough, so she can sleep better at home. The nurse states that there are a few medications that will be effective in suppressing the cough.

EXERCISE 6.81 Select all that apply:

Choose the ingredients in many cough and cold medicines that suppress coughing:

A. Codeine
B. Acetaminophen
C. Diphenhydramine
D. Dextromethorphan
E. Pseudoephedrine

The answer can be found on page 472

Joyce is discharged to home. A week later she calls the health center and states that she is experiencing nausea after taking prednisone. She states the wheezing is improving. She asks whether she can stop taking prednisone at this time.

EXERCISE 6.82 Fill in the blank:

How should the nurse respond to Joyce's concern about nausea?

____

The answer can be found on page 472

eRESOURCE

To review the patient teaching required for these new medications, refer to Epocrates Online. [Pathway: http://online.epocrates.com ➔ under the "Drugs" tab, enter "Prednisone" in the search field ➔ select "Prednisone" ➔ select "Patient Education" and review content—focusing on content under "What is the most important information I should know about prednisone?"]

Joyce arrives at her primary care provider's office a month later after completing the prednisone taper. She is now experiencing an increased frequency of wheezing and shortness of breath. She reports needing to use the albuterol HFA metered-dose inhaler several times a day. The health care provided decides to add a combination inhaled fluticasone and salmeterol to her daily medication regimen.

EXERCISE 6.83 Multiple-choice:

The nurse provides teaching about inhaled corticosteroids. Which statement, if made by Joyce, indicates the need for further teaching?

A. "I will be sure to rinse my mouth with water before using the inhaled steroid."
B. "If I become short of breath, I will use the albuterol HFA inhaler and not the inhaled steroid."
C. "I should take the inhaled steroid after I use the albuterol HFA inhaler."
D. "I will notify my physician if I notice any white spots in my mouth or on my tongue."

The answer can be found on page 472

Joyce makes an appointment to see her gynecologist because she has experienced heavy bleeding with her menses for the past several months. She tells the gynecologist that she feels fatigued. On initial examination her skin appears pale. A hemoglobin and hematocrit are prescribed and reveal the values indicated in Table 6.4.

The gynecologist diagnoses Joyce with iron-deficiency anemia secondary to menstrual blood loss and prescribes oral ferrous sulfate. The gynecologist also prescribes an oral hormonal contraceptive to regulate Joyce's menstrual cycles.

TABLE 6.4 Joyce's Hemoglobin and Hematocrit Results

Hemoglobin: 9.1 g/dL
Hematocrit: 27%

EXERCISE 6.84 List:

The nurse provides instructions about the adverse effects of oral ferrous sulfate. List three or more gastrointestinal adverse effects of ferrous sulfate.

1. ______
2. ______
3. ______
4. ______
5. ______
6. ______

The answer can be found on page 473

eRESOURCE

To review the patient teaching required for ferrous sulfate, refer to Epocrates Online. [Pathway: http://online.epocrates.com → under the "Drugs" tab, enter "Ferrous Sulfate" in the search field → select "Ferrous Sulfate" → select "Patient Education" and review content.]

On performing a pelvic examination, the gynecologist notes a thick white vaginal discharge. In addition, two red vesicles are noted on the labia. Joyce is diagnosed with genital herpes and vulvovaginal candidiasis. Joyce has no previous history of herpes infections or vulvovaginal candidiasis. The gynecologist writes a prescription for one dose of miconazole 1,200-mg vaginal suppositories.

EXERCISE 6.85 Ordering:

Place in priority order from 1 to 6 the procedures used to administer a vaginal suppository.

______ Use the lubricated finger to insert the rounded end of the suppository 3 to 4 inches into the vaginal canal along the posterior wall

______ Verify the medication prescription and don clean gloves

______ Instruct the patient to remain in a supine position for 10 minutes

______ Lubricate the rounded end of suppository and the index finger of the dominant hand with water-based lubricant

______ Remove the suppository from the wrapper

______ Document administration of the medication

The answer can be found on page 473

eRESOURCE

To review the patient teaching required to administer a vaginal suppository, refer to Epocrates Online. [Pathway: http://online.epocrates.com → under the "Drugs" tab, enter "Miconazole" in the search field → select "Miconazole Vaginal" → select "Patient Education" and review content—focusing on content under "How should I use miconazole vaginal?"]

The gynecologist also writes a prescription for acyclovir 400 mg PO every 8 hours for 10 days.

EXERCISE 6.86 Select all that apply:

When providing medication education about acyclovir, which of the following instructions should the nurse include in the discharge instructions?

A. Nausea, vomiting, and diarrhea are common adverse effects of acyclovir.
B. Long-term acyclovir treatment will cure the herpes infection.
C. Condoms should be used even when the lesions are not present.
D. Acyclovir decreases the duration of the herpetic lesions.

The answer can be found on page 473

The vulvovaginal candidiasis and initial infection of genital herpes improve and Joyce has no adverse reactions to the medications. Her menses are well regulated with the use of the oral hormonal contraceptive agent and her hemoglobin and hematocrit are within normal limits after completing her regimen of oral ferrous sulfate.

The gynecologist recommended additional sexually transmitted infection (STI) diagnostic screenings for Joyce and her male partner. Testing for human immunodeficiency virus (HIV) determined that Joyce was HIV negative and her partner HIV positive. Joyce informs her gynecologist that she wishes to remain in a relationship with her partner, but is concerned that he has HIV. Joyce and her gynecologist determine that she is a candidate for long-term emtricitabine/tenofovir treatment as HIV preexposure prophylaxis. Emtricitabine/tenofovir is a combination nucleoside/nucleotide reverse transcriptase inhibitor (NRTI).

EXERCISE 6.87 Multiple-choice

The nurse provides teaching regarding use of emtricitabine/tenofovir as HIV pre-exposure prophylaxis. Which statement, if made by Joyce, indicates need for further instruction?

A. "I won't need to use condoms because this will prevent HIV transmission."
B. "I should contact the physician if I get abdominal pain or repeated vomiting."
C. "I will need to be routinely screened for HIV infection."
D. "I plan to take the medication each day with my breakfast."

The answer can be found on page 474

---

eRESOURCE

To review the patient teaching required for this medication, refer to Epocrates Online. [Pathway: http://online.epocrates.com ➔ under the "Drugs" tab, enter "Emtricitabine" in the search field ➔ select "Emtricitabine/Tenofovir" ➔ select "Patient Education" and review content.]

Three months later, Joyce presents to her primary care provider reporting a fever and sore throat. Joyce also reports only minimal improvement of her asthma symptoms since beginning the inhaled corticosteroid. Her vital signs are: BP: 106/68 mmHg, HR: 100 bpm, RR: 16 breaths per minute, temperature: 100.6°F (38.1°C), pulse oximetry: 95% on room air.

Joyce's current medication regimen is:

- Loratadine daily
- Fluticasone and salmeterol inhaler daily
- Albuterol sulfate metered dose inhaler, as needed
- Oral hormonal contraceptive
- Emtricitabine/tenofovir daily

Joyce states that she has also been taking over-the-counter ibuprofen 400 mg every 6 hours to treat her fever and sore throat. On physical examination, pharyngeal erythema and tonsillar swelling with white exudate are noted. Inspiratory wheezes are present in both upper lobes.

The health care provider orders a rapid culture to detect the presence of group A *Streptococcus*. This diagnostic test is positive for the presence of group A *Streptococcus* and the provider chooses to treat Joyce with penicillin V 500 mg every 8 hours for 10 days.

EXERCISE 6.88 Fill in the blank:

After reviewing Joyce's current medication list, the nurse notes a potential drug–drug interaction between penicillin V and one of Joyce's routine medications. Which of her routine medications may have a drug–drug interaction with penicillin V and what teaching should the nurse provide about this potential interaction? ______________________________

The answer can be found on page 474

eRESOURCE

To check your answer, refer to Epocrates Online. [Pathway: http://online.epocrates.com ➔ under the "Drugs" tab, select "Interaction Check" and enter all of Joyce's medications.]

The health care provider tells Joyce that she can continue her current dosing of over-the-counter ibuprofen, as needed, as she has been doing at home.

EXERCISE 6.89 Multiple-choice:

The nurse explains that ibuprofen may be a better medication choice than acetaminophen for the treatment of the throat pain because:

A. Ibuprofen causes less gastrointestinal (GI) disturbances than acetaminophen.
B. Acetaminophen does not have an anti-inflammatory action.
C. Acetaminophen increases the risk of bleeding.
D. Ibuprofen can be taken more frequently than acetaminophen.

The answer can be found on page 474

The health care provider prescribes theophylline to improve the asthma symptoms.

EXERCISE 6.90 Fill in the blank:

What types of beverages should Joyce be instructed to avoid while taking theophylline?

____

The answer can be found on page 474

eRESOURCE

To review the patient teaching required for this medication, refer to Epocrates Online. [Pathway: http://online.epocrates.com ➔ under the "Drugs" tab, enter "Theophylline" in the search field ➔ select "Theophylline" ➔ select "Patient Education" and review content.]

Joyce talks to her friends and realizes that many young people have the same health problems. One of her friends, Alecia, takes the following medications daily to prevent an exacerbation of asthma.

EXERCISE 6.91 Matching:

Match the medication in Column A with the category and action in Column B:

Column A	Column B
A. Montelukast	_____ Antihistamine, second generation: blocks action of histamine
B. Beclomethasone dipropionate	_____ Glucocorticoid, inhaled: decreases release of inflammatory mediators
C. Cetirizine	_____ Glucocorticoid, intranasal: prevents inflammatory response to allergens
D. Mometasone	_____ Leukotriene modifier: suppresses bronchoconstriction, eosinophil infiltration, mucus production, airway edema

The answer can be found on page 475

Joyce's streptococcal pharyngitis improves a week after she began taking the penicillin V. The wheezing and shortness of breath also improve with the addition of theophylline to her medication regimen. One month later, Joyce arrives at the triage area at the ED. She reports feeling anxious, restless, nauseous, and as if her heart is racing.

EXERCISE 6.92 Fill in the blank:

The nurse takes a brief history and initially suspects that Joyce may be having a reaction to which of her medications?

The answer can be found on page 475

Joyce's BP is 90/52 mmHg and her HR is 200 bpm. She is taken immediately to a treatment room where a stat 12-lead EKG is performed. This reveals that Joyce is experiencing paroxysmal supraventricular tachycardia (SVT). The health care provider prescribes adenosine 6 mg IV, stat.

EXERCISE 6.93 Multiple-choice:

On receiving this prescription, the nurse should:

A. Question the medication route prescribed by the provider
B. Dilute the adenosine in 100 mL normal saline and infuse over 15 minutes
C. Administer the adenosine slowly as an intravenous (IV) push
D. Rapidly inject the medication via the IV then quickly flush with normal saline

The answer can be found on page 475

After the initial bolus of IV adenosine, Joyce's cardiac rhythm converts to sinus tachycardia with an HR of 104 bpm. Her BP increases to 116/80 mmHg. Joyce reports feeling improved after her cardiac rhythm is converted to sinus tachycardia. The following laboratory value is received from the lab: serum theophylline: 9 mcg/mL. The health care team decides to admit Joyce to the telemetry unit for observation. The initial suspicion of theophylline toxicity has been ruled out, so additional studies are prescribed.

The following day Joyce's heart rhythm remains sinus tachycardia at a rate of 120 bpm. Joyce reports a 15-lb weight loss over the past 2 months despite experiencing increased hunger. In addition, she reports frequent diarrhea and hot flashes. Further physical examination reveals an enlarged thyroid. The laboratory values received are indicated in Table 6.5.

TABLE 6.5 Joyce's Thyroid Study Results

Lab Test	Lab Value
Thyroid-stimulating hormone	0.3 mIU/L
T4	19 mcg/dL
T3	250 ng/dL

Joyce is diagnosed with thyrotoxicosis secondary to Graves' disease. The health care team decides to place Joyce on a beta-adrenergic antagonist to control her heart rate. In addition, the health care provider prescribes propylthiouracil (PTU) 600 mg PO daily.

EXERCISE 6.94 Multiple-choice:

The health care provider prescribes propranolol 40 mg PO twice daily. On receiving this prescription, the nurse contacts the health care provider and questions it because:

A. There are other preferred beta-adrenergic blockers to treat thyrotoxicosis.
B. The dose is too large and may cause severe bradycardia.
C. The patient has frequent exacerbations of asthma.
D. The nonselective beta-adrenergic blocker is contraindicated for the treatment of supraventricular tachycardia (SVT).

The answer can be found on page 475

eRESOURCE

To check your answer, refer to Medscape on your mobile device. [Pathway: Medscape → enter "Propranolol" into the search field → select "Propranolol (Rx)" → select "Warnings" and review content.]

The health care provider agrees with the nurse and changes the prescription to atenolol 50 mg PO daily. Joyce is discharged home 3 days later. She remains on PTU and atenolol. The health care provider discontinues the theophylline and oral hormonal contraceptive and also instructs her to continue the albuterol sulfate metered-dose inhaler, as needed, loratadine, and inhaled fluticasone/salmeterol. Follow-up is arranged with endocrinology on an outpatient basis. Two weeks later Joyce calls the nurse at the endocrinology clinic.

EXERCISE 6.95 Multiple-choice:

Joyce tells the nurse that she has an oral temperature of 101.2°F (38.4°C) and a cough. What action should the nurse take?

A. Schedule Joyce an appointment with the endocrinologist for the next day
B. Tell Joyce she needs to contact her primary care provider for a routine sick visit
C. Recommend that Joyce take acetaminophen, increase intake of PO fluids, and rest
D. Advise Joyce to go immediately to the emergency department (ED)

The answer can be found on page 476

Laboratory studies are prescribed in the ED and indicate that Joyce is not experiencing agranulocytosis. She is discharged with a diagnosis of viral infection and given instructions to take acetaminophen as needed and to rest. Ultimately Joyce and the health care team decide that a subtotal thyroidectomy is the best treatment option to treat the hyperthyroidism. Joyce is admitted to the hospital and has the surgery without any complications. Joyce is started on levothyroxine.

EXERCISE 6.96 Multiple-choice:

When planning Joyce's care, the nurse anticipates that levothyroxine should be administered:

A. Before breakfast

B. With the evening meal

C. At bedtime

D. With food

The answer can be found on page 476

EXERCISE 6.97 Fill in the blank:

In preparing Joyce for levothyroxine use at home, the nurse teaches Joyce how to assess which vital sign?

___

The answer can be found on page 476

Two days after surgery, Joyce develops a fever and the nurse notes purulent drainage from her incision. The health care provider prescribes gentamicin 75 mg IV every 8 hours.

EXERCISE 6.98 Fill in the blanks:

In addition to a serum creatinine and blood urea nitrogen (BUN), the nurse ensures which blood test is added to Joyce's routine laboratory studies?

___

Why?

___

The answer can be found on page 476

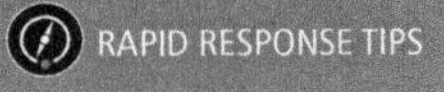
RAPID RESPONSE TIPS

Peak and trough levels

Peak level is drawn 30 minutes after the completion of the IV infusion.
Trough is drawn before administration of the next dose of IV medication.

eRESOURCE

To review the monitoring required for this medication, refer to Epocrates Online. [Pathway: http://online.epocrates.com ➔ under the "Drugs" tab, enter "Gentamicin" in the search field ➔ select "Gentamicin" ➔ select "Safety/Monitoring" and review content.]

Joyce reports feeling nauseous. The health care provider prescribes prochlorperazine 10 mg IV, one dose now.

EXERCISE 6.99 Multiple-choice:

Twenty minutes after administering prochlorperazine, the nurse enters Joyce's room and finds that she is anxious, restless, and agitated. The nurse should prepare to administer an intravenous (IV) dose of:

A. Naloxone
B. Flumazenil
C. Diphenhydramine
D. Protamine sulfate

The answer can be found on page 476

One week later, the wound infection is improved and a euthyroid state has been achieved with the levothyroxine. Joyce manages her thyroid levels at home with the effective use of pharmacological agents and a healthy lifestyle.

Answers

EXERCISE 6.1 Matching:

Match the antihypertensive classes in Column A with the mechanisms in Column B:

Column A	Column B
Antihypertensive Class	**Mechanism by Which It Decreases Blood Pressure (BP)**
A. Diuretics B. Beta blockers C. Calcium channel blockers	<u>G</u> Decreases sympathetic stimulation from the central nervous system (CNS), resulting in decreased heart rate, decreased vasoconstriction, and decreased vascular resistance within the kidneys. <u>D</u> Causes vasodilation by blocking the receptor sites of alpha-1 adrenergic receptors. <u>I</u> Blocks the receptor sites of angiotensin II, thus preventing the vasoconstricting effects. Prevents the release of aldosterone, which causes increased sodium and water reabsorption.

(*continued*)

Column A	Column B
D. Angiotensin-converting enzyme inhibitors (ACE inhibitors) E. Angiotensin II receptor antagonists F. Centrally acting alpha-2 stimulators G. Peripherally acting alpha-1 blockers H. Alpha-1 beta blockers I. Direct vasodilators	F Decreases heart rate, resulting in decreased cardiac output. C Causes direct relaxation to arterioles, resulting in decreased peripheral resistance. A Inhibits the conversion of angiotensin I to angiotensin II, thereby preventing the vasoconstrictive actions of angiotensin II. Prevents the release of aldosterone, which causes increased sodium and water reabsorption. B Decreases reabsorption of water in the kidneys, resulting in decreased circulating volume and decreased peripheral resistance. H Decreases heart rate, resulting in decreased cardiac output, and causes dilation of peripheral vessels resulting in decreased vascular resistance. E Decreases the mechanical contraction of the heart by inhibiting the movement of calcium across cell membranes. Also dilates coronary vessels and peripheral arteries.

EXERCISE 6.2 List:

The health care provider prescribes labetalol 10 mg intravenous (IV) push as a stat, one-time prescription. After preparing the medication using aseptic technique, the nurse enters Robert's room and prepares to administer the medication. On entering the room the nurse first pauses to check the "six rights" of medication administration. List these rights, which the nurse must check before medication administration.

1. **Right patient**
2. **Right medication**
3. **Right dose**
4. **Right time**
5. **Right route**
6. **Right documentation**

EXERCISE 6.3 Multiple-choice:

After identifying the six rights, the nurse notes Robert's blood pressure (BP), heart rate (HR), and cardiac rhythm. Robert's BP is 218/108 mmHg, and his cardiac rhythm is sinus bradycardia at a rate of 50 beats per minute (bpm). What action should the nurse take?

A. Administer the medication as prescribed—NO; labetalol blocks beta-1 adrenergic receptors, causing a decrease in heart rate, and should not be administered to a patient with bradycardia.

B. Ask the physician to change the prescription to PO (oral) labetalol—NO; PO labetalol also blocks beta-1 adrenergic receptors, causing a decrease in heart rate and should not be administered to a patient with bradycardia.

C. Obtain a 12-lead electrocardiogram (EKG) before administering the medication—NO; a 12-lead EKG is not required to administer intravenous (IV) labetalol.

D. Hold the medication and request a different antihypertension medication—**YES; labetalol should be held because of the bradycardia and an alternate antihypertensive medication should be prescribed.**

EXERCISE 6.4 Select all that apply:

The nurse understands that labetalol was discontinued for this patient because of the adverse effect of:

A. Agranulocytosis—NO; the medication decreases white blood cells, but this is not a concern for this patient.

B. Heart block—**YES; the patient's heart rate is 50 beats per minute (bpm) and decreasing the heart rate could cause atrioventricular (AV) block.**

C. Bradycardia—**YES; bradycardia is an adverse effect and the patient's heart rate is 50 bpm.**

D. Hypotension—NO; hypotension can occur, but this is not the concern with this patient.

EXERCISE 6.5 Calculation:

Hydralazine is available in a concentration of 20 mg/mL. How many milliliters of medication must be withdrawn from the vial to administer 10 mg?

0.5 mL

10 mg/20 mg × 1 mL = 0.5 mL

EXERCISE 6.6 Ordering:

In what order should the following be done? Place a number next to each.

__4__ Administer the medication over a 1-minute period

__2__ Clean the hub of the intravenous (IV) port using an alcohol pad

__3__ Flush the IV with 3 mL of normal saline to assess its patency

__1__ Identify the patient per hospital policy

__5__ Flush the IV with 3 mL of normal saline to clear site of medication

EXERCISE 6.7 Multiple-choice:

Which of the following medications would the nurse anticipate administering to Robert next?

A. PO hydrochlorothiazide—NO; this is not indicated to treat hypertensive emergency.

B. Intravenous (IV) sodium nitroprusside infusion—**YES; nitroprusside causes a rapid decrease in blood pressure (BP) and is the medication of choice for the treatment of hypertensive emergency.**

C. PO clonodine—NO; this is not indicated to treat hypertensive emergency.

D. IV metoprolol—NO; nitroprusside would most likely be given in this situation, as it is the medication of choice to treat hypertensive emergency.

EXERCISE 6.8 Multiple-choice:

Furosemide is prescribed in combination with the vasodilator in order to:

A. Decrease cardiac workload by decreasing afterload—NO; this is not the indication for furosemide in this situation.

B. Increase potassium excretion by the kidneys to prevent hyperkalemia—NO; this is not the indication for furosemide in this situation.

C. Decrease systolic blood pressure (BP) by decreasing preload—NO; this is not the indication for furosemide in this situation.

D. Prevent sodium and water retention caused by sodium nitroprusside—**YES; furosemide is usually given in combination with sodium nitroprusside to prevent excess fluid retention caused by sodium nitroprusside.**

EXERCISE 6.9 Multiple-choice:

The nurse understands that the intravenous (IV) sodium nitroprusside solution must be protected from light with an opaque sleeve to:

A. Prevent the medication from being degraded by light—**YES; light exposure causes decomposition of nitroprusside and increases the risk of cyanide toxicity.**

B. Decrease replication of any bacterial contaminants—NO; decreasing exposure to light does not decrease bacterial replication.

C. Increase the vasodilatory properties of the medication—NO; decreasing exposure to light does not increase the vasodilatory properties of the medication.

D. Prevent the solution from developing crystallized precipitates—NO; light exposure does not cause formation of crystallized precipitates.

EXERCISE 6.10 Multiple-choice:

Ten minutes after the sodium nitroprusside infusion is initiated, Robert's blood pressure (BP) is 240/120 mmHg and the mean arterial pressure (MAP) is 160 mmHg. Which action by the nurse is most appropriate?

A. Notify the health care provider of the BP—NO; this is not an appropriate action, as the health care provider is already aware of the BP and that the medication prescription is to titrate dose to a MAP of 125 mmHg.

B. Stop the sodium nitroprusside infusion and request a change in medication—NO; this is not an appropriate action because an increase in dose has not yet been attempted.

C. Increase the sodium nitroprusside infusion to 1 mcg/kg/min—**YES; sodium nitroprusside has a short half-life (2 minutes) and its effects should have been noted within 10 minutes. It is appropriate to increase the dose per the prescription.**

D. Continue the infusion at the same rate allowing more time for medication to work—NO; an effect should have been noted within 10 minutes. This indicates the need for a higher dose.

EXERCISE 6.11 Multiple-choice:

In managing Robert's care at this time, which task can the nurse delegate to an experienced unlicensed assistive personnel (UAP)?

A. Measure the blood pressure (BP)—NO; this should be done by the nurse because the patient is receiving a continuous vasodilator for treatment of hypertensive emergency.

B. Assess pain level on 0 to 10 scale—NO; the nurse must assess the headache because of the risk for cardiovascular complications.

C. Empty the urinal and document output—**YES; an experienced UAP is qualified to empty the urinal and record the output as the patient is not having urinary complications at this time.**

D. Silence the alarm on the volumetric pump—NO; any alarms from the volumetric pump should be promptly investigated by the nurse.

EXERCISE 6.12 Multiple-choice:

The hospital's standard concentration is 100 units of insulin in 100 mL of 0.9% normal saline (NS) (1 unit/mL concentration). What type of insulin would the nurse add to the bag of normal saline (NS)?

A. Neutral protamine Hagedorn (NPH) insulin—NO; this cannot be given intravenously.

B. Insulin glargine—NO; this cannot be given intravenously.

C. Mixed NPH/regular insulin 70/30—NO; this cannot be given intravenously.

D. Regular insulin—**YES; regular insulin can be administered intravenously.**

EXERCISE 6.13 Multiple-choice:

Which of the following measures should the nurse implement in order to ensure patient safety when using a continuous insulin infusion?

A. Check capillary blood glucose every 8 hours—NO; more frequent blood glucose assessments will be required.

B. Administer the insulin as a piggyback to 0.9% normal saline—NO; this will not increase the safety of the infusion.

C. Infuse the insulin using an intravenous (IV) volumetric pump—**YES; a volumetric pump should be used to regulate the rate of the infusion.**

D. Have the unlicensed assistive personnel (UAP) perform a double check of the infusion rate—NO; another registered nurse should independently double check the infusion. This is not within the UAP's scope of practice.

EXERCISE 6.14 Fill in the blank:

Robert's initial medication prescriptions include famotidine 20 mg intravenous (IV) every 12 hours. The nurse reviews the medication prescriptions with Robert before administering. Robert asks, "Why am I taking that heartburn medicine? I don't have any heartburn and I never had stomach problems." How should the nurse respond to Robert's question?

Histamine-2 receptor blockers or proton pump inhibitors are prescribed during a physiological insult to prevent stress-related mucosal disease.

EXERCISE 6.15 Multiple-choice:

In preparation for discharge, what teaching should the nurse include regarding use of hydrochlorothiazide?

A. Decrease intake of foods high in potassium—NO; increased potassium intake is needed to replace losses from increased diuresis.

B. Take this medication upon waking in the morning—**YES; it should be taken in the morning to prevent nocturesis.**

C. Expect to gain weight while taking this medication—NO; weight gain is not an adverse effect.

D. Report impaired hearing to health care provider immediately—NO; ototoxicity is associated with loop diuretics, not thiazide diuretics.

EXERCISE 6.16 Fill in the blank:

Based on the pharmacokinetics of insulin glargine, how should the nurse respond to Robert's question?

Insulin glargine has a duration of 24 hours. The medication is steadily released over an extended period of time, thus preventing a peak from occurring.

EXERCISE 6.17 Fill in the blank:

At 11:30 a.m., Robert's finger-stick blood glucose is 257 mg/dL. Based on the prescription in Table 6.1, what action should the nurse take?

Administer 7 units of insulin aspart subcutaneously.

EXERCISE 6.18 Fill in the blanks:

Based on the pharmacokinetics of insulin aspart, the nurse should expect to note a decrease in capillary glucose within what period of time after administering subcutaneous insulin aspart?

Insulin aspart is a short-duration/rapid-acting insulin. A decrease in capillary glucose would be expected 10 to 20 minutes after subcutaneous administration.

During what period after administration of subcutaneous insulin aspart is Robert most likely to experience a hypoglycemic event?

A hypoglycemic event is most likely to occur when the insulin reaches its peak action. A hypoglycemic event would be most likely to occur 1 to 3 hours after subcutaneous administration of insulin aspart.

EXERCISE 6.19 Multiple-choice:

Ninety minutes after the subcutaneous insulin aspart is administered, Robert rings his call light. The nurse enters the room and observes that Robert is awake and oriented but anxious and diaphoretic. Robert reports a headache and feelings of fatigue. His capillary blood glucose is 51 mg/dL. What action should the nurse take *first*?

A. Contact the health care provider—NO; the nurse should take action first.

B. Prepare intravenous (IV) dextrose 50%—NO; if the patient is alert and able to have PO intake, IV dextrose is not the preferred intervention, but should be readily available.

C. Have the patient drink orange juice—**YES; fruit juice should be given PO to quickly increase blood glucose.**

D. Ensure the patency of the peripheral IV—NO; this is an important action in case IV dextrose must be given, but a different action should be taken first.

EXERCISE 6.20 Multiple-choice:

Before Robert can finish drinking the orange juice he becomes confused, tachycardic, and increasingly diaphoretic. Robert then becomes unresponsive to verbal and painful stimuli. Robert has a patent airway and has an respiratory rate (RR) of 12 breaths per minute. The nurse understands that the best intervention for this patient is to:

A. Call a Code Blue (cardiac arrest/emergency response)—NO; the nurse should take action first.

B. Place oral glucose under the patient's tongue—NO; this may occlude the airway or cause aspiration.

C. Administer intravenous (IV) glucagon—NO; glucagon has a slower onset and should be used if administration of IV dextrose is not possible. Generally, glucagon is given via an intramuscular (IM) route if IV access is not readily available.

D. Administer IV dextrose 50%—**YES; Robert is exhibiting signs of severe hypoglycemia. IV dextrose 50% should be given to rapidly increase blood glucose.**

EXERCISE 6.21 Matching:

Match the classes of oral hypoglycemic agents for type 2 diabetes mellitus in Column A with the actions and prototypes in Column B:

Column A	Column B	
A. Meglitinides	E	Increases insulin secretion by pancreas. Prototype: glipizide
B. Thiazolidinediones	A	Increases insulin secretion by pancreas. Prototype: repaglinide
C. Alpha-glucosidase inhibitors	C	[Inhibitors]. Inhibits the digestion and absorption of carbohydrates. Prototype: acarbose
D. Biguanides	D	Increases muscle utilization of glucose, decreases glucose production by liver. Prototype: metformin
E. Sulfonylureas	B	Decreases cellular resistance to insulin. Prototype: rosiglitazone

EXERCISE 6.22 Multiple-choice:

The nurse provides education about the glipizide/metformin tablet. Which statement, if made by Robert, indicates correct understanding of the education?

A. "I will need to temporarily stop this medication if I need a radiological study with intravenous (IV) dyes."—**YES; lactic acidosis can develop if metformin is taken after receiving IV radiographic contrast.**

B. "Excessive thirst may indicate that my blood sugar has dropped too low."—NO; excessive thirst is a sign of hyperglycemia.

C. "I will need to have my complete blood count (CBC) tested regularly while taking this."—NO; hematologic side effects are not commonly associated with glipizide or metformin.

D. "If I forget to take a dose one day, I should double my dose the following day."—NO; doubling the dose could potentially cause dangerous hypoglycemia.

EXERCISE 6.23 Select all that apply:

Which of the following are therapeutic uses for rosuvastatin?

A. Decreases low-density lipoproteins (LDLs)—**YES; this is a therapeutic effect of rosuvastatin.**

B. Increases high-density lipoprotein—**YES; this is a therapeutic effect of rosuvastatin.**

C. Decreases risk of a heart attack or stroke—**YES; this is a therapeutic effect of rosuvastatin.**

D. Helps to maintain blood glucose within normal limits—NO; this is not a therapeutic effect of rosuvastatin.

EXERCISE 6.24 Multiple-choice:

The following are known adverse effects of rosuvastatin. Which of these should the patient be instructed to report to the health care provider immediately if noted?

A. Flatus—NO; this is a common, non-life-threatening adverse effect of rosuvastatin.

B. Abdominal cramps—NO; this is a common, non-life-threatening adverse effect of rosuvastatin.

C. Muscle tenderness—**YES; this may be a sign of rhabdomyolysis, a potentially life-threatening complication of rosuvastatin therapy.**

D. Diarrhea—NO; this is a common, non-life-threatening adverse effect of rosuvastatin.

EXERCISE 6.25 Multiple-choice:

The nurse is providing medication education about metronidazole. Which statement from Robert indicates a need for additional teaching?

A. "I can continue to eat yogurt each morning."—NO; this is a correct statement; this will not cause an interaction with metronidazole.

B. "I am able to continue taking acetaminophen for headaches."—NO; this is a correct statement; this will not cause an interaction with metronidazole

C. "I can still have a few beers with my friends on Friday."—**YES; a disulfiram-like reaction may occur with concurrent ingestion of alcohol and metronidazole. Further teaching is needed.**

D. "I can eat cooked or raw fruits and vegetables while taking this."—NO; this is a correct statement. Fruits and vegetables will not cause an interaction with metronidazole.

EXERCISE 6.26 Fill in the blanks:

Describe why each of the following medications may be given in the treatment of hyperkalemia.

Intravenous (IV) regular insulin and IV dextrose 50%

The action of insulin causes potassium to move into cells. Dextrose is given concurrently to prevent hypoglycemia (depending on patient's baseline serum glucose value). Insulin will only temporarily keep potassium ions within the cells.

IV calcium gluconate

This increases the threshold of cardiac tissue to decrease threat of lethal arrhythmias from hyperkalemia.

IV sodium bicarbonate

This causes potassium to move into cells and also concurrently corrects acidosis.

PO or retention enema of sodium polystyrene sulfonate

This causes sodium to exchange with potassium within the bowel. Then it causes an osmotic diarrhea to remove potassium from the bowel.

EXERCISE 6.27 Multiple-choice:

After noting the change in Robert's medication prescriptions, which of the following is the priority nursing diagnosis for Robert?

A. Activity intolerance—NO; this is not the priority nursing diagnosis at this time.

B. Chronic pain—NO; this is not the priority nursing diagnosis at this time.

C. Risk for infection—**YES; the immunosuppresive agents used to prevent transplant rejection put Robert at risk for infection.**

D. Risk for unstable glucose level—NO; this is not the priority nursing diagnosis at this time.

EXERCISE 6.28 Calculation:

Robert weighs 75 kg; calculate the hourly dosage of tacrolimus given this prescription (Tacrolimus, 0.1 mg/kg/d IV, given as a continuous infusion over 24 hours; round to the nearest hundredth of a milligram).

0.1 mg × 75 kg = 7.5 mg/d; 7.5/24 hr = 0.31 mg/hr

EXERCISE 6.29 Select all that apply:

What would the nurse check before administering the prescribed morphine?

A. Temperature—NO; temperature is not a necessary assessment to complete before morphine administration.

B. Respiratory rate (RR)—**YES; morphine can cause respiratory depression, so the RR must be assessed before and after administration.**

C. Blood pressure (BP)—**YES; morphine can cause a drop in BP, so BP must be assessed before and after administration.**

D. Pulse—**YES; morphine can cause decreased cardiac output, so the pulse must be assessed before and after administration.**

EXERCISE 6.30 Multiple-choice

Ten minutes after administering the intravenous (IV) morphine, the nurse returns to Robert's room in response to an alarm from the heart rate (HR) monitor. The nurse finds that Robert has an HR of 58 beats per minute (bpm), prolonged apnea, and constricted pupils. What is the priority nursing intervention?

A. Check pulse oximeter—NO; the patient is presently not breathing; therefore, this is not the priority action.

B. Listen to breath sounds—NO; the patient is presently not breathing; the apnea must be corrected in order to hear breath sounds.

C. Provide supplemental oxygen—NO; the patient is presently not breathing; a different action must be taken first.

D. Administer naloxone—**YES; this patient exhibits signs of opioid toxicity. Naloxone is the antidote and should be given as soon as possible. In addition, airway and ventilatory support should be provided until the patient begins breathing again.**

EXERCISE 6.31 Select all that apply:

Nurses administer naloxone to patients to reverse the effects of opioids. After administration, what symptoms of naloxone would the nurse report immediately?

A. Dilated pupils—NO; pupillary constriction is associated with opioid overdose. Increased pupil size after naloxone administration is not a concern.

B. Rhinorrhea—**YES; this is an indication of acute withdrawal after the naloxone is administered.**

C. Abdominal aches—**YES; this is an indication of acute withdrawal after the naloxone is administered.**

D. Perspiration—**YES; this is an indication of acute withdrawal after the naloxone is administered. Patients in acute withdrawal need to be treated immediately.**

EXERCISE 6.32 Fill in the blank:

What effects will naloxone have on Robert's incisional pain at this time?

Naloxone not only decreases the respiratory depression caused by opioid medications but also reverses the analgesic effects of all opioid medications. An alternate method of pain management will be required until the antagonistic effects of naloxone cease (half-life: 60–90 minutes).

EXERCISE 6.33 Select all that apply:

Which statement(s) made by Robert indicate that medication discharge teaching has been successful?

A. "I should avoid contact with anyone who is ill to the best of my ability."—**YES; immunosuppressants used to prevent rejection place Robert at increased risk for infection.**

B. "My blood count will need to be monitored regularly."—**YES; tacrolimus and mycophenolate mofetil both have hematological adverse effects. Complete blood counts (CBCs) must be monitored.**

C. "My serum tacrolimus level will need to be monitored."—**YES; serum tacrolimus levels should be monitored to prevent rejection and toxicity.**
D. "I should take an oxycodone/acetaminophen before driving to my follow-up appointment."—NO; Robert should be instructed not to operate a vehicle or dangerous machinery while taking opioid analgesics.
E. "I should notify the health care provider if my blood pressure is elevated."—**YES; hypertension is a potential adverse reaction to tacrolimus.**
F. "I will immediately stop taking the prednisone if I develop nausea."—NO; nausea is not an indication to stop taking prednisone. Sudden cessation of prednisone may increase the risk of organ transplant rejection and/or cause adrenocortical insufficiency.

EXERCISE 6.34 Multiple-choice:

Which statement, if made by Robert, indicates the need for further teaching about cyclobenzaprine?

A. "I should chew gum if I develop dry mouth."—NO; this indicates correct understanding of managing anticholinergic adverse effects.
B. "I will return to the ED if I cannot urinate."—NO; this indicates correct understanding of managing anticholinergic adverse effects.
C. "I should not take this medication before going to sleep."—**YES; this statement requires further teaching. Drowsiness is a common adverse effect; therefore, cyclobenzaprine can ideally be taken at bedtime.**
D. "This medication relaxes the muscle spasm."—NO; this indicates a correct understanding of the therapeutic actions of cyclobenzaprine.

EXERCISE 6.35 Fill in the blank:

Robert asks the nurse whether he can take over-the-counter nonsteroidal anti-inflammatory drugs (NSAIDs), such as ibuprofen or naproxen, to treat the back pain. How should the nurse respond to this question?

NSAIDs should be avoided as they can increase the nephrotoxic effects of medications such as tacrolimus. In addition, taking NSAIDs with glucocorticoids can increase the risk of gastrointestinal bleeding.

EXERCISE 6.36 Fill in the blank:

Review the following medication prescriptions that are initially written for Wanda. Describe the pharmacological rationale for each of these medications for a patient having a myocardial infarction.

Clopidogrel 300 mg orally, one dose now

This inhibits platelet aggregation.

Nitroglycerin 0.4 mg sublingual every 5 minutes, three times now

This increases coronary blood flow.

Metoprolol 5 mg intravenous (IV) push, one dose now

This decreases myocardial demands for oxygen.

EXERCISE 6.37 Select all that apply:

Sublingual nitroglycerin has an onset of 1 to 3 minutes. Before and after each dose of sublingual nitroglycerin, the nurse should assess which of the following?

A. Blood pressure (BP)—**YES; hypotension is a common adverse effect of nitroglycerin.**
B. Pupil size—NO; this is not a priority assessment.
C. Deep tendon reflexes (DTR)—NO; this is not a priority assessment.
D. Heart rate (HR)—**YES; tachycardia is a common adverse effect of nitroglycerin.**
E. Location, severity of pain—**YES; this evaluates the effectiveness of the medication.**
F. Temperature—NO; this is not a priority assessment.

EXERCISE 6.38 Fill in the blanks:

Explain the rationale for administering intravenous (IV) nitroglycerin.

Because of its very short half-life (1–4 minutes), nitroglycerin has a rapid onset but a very short duration.

How would you respond to the family's concerns about a potential overdose of nitroglycerin?

Additional nitroglycerin can be administered via IV without fear of toxicity as the sublingual doses have already been metabolized.

Briefly summarize the difference in pharmacokinetics between IV and sublingual nitroglycerin.

A continuous infusion of nitroglycerin is necessary to maintain its therapeutic action.

EXERCISE 6.39 Calculation:

After administering the intravenous (IV) heparin bolus, the nurse prepares the continuous IV heparin infusion. The concentration of heparin is 25,000 units/250 mL 0.9% normal saline (NS). At what rate would the volumetric pump be set to administer 1,000 units/hr?

250 mL/25,000 units × 1,000 units/hr = 10 mL/hr

EXERCISE 6.40 Calculation:

The nitroglycerin is set to infuse at 9 mL/hr. The concentration is 25 mg of nitroglycerin in 250 mL 0.9% normal saline (NS). Calculate the micrograms per hour.

25 mg : 250 mL = *x* mg : 9 mL
250*x*/250 = 225/250
***x* = 0.9 mg/hr**
Convert to micrograms (1,000 mcg = 1 mg)
0.9 × 1,000 = 900 mcg/hr

EXERCISE 6.41 Multiple-choice:

Ten minutes after the nitroglycerin infusion is initiated, Wanda reports a headache of moderate severity. Her blood pressure (BP) is 105/68 mmHg, heart rate (HR) is 80 beats per minute (bpm), sinus rhythm. What action should the nurse take?

A. Immediately notify the cardiologist—NO; this is an expected adverse effect and not a reason to contact the cardiologist.

B. Decrease the infusion in 5 mcg/min increments until headache improves—NO; this is not a reason to decrease the dose.
C. Turn off the nitroglycerin infusion—NO; this is not an indication to stop the infusion.
D. Reassure Wanda that a headache is an expected adverse effect—**YES; Wanda should be reassured that this is an expected adverse effect of nitroglycerin.**

EXERCISE 6.42 Multiple-choice:

Shortly after being reassured, Wanda complains of feeling dizzy and light-headed. Her blood pressure (BP) is 70/30 mmHg, heart rate (HR) is 88 beats per minute (bpm), sinus rhythm. Which of the following actions would be the initial priority?

A. Place the patient in a supine position—NO; this is an important intervention, but another action should be taken first.
B. Administer a bolus of intravenous (IV) normal saline—NO; this is an important intervention, but another action should be taken first.
C. Stop the nitroglycerin infusion—**YES; the nitroglycerin is likely the cause of hypotension and the infusion should be stopped immediately.**
D. Notify the physician—NO; this is an important intervention, but another action should be taken first.

EXERCISE 6.43 Fill in the blank:

What class of medication would the nurse expect to be prescribed for Wanda?

Antidysrhythmics

EXERCISE 6.44 Calculation:

An amiodarone bolus of 150 mg intravenous (IV) × 1 dose now is prescribed, followed by an amiodarone infusion of 1 mg/hr × 6 hours. The initial amiodarone bolus of 150 mg is prepared in a 100-mL bag of 0.9% normal saline solution (NSS) and should be infused over 10 minutes. At what rate (mL/hr) should the bolus infuse?

100 mL/10 minutes = 10 mL/min × 60 min/hr = 600 mL/hr

EXERCISE 6.45 Multiple-choice:

The nurse continues to monitor Wanda while she receives the amiodarone infusion. Which assessment finding should be reported to the health care provider immediately?

A. Normal sinus rhythm with 4 premature ventricular contractions (PVCs) per minute—NO; occasional PVCs would be expected at this time.
B. Generalized weakness and slight tremor to both hands—NO; CNS side effects are common with amiodarone. The patient may also have generalized weakness because of the underlying cardiac dysfunction.
C. Nausea and one episode of vomiting with tan-colored emesis—NO; nausea and vomiting are commonly associated with amiodarone and may also be associated with the underlying cardiac dysfunction. One episode of vomiting with tan-colored emesis is not the most concerning option.
D. Cough with white sputum and crackles in both lung fields—**YES; pulmonary toxicity, including acute respiratory distress syndrome, is associated with amiodarone use. In addition, amiodarone can precipitate heart failure, which also may be manifested by a productive cough and crackles.**

EXERCISE 6.46 Multiple-choice:

Which of the following would be a priority nursing assessment for Wanda?

A. Deep tendon reflexes (DTR)—NO; this is not a priority assessment at this time.
B. Monitor urine specific gravity—NO; this is not a priority assessment at this time.
C. Assess percutaneous coronary intervention (PCI) insertion site—**YES; both abciximab and heparin increase the risk of bleeding and the PCI insertion site must be carefully monitored.**
D. Strict intake and output measurement—NO; this is not a priority assessment at this time.

EXERCISE 6.47 Fill in the blank:

Why has Wanda been excluded as a candidate for intravenous (IV) thrombolytic treatment?

Wanda is at high risk of hemorrhage as a result of anticoagulant therapy and recent percutaneous coronary intervention (PCI). Risks of bleeding outweigh the potential benefit of thrombolytic treatment in this scenario.

EXERCISE 6.48 Multiple-choice:

Wanda starts having a tonic–clonic seizure. What medication should the nurse prepare to administer first?

A. Phenytoin—NO; phenytoin is not indicated as the initial treatment for active seizures.
B. Carbamazepine—NO; this is not indicated for the treatment of active seizures.
C. Lorazepam—**YES; lorazepam is indicated as the initial medication to treat active seizures.**
D. Hydromorphone—NO; this is an opioid analgesic.

EXERCISE 6.49 Select all that apply:

The nurse recognizes that intravenous (IV) phenytoin must be given slowly (no faster than 50 mg/min), as more rapid administration can cause what serious complications?

A. Cardiac dysrhythmias—**YES; cardiac dysrhythmias can result from rapid injection of IV phenytoin.**
B. Coma—NO; this is not a cardiac complication of IV phenytoin.
C. Cough—NO; this is not a cardiac complication of IV phenytoin.
D. Mania—NO; this is not a cardiac complication of IV phenytoin.
E. Hypotension—**YES; hypotension can result from rapid injection of IV phenytoin.**

EXERCISE 6.50 Fill in the blank:

What is the rationale for not mixing phenytoin with other medications?

Mixing intravenous (IV) phenytoin with other solutions, dextrose in particular, causes formation of precipitates.

EXERCISE 6.51 Fill in the blank:

What action can the nurse take to reduce venous irritation when administering intravenous (IV) phenytoin?

Flush IV site with 0.9% normal saline immediately after the infusion has been completed.

EXERCISE 6.52 Fill in the blanks:

What is the rationale for giving etomidate to Wanda?

It is an anesthetic and it produces loss of consciousness.

What type of medication should always be given in combination with neuromuscular blockers, such as succinylcholine (Anectine)?

It is an anesthetic; neuromuscular blockers do not enter the central nervous system (CNS), therefore the patient is only paralyzed. The ability to hear, to think, and feel pain is still present after administering a neuromuscular blocking agent.

What laboratory value should be monitored carefully with use of succinylcholine?

Potassium; the medication can cause release of potassium from tissues resulting in hyperkalemia.

EXERCISE 6.53 Exhibit-format:

The nurse sets up the infusion and a second nurse independently confirms the medication. Wanda has two peripheral intravenous (IV) sites and a triple-lumen subclavian central venous line.

A. Which IV access site would be the ***best*** to use for IV administration of dopamine?
B. Which IV access site would ***not be appropriate*** for IV administration of dopamine?

Explain your rationale.

IV site A: Right subclavian triple-lumen central venous line—**Best choice.**
IV site B: Distal left-hand 22-gauge peripheral IV—**Not an appropriate site.**
IV site C: Right antecubital 18-gauge peripheral IV—NO; patient will not be able to bend arm.

Extravasation of IV dopamine can cause severe irritation and necrosis. To prevent this from occurring, the best action is to administer via a central venous access. If a peripheral IV access is used, the drug should be given through a large vein and the site must be assessed frequently for signs of extravasation.

EXERCISE 6.54 Fill in the blank:

Five minutes after the dopamine infusion is initiated, Wanda's vital signs and physical assessment are unchanged. What action should the nurse anticipate taking?

Notify the health care provider. Anticipate increasing the rate of the dopamine infusion. If hypotension persists, the nurse should anticipate adding the administration of a potent vasoconstrictor such as norepinephrine.

EXERCISE 6.55 Select the correct response:

As dopamine in higher doses (such as 5–10 mcg/kg/min) stimulates beta-1 adrenergic receptors, the nurse would anticipate an ***increase*** in heart rate as an expected effect.

EXERCISE 6.56 Fill in the blank:

The nurse notices a nursing student crushing the carbamazepine (Tegretol XR) extended-release tablet in applesauce. What action, if any, should the nurse take?

The nurse should instruct the nursing student to dispose of the crushed tablet and call pharmacy for a new tablet. The nurse should explain that crushing an extended-release tablet will prevent the medication from being appropriately absorbed over an extended period of time.

EXERCISE 6.57 Fill in the blank:

The nurse must carefully monitor the complete blood count (CBC) when a patient is on carbamazepine. Explain why.

There are possible life-threatening adverse effects of carbamazepine, including agranulocytosis, aplastic anemia, and thrombocytopenia.

EXERCISE 6.58 Multiple-choice:

Before administering vancomycin, the nurse should be sure to assess which of the following laboratory values?

A. Hemoglobin and hematocrit—NO; this is not a priority laboratory assessment for use of cefepime and vancomycin.
B. Prothrombin time (PT) and international normalized ratio (INR)—NO; this is not a priority laboratory assessment for use of cefepime and vancomycin.
C. Albumin and glucose—NO; this is not a priority laboratory assessment for use of cefepime and vancomycin.
D. Serum creatinine and blood urea nitrogen (BUN)—**YES; vancomycin can cause nephrotoxicity.**

EXERCISE 6.59 Multiple-choice:

Wanda is also receiving intravenous (IV) furosemide when the vancomycin is added to her medication profile. Which of the following symptoms should the nurse advise Wanda to report immediately?

A. Urinary urgency—NO; this is not a complication of this medication combination.
B. Tinnitus—**YES; both vancomycin and loop diuretics can cause ototoxicity. Patients should be instructed to report hearing loss and/or tinnitus while taking either medication.**
C. Diarrhea—NO; this is not a complication of this medication combination.
D. Chills—NO; this is not a complication of this medication combination.

EXERCISE 6.60 Select all that apply:

Too rapid administration of intravenous (IV) vancomycin may place the patient at increased risk for an adverse reaction such as:

A. Nausea and vomiting—NO; this is not associated with too rapid administration of vancomycin.
B. Red man syndrome—**YES; red man syndrome is a possible adverse effect of vancomycin resulting from too rapid administration of the medication.**
C. Superinfection—NO; this is not associated with too rapid administration of vancomycin.
D. Phlebitis—**YES; phlebitis is a possible adverse effect of vancomycin resulting from too rapid administration of the medication.**

EXERCISE 6.61 Multiple-choice:

Which action should be taken by the nurse *first*?

A. Administer a 500-mL bolus of normal saline intravenous (IV)—NO; this is an important intervention, but another action should be taken first.

B. Give 50 mg of diphenhydramine IV push—NO; this is an important intervention, but another action should be taken first.

C. Page the health care provider to the unit, stat—NO; this is an important intervention, but another action should be taken first.

D. Discontinue the vancomycin infusion—**YES; Wanda is exhibiting signs and symptoms of red man syndrome. The vancomycin infusion should be discontinued immediately.**

EXERCISE 6.62 Fill in the blank:

What most common central nervous system (CNS) adverse effect of diphenhydramine should the nurse explain to Wanda when she is administering this medication?

Drowsiness is the most common CNS adverse effect of diphenhydramine. Geriatric patients may be at high risk for sedation and confusion when treated with diphenhydramine. Precautions to minimize the risk of falls should be implemented with geriatric patients.

EXERCISE 6.63 Fill in the blank:

Before administering cefepime, the nurse should be certain that Wanda does not have a history of serious allergic reactions to cephalosporins and what other class of anti-infectives?

Penicillins; cephalosporins may be contraindicated in patients with a history of serious hypersensitivity to penicillins owing to risk of a cross-sensitivity reaction.

EXERCISE 6.64 Fill in the blank:

Wanda has now been on intravenous (IV) heparin therapy for 7 days. In addition to monitoring the activated partial thromboplastin time (aPTT), the nurse should very carefully monitor which other hematological laboratory value?

Platelet count; heparin-induced thrombocytopenia (HIT) is a potentially serious complication of heparin therapy and usually has an onset around the eighth day of heparin therapy.

EXERCISE 6.65 Calculation:

If diltiazem is available in vials of 25 mg/5 mL, how many milliliters of diltiazem must the nurse give via intravenous (IV) push?

154 lb/2.2 = 70 kg

70 kg × 0.25 = 17.5 mg

17.5 mg/25 mg × 5 mL = 3.5 mL

EXERCISE 6.66 Calculation:

The diltiazem infusion is prepared as 125 mg in 250 mL normal saline solution (NSS). At what rate should the diltiazem be infused?

125 mg/250 mL = 0.5 mg/mL

10 mg/hr/0.5 mg/hr = 20 mL/hr

EXERCISE 6.67 List:

What three cardiac assessments must be done periodically while Wanda is on the diltiazem infusion?

1. **Pulse**
2. **Blood pressure (BP)**
3. **Cardiac rhythm**

EXERCISE 6.68 Fill in the blank:

Before administering digoxin, the nurse listens to the apical heart rate for 1 minute. If the apical heart rate is less than 60, what action should the nurse take?

Hold the medication and notify the health care provider. Digoxin has a negative chronotropic effect and therefore slows the heart rate. Administering it to a patient with a heart rate (HR) below 60 beats per minute (bpm) may cause dangerous bradycardia.

EXERCISE 6.69 Fill in the blanks:

As Wanda remains on a loop diuretic, what laboratory value must be carefully monitored to prevent a serious complication from digoxin therapy?

Potassium; hypokalemia significantly increases the risk of digoxin toxicity. Loop diuretics, such as furosemide, cause increased loss of potassium.

What is the therapeutic serum range for digoxin?

0.5 to 2 ng/mL

EXERCISE 6.70 List:

Name five signs/symptoms of digoxin toxicity:

1. **Abdominal pain**
2. **Nausea**
3. **Vomiting**
4. **Anorexia**
5. **Visual disturbances**

EXERCISE 6.71 Fill in the blank:

What is the antidote to digoxin?

Digoxin immune Fab.

EXERCISE 6.72 Fill in the blank:

Explain why Wanda is able to receive both warfarin and heparin concurrently.

Heparin and warfarin inhibit clotting at different areas on the coagulation cascade; therefore, receiving heparin and warfarin concurrently does not create a synergistic effect. PO warfarin takes 3 to 5 days to reach a therapeutic level and, therefore, heparin must be concurrently administered to maintain adequate anticoagulation until a therapeutic international normalized ratio (INR) is achieved with warfarin.

EXERCISE 6.73 List:

In order to provide medication teaching to Wanda, list four or more foods rich in vitamin K:

1. **Asparagus**
2. **Broccoli**
3. **Beans**
4. **Cabbage**
5. **Cauliflower**
6. **Kale**
7. **Spinach**
8. **Turnips**

EXERCISE 6.74 Matching:

Match the drug classes in Column A with the functions in Column B:

Column A	Column B
A. Proton pump inhibitors (PPIs)	B Inhibits parietal cells from secreting gastric acid. Prototype: famotidine
B. Histamine 2 (H2) receptor blockers	D Neutralizes gastric contents. Prototype: magnesium hydroxide/aluminum hydroxide
C. Gastrointestinal protectants	A Prevents hydrogen ions from being transported into the gastric lumen. Prototype: pantoprazole
D. Antacids	C Forms a paste when exposed to gastric acid which then covers the surface of peptic ulcers. Prototype: sucralfate

EXERCISE 6.75 Fill in the blank:

What might be the cause of Wanda's diarrhea?

Diarrhea is a possible adverse effect of proton pump inhibitors (PPIs). Diarrhea may also be caused by magnesium hydroxide, although this is usually counteracted by the constipating effects of aluminum hydroxide.

EXERCISE 6.76 Fill in the blank:

Which of the medications prescribed for Wanda should not be taken within 1 to 3 hours of doxycycline, and why?

Magnesium hydroxide/aluminum hydroxide (Maalox) should not be taken within 1 to 3 hours of doxycycline. Antacids, calcium, magnesium, sodium bicarbonate, and iron supplements will cause decreased absorption of PO doxycycline.

EXERCISE 6.77 Fill in the blank:

What change in the appearance of her stools should Wanda be instructed to expect while taking bismuth subsalicylate?

Stool may appear gray-black in color while taking bismuth subsalicylate.

EXERCISE 6.78 Fill in the blanks:

What is the rationale for administering albuterol and ipratropium to Joyce?

Joyce is presently experiencing bronchoconstriction as evidenced by wheezing, cough, and dyspnea. Albuterol and ipratropium have been prescribed for their bronchodilating effects.

Describe the basic mechanism by which albuterol and ipratropium will improve Joyce's symptoms.

Albuterol: selectively activates the beta-2 receptor cells of smooth muscles in lung, causing bronchodilation.

Ipratropium: causes bronchodilation by blocking cholinergic receptors in bronchi.

EXERCISE 6.79 Multiple-choice:

What action should the nurse take?

A. Immediately notify the health care provider of this potential complication—NO; this is an expected adverse effect of the medication and does not require immediate notification of the health care provider.

B. Position the patient in a modified Trendelenburg position—NO; Trendelenburg positioning is not indicated.

C. Place the patient on telemetry and prepare to administer a beta-2 receptor antagonist—NO; this is not necessary as her symptoms are an expected adverse effect and her physical examination indicates adequate perfusion.

D. Reassure the patient that this is an expected adverse effect from albuterol—**YES; nervousness, tremors, restlessness, and tachycardia are common adverse effects of Ventolin HFA.**

EXERCISE 6.80 Multiple-choice:

What instructions should the nurse include for Joyce when providing discharge teaching about erythromycin stearate?

A. "Discontinue the medication and notify the health care provider if you have multiple loose stools."—**YES; this is a sign of a suprainfection.**

B. "Take the medication on an empty stomach with a glass of water."—NO; erythromycin stearate can be taken with food.

C. "Discontinue the medication once presenting symptoms have completely improved to reduce side effects."—NO; antibiotics should not be stopped early even if symptoms have resolved.

D. "Vaginal itching is common while taking this medication, but it is expected and not a concern."—NO; this is a sign of a suprainfection.

EXERCISE 6.81 Select all that apply:

Choose the ingredients in many cough and cold medicines that suppress coughing.

A. Codeine—**YES; codeine in low doses is used as an antitussive.**

B. Acetaminophen—NO; acetaminophen is an analgesic and antipyretic agent.

C. Diphenhydramine—NO; diphenhydramine is a first-generation antihistamine and is not indicated to treat cough.

D. Dextromethorphan—**YES; dextromethorphan is an antitussive agent commonly used in over-the-counter cold medications.**

E. Pseudoephedrine—NO; pseudoephedrine is a decongestant.

EXERCISE 6.82 Fill in the blank:

How should the nurse respond to Joyce's concern about nausea?

Nausea is an expected adverse effect of prednisone and is not an indication to stop the medication early. The prednisone dose is tapered because of the risk for adrenal suppression; it should not be stopped abruptly.

EXERCISE 6.83 Multiple-choice:

The nurse provides teaching about inhaled corticosteroids. Which statement, if made by Joyce, indicates the need for further teaching?

A. "I will be sure to rinse my mouth with water before using the inhaled steroid."—**YES; this statement indicates a need to further teaching. Patients should be advised to rinse their mouths with water after using inhaled corticosteroids to decrease risk of oropharyngeal fungal infections.**

B. "If I become short of breath I will use the albuterol HFA inhaler and not the inhaled steroid."—NO; this is a correct statement. Acute shortness of breath should be treated with her albuterol HFA metered-dose inhaler.

C. "I should take the inhaled steroid after I use the albuterol HFA inhaler."—NO; this is a correct statement. Taking the inhaled corticosteroid after using a bronchodilator improves absorption.

D. "I will notify my physician if I notice any white spots in my mouth or on my tongue."—NO; this is a correct statement. White spots should be reported as this may be a sign of an oropharyngeal fungal infection.

EXERCISE 6.84 List:

The nurse provides instructions about the adverse effects of oral ferrous sulfate. List three or more gastrointestinal adverse effects of ferrous sulfate.

1. **Nausea**
2. **Vomiting**
3. **Epigastric pain**
4. **Constipation**
5. **Dark stools**
6. **GI bleeding**

EXERCISE 6.85 Ordering:

Place in priority order from 1 to 6 the procedures used to administer a vaginal suppository.

4 Use the lubricated finger to insert the rounded end of suppository 3 to 4 inches into the vaginal canal along the posterior wall

1 Verify the medication prescription and don clean gloves

5 Instruct the patient to remain in a supine position for 10 minutes

3 Lubricate the rounded end of suppository and the index finger of dominant hand with water-based lubricant

2 Remove the suppository from the wrapper

6 Document administration of the medication

EXERCISE 6.86 Select all that apply:

When providing medication education about acyclovir, which of the following instructions should the nurse include in the discharge instructions?

A. Nausea, vomiting, and diarrhea are common adverse effects of acyclovir.—**YES; nausea, vomiting, and diarrhea are common adverse effects of PO acyclovir.**

B. Long-term acyclovir treatment will cure the herpes infection.—NO; acyclovir can decrease the duration and frequency of herpes outbreaks, but does not cure the infection.

C. Condoms should be used even when the lesions are not present.—**YES; the herpes virus can still be spread when lesions are not present, so condoms should be used to decrease the possibility of transmission to sexual partners.**

D. Acyclovir decreases the duration of the herpetic lesions.—**YES; acyclovir decreases the duration and severity of the herpetic lesions during the initial infection.**

EXERCISE 6.87 Multiple-choice:

The nurse provides teaching regarding use of emtricitabine/tenofovir as HIV pre-exposure prophylaxis. Which statement, if made by Joyce, indicates need for further instruction?

A. "I won't need to use condoms because this will prevent HIV transmission."—**YES; condoms should be used in combination with antiretroviral therapy to prevent HIV transmission.**

B. "I should contact the physician if I get abdominal pain or repeated vomiting."—NO; this is a correct statement. This is a sign of lactic acidosis, a less common, but very serious adverse effect, of NRTIs.

C. "I will need to be routinely screened for HIV infection."—NO; this is a correct statement. Routine screening for HIV is necessary. Medication regimens differ between treatment of HIV and prophylaxis of HIV.

D. "I plan to take the medication each day with my breakfast."—NO; this is a correct statement. Prophylaxis works best when taken daily without missed doses. This medication can be taken with or without food. Associating the medication with breakfast may prevent missed doses.

EXERCISE 6.88 Fill in the blank:

After reviewing Joyce's current medication list, the nurse notes a potential drug–drug interaction between penicillin V and one of Joyce's routine medications. Which of her routine medications may have a drug–drug interaction with penicillin V and what teaching should the nurse provide about this potential interaction?

Penicillin may decrease the effectiveness of oral hormonal contraceptives. If such a contraceptive is being used to prevent pregnancy, a second method of birth control should be added.

EXERCISE 6.89 Multiple-choice:

The nurse explains that ibuprofen may be a better medication choice than acetaminophen for the treatment of the throat pain because:

A. Ibuprofen causes less gastrointestinal (GI) disturbances than acetaminophen.—NO; ibuprofen causes more frequent GI adverse effects than acetaminophen.

B. Acetaminophen does not have an antiinflammatory action.—**YES; acetaminophen does not have an antiinflammatory effect. Ibuprofen has anti-inflammatory, analgesic, and antipyretic effects.**

C. Acetaminophen increases the risk of bleeding.—NO; ibuprofen does have some platelet aggregation inhibitory effects, whereas acetaminophen does not.

D. Ibuprofen can be taken more frequently than acetaminophen.—NO; acetaminophen can be taken every 4 hours and ibuprofen can be taken every 6 to 8 hours.

EXERCISE 6.90 Fill in the blank:

What types of beverages should Joyce be instructed to avoid while taking theophylline?

Joyce should avoid beverages containing caffeine such as coffee, cola, and tea. Both caffeine and theophylline are methylxanthines and ingestion of both substances will increase neurological and cardiovascular adverse effects.

EXERCISE 6.91 Matching:

Match the medication in Column A with the category and action in Column B:

Column A	Column B
A. Montelukast	__C__ Antihistamine, second generation: blocks action of histamine
B. Beclomethasone dipropionate	__B__ Glucocorticoid, inhaled: decreases release of inflammatory mediators
C. Cetirizine	__D__ Glucocorticoid, intranasal: prevents inflammatory response to allergens
D. Mometasone	__A__ Leukotriene modifier: suppresses bronchoconstriction, eosinophil infiltration, mucus production, airway edema

EXERCISE 6.92 Fill in the blank:

The nurse takes a brief history and initially suspects that Joyce may be having a reaction to which of her medications?

Theophylline; Joyce is exhibiting signs of theophylline toxicity.

EXERCISE 6.93 Multiple-choice:

On receiving this prescription, the nurse should:

A. Question the medication route prescribed by the provider—NO; because of its very short half-life, adenosine is only given via intravenous (IV).

B. Dilute the adenosine in 100 mL normal saline and infuse over 15 minutes—NO; because of its very short half-life, adenosine is only given as a rapid IV push.

C. Administer the adenosine slowly as an intravenous (IV) push—NO; because of its very short half-life, adenosine is only given as a rapid IV push.

D. Rapidly inject the medication via the IV then quickly flush with normal saline—**YES; because of its very short half-life, adenosine is given as a rapid IV push followed immediately by a normal saline flush. Adenosine should be given via an IV access as close to the heart as possible.**

EXERCISE 6.94 Multiple-choice:

The health care provider prescribes propranolol 40 mg PO twice daily. On receiving this prescription, the nurse contacts the health care provider and questions it because:

A. There are other preferred beta-adrenergic blockers to treat thyrotoxicosis.—NO; propranolol is the preferred beta blocker to treat symptoms of thyrotoxicosis.

B. The dose is too large and may cause severe bradycardia.—NO; this is an appropriate dose for this indication.

C. The patient has frequent exacerbations of asthma.—**YES; propranolol is a nonselective beta blocker and may cause bronchoconstriction, which may cause further complications for those with asthma.**

D. A nonselective beta-adrenergic blocker is contraindicated for the treatment of supraventricular tachycardia (SVT).—NO; SVT is not a contraindication to using nonselective beta-adrenergic blockers.

EXERCISE 6.95 Multiple-choice:

Joyce tells the nurse that she has an oral temperature of 101.2°F (38.4°C) and a cough. What action should the nurse take?

A. Schedule Joyce an appointment with the endocrinologist for the next day—NO; Joyce may have agranulocytosis and requires immediate treatment.

B. Tell Joyce she needs to contact her primary care provider for a routine sick visit—NO; Joyce may have agranulocytosis and requires immediate treatment.

C. Recommend that Joyce take acetaminophen, increase intake of PO fluids, and rest—NO; Joyce may have agranulocytosis and requires immediate treatment.

D. Advise Joyce to go immediately to the emergency department (ED)—**YES; agranulocytosis is a potentially life-threatening adverse effect of propylthiouracil (PTU). She should be immediately referred to an ED for treatment.**

EXERCISE 6.96 Multiple-choice:

When planning Joyce's care, the nurse anticipates that levothyroxine should be administered:

A. Before breakfast—**YES; levothyroxine should be given in the morning to prevent insomnia and on an empty stomach to improve absorption.**

B. With the evening meal—NO; see aforementioned rationale.

C. At bedtime—NO; see aforementioned rationale.

D. With food—NO; see aforementioned rationale.

EXERCISE 6.97 Fill in the blank:

In preparing Joyce for levothyroxine use at home, the nurse teaches Joyce how to assess which vital sign?

Assess the radial pulse. Patients on levothyroxine should assess their pulse rate before taking this medication. Tachycardia may indicate elevated thyroid levels.

EXERCISE 6.98 Fill in the blanks:

In addition to a serum creatinine and blood urea nitrogen (BUN), the nurse ensures which blood test is added to Joyce's routine laboratory studies?

Gentamicin peak and trough levels.

Why?

The dose is adjusted in relation to the plasma drug levels.

EXERCISE 6.99 Multiple-choice:

Twenty minutes after administering prochlorperazine, the nurse enters Joyce's room and finds that she is anxious, restless, and agitated. The nurse should prepare to administer an intravenous (IV) dose of:

A. Naloxone—NO; this is the antidote to opioid medications.

B. Flumazenil—NO; this is the antidote to benzodiazepines.

C. Diphenhydramine—**YES; Joyce is likely having akathisia, an extrapyramidal side effect, from the prochlorperazine and will be treated with an anticholinergic agent.**

D. Protamine sulfate—NO; this is the antidote to heparin.

Resource

Lewis, S. L., Dirksen, S. R., Heitkemper, M. M., & Bucher, L. (Eds.). (2014). *Medical–surgical nursing: Assessment and management of clinical problems* (9th ed.). St. Louis, MO: Mosby–Elsevier.

CHAPTER 7

Community Health Nursing

Mary Gallagher Gordon

Nursing is love in action, and there is no finer manifestation of it than the care of the poor and disabled in their own homes.—Lillian Wald

UNFOLDING CASE STUDY 1: Sara

Sara is a public health nurse with a community focus. A public health nurse is someone who has obtained an advanced degree specializing in a public health/community curriculum. A public health nurse has a focus on population-based care to improve the health of individuals, communities, and populations. Sara has moved to the suburbs of a new city and investigates the community health concerns of the surrounding area to determine the challenges of any of the jobs that she may choose. She is aware that within the city there is public transportation access. The city is an average large, urban city in the United States. Neighborhoods consist of a wide swath of high- to low-income households. In one low-income neighborhood, there is a federally funded nurse-run clinic that, in addition to office health care, makes house calls, has home hospice service, and sponsors community outreach activity to promote health in the population. Sara understands that because of escalating hospital costs, community-based health care is very important to the well-being of the nation.

EXERCISE 7.1 Matching:

Match the terms in Column A with the definitions in Column B:

Column A	Column B
A. Community-based nursing (CBN)	___ Health care of populations
B. Community-oriented nursing	___ Health care focus is the aggregate or community group
C. Public health nursing (PHN)	___ Illness care of individuals across the life span

The answer can be found on page 509

Sara knows that the core functions of community health nursing include:

- Assessment of the community's health status
- Policy development by agencies and government to support the health of a community
- Assurance that health care is available and accessible

eRESOURCE

To review the essential competencies for a public health nurse, access:

- Quad Council's Public Health Nurse (PHN) Competencies. [Pathway: www.phnurse.org ➔ select "Resources" ➔ "Documents" ➔ "Current" and scroll down to select "Quad Council PHN Competencies 2011."]
- School of Public Health at University of Albany, which provides an overview of Public Health Nursing Competencies. [Pathway: http://goo.gl/zyoeR]
- *Core Competencies for Public Health Professionals—Background and Tools* by Ron Bialek, President, Public Health Foundation National. [Pathway: http://goo.gl/C7mPR]

RAPID RESPONSE TIPS

Community health comprises three levels of care

- Primary health care services, to promote health and prevent diseases
- Secondary health care services, which involve health screening for the detection and treatment of diseases
- Tertiary health care services, which are aimed at the prevention of complications from a disease as well as rehabilitation after a diagnosis

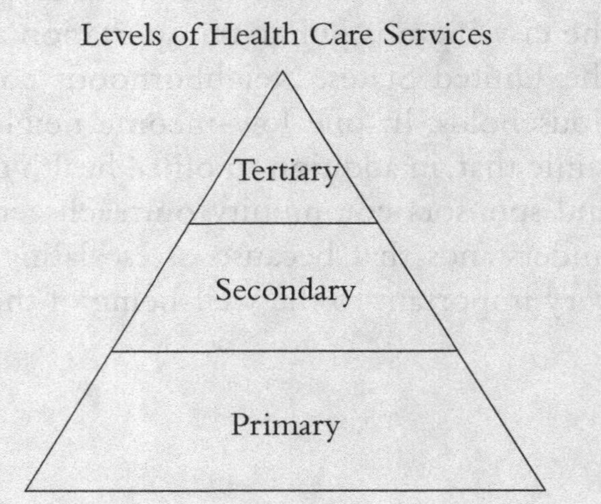

EXERCISE 7.2 Matching:

Using the following list, add to Column B the type of prevention found in Column A:

- 1 for primary prevention
- 2 for secondary prevention
- 3 for tertiary prevention

Column A	Column B
Disease prevention	______
Health promotion	______
Admission for cardiac rehab	______
Prenatal group education	______
Outpatient mental health treatment	______
Exercise programs for seniors	______

The answer can be found on page 509

eRESOURCE

To review levels of prevention, view this online tutorial from the Wisc-Online Digital Library: http://goo.gl/2blsz

Sara decides to accept a position at a community health center that is open 6 days a week and provides culturally competent, family-centered community care. The center also has a home visiting nurse component, mental health services, and an in-home hospice component for end-of-life care. As a public health nurse, Sara uses the nursing process when engaging with her clients, the community, and systems while also using critical-thinking skills. This process allows her to identify factors that may be impeding health and to develop a process to make improvements (American Nurses Association [ANA], 2013).

EXERCISE 7.3 True/False:

Sara accesses the following demographic trends for the population:

A. *Replacement* means that for every person who dies another is born.

______True

______False

B. Immigration does not impact the U.S. population.

______True

______False

C. Women are beginning to have babies at later ages in this society.

______True

______False

D. The average age of the population is increasing.

______True

______False

E. Large numbers of baby boomers are dying off.

______True

______False

F. Asians comprise the fastest growing immigrant population.

______True

______False

The answer can be found on page 510

As a public health nurse, Sara is aware that there are many factors called *health determinants* that play a role in the health of an individual. According to the *Healthy People 2020* report, of the 26 leading health indicators, there are still 12 that have been identified as showing little change, or getting worse in the U.S. population. Three indicators showing little change are people with health care insurance and a primary provider, and obesity. These have been identified at the health center as critical and the staff is working with each of the clients to assist them with access to care. The center has physical therapy (PT) staff who work with the community with regard to mobility, improved physical activity, as well as education related to obesity. The number of suicides and adolescents with depression have not improved, according to the current report, and the health center also offers behavioral health counseling services to the community (Healthy People, 2016).

EXERCISE 7.4 Select all that apply:

Select all the social and economic factors that affect health care trends in the community setting:

A. Cost
B. Age distribution of the population
C. Workforce trends
D. Season
E. Access
F. Technology
G. Attitude

The answer can be found on page 510

eRESOURCE

To reinforce your understanding of these trends, visit: Health Indicators Warehouse (HIW). [Pathway: http://healthindicators.gov.]

Sara completes a community assessment of the neighborhood surrounding the clinic. This may be known as a *windshield assessment*, in which the nurse uses all five senses to learn about the community, its specific characteristics, and available resources to promote health. In addition to the positives of the community, the nurse also needs to evaluate the environmental hazards and living spaces in the surrounding area (Garcia, Schaffer, & Schoon, 2014).

EXERCISE 7.5 Select all that apply:

Select all the factors that the nurse looks at when completing a community assessment:

A. Environment
B. Perceptions of health needs within the community
C. Cost to complete the assessment
D. Housing and conditions
E. Barriers to health care
F. Playgrounds and open spaces
G. Services offered

The answer can be found on page 511

Sara has experience working with interdisciplinary teams in previous community agencies, including members with expertise in behavioral health, PT, dentistry, and creative arts. She is well oriented to the clinic and is ready to volunteer for home health visits as needed.

EXERCISE 7.6 Select all that apply:

Select the skills performed by the home care nurse:

A. Skilled assessments
B. Wound care
C. Simple well-child care
D. Coordination of care
E. Wellness teaching

The answer can be found on page 511

Sara knows that when home care is initiated with a client, there are components that are important to consider.

EXERCISE 7.7 Select all that apply:

The components of home care that must be considered by the nurse are:

A. Development of a personal relationship
B. Contracting
C. No goals or outcomes established

The answer can be found on page 511

Sara schedules a visit to Mrs. Hernandez, a Spanish-speaking woman, during the dinner hour. Sara is there to check on a healing leg ulcer. Mrs. Hernandez lives alone in a two-story walk-up apartment near the center of town. There are neighbors in her apartment complex who assist Mrs. Hernandez. Sara knows that developing a trusting relationship is key for home visits, as she will be asking personal questions that people rarely share with strangers who come to their home (Garcia et al., 2014).

EXERCISE 7.8 Multiple-choice:

In order to communicate with Mrs. Hernandez, what should Sara do?

A. Ask a neighbor to interpret
B. Use picture books
C. Write the instructions down in English for later interpretation
D. Use an approved interpreter

The answer can be found on page 511

EXERCISE 7.9 Multiple-choice:

Mrs. Hernandez's leg wound is draining. What is the priority precaution Sara should use with the dressing change?

A. Cleanse the wound with hydrogen peroxide
B. Continue to assess for potential problems with infection control
C. Cleanse the wound beginning at the outer aspect
D. Keep the leg in a dependent position during dressing change

The answer can be found on page 512

---

eRESOURCE

To reinforce your understanding of wound care, refer to Medscape on your mobile device. [Pathway: Medscape ➔ enter "Wound" into the search field ➔ select "Wound Care" and review content.]

Mrs. Hernandez was recently started on oral medication for her diabetes. Sara asks Mrs. Hernandez if she knows the signs and symptoms of hyperglycemia and hypoglycemia. Mrs. Hernandez is not proficient with the different signs and symptoms.

EXERCISE 7.10 Matching:

Match the symptom in Column A with the condition in Column B using the following choices:

A. Hypoglycemia
B. Hyperglycemia

Column A	Column B
Hunger, pallor	______
Increased frequency of urination	______
Increased thirst	______
Also called *insulin reaction*	______
Sweating, anxiety	______
Headache	______
Diabetic ketoacidosis (DKA)	______
Increased incidence with insulin versus oral medication	______
Hypotensive, tachycardia	______
Decreased reflexes	______
Caused by unplanned exercise	______
Too little food	______
Consuming too much food or too many calories	______

The answer can be found on page 512

While Sara is visiting Mrs. Hernandez, she is offered a piece of pie that Mrs. Hernandez baked herself. Sara accepts it because she knows that Mrs. Hernandez would be insulted if she did not. It is a sign of gratitude and friendship to accept the slice of pie. Sara knows that as a community health nurse, she must assess the cultural beliefs and values of the community in which she is working. An important aspect of cultural competency is the ability to maintain an open mind and attitude regarding other cultures.

EXERCISE 7.11 Matching:

Match the terms in Column A with the cultural competencies explained in Column B:

Column A	Column B
A. Cultural awareness	___ The process in which one can communicate and interact with others, taking into account their cultural background
B. Cultural knowledge	___ The internal motivation to provide care that is culturally competent
C. Cultural skill	___ The process of evaluating one's own beliefs and values
D. Cultural encounter	___ The ability to gather information about other cultures and ethnicities
E. Cultural desire	___ The ability to gather and assess information to meet the needs of a group

Source: Stanhope and Lancaster (2013).

The answer can be found on page 513

While Sara is in Mrs. Hernandez's apartment, she assesses it for safety and security to further ensure positive health care outcomes. She notes that there is a parking garage on the basement level of the apartment complex.

EXERCISE 7.12 Multiple-choice:

Because there is a parking garage under the apartment, what is the first environmental concern?

A. Fire
B. Carbon monoxide
C. Ozone
D. Allergens

The answer can be found on page 513

EXERCISE 7.13 Multiple-choice:

Because Mrs. Hernandez lives in a two-story walk-up, what is the first safety concern?

A. Doors
B. Social isolation
C. No handrails on the outside stairs
D. Ability to drive

The answer can be found on page 513

Mrs. Hernandez has a battery-powered fire alarm but not a carbon monoxide detector. Sara calls Emmanuel, a nurse at the clinic, who is an expert in the environmental health of the community where Mrs. Hernandez lives. Emmanuel knows the community well; he was born and reared there. After nursing school, he earned his master's in nursing science (MSN) in environmental health. He understands the environmental epidemiology of the community and explains to Sara that she is correct in being concerned about toxicology or chemical exposure within the community. He goes on to tell Sara that there is a bathing suit manufacturer located in the community. This company provides many within the community with jobs but uses latex in the production of bathing suits. This community has a larger than normal number of people with latex allergies.

Emmanuel further explains to Sara that although the Environmental Protection Agency (EPA) tests the community often for the presence of latex allergies and contamination, latex can be airborne and, therefore, it can get into the water and food supply. He teaches her the four basic principles of environmental health:

1. Everything is *connected*; therefore one thing, such as a factory, affects everything else in the community.
2. Everything *goes somewhere* because matter cannot be destroyed, therefore airborne particles settle on other things.

3. *Dilution* helps pollution and even though the waste from the factory is now diluted, in years past it was not because there were no governing agencies supervising the environment.
4. *Today's habits* will impact tomorrow, so by diluting the latex particles we may actually affect tomorrow's health by disseminating the latex particles further.

Emmanuel then goes on to discuss the need for referral if Sara notices anything within the environment that may affect the health of the community. Emmanuel teaches Sara to recall this information using the "IPREPARE" mnemonic:

I Investigate potential exposures

P Present work

R Residence

E Environmental concerns

P Past work

A Activities

R Referrals and resources

E Educate (Stanhope & Lancaster, 2013)

EXERCISE 7.14 Multiple-choice:

Sara knows that the people in her community have the right to know about hazardous materials in their community environment. Where would Sara find this information?

A. Hazard Communication Standard
B. Task Force on the Environment
C. Environmental Protection Agency (EPA) Envirofacts
D. Consumer Confidence Report

The answer can be found on page 513

Sara uses the nursing center interpreter to translate health teaching to Mrs. Hernandez after she redresses her leg wound. Sara knows that it is important to use words that Mrs. Hernandez will understand, and to give her the opportunity to ask questions after she is done with the teaching.

EXERCISE 7.15 Select all that apply:

Sara should bear which of the following in mind when using an interpreter?

A. Use anyone who is around; anyone will do
B. Observe the client for nonverbal cues as the information is being delivered
C. Select an interpreter who has knowledge of medical terminology
D. Let the interpreter summarize the client's own words

The answer can be found on page 514

In the discussion with Mrs. Hernandez, Sara learns that one of the current community concerns is food-borne illness.

EXERCISE 7.16 Multiple-choice:

Mrs. Hernandez is instructed to wash her greens well to prevent which two preventable food contaminants?

A. Methacillin-resistant *Staphylococcus aureus* (MRSA) and *Salmonella*
B. *Escherichia coli* (*E. coli*) and *Clostridium difficile* (*C. diff*)
C. *C. diff* and MRSA
D. *E. coli* and *Salmonella*

The answer can be found on page 514

Mrs. Hernandez is concerned about her vaccines. She questions Sara about whether or not she will need to get her yearly "shots" with the winter season coming up.

EXERCISE 7.17 Select all that apply:

Sara knows that Mrs. Hernandez is 72 years old and should receive the following yearly immunization:

A. Influenza
B. Varicella
C. Pneumococcal polysaccharide
D. Meningococcal vaccine

The answer can be found on page 514

---

eRESOURCE

To review recommended immunization schedules, refer to:

- Centers for Disease Control and Prevention (CDC) adult immunization schedule. [Pathway: http://goo.gl/Pm4cd]
- WHO immunization schedule. [Pathway: http://goo.gl/8XvLc7]

EXERCISE 7.18 Multiple-choice:

Which would be the appropriate needle gauge, needle size, and site to administer an intramuscular (IM) immunization to Mrs. Hernandez, who weighs 148 lb?

A. Anterolateral site, 22–25 gauge, 1 in. needle size
B. Deltoid or anterolateral site, 22–25 gauge, 1–1¼ in. needle size
C. Deltoid site, 22–25 gauge, 1–1½ in. needle size
D. Anterolateral site, 22–25 gauge, 5/8 in. needle size

The answer can be found on page 514

EXERCISE 7.19 True/False:

Shake the vial vigorously to obtain uniform suspension of solution.

_____True

_____False

The answer can be found on page 515

EXERCISE 7.20 Fill in the blanks:

Discuss what criteria must be documented after administration of a vaccine:

____

____

____

____

____

____

____

The answer can be found on page 515

Sara discusses the immunizations with Mrs. Hernandez, completes her visit, and returns home. She is off the following day.

When she returns to the nursing center, Sara is scheduled to work with Marianna. Marianna is a new nurse who is shadowing the school nurse at the high school to understand the community dynamics because she is from out of the area. Marianna, who speaks Spanish, is an asset to the clinic. School nursing has a health education focus to promote the concept of making healthy choices. When planning a health education program, Marianna recalls the three domains of learning.

EXERCISE 7.21 Matching:

Match the explanations in Column B that are used to describe the three domains of learning in Column A:

Column A	Column B
A. Affective domain	____ In this domain, the learner performs a learned skill using motor skills
B. Cognitive domain	____ In this domain, the learner gets the information, integrates this into his or her values system, and adopts these values to change his or her attitude; a person needs much support to develop these new behaviors
C. Psychomotor domain	____ In this domain, the learner recalls the information, can use the information, and understands the value of what has been learned

The answer can be found on page 515

In the school health office, Sara, Marianna, and the school nurse see three cases of community-associated methicillin-resistant *S. aureus* (CA-MRSA) on the skin of teenagers. After careful assessment of all three cases, it is determined that all three students were using the exercise equipment in the gym during the past week.

Marianna asks Sara to assess the high school population's knowledge about CA-MRSA. Sara gives the students a questionnaire in order to develop an educational program. The questionnaire is as follows.

EXERCISE 7.22 Riveredge High School Health Questionnaire (Multiple-choice):

Hello Students and Faculty,

This is an anonymous questionnaire to find out how much we all know about community-associated methicillin-resistant *S. aureus* (CA-MRSA), as it has become a common community health issue.

Please feel free to make comments on the back of the paper. We look forward to developing an educational program suited to your needs.

Please return your completed questionnaire to the locked box located outside the health office on the first floor of the high school.

Thank you, Riveredge Community Care School Nurses

1. What is MRSA?
   A. A skin infection
   B. A parasitic infection
   C. A food-borne disease
   D. A vector-borne disease
2. How long can MRSA live on surfaces?
   A. Less than 1 hour
   B. More than 1 hour
   C. One day
   D. Days, weeks, or months
3. What are some of the health care practices that would reduce the spread of MRSA? Select all that apply:
   A. Washing hands
   B. Spraying rooms with disinfectant
   C. Washing floors
   D. Washing equipment surfaces
   E. Covering lesions on your skin
   F. Sharing sports gear
4. What does MRSA look like?
   A. Looks like a scab
   B. Looks like a pimple or boil
   C. Looks like a scratch
   D. Looks like a blackhead

5. Do I have to launder my school clothes separately?
   A. Yes
   B. No
6. Please list any comments or concerns!

The answer can be found on page 515

---

eRESOURCE

To reinforce your understanding of MRSA, refer to Medscape on your mobile device. [Pathway: Medscape ➔ enter "Staphylococcal" into the search field ➔ select "Staphylococcal Infections" and review content.]

Marianna knows that the rate or incidence of CA-MRSA is increasing, so she calculates the risk for the high school population.

EXERCISE 7.23 Multiple-choice:

A *risk factor* is defined as:

A. Probability that the event will occur over a specified period of time
B. Measurement of the frequency of an event over time
C. Measurement of an existing disease currently in a population
D. The rate of disease is unusually high in a population

The answer can be found on page 516

Marianna calculates an increased risk for CA-MRSA in the school because of its past prevalence compared with the current trends. She and Sara then develop an educational program for both students and faculty: they approach this with an epidemiological point of view using the epidemiological triangle.

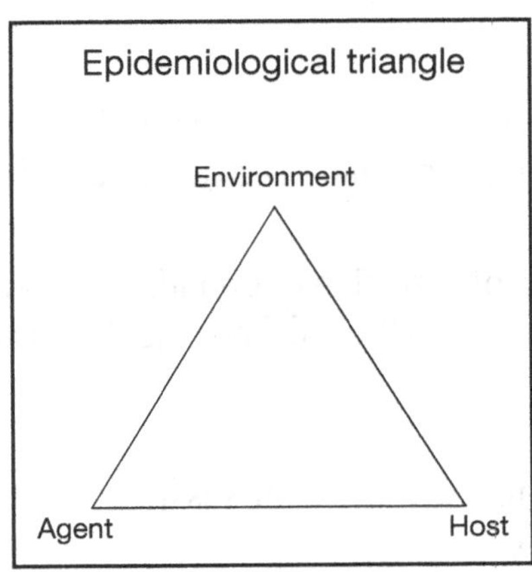

EXERCISE 7.24 Matching:

Match the infections in Column B that are used to describe the four main categories of infectious agents in Column A:

Column A	Column B
A. Bacteria	___ Pinworm
B. Fungi	___ West Nile
C. Parasite	___ Ringworm
D. Viruses	___ Salmonellosis

The answer can be found on page 517

Marianna knows there are three levels of prevention in public health: primary, secondary, and tertiary.

EXERCISE 7.25 Matching:

Match the level of prevention in Column A with the goal of each level in Column B:

Column A	Column B
A. Primary	___ Reduces complications or disabilities with rehabilitation and optimal function
B. Secondary	___ Reduces the incidence of disease by focusing on health education and health promotion
C. Tertiary	___ Uses screening to prevent the severity of disease once it has happened, treating the problem

The answer can be found on page 517

eRESOURCE

To reinforce your understanding of the levels of prevention, refer to:

- An online tutorial from the Wisc-Online Digital Library: *Levels of Prevention.* [Pathway: http://goo.gl/2blsz]
- The Association of Faculties of Medicine of Canada's Primer on Population Health, Stages of Prevention. [Pathway: http://goo.gl/yOtmkO] from the Wisc-Online Digital Library. [Pathway: http://goo.gl/brPNE]

Marianna and Sara approach the educational session from a perspective of primary, secondary, and tertiary disease prevention.

EXERCISE 7.26 Matching:

Match the level of prevention in Column A with the effort of each level in Column B:

Column A	Column B
A. Primary	___ Checking all student athletes for lesions
B. Secondary	___ Cleaning the wrestling mats
C. Tertiary	___ Sending home information in a handout
	___ Referring students with lesions to their primary care provider (PCP)
	___ Developing a poster to hang in the cafeteria for information

The answer can be found on page 517

When Marianna makes the pamphlet to send home with each student, she considers the educational process needed to get the information to people in the most appropriate manner.

EXERCISE 7.27 Exhibit-format:

The nurse accesses the parental population through school records and finds the following facts and statistics:

- Only 55% of the homes have an Internet connection
- 36% speak Spanish in the home
- 82% of the parents have a high school diploma
- 15% of the parents are college educated
- 65% are working, single-parent families

According to this information, what format would you choose to educate families about community-associated methicillin-resistant *S. aureus* (CA-MRSA)?

A. Internet tutorial
B. Phone call during school hours
C. DVD that can be played in any computer
D. Take-home information sheet written at a fourth- to sixth-grade level

The answer can be found on page 518

Marianna and Sara have good results with the educational information sent home and the school nurse continues to monitor the incidence of CA-MRSA.

In the following week, Sara has become oriented to the case management role at the health clinic. Case management involves assessing, planning for the client, monitoring change in status and needs, as well as coordination of service among all disciplines that are involved in the client's care. Sara is stationed at the telehealth phone and is responsible for coordinating multiple services for the nurse-run health clinic population as needed. Sara agrees it is a great way to "learn" about the community and its resources. The nursing preceptor asks Sara whether she is aware of the various components of case management.

EXERCISE 7.28 Fill in the blanks:

Understanding case management.

Case management uses the ________ process to help the client obtain the necessary services.

Case management is a ________ between the client and all disciplines that are involved in the client's care.

A case manager acts as a ________ by providing scientific and necessary information and supporting client decisions.

Good _____________are necessary for case managers to interact with others.

The answer can be found on page 518

The Nevel family are some of Sara's clients. Mr. Nevel has recently been discharged from the hospital and is now on hospice care. The clinic coordinates hospice care for its population. Sara has a chance to visit the Nevels the following week.

EXERCISE 7.29 Select all that apply:

Mrs. Nevel tells Sara that if she gives Mr. Nevel morphine for his pain she feels as if she is killing him. How should Sara respond?

A. "Yes, you are just hurrying the inevitable along."
B. "No, that is what lots of people believe but it is not true."
C. "Yes, it will cause quicker organ shut down."
D. "No, it will just keep him comfortable during this time."

The answer can be found on page 518

eRESOURCE

To reinforce your understanding of morphine, refer to Epocrates Online. [Pathway: http://online.epocrates.com ➔ under the "Drugs" tab, enter "Morphine" in the search field ➔ select "Morphine Sulfate" ➔ review "Patient Education."]

EXERCISE 7.30 Calculation:

Mr. Nevel is receiving morphine 15 mg by mouth every 4 hours as needed for pain. The oral solution that is in the home is 20 mg/5 mL. How much does Mrs. Nevel pour into the medication cup to administer to Mr. Nevel for one dose?

The answer can be found on page 518

EXERCISE 7.31 Calculation:

Mr. Nevel is receiving another medication and he needs to take two teaspoons four times a day as ordered. The container holds 500 mL of the medication. Mrs. Nevel asks you how long the bottle will last. What would be the correct response? Two teaspoons is how many mL?

The answer can be found on page 519

While in hospice care, Mrs. Nevel is having difficulty turning Mr. Nevel every 2 hours as there is no one else available and he is in a standard hospital bed. Sara calls the clinic to coordinate delivery of an air mattress. She teaches Mrs. Nevel how to place bed rolls in different spots to change the pressure points and provide comfort to Mr. Nevel.

Hospice care helps Mrs. Nevel with physical and emotional care of her husband. One of the goals of hospice nursing is to increase the quality of the client's remaining life. Working with the family to find ways to comfort their loved one is part of the role of the hospice nurse.

Sara asks Mrs. Nevel whether the family has advance directives.

EXERCISE 7.32 Fill in the blank:

What is the purpose of an advance directive?

The answer can be found on page 519

The staff at the health clinic is enlisted by the state-wide emergency system to develop a community disaster plan. The first part of the plan is staff education, which Sara volunteers to assist with. Martin is the regional representative for the state and an effective disaster educator. He holds conferences with the staff that include education, identification photos for emergency personal, and setting up practice disasters.

eRESOURCE

To reinforce your understanding of the clinic's role in disaster planning, view the video provided by Wellington-Dufferin-Guelph Public Health: *Public Health's Role in Emergency Preparedness and Management.* [Pathway: http://youtu.be/R0z6FRH4dYY]

EXERCISE 7.33 Matching:

Match the disaster in Column A with the type of disaster in Column B:

Column A	Column B
A. Toxic material	_______ Man made
B. Earthquake	_______ Natural
C. Floods	
D. Structural collapse	
E. Communicable disease epidemics	

The answer can be found on page 519

EXERCISE 7.34 Select all that apply:

Which of these terms are considered the three levels of a disaster?

A. Disaster identification
B. Disaster preparedness
C. Disaster recovery
D. Disaster isolation
E. Disaster response
F. Disaster aftermath

The answer can be found on page 519

eRESOURCE

As part of their training, the staff reviews the following materials:

- Disaster Preparedness from Ready.gov [Pathway: http://youtu.be/7CTj5KZk7eg]
- The Red Cross's *Prepare Your Home and Family* program. [Pathway: http://arcbrcr.org/#SITE]
- The Federal Emergency Management Agency's (FEMA) manual, *Are You Ready?* [Pathway: http://goo.gl/FTWGJ]

After a disaster, Martin explains to the staff at the center that there are populations in the community at high risk for disruption.

EXERCISE 7.35 Select all that apply:

The populations that are at *high* risk for disruptions post-disaster are:

A. Migrant workers
B. Families
C. People with chronic illness
D. Working adults
E. People new to the area

The answer can be found on page 520

The staff recognizes that it is important to provide culturally competent care even in emergency situations, so they are interested in becoming more culturally competent and better able to work effectively in high-stress, cross-cultural situations.

eRESOURCE

To provide culturally competent care in emergencies, review the U.S. Department of Heath & Human Services Office of Minority Health's resources:

- Cultural Competency Curriculum for Disaster Preparedness. [Pathway: http://goo.gl/cwb0a]
- RESPOND TOOL for emergency responders: Culturally Competent History Taking in a Crisis. [Pathway: http://goo.gl/1xazu5]

Martin explains the use of the triage system in disaster nursing.

EXERCISE 7.36 Matching:

Match the color in Column A with the definition of its use in Column B:

Column A	Column B
A. Red	___ Dying or dead. Catastrophic injuries. No hope for survival.
B. Yellow	___ Third priority. Minimal injuries with no systemic complications. Treatment delayed several hours.
C. Green	___ First priority for nursing care. Life-threatening injuries. No delay in treatment.
D. Black	___ Urgent, second priority. Injuries with complications. Treatment delayed 30 to 60 minutes.

The answer can be found on page 520

eRESOURCE

To reinforce your understanding of disaster triage, view:

- University of Nebraska Medical Center's *START Triage Basics video*. [Pathway: http://youtu.be/9QHDs10e-G0]
- The National Institute of Health's Web Information System for Emergency Responders (WISER) *JumpSTART*:
  - Adult Triage Algorithm. [Pathway: http://goo.gl/kEvmF]
  - Pediatric Triage Algorithm. [Pathway: http://goo.gl/u8gu7]

The second part of the staff training is a day spent at the local airport doing a mock disaster with participants from the community. The disaster simulation was of a large plane making a crash landing with an emergency evacuation. The passengers and crew sustained multiple injuries and the triage nurses had to categorize them correctly to save lives and expedient appropriate care.

EXERCISE 7.37 Matching:

Match the situation in Column A to the red, yellow, green, or black triage label in Column B:

Column A	Column B
A. Child unconscious with a head injury	________ Red
B. Adult male with a broken femur	________ Yellow
C. Adult male with chest pain	________ Green
D. Adult female crying with hysteria	________ Black
E. Adult female with extensive internal injuries and a weak pulse who is unconscious with no respirations	
F. Young adult male with profuse bleeding from the femoral artery	
G. Child with 40% burns	
H. A child who is cyanotic with no pulse or respirations	

The answer can be found on page 521

Another important aspect of disaster nursing is understanding bioterrorism in the form of *biological* or *chemical* agents. Rapid identification of the agent is critical to the triage and protection of first responders.

EXERCISE 7.38 Fill in the blanks:

This is when there is an intentional release of an agent used to cause death or disability to others.

____

Bacteria that form spores that can be cutaneous, inhaled, or digested. There is a vaccine available that has not been made available to the general public to date. ________________

Bacteria found in rodents and fleas spread in droplets from which pneumonia develops. There is no vaccine but treatment is available with antibiotics. ________________

A toxin made by bacteria that is food borne; it produces muscle weakness; there is no vaccine; supportive care is the available treatment. ________________

Variola virus aerosol that when released with close contact will spread the disease. High fever and body aches with raised bumps and scabs result. ________________

Francisella tularensis, a highly infectious bacterium from animals that produces skin ulcers and pneumonia in humans. ________________

Causes bleeding under the skin and in organs; transmitted by rodents and person to person. It consists of four families of viruses such as Ebola. ________________

Poison made from waste of processing castor beans. Miniscule amount can kill if inhaled or injected.

____

A chemical made by humans that is odorless, tasteless, and produces a clear liquid similar to a pesticide. This chemical can be spread in the air, water, or on clothing. ________________

Manufactured or natural, high doses can cause a syndrome with nausea, vomiting, and diarrhea; can lead to cancer. ________________

This product causes blistering of the mucous membranes and the skin. It may smell like garlic or mustard when it is released as a vapor. ______________

This weapon, when set off, releases a mix of explosives with radioactive dust. ______________

The answer can be found on page 521

---

eRESOURCE

To verify your answers, consult Wireless Information System for Emergency Responders (WISER) on your mobile device. [Pathway: http://wiser.nlm.nih.gov ➔ select "Help Identify" and enter characteristics of unknown substances.]

According to Martin, nurses who are working in a disaster situation should look at strategies for dealing with stress.

EXERCISE 7.39 Select all that apply:

Select the strategies for dealing with stress:

A. Avoid humor
B. Keep a hourly log
C. Get enough sleep
D. Stay in touch with family
E. Provide peer support

The answer can be found on page 522

Sara returns to work after a day off and on her drive to the clinic observed a correctional facility as well as the bathing suit manufacturer. Community health nursing looks at the community as a partner. She discusses her findings with Kendra, a nurse practitioner at the nurse-run health center.

Kendra, a long-time local resident of the community as well as a nurse practitioner at the health center, explains to Sara that the penitentiary, which presently houses women prisoners, has been part of the fabric of the community since the 1800s. There are correctional nurses who are employed full time at the penitentiary. Kendra has worked for the penitentiary providing nursing services to both the inmates as well as the penitentiary staff. Kendra explains to Sara that the number of women who are incarcerated is increasing at a higher rate than that for men. These women may experience some additional health care needs such as pregnancy and childbirth as well as routine gynecological care.

EXERCISE 7.40 Select all that apply:

Select the roles of the nurse working in a prison system:

A. Health education
B. Dependent care

C. Self-care
D. Policy development
E. Self-care and safety education

The answer can be found on page 522

EXERCISE 7.41 Multiple-choice:

What would be an example of primary prevention in the correctional facility?

A. Suicide prevention
B. Providing first aid
C. Gynecological examination
D. Counseling

The answer can be found on page 522

Sara realizes that the women in the prison represent part of the vulnerable populations found within the U.S. population.

EXERCISE 7.42 Multiple-choice:

Which of the following correctly defines *vulnerability*?

A. Higher probability of an illness
B. Susceptibility to a negative occurrence
C. Lack of resources to meet basic needs
D. Lack of adequate resources over an extended period of time

The answer can be found on page 522

Sara recalls another important section of vulnerability, a facet called *disenfranchisement.*

EXERCISE 7.43 Fill in the blank:

***Disenfranchisement* is defined as:**

The answer can be found on page 522

Kendra explained to Sara that the bathing suit factory has a full-time occupational nurse. Sara recalls that occupational health has been a profession since Ada Stewart was hired by the Vermont Marble Company in 1895.

EXERCISE 7.44 Select all that apply:

When doing an assessment of the work environment, which of the following should the occupational health nurse focus on?

A. Type of work performed by each employee
B. Safety policy and procedures
C. Suicide procedures
D. Personal health care insurance utilization
E. Exposure to toxins in the workplace

The answer can be found on page 523

EXERCISE 7.45 Matching:

Match the terms in Column A with the definitions in Column B:

Column A	Column B
A. OSHA	___ Compensation that is given after a work injury
B. Occupational health hazards	___ Occupational Safety and Health Administration
C. Workers' compensation	___ Conditions or a process that may put the worker at risk
D. Hazards	___ In the epidemiologic triangle, this would be a host
E. Worker	___ In the epidemiologic triangle, this would be an agent

The answer can be found on page 523

One group of workers that may be overlooked in the United States is the migrant worker. These workers move from place to place as the work becomes available. They have the same basic health needs as others, as well as some that are specific to the type of job being performed.

EXERCISE 7.46 Select all that apply:

When doing a health assessment with a migrant worker, what should the nurse be sure to include?

A. Type of work performed
B. Hours worked each day
C. Housing conditions
D. Cultural considerations
E. Disease-prevention education
F. Availability for telehealth
G. Exposures to toxins in the workplace

The answer can be found on page 523

Now that Sara has a better understanding of the community surrounding the health center, she begins to look at the people who live in the neighborhood. On her list of home visits today are Ms. Jackson, a single mother, and her 2-year-old daughter, Wanda. The child has been diagnosed with an elevated lead level and will need follow-up care. Sara introduces herself and begins with a family assessment.

EXERCISE 7.47 Select the correct response:

An assessment drawing using circles, squares, and line connections that shows the family health history over the past generations is called an (*ecomap/genogram*)?

The answer can be found on page 524

EXERCISE 7.48 Fill in the blank:

Lead intoxication is highest in children younger than ________________.

The answer can be found on page 524

EXERCISE 7.49 Fill in the blanks:

The common sources of lead intoxication in children:

____

____

____

____

____

____

____

The answer can be found on page 524

EXERCISE 7.50 Multiple-choice:

Wanda had her blood lead levels checked. A diagnosis of lead intoxication is confirmed when the blood lead level is higher than?

A. 8 mcg/dL
B. 9 mcg/dL
C. 10 mcg/dL
D. 11 mcg/dL

The answer can be found on page 524

EXERCISE 7.51 Fill in the blanks:

Make two nutritional recommendations for a child with a high lead level:

1. ______________________________
2. ______________________________

The answer can be found on page 525

Wanda's repeat lead level was 10 mcg/dL. When Sara arrives at the home she discusses with Ms. Jackson ways to prevent Wanda from having further exposure to lead.

EXERCISE 7.52 Fill in the blanks:

List at least two recommendations to prevent lead exposure in a child:

1. ______________________________
2. ______________________________

The answer can be found on page 525

---

eRESOURCE

To reinforce your understanding of lead poisoning, refer to Medscape on your mobile device. [Pathway: Medscape → enter "Lead" into the search field → select "Lead Toxicity" and review content.]

EXERCISE 7.53 Select all that apply:

Safety is another concern when rearing a 2-year-old. Which of the following are appropriate parent teaching safety guides for this age group?

A. Lock the cabinets
B. Wear seat belts
C. Cover electrical outlets
D. Cross the street at cross-walks
E. Use safety gates on stairs
F. Bicycle safety on the street

The answer can be found on page 525

---

eRESOURCE

To reinforce her teaching, Sarah uses the following:

- *Lead Poisoning: Words to Know from A to Z.* [Pathway: http://goo.gl/YO4wx]
- A short video, Lead Awareness for Parents. [Pathway: http://youtu.be/C0HnWFrQlo4]
- The Lead Safety Video. [Pathway: http://youtu.be/WQmrYudUloQ]
- A pamphlet *Know the Facts:* A fact sheet with general lead poisoning prevention information. [Pathway: http://www.cdc.gov/nceh/lead/tools/Know_the_Facts.pdf]

- Additional educational materials are available from the CDC. [Pathway: www.cdc.gov/nceh/lead/tips.htm]

Sara discusses with Ms. Jackson follow-up for Wanda and the normal health and safety needs of a 2-year-old. After listening intently, Ms. Jackson states she is having problems making ends meet and is fearful she will lose her apartment and have no home. Ms. Jackson explains to Sara that she has extended family, and had been living with them but it was so crowded she moved into her own place more than a year ago. Sara places a call to Sierra, one of the community outreach workers to see whether she can help Ms. Jackson.

EXERCISE 7.54 Fill in the blank:

Poverty is defined as ________________________________

The answer can be found on page 525

eRESOURCE

To reinforce your understanding of the impact of poverty on vulnerable populations, view:

- The current federal poverty income guidelines. [Pathway: http://goo.gl/n2VhO or http://goo.gl/Jiabq]
- Download the U.S. Census Bureau's mobile app. [Pathway: www.census.gov/mobile]

EXERCISE 7.55 Matching:

Match the terms in Column A with the definitions in Column B:

Column A	Column B
A. Family	___ A state of being that evolves and includes all aspects of human living, such as emotional, biological, social, and cultural
B. Empowerment	___ The configuration and makeup of the family unit, including gender and age
C. Family structure	___ Situations in which the demands on the family exceed the family's available resources and coping capabilities
D. Family crisis	___ The events that alter the structure of the family, such as marriage, birth, and death
E. Family health	___ Self-defined group of two or more people who depend on each other to meet physical, emotional, and financial needs
F. Family interactions	___ The process of assisting others to gain the knowledge and authority to make informed decisions

The answer can be found on page 526

Sierra identifies options to assist Ms. Jackson with her housing needs. Ms. Jackson is presently on welfare and is participating in the Special Supplemental Nutrition Program for Women, Infants, and Children (WIC). Her concern is that she may not be able to afford to live in her apartment much longer. Ms. Jackson is scared she will be forced to live on the streets with her small daughter.

EXERCISE 7.56 Fill in the blank:

WIC stands for ______________________________

The answer can be found on page 526

Sierra and Sara discuss the issue of homelessness in the neighborhood. With the upcoming cold months, Sierra explains about the potential health problems that are commonly seen in this population. Within the city, if the weather is going to be very cold and severe, a Code Winter will be called. At that time, the homeless will be helped into shelters and will be mandated not to leave the shelter during the day until after the code has been deactivated.

Sara volunteers at the local shelter and is scheduled to work during the middle of a winter storm. During this Code Winter experience, Sara has the opportunity to meet many of the clients who come into the shelter seeking warmth and food. One of the clients, Ava, often comes to the nurse's office seeking help for her young daughter. Emma is a 3-year-old child who lives with her mother, moving from shelter to shelter or living on the streets. Emma has crusty, honey-colored drainage from a sore under her nose.

EXERCISE 7.57 Matching:

Match the terms in Column A with the definitions in Column B:

Column A	Column B
A. Eczema	___ Usually appear as burrows in the skin
B. Head lice	___ Bright red rash
C. Periorbital cellulitis	___ Can return to school 48 hours after treatment has begun
D. Impetigo	___ A chronic, superficial skin problem with severe itching
E. Acne vulgaris	___ Diffuse redness at the site with pitting edema usually present
F. Diaper rash	___ Also called *pediculosis capitis*
G. Scabies	___ Usually caused by inflammation of the sebaceous glands

The answer can be found on page 526

Emma is referred to the nurse practitioner (NP) for treatment of her impetigo. Sara follows up with the mother regarding her needs.

eRESOURCE

To reinforce your understanding of impetigo, refer to Medscape on your mobile device. [Pathway: Medscape ➔ enter "Impetigo" into the search field ➔ select "Impetigo" and review content.]

EXERCISE 7.58 Multiple-choice:

Which homeless population is the fastest growing?

A. Young men
B. Elders
C. Families
D. Older women

The answer can be found on page 527

EXERCISE 7.59 Select all that apply:

What are the causes of homelessness?

A. Living above the poverty line
B. An increase in the availability of affordable housing
C. Addiction to substances such as drugs or alcohol
D. Loss of affordable rentals
E. Job losses and changes in the financial market
F. Mental illness

The answer can be found on page 527

Ava is complaining of problems with her feet. Sara and Ava sit down to look at what may be the problem. Sara assesses not only Ava's feet, but her overall health status. Sara completes her assessment of Ava and Emma, and ends her shift at the shelter.

EXERCISE 7.60 Select all that apply:

What are some of the common health problems that are seen with the homeless population?

A. Mental health problems
B. Trauma to the skin
C. Regular screenings
D. Respiratory problems

The answer can be found on page 528

Members of vulnerable populations, such as Ava and Emma, may also be at risk for potential violence and abuse.

EXERCISE 7.61 Fill in the blank:

Violence is defined as ______________________________

The answer can be found on page 528

Examples of violent acts or behaviors would be homicide, rape, assault, child abuse and neglect, as well as suicide. Nurses need to recognize potential factors in order to intervene when necessary. When looking at abuse and the family structure, the nurse needs to be aware of the potential for elder, child, sexual, physical, and emotional abuse that may occur and also be cognizant of the responsibility to report suspected abuse.

eRESOURCE

For current information on state laws regarding mandatory reporters of child abuse and neglect, visit the U.S. Department of Health & Human Services Child Welfare Information Gateway. [Pathway: http://goo.gl/avVnR]

EXERCISE 7.62 Fill in the blanks:

The two categories of child neglect are ______________ and ____________________.

The answer can be found on page 528

The following week, Sara volunteers at a community resource center located two blocks from the nurse-centered clinic. Here she is working with Mark, a volunteer nurse at the facility. This site offers health services on a walk-in basis, which allows access for all in the community. Mark explains to Sara that the number of walk-in clients will vary depending on both the weather and the activities that may be going on within the community. Mark explains that some of the frequently requested services are sexually transmitted infection (STI) testing, HIV testing, and vaccinations. He explains that many of the clients would like testing for both HIV and hepatitis. Mark asks Sara to offer some health-promotion education to the clients who come in today.

Sara meets Jorge, who has come in to get tested for HIV. Sara does a cheek swab and while they are waiting for the results discusses HIV prevention with Jorge.

EXERCISE 7.63 Select all that apply:

Select the common routes by which HIV can be transmitted:

A. Contact with someone who has nausea and is HIV positive
B. Casual contact with an HIV-positive person
C. Perinatal transmission for previous children of a now-positive HIV mother
D. Sexual contact with an HIV-positive person
E. Contact with blood infected with HIV

The answer can be found on page 528

Jorge's results come back positive. Further lab work is ordered to verify the findings, as well as to evaluate Jorge's hepatitis status. Mark further discusses with Jorge some various aspects of his HIV status, beginning with medications. Jorge asks whether there are certain things he should avoid with his HIV status.

EXERCISE 7.64 Multiple-choice:

To decrease the risk of developing resistance to the antiretroviral medication, the client should:

A. Take at least two different antiretroviral medications at one time
B. Take at least three different antiretroviral medications at one time
C. Take at least four different antiretroviral medications at one time
D. Take at least five different antiretroviral medications at one time

The answer can be found on page 529

EXERCISE 7.65 Select the correct response:

A live vaccine, such as rubella or varicella, (*should/should not*) be given to an HIV-positive person who has a low CD4 cell count.

The answer can be found on page 529

EXERCISE 7.66 Multiple-choice:

For an HIV-positive client, toxoplasmosis is an opportunistic infection. One way to prevent this infection is to avoid:

A. Raking leaves
B. Cleaning cat litter
C. Cutting the grass
D. Emptying the vacuum bag

The answer can be found on page 529

---

eRESOURCE

To reinforce your understanding of HIV, refer to Medscape on your mobile device. [Pathway: Medscape → enter "HIV" into the search field → select "HIV Disease" and review content.]

Jorge asks Mark how he will know when his HIV is under control. Mark explains that they would like his viral load to be undetectable.

EXERCISE 7.67 Multiple-choice:

An undetectable viral load means:

A. The client can say that the virus is gone.
B. The amount of virus in the clients blood is so low it cannot be found using the current lab tests.
C. The client can no longer transmit the virus.
D. The client will no longer need to use any protection when having sex.

The answer can be found on page 529

Jorge has no further questions for Mark and Sara. But before he leaves, Sara instructs him on how to clean up if he has any blood spills.

EXERCISE 7.68 Select the correct response:

A dilution of bleach is an inexpensive and effective way to clean up and disinfect. The dilution should be (*1:1/1:10*) dilution of household bleach.

The answer can be found on page 529

Sara completes her time at the community resource center for the day.

Answers

EXERCISE 7.1 Matching:

Match the terms in Column A with the definitions in Column B:

Column A	Column B
A. Community-based nursing (CBN)	C Health care of populations
B. Community-oriented nursing	B Health care focus is the aggregate or community group
C. Public health nursing (PHN)	A Illness care of individuals across the life span

EXERCISE 7.2 Matching:

Using the following list, add to Column B the type of prevention found in Column A:

- 1 for primary prevention
- 2 for secondary prevention
- 3 for tertiary prevention

Column A	Column B
Disease prevention	1
Health promotion	1
Admission for cardiac rehab	3
Prenatal group education	1
Outpatient mental health treatment	2
Exercise programs for seniors	1

EXERCISE 7.3 True/False:

Sara accesses the following demographic trends for the population:

A. *Replacement* means that for every person who dies another is born.

__X__ **True**

B. Immigration does not impact the U.S. population.

__X__ **False**

C. Women are beginning to have babies at later ages in this society.

__X__ **True**

D. The average age of the population is increasing.

__X__ **True**

E. Large numbers of baby boomers are dying off.

__X__ **False**

F. Asians comprise the fastest growing immigrant population.

__X__ **True**

EXERCISE 7.4 Select all that apply:

Select all the social and economic factors that affect health care trends in the community setting:

A. Cost—**YES; this is an important consideration for most people.**
B. Age distribution of the population—**YES; this will help health care providers decide the correct approach.**
C. Workforce trends—**YES; this will clue health care providers to occupational hazards.**
D. Season—NO; all seasons have concerns.
E. Access—**YES; health care access is a concern for many populations.**
F. Technology—**YES; appropriate technology can increase health care literacy and information.**
G. Attitude—NO; attitude should not decrease access to health care.

EXERCISE 7.5 Select all that apply:

Select all the factors that the nurse looks at when completing a community assessment:

A. Environment—**YES; document any areas of pollution, health hazards, physical barriers, and hangout areas that may impact the residents.**

B. Perceptions of health needs within the community—**YES; this can be gathered from key informants while completing a community assessment.**

C. Cost to complete the assessment—NO; it is important that the nurse has completed an assessment of the community in order to begin to understand the needs of the residents.

D. Housing and conditions—**YES; the nurse must determine what are the conditions of housing, the types of housing, and the problems related to housing and zoning in the community.**

E. Barriers to health care—**YES; this may be observed with handicapped individuals who are unable to access the health center or access health care options.**

F. Playgrounds and open spaces—**YES; the nurse needs to assess where these are, their conditions, how many there are, their quality, whether they offer shade, and assess any safety concerns.**

G. Services offered—**YES; the nurse needs to assess the services offered, such as recreation centers, health care providers, dentists, availability of a pharmacy, food markets, and availability of public transportation.**

EXERCISE 7.6 Select all that apply:

Select the skills performed by the home care nurse:

A. Skilled assessments—**YES; this is a skill completed by the home health nurse.**

B. Wound care—**YES; this is a skill completed by the home health nurse.**

C. Simple well-child care—NO; this is not a routine service of a home health nurse.

D. Coordination of care—**YES; this is a skill completed by the home health nurse.**

E. Wellness teaching—NO; this is not a routine service of a home health nurse.

EXERCISE 7.7 Select all that apply:

The components of home care that must be considered by the nurse are:

A. Development of a personal relationship—NO; the relationship is a professional one between the nurse and the client.

B. Contracting—**YES; this is vital to the professional nurse–client relationship.**

C. No goals or outcomes established—NO; goals must be established with the client to meet both short- and long-term needs.

EXERCISE 7.8 Multiple-choice:

In order to communicate with Mrs. Hernandez, what should Sara do?

A. Ask a neighbor to interpret—NO; this is against confidentiality rules and you are never sure of the level of interpretation of health care terms.

B. Use pictures books—NO; this is developmentally inappropriate.

C. Write the instructions down in English for later interpretation—NO; this is not culturally sensitive.

D. Use an approved interpreter—**YES; you must use an interpreter with an understanding of the medical terminology. Bear in mind that the gender, age, and relationship of the interpreter may be important when interacting with the client.**

EXERCISE 7.9 Multiple-choice:

Mrs. Hernandez's leg wound is draining. What is the priority precaution Sara should use with the dressing change?

A. Cleanse the wound with hydrogen peroxide—NO; this causes irritation to healthy tissue.

B. Continue to assess for potential problems with infection control—**YES; this is a priority for Sara while caring for Mrs. Hernandez.**

C. Cleanse the wound beginning at the outer aspect—NO; begin cleansing from the inner aspect and move outward.

D. Keep the leg in a dependent position during dressing change—NO; ideally, place the leg in a position that allows for good visibility and assessments.

EXERCISE 7.10 Matching:

Match the symptom in Column A with the condition in Column B using the following choices:

A. Hypoglycemia

B. Hyperglycemia

Column A	Column B
Hunger, pallor	A
Increased frequency of urination	B
Increased thirst	B
Also called *insulin reaction*	A
Sweating, anxiety	A
Headache	B
Diabetic ketoacidosis (DKA)	B
Increased incidence with insulin versus oral medication	A
Hypotensive, tachycardia	B
Decreased reflexes	B
Caused by unplanned exercise	A
Too little food	A
Consuming too much food or too many calories	B

EXERCISE 7.11 Matching:

Match the terms in Column A with the cultural competencies explained in Column B:

Column A	Column B
A. Cultural awareness	D The process in which one can communicate and interact with others, taking into account their cultural background
B. Cultural knowledge	E The internal motivation to provide care that is culturally competent
C. Cultural skill	A The process of evaluating one's own beliefs and values
D. Cultural encounter	B The ability to gather information about other cultures and ethnicities
E. Cultural desire	C The ability to gather and assess information to meet the needs of a group

Source: Stanhope and Lancaster (2013).

EXERCISE 7.12 Multiple-choice:

Because there is a parking garage under the apartment, what is the first environmental concern?

A. Fire—NO; this is important, but not the first concern.
B. Carbon monoxide—**YES; client education would include the knowing signs and symptoms of carbon monoxide poisoning. These include dizziness, nausea, vomiting, headache, fatigue, and loss of consciousness.**
C. Ozone—NO; this is important, but not the first concern.
D. Allergens—NO; this is important, but not the first concern.

EXERCISE 7.13 Multiple-choice:

Because Mrs. Hernandez lives in a two-story walk up, what is the first safety concern?

A. Doors—NO; this is not the first concern.
B. Social isolation—NO; not a safety concern.
C. No handrails on the outside stairs—**YES; this is a priority safety concern.**
D. Ability to drive—NO; not the first concern.

EXERCISE 7.14 Multiple-choice:

Sara knows that the people in her community have the right to know about hazardous materials in their community environment. Where would Sara find this information?

A. Hazard Communication Standard—NO; this provides information to ensure safety in the workplace.
B. Task Force on the Environment—NO; there is no such organization.
C. Environmental Protection Agency (EPA) Envirofacts—**YES; here one can view environmental information by zip code (EPA Envirofacts found at http://www.epa.gov).**
D. Consumer Confidence Report—NO; this provides water information to customers.

EXERCISE 7.15 Select all that apply:

Sara should bear which of the following in mind when using an interpreter?

A. Use anyone who is around; anyone will do—NO; this may cause misinterpretation of information as well as a breach of confidentiality.

B. Observe the client for nonverbal cues as the information is being delivered—**YES; this will help in the understanding of what is being discussed.**

C. Select an interpreter who has knowledge of medical terminology—**YES; this will help ensure that the correct information is being relayed.**

D. Let the interpreter summarize the client's own words—NO; have the interpreter repeat exactly what the client stated, for exactness.

EXERCISE 7.16 Multiple-choice:

Mrs. Hernandez is instructed to wash her greens well to prevent which two preventable food contaminants?

A. Methacillin-resistant *Staphylococcus aureus* (MRSA) and *Salmonella*—NO; *Salmonella* is usually a food contaminant but MRSA is a bacteria that lives on people's skin and in their nasal cavity.

B. *Escherichia coli* (E. coli) and *Clostridium difficile* (C. diff)—NO; *C. diff* is usually a gastrointestinal bacterium that is caused by antibiotic use and is prevalent in the elderly in extended care facilities. *E. coli* is usually found in the gastrointestinal tract, but it may cause food poisoning in humans.

C. *C. diff* and MRSA—NO; this is usually not the reason.

D. *E. coli* and *Salmonella*—**YES; both organisms can be transmitted by contact.**

EXERCISE 7.17 Select all that apply:

Sara knows that Mrs. Hernandez is 72 years old and should receive the following yearly immunization:

A. Influenza—**YES; this should be received annually in the fall.**

B. Varicella—NO; this is not a yearly vaccine, but one that is done in two separate doses in 4- to 8-week intervals for susceptible individuals.

C. Pneumococcal polysaccharide—NO; this vaccine would be given if it has been more than 5 years since the last vaccination or if it was given before the age of 65 years. It would be important to document when this vaccine was last given.

D. Meningococcal vaccine—NO; not usually given at this age.

EXERCISE 7.18 Multiple-choice:

Which would be the appropriate needle gauge, needle size, and site to administer an intramuscular (IM) immunization to Mrs. Hernendez, who weighs 148 lb?

A. Anterolateral site, 22–25 gauge, 1 in. needle size—NO; this is for a 1- to 12-month-old infant.

B. Deltoid or anterolateral site, 22–25 gauge, 1–1¼ in. needle size—NO; this is for a 3- to 18-year-old person.

C. Deltoid site, 22–25 gauge, 1–1½ in. needle size—**YES; this is the appropriate choice for an adult who weighs between 130 and 200 lb.**

D. Anterolateral site, 22–25 gauge, 5/8 in. needle size—NO; this is for a newborn younger than 28 days.

EXERCISE 7.19 True/False:

Shake the vial vigorously to obtain uniform suspension of solution.

_X_ True; you do shake the vial to obtain a uniform solution, do not use if discolored or if particulates are in the vaccine. Always refer to the packaging instructions with each vaccine administration.

EXERCISE 7.20 Fill in the blanks:

Discuss what criteria must be documented after administration of a vaccine:

Type of vaccine
Date given
Vaccine lot number and manufacturer information
Source: either, federal, state, or private supported
Site administered, RA (right arm), LA (left arm), LT (left thigh), RT (right thigh), IN (intranasal)
Vaccine information statement with publication date of the information sheet documented as well as the date given
Signature of the person administering the vaccine

EXERCISE 7.21 Matching:

Match the explanations in Column B that are used to describe the three domains of learning in Column A:

Column A	Column B
A. Affective domain	_C_ In this domain, the learner performs a learned skill using motor skills
B. Cognitive domain	_B_ In this domain, the learner gets the information, integrates this into his or her values system, and adopts these values to change his or her attitude; a person needs much support to develop these new behaviors
C. Psychomotor domain	_A_ In this domain, the learner recalls the information, can use the information, and understands the value of what has been learned

EXERCISE 7.22 Riveredge High School Health Questionnaire (Multiple-choice):

Hello Students and Faculty,

This is an anonymous questionnaire to find out how much we all know about community-associated methicillin-resistant *S. aureus* (CA-MRSA), as it has become a common community health issue.

Please feel free to make comments on the back of the paper. We look forward to developing an educational program suited to your needs.

Please return your completed questionnaire to the locked box located outside the health office on the first floor of the high school.

Thank you, Riveredge Community Care School Nurses

1. What is MRSA?
   A. A skin infection—**YES; it is a skin infection that can turn systemic.**
   B. A parasitic infection—NO; it is not a parasite, it is a bacteria.
   C. A food-borne disease—NO; it is spread by contact.
   D. A vector-borne disease—NO; it is spread by contact.
2. How long can MRSA live on surfaces?
   A. Less than 1 hour—NO; it can live on surfaces longer.
   B. More than 1 hour—NO; it can live on surfaces longer.
   C. One day—NO; it can live on surfaces longer.
   D. Days, weeks, or months—**YES; depending on the surface.**
3. What are some of the health care practices that would reduce the spread of MRSA? Select all that apply:
   A. Washing hands—**YES.**
   B. Spraying rooms with disinfectant—NO; studies show this is not helpful.
   C. Washing floors—NO; studies show this is not helpful.
   D. Washing equipment surfaces—**YES; wash any equipment that touches bare skin.**
   E. Covering lesions on your skin—**YES; covering lesions makes them less likely to be contaminated.**
   F. Sharing sports gear—NO; this may spread the infection.
4. What does MRSA look like?
   A. Looks like a scab
   B. **Looks like a pimple or boil**
   C. Looks like a scratch
   D. Looks like a blackhead
5. Do I have to launder my school clothes separately?
   A. Yes—NO; regular laundering is sufficient.
   B. **No**
6. Please list any comments or concerns!

EXERCISE 7.23 Multiple-choice:

A *risk factor* is defined as:

A. Probability that the event will occur over a specified period of time—**YES; an event that very well may occur.**
B. Measurement of the frequency of an event over time—NO; this is the *rate*.
C. Measurement of an existing disease currently in a population—NO; this is the *prevalence*.
D. The rate of disease is unusually high in a population—NO; this is an *epidemic* because it exceeds the usual or *endemic* rate.

EXERCISE 7.24 Matching:

Match the infections in Column B that are used to describe the four main categories of infectious agents in Column A:

Column A	Column B
A. Bacteria	C Pinworm—itching around anus, usually seen in small children
B. Fungi	D West Nile—mild flu-like symptoms
C. Parasite	B Ring worm—red, round, raised bumpy patch on the skin
D. Viruses	A Salmonellosis—sudden onset of headache, abdominal pain, diarrhea, nausea, and fever; onset 48 hours after ingestion

EXERCISE 7.25 Matching:

Match the level of prevention in Column A with the goal of each level in Column B:

Column A	Column B
A. Primary	C Reduces complications or disabilities with rehabilitation and optimal function
B. Secondary	A Reduces the incidence of disease by focusing on health education and health promotion
C. Tertiary	B Uses screening to prevent the severity of disease once it has happened, treating the problem

EXERCISE 7.26 Matching:

Match the level of prevention in Column A with the effort of each level in Column B:

Column A	Column B
A. Primary	B Checking all student athletes for lesions
B. Secondary	A Cleaning the wrestling mats
C. Tertiary	A Sending home information in a handout
	C Referring students with lesions to their primary care provider (PCP)
	A Developing a poster to hang in the cafeteria for information

EXERCISE 7.27 Exhibit-format:

The nurse accesses the parental population through school records and finds the following facts and statistics:

- Only 55% of the homes have an Internet connection
- 36% speak Spanish in the home
- 82% of the parents have a high school diploma
- 15% of the parents are college educated
- 65% are working, single-parent families

According to this information, what format would you choose to educate families about community-associated methicillin-resistant *S. aureus* (CA-MRSA)?

A. Internet tutorial—NO; you may only reach 55%.
B. Phone call during school hours—NO; 65% work.
C. DVD that can be played in any computer—NO; they may not take it outside the house if they do not have a computer.
D. Take-home information sheet written at a fourth- to sixth-grade level—**YES; for this population, this is the best choice.**

EXERCISE 7.28 Fill in the blanks:

Understanding case management.

Case management uses the **nursing** process to help the client obtain the necessary services.

Case management is a **liaison** between the client and all disciplines that are involved in the client's care.

A case manager acts as a **patient advocate** by providing scientific and necessary information and supporting client decisions.

Good **communication skills** are necessary for case managers to interact with others.

EXERCISE 7.29 Select all that apply:

Mrs. Nevel tells Sara that if she gives Mr. Nevel morphine for his pain she feels as if she is killing him. How should Sara respond?

A. "Yes, you are just hurrying the inevitable along."—NO; morphine is used for comfort.
B. "No, that is what lots of people believe but it is not true."—**YES; this is true but not very therapeutic; it won't alter her current knowledge about it.**
C. "Yes, it will cause quicker organ shut down."—NO; this is untrue.
D. "No, it will just keep him comfortable during this time."—**YES; the objective of the intervention should be kept in the forefront of care.**

EXERCISE 7.30 Calculation:

Mr. Nevel is receiving morphine 15 mg by mouth every 4 hours as needed for pain. The oral solution that is in the home is 20 mg/5 mL. How much does Mrs. Nevel pour into the medication cup to administer to Mr. Nevel for one dose?

$$\frac{20\text{ mg}}{5\text{ mL}} = \frac{15\text{ mg}}{\times}$$

Cross multiply the 5 × 15 = 75

Divide the 75 by 20 for a result of 3.75 mL that Mrs. Nevel will pour out for Mr. Nevel. For accuracy of the dose, this may be easier for Mrs. Nevel to pull up into an oral medication syringe.

EXERCISE 7.31 Calculation:

Mr. Nevel is receiving another medication and he needs to take two teaspoons four times a day as ordered. The container holds 500 mL of the medication. Mrs. Nevel asks you how long the bottle will last. What would be the correct response? Two teaspoons is how many mL?

One teaspoon = 5 mL, therefore two teaspoons = 10 mL

10 mL four times a day = 40 mL/d

500 mL divided by 40 mL = 12.5 days that the bottle of medication will last

EXERCISE 7.32 Fill in the blank:

What is the purpose of an advance directive?

An advance directive allows the client to convey his or her medical wishes if he or she is unable to do so. Depending on the type of illness, this can be a multilevel directive. One type is a living will; another is durable power of attorney for health care (from http://www.nlm.nih.gov/medlineplus/advancedirectives.html).

EXERCISE 7.33 Matching

Match the disaster in Column A with the type of disaster in Column B:

Column A	Column B
A. Toxic material	A, D Man made
B. Earthquake	B, C, E Natural
C. Floods	
D. Structural collapse	
E. Communicable disease epidemics	

EXERCISE 7.34 Select all that apply:

Which of these terms are considered the three levels of a disaster?

A. Disaster identification—NO; disasters are usually easy to identify.

B. Disaster preparedness—**YES; this is the first stage in disaster planning. The plan must be simple and realistic as well as flexible to work with during a multitude of potential disasters. Health care professionals must also have a personal plan in place to avoid conflicts with family and workplace.**

C. Disaster recovery—**YES; this is the third and final stage in disaster planning in which all agencies join together to help rebuild the community involved. Lessons learned need to be identified at this level to prepare for any future events.**
D. Disaster isolation—NO; relief workers contain disasters but this is not always necessary.
E. Disaster response—**YES; this is the second stage in disaster planning with the goal of minimizing death and injury. Depending on the level and scope of the disaster, resources are allocated to assist responders.**
F. Disaster aftermath—NO; this is the same as recovery.

EXERCISE 7.35 Select all that apply:

The populations that are at *high* risk for disruptions post-disaster are:

A. Migrant workers—**YES; home and jobs are temporary, language may be a problem and this population may not know the resources that are available.**
B. Families—NO; they may be at risk, but not at high risk, as they usually have support systems in place as part of the community.
C. People with chronic illness—**YES; there may be difficulty controlling the disease process, they may not have access to their medications and storage of medications, such as refrigeration, or they may need power for ventilator or equipment.**
D. Working adults—NO; they are not usually at high risk.
E. People new to the area—**YES; they may not be aware of all the resources that are available.**

EXERCISE 7.36 Matching:

Match the color in Column A with the definition of its use in Column B:

Column A	Column B
A. Red	__D__ Dying or dead. Catastrophic injuries. No hope for survival.
B. Yellow	__C__ Third priority. Minimal injuries with no systemic complications. Treatment delayed several hours.
C. Green	__A__ First priority for nursing care. Life-threatening injuries. No delay in treatment.
D. Black	__B__ Urgent, second priority. Injuries with complications. Treatment delayed 30 to 60 minutes.

EXERCISE 7.37 Matching:

Match the situation in Column A to the red, yellow, green, or black triage label in Column B:

Column A	Column B
A. Child unconscious with a head injury	C, F Red
B. Adult male with a broken femur	A, G Yellow
C. Adult male with chest pain	B, D Green
D. Adult female crying with hysteria	E, H Black
E. Adult female with extensive internal injuries and a weak pulse who is unconscious with no respirations	
F. Young adult male with profuse bleeding from the femoral artery	
G. Child with 40% burns	
H. A child that is cyanotic with no pulse or respirations	

EXERCISE 7.38 Fill in the blanks:

This is when there is an intentional release of an agent used to cause death or disability to others. **Bioterrorism attack**

Bacteria that form spores that can be cutaneous, inhaled, or digested. There is a vaccine available that has not been made available to the general public to date. **Anthrax**

Bacteria found in rodents and fleas spread in droplets from which pneumonia develops. There is no vaccine but treatment is available with antibiotics. **Pneumonic plague**

A toxin made by bacteria that is food borne; it produces muscle weakness; there is no vaccine; supportive care is the available treatment. **Botulism**

Variola virus aerosol that when released with close contact will spread the disease. High fever and body aches with raised bumps and scabs result. **Smallpox**

Francisella tularensis, a highly infectious bacterium from animals that produces skin ulcers and pneumonia in humans. **Inhalation tularemia**

Causes bleeding under the skin and in organs; transmitted by rodents and person to person. It consists of four families of viruses such as Ebola. **Viral hemorrhagic fever**

Poison made from waste of processing castor beans. Miniscule amount can kill if inhaled or injected. **Ricin**

A chemical made by humans that is odorless, tasteless, and produces a clear liquid similar to a pesticide. This chemical can be spread in the air, water, or on clothing. **Sarin**

Manufactured or natural, high doses can cause a syndrome with nausea, vomiting, and diarrhea; can lead to cancer. **Radiation**

This product causes blistering of the mucous membranes and the skin. It may smell like garlic or mustard when it is released as a vapor. **Mustard gas**

This weapon, when set off, releases a mix of explosives with radioactive dust. **Dirty bomb**

EXERCISE 7.39 Select all that apply:

Select the strategies for dealing with stress:

A. Avoid humor—NO; humor has been shown to decrease stress if used appropriately.
B. Keep an hourly log—NO; journaling may help but by doing it every hour it may cause more stress.
C. Get enough sleep—**YES; this will decrease the stress reaction.**
D. Stay in touch with family—**YES; this will decrease the stress reaction.**
E. Provide peer support—**YES; this will decrease the stress reaction.**

EXERCISE 7.40 Select all that apply:

Select the roles of the nurse working in a prison system:

A. Health education—**YES; prisoners should be taught to care for themselves.**
B. Dependent care—NO; this is not part of the duty of the nurse, as the dependents are not housed within the prison system.
C. Self-care—**YES; prisoners should be able to care for themselves.**
D. Policy development—**YES; to maintain a safe and fair environment.**
E. Self-care and safety education—**YES; so everyone knows the safety rules.**

EXERCISE 7.41 Multiple-choice:

What would be an example of primary prevention in the correctional facility?

A. Suicide prevention—**YES; so everyone is aware of what signs to observe.**
B. Providing first aid—NO; secondary prevention.
C. Gynecological examination—NO; secondary prevention.
D. Counseling—NO; secondary prevention, possibly tertiary.

EXERCISE 7.42 Multiple-choice:

Which of the following correctly defines *vulnerability*?

A. Higher probability of an illness—NO; this is a risk, the possibility that some incident will occur within a period of time.
B. Susceptibility to a negative occurrence—**YES; vulnerability results from both internal and external influences that may increase the risk of developing undesirable health problems.**
C. Lack of resources to meet basic needs—NO; this is poverty.
D. Lack of adequate resources over an extended period of time—NO; this is persistent poverty.

EXERCISE 7.43 Fill in the blank:

Disenfranchisement is defined as:

A separation from the mainstream population through which the person may not have an emotional connection with any one social group. Some examples may be people who are homeless or who are migrant workers. Many people in the mainstream may not even notice these people as they walk by them on the streets.

EXERCISE 7.44 Select all that apply:

When doing an assessment of the work environment, which of the following should the occupational health nurse focus on?

A. Type of work performed by each employee—**YES; this is baseline data needed to assess the work environment.**
B. Safety policy and procedures—**YES; this will keep employees safe.**
C. Suicide procedures—NO; this may be a concern for a client in the prison system.
D. Personal health care insurance utilization—NO; this does not apply.
E. Exposure to toxins in the workplace—**YES; this is important for employee health.**

EXERCISE 7.45 Matching:

Match the terms in Column A with the definitions in Column B:

Column A	Column B
A. OSHA	C Compensation that is given after a work injury
B. Occupational health hazards	A Occupational Safety and Health Administration
C. Workers' compensation	B Conditions or a process that may put the worker at risk
D. Hazards	E In the epidemiologic triangle, this would be a host
E. Worker	D In the epidemiologic triangle, this would be an agent

EXERCISE 7.46 Select all that apply:

When doing a health assessment with a migrant worker, what should the nurse be sure to include?

A. Type of work performed—**YES; the exposure to any chemicals, the physical component of the job, the length of exposure to the repetition of the job all should be evaluated.**
B. Hours worked each day—**YES; this is important, as are how many days worked each week. The lifestyle of the worker may predispose him or her to added stress from the unknown, the housing, or the type of work he or she is performing.**
C. Housing conditions—**YES; the availability, conditions, sanitation, and crowding need to be evaluated. Many workers live in a trailer, or even in their cars if necessary to earn a living. Questions need to be raised about the location of the housing in relation to fields where pesticides are being used. Where are their children living? Where is the field equipment and pesticide storage in relation to the children and their play area?**
D. Cultural considerations—**YES; the nurse must be culturally competent when working with clients.**
E. Disease-prevention education—**YES; anticipatory guidance is critical when caring for a population that frequently travels. Other issues, such as dental care, childcare, and schooling concerns for the children, should also be addressed.**

F. Availability for telehealth—NO; this is not critical for the migrant worker.
G. Exposures to toxins in the workplace—**YES; having an understanding of the potential exposures that the worker may experience will assist the nurse in education. It will also assist in diagnosis by the practitioner.**

EXERCISE 7.47 Select the correct response:

An assessment drawing using circles, squares, and line connections that shows the family health history over the past generations is called an *ecomap*?

An ecomap is a drawing that looks at the social interactions that the family has with the outside environment and organizations. This may be helpful when looking at where Wanda may have had exposure to the lead.

EXERCISE 7.48 Fill in the blank:

Lead intoxication is highest in children younger than **6 years.**

EXERCISE 7.49 Fill in the blanks:

The common sources of lead intoxication in children:

Lead-based paint
Dust from lead-based paint
Lead-based solder
Lead in the soil
Painted toys and furniture made before 1978
Foreign pottery
Leaded crystal

EXERCISE 7.50 Multiple-choice:

Wanda had her blood lead levels checked. A diagnosis of lead intoxication is confirmed when the blood lead level is higher than?

A. 8 mcg/dL—NO; this is incorrect.
B. 9 mcg/dL—NO; this is incorrect.
C. 10 mcg/dL—**YES; this is correct, when there are two successive blood lead levels (1 month apart) greater than 10 mcg/dL, a diagnosis of lead poisoning is made. Levels need to be rechecked within 2 to 3 months for levels less than 19. For levels higher than 19, a repeat test is done within the week and the health department is referred to help with the home environment. With levels greater than 44 mcg/dL, the test is repeated within days and chelation therapy is begun.**
D. 11 mcg/dL—NO; this is incorrect.

EXERCISE 7.51 Fill in the blanks:

Make two nutritional recommendations for a child with a high lead level:

1. **Increase the intake of iron and calcium with foods such as eggs and dairy products, beans and red meats, broccoli, collard greens, and chicken and turkey.**
2. **Keep food out of lead crystal or imported pottery.**

EXERCISE 7.52 Fill in the blanks:

List at least two recommendations to prevent lead exposure in a child:

1. **Wash toys, hands, and objects that come in contact with lead dust.**
2. **Work with the child to keep objects and fingers out of the child's mouth.**
3. **Run tap water for 2 minutes in the morning before drinking or using water to make formula.**
4. **Eat a well-balanced diet.**
5. **Wash off any item that falls on the floor, such as spoons, bottles, cups, or pacifiers.**

EXERCISE 7.53 Select all that apply:

Safety is another concern when rearing a 2-year-old. Which of the following are appropriate parent teaching safety guides for this age group?

A. Lock the cabinets—**YES; any cabinet that stores chemicals, sharp objects, medication, or has objects that pose a safety risk should be locked. Anticipatory guidance is critical when working with families to address the next level of growth and development.**

B. Wear seat belts—NO; this would be for the child who is no longer in a child safety seat, and a 2-year-old should still be in a child safety seat.

C. Cover electrical outlets—**YES; covering outlets is necessary to prevent injury. Injuries are the number-one cause of death for individuals between the age of 1 and 34 years.**

D. Cross the street at cross-walks—NO; toddlers should not be crossing the street or going near the street alone. This age requires direct observation.

E. Use safety gates on stairs—**YES; gates are needed to prevent injury.**

F. Bicycle safety on the street—NO; this would begin with the preschooler who is just learning how to ride a bike; also the child should be riding the bike on the sidewalk.

EXERCISE 7.54 Fill in the blank:

Poverty is defined as **not having the means to support oneself. In the United States, poverty would be defined as an income that falls below the government-determined poverty line.**

EXERCISE 7.55 Matching:

Match the terms in Column A with the definitions in Column B:

Column A	Column B
A. Family	__E__ A state of being that evolves and includes all aspects of human living, such as emotional, biological, social, and cultural
B. Empowerment	__C__ The configuration and makeup of the family unit, including gender and age
C. Family structure	__D__ Situations in which the demands on the family exceed the family's available resources and coping capabilities
D. Family crisis	__F__ The events that alter the structure of the family, such as marriage, birth, and death
E. Family health	__A__ Self-defined group of two or more people who depend on each other to meet physical, emotional, and financial needs
F. Family interactions	__B__ The process of assisting others to gain the knowledge and authority to make informed decisions

EXERCISE 7.56 Fill in the blank:

WIC stands for **the Women, Infants, and Children program. This program is a government program that offers nutritional support assistance to pregnant or breastfeeding women, infants, and children up to the age of 5 years who may be at risk for nutritional deficits. There are income guidelines to be met to participate in this program.**

EXERCISE 7.57 Matching:

Match the terms in Column A with the definitions in Column B:

Column A	Column B
A. Eczema	__G__ Usually appear as burrows in the skin. **This is a contagious skin disorder. The mites burrow and their secretions are what causes the itch. They appear as linear gray burrows that may be difficult to see if the person has been scratching and irritation has occurred. To treat, scabicidal lotion is applied to cool, dry skin.**
B. Head lice	__F__ Bright red rash. **Inflammation in the diaper area usually in response to skin irritation. Most common cause is exposure to urine and stool.**
C. Periorbital cellulitis	
D. Impetigo	
E. Acne vulgaris	
F. Diaper rash	
G. Scabies	

(*continued*)

Column A	Column B
	__D__ Can return to school 48 hours after treatment has begun. **Usual treatment is application of a topical antibiotic ointment for 5 to 7 days. Good hand washing is critical as this is a highly contagious condition. Usually presents as a bullae, a fluid-filled lesion. When this bullae ruptures, a honey-like crusting occurs. This is usually secondary to a skin trauma.**
	__A__ A chronic, superficial skin problem with severe itching. **May be called atopic dermatitis. There are no lab tests for eczema, and treatment is usually with creams, topical steroids, and, if any skin breakdown, be aware of potential for infection.**
	__C__ Diffuse redness at the site with pitting edema usually present **with this acute inflammation.**
	__B__ Also called *pediculosis capitis.* **Head lice is a highly communicable parasite that is spread through direct contact. Usually seen on the hair shaft, close to the skin around the neck and ear.**
	__E__ Usually caused by inflammation of the sebaceous glands. **Skin should be cleaned twice a day, and medication therapy may be an option.**

EXERCISE 7.58 Multiple-choice:

Which homeless population is the fastest growing?

A. Young men—NO; this is not the fastest growing group, although older men and military veterans are populations that comprise the homeless population.
B. Elders—NO; this is not the fastest growing group.
C. Families—**YES; this is the fastest growing group of the homeless population.**
D. Older women—NO; this is not the fastest growing group.

EXERCISE 7.59 Select all that apply:

What are the causes of homelessness?

A. Living above the poverty line—NO; living below the poverty line is a cause.
B. An increase in the availability of affordable housing—NO; a decrease in affordable housing causes homelessness.

C. Addiction to substances such as drugs or alcohol—**YES; this is often linked to lack of funds, family, and home.**
D. Loss of affordable rentals—**YES; this happens in areas that are being revitalized.**
E. Job losses and changes in the financial market—**YES; this occurs in high-unemployment markets.**
F. Mental illness—**YES; this is a major cause of homelessness.**

EXERCISE 7.60 Select all that apply:

What are some of the common health problems that are seen with the homeless population?

A. Mental health problems—**YES; this population is at risk or may have a previous diagnosis of a mental health problem.**
B. Trauma to the skin—**YES; such as injuries or wounds are common.**
C. Regular screenings—NO; this is not a common health problem.
D. Respiratory problems—**YES; respiratory problems, such as tuberculosis, asthma, pneumonia, and infectious illnesses, affect the homeless population.**

EXERCISE 7.61 Fill in the blank:

Violence is defined as **a behavior or act that is often predictable and results in injury that is either physical or psychological to a person.**

EXERCISE 7.62 Fill in the blanks:

The two categories of child neglect are **physical** and **emotional**.

In the area of physical neglect, this is defined as not providing for the basic needs of the child in areas such as food, shelter, and medical care. In the area of emotional neglect, this involves not providing nurture, care, and helping the child meet the basic levels of growth and development.

EXERCISE 7.63 Select all that apply:

Select the common routes by which HIV can be transmitted:

A. Contact with someone who has nausea and is HIV positive—NO; HIV is not spread through casual contact such as someone who has nausea.
B. Casual contact with an HIV-positive person—NO; HIV is not spread through casual contact.
C. Perinatal transmission for previous children of a now-positive HIV mother—NO; HIV is not spread from a now-positive HIV mother to her previous children, with the understanding that she was HIV negative with the previous pregnancies. HIV transmission when pregnant is one of the most common routes of transmission for newborns.
D. Sexual contact with an HIV-positive person—**YES; this is a common route of transmission of HIV. This contact exposes a person to semen, vaginal secretions, and blood.**
E. Contact with blood infected with HIV—**YES; this can be either accidental, such as a splash with contaminated blood, sharing a contaminated needle, or unprotected sex.**

EXERCISE 7.64 Multiple-choice:

To decrease the risk of developing resistance to the antiretroviral medication, the client should:

A. Take at least two different antiretroviral medications at one time—NO; taking at least three different antiretroviral medications at one time will decrease the drug resistance for the client.
B. Take at least three different antiretroviral medications at one time—**YES; taking at least three different antiretroviral medications at one time will decrease the drug resistance for the client.**
C. Take at least four different antiretroviral medications at one time—NO; taking at least three different antiretroviral medications at one time will decrease the drug resistance for the client.
D. Take at least five different antiretroviral medications at one time—NO; taking at least three different antiretroviral medications at one time will decrease the drug resistance for the client.

EXERCISE 7.65 Select the correct response:

A live vaccine, such as rubella or varicella, ***should not*** be given to an HIV-positive person who has a low CD4 cell count.

Live vaccines should be avoided in an HIV-positive person who has a low CD4 cell count.

EXERCISE 7.66 Multiple-choice:

For an HIV-positive client, toxoplasmosis is an opportunistic infection. One way to prevent this infection is to avoid:

A. Raking leaves—NO; but it may be a good idea to wear gloves if one is bagging the leaves.
B. Cleaning cat litter—**YES; cleaning cat litter should be avoided as the cat feces may carry the parasite *Toxoplasma gondii*.**
C. Cutting the grass—NO; but one should wear gloves if gardening or digging in the soil.
D. Emptying the vacuum bag—NO; this should not be a means to be exposed to toxoplasmosis.

EXERCISE 7.67 Multiple-choice:

An undetectable viral load means:

A. The client can say that the virus is gone.—NO; although the viral load is undetectable, the client still has HIV.
B. The amount of virus in the client's blood is so low it cannot be found using the current lab tests. —**YES; an undetectable viral load means that the amount of virus in the blood is too low to be detected with present technology.**
C. The client can no longer transmit the virus.—NO; once the viral load is undetectable, the client will still have HIV and therefore the virus can be transmitted.
D. The client will no longer need to use any protection when having sex.—NO; the client will still have to use protection because the client still has HIV.

EXERCISE 7.68 Select the correct response:

A dilution of bleach is an inexpensive and effective way to clean up and disinfect. The dilution should be ***1:10*** dilution of household bleach.

A 1:10 dilution of household bleach is correct; one part bleach to 10 parts of water can be used to clean and disinfect.

Resources

American Nurses Association. (2013). *Public health nursing: Scope and standards of practice.* Silver Spring, MD: Nursesbooks.org.

Centers for Disease Control and Prevention. (n.d.). *Vaccines and immunizations.* Retrieved from http://www.cdc.gov/vaccines

Clark, M. J. (2008). *Community health nursing* (5th ed.). Upper Saddle River, NJ: Prentice Hall.

Garcia, C., Schaffer, M., & Schoon, P. (2014). *Population-based public health clinical manual: The Henry Street model for nurses* (2nd ed.). Indianapolis, IN: Sigma Theta Tau International.

Stanhope, M., & Lancaster, J. (2013). *Foundations of nursing in the community: Community-oriented practice* (4th ed.). St. Louis, MO: Mosby.

U.S. Department of Health and Human Services. (n.d.). *Healthy People 2020: About Healthy People 2020: Leading health indicators.* Retrieved from http://healthypeople.gov/2020/default.aspx

CHAPTER 8

Leadership and Management in Nursing

Cheryl Portwood

Nurses don't wait until October to celebrate Make a Difference Day—they make a difference every day!—Author Unknown

UNFOLDING CASE STUDY 1: Mark

Mark is a new "grad" who was successful on his first NCLEX-RN® try! He started his new job last year and completed the 6-week hospital orientation. Mark has good critical thinking skills and is the night charge nurse of a large 30-bed mixed medical–surgical unit. One of Mark's assets is that early in his career he was recognized as a patient advocate.

EXERCISE 8.1 Select all that apply:

The following are characteristics of advocacy:

A. Telling the patient his or her rights
B. Telling visitors the patient's rights
C. Directing patients' decisions to the best health care option
D. Explaining to patients that access to health is their responsibility
E. Providing the patient with information about his or her condition

The answer can be found on page 550

Mark usually has a reduced patient assignment when he works so that he can assist the other staff members to provide the central nursing office with bed availability updates and provide assistance to the staff in troubleshooting.

Mark listens to a conversation between two staff members; they are discussing the American Hospital Association (AHA) Patient Bill of Rights. Sara states that it has a new name and has been published in a plain-language document.

EXERCISE 8.2 Multiple-choice:

The Patient Bill of Rights is now titled:

A. The Family Bill of Rights
B. The Advocacy Document
C. The Patient Care Partnership
D. The Family Care Consensus

The answer can be found on page 550

On this particular night, Mr. B calls Mark into his room because he and his wife of 35 years are having difficulty deciding on treatment. Mr. B has stage IV lung cancer and does not want further chemotherapy or radiation. Mark understands Mrs. B's concerns and provides them with important information.

EXERCISE 8.3 Fill in the blank:

Mark understands that under the Patient Self-Determination Act that was passed in 1991 he should ask Mr. B if he has what important document completed?

____

The answer can be found on page 550

Mark leaves a message for the legal department of the hospital to visit Mr. B because he has voiced his preference to have a living will. One of the things that Mr. B would like on his living will is the ability to refuse specific treatments if his disease process gets to the point at which he cannot speak for himself.

EXERCISE 8.4 Multiple-choice:

The following things might be found on a living will *except*:

A. Refusal of cardiopulmonary resuscitation
B. Refusal of artificial nutrition
C. Refusal of a ventilator
D. Refusal of pain medication

The answer can be found on page 550

Paula, the charge nurse the following day, notifies the legal department and they assist Mr. and Mrs. B in filling out the proper paperwork. Mrs. B is given *durable power of attorney* in the event Mr. B cannot advocate for himself. Mr. B does consent to have a peripherally inserted central catheter (PICC) line for antibiotics. Mr. B signs an *informed consent.*

eRESOURCE

To reinforce your understanding of durable power of attorney and informed consent, refer to:

- University of California San Francisco's (UCSF) publication, *Ethics Fast Facts.* [Pathway: http://goo.gl/uVme7 and review content.]
- What Are Advance Directives? [Pathway: http://youtu.be/OaQ8Z9XFK8E]

EXERCISE 8.5 True/False:

In most cases, nurses can obtain a patient's informed consent.

___True

___False

The answer can be found on page 550

---

eRESOURCE

To get a deeper understanding of informed consent, review:

- American College of Physicians' *ACP Ethics Manual,* Sixth Edition. [Pathway: http://goo.gl/5qvPt → scroll down and select "Informed Decision Making and Consent" and review content.]
- University of California San Francisco's (UCSF) publication, *Ethics Fast Facts.* [Pathway: http://goo.gl/uVme7 → select "Informed Consent" and review content.]

Paula assisted Mr. and Mrs. B to arrive at their decision to have the antibiotics by using the process of ethical decision making, which included the following steps:

- Clearly identify the problem at hand
- Discuss the consequences of the problem
- Look at all the options
- Evaluate the risk/benefit ratio of each option and its effect on Mr. B
- Choose
- Implement and evaluate

eRESOURCE

To supplement your understanding of the decision-making process, view:

- A brief video presentation: *Tips to Improve the Decision Making Process.* [Pathway: http://goo.gl/guvW1]
- Two interactive learning activities:
  - Decision Making Methods. [Pathway: http://goo.gl/rZ0Qo]
  - Problem Solving and Decision Making. [Pathway: http://goo.gl/2MeAk]

After the procedure is completed, Mrs. B goes home to rest and Paula takes a phone call at the nurses' station from Mr. B's son-in-law. The son-in-law demands to know why things were done when the patient told him that he did not want any more treatments.

EXERCISE 8.6 Multiple-choice:

The proper response to Mr. B's son-in-law is:

A. "The peripherally inserted central catheter (PICC) line was discussed with your mother-in-law and she agreed."
B. "The PICC line was decided on by the doctor, please call her."
C. "This cannot be discussed because it would violate patient confidentiality."
D. "This happens many times once things are discussed and the PICC line is explained."

The answer can be found on page 551

At the change of shift, Mark returns and is again assigned to four patients, one of whom is Mr. B. Paula gives Mark the report in a private area because walking rounds also breach confidentiality.

During a quiet time in the shift, Mark reads his e-mail and catches up on the mandatory competencies that are computer based, such as fire safety. One of his e-mails is from the director of the Nursing Education Department at the hospital. She is requesting Mark speak to the new orientees who are starting next month. The topic she would like him to cover is legal responsibilities of professional nursing. Mark agrees to do this and verifies that he will have an hour available to present the basic legal concepts that every professional nurse should be aware of. Mark decides he will use a combination of a PowerPoint presentation and gaming to hold the interest of the orientees.

Using a matching format in his first PowerPoint slide, Mark reviews the standards of practice.

EXERCISE 8.7 Matching:

Match the standards of practice in Column A with the organizational levels that they originate from in Column B:

Column A	Column B
A. The Nurse Practice Act	_______ Facility
B. Standards of Practice	_______ Professional organization
C. Policies and Procedures	_______ State

The answer can be found on page 551

Next Mark tells the group about *professional negligence* and he asks the group to pick up the words that are associated with negligence from the words listed on his next slide.

EXERCISE 8.8 Select all that apply:

Which of the following words are often used in conjunction with negligence?

A. Acceptable
B. Best
C. Reasonable
D. Action
E. Demonstrate
F. Prudent
G. Conscientious

The answer can be found on page 551

Mark explains that there are five concepts associated with negligence that are easy to understand and they are:

1. Duty—what a reasonably prudent nurse would do
2. Breach of duty—not providing a standard of care
3. Foreseeability of harm—knowing that not doing something could cause your patient harm
4. Breach of duty has potential to cause harm—something was not done and the person knew it may cause harm
5. Harm occurs—patient is hurt in some way

EXERCISE 8.9 Select all that apply:

Select the things that nurses can do to avoid negligence:

A. Follow the standard of care
B. Give competent care
C. Follow the family's wishes
D. Do not get too close to your patients
E. Develop a caring rapport
F. Document only what someone tells you
G. Document fully

The answer can be found on page 551

Mark also explains to the students what *an intentional tort* is and that there are usually three kinds; he asks the students to provide an example of each:

EXERCISE 8.10 Fill in the blanks:

Write an example of each of the following terms:

Assault ______________________

Battery______________________

False imprisonment______________________

The answer can be found on page 552

Scope of practice is the next area that Mark speaks about with a PowerPoint slide; he asks the orientees what is in their scope of practice:

EXERCISE 8.11 Multiple-choice:

Which scenario is within the nurse's scope of practice?

A. Nurse A is caring for a patient who is out of surgery and no longer needs his epidural catheter. She removes it and makes sure the tip is intact.

B. Nurse B is caring for a client who is out of surgery and no longer needs his epidural catheter. She calls the certified nursing assistant (CNA) to remove it.

C. Nurse C is caring for a patient who is out of surgery and no longer needs his epidural catheter. She calls the nurse anesthetist to remove it.

D. Nurse D is caring for a patient who is out of surgery and no longer needs his epidural catheter. She transfers him to the medical–surgical unit with the catheter in place.

The answer can be found on page 552

---

eRESOURCE

To supplement your understanding of the scope of practice, review:

- Standards of Nursing Practice. [Pathway: http://goo.gl/Rnw2z]
- American Nurses Association's (ANA) *Code of Ethics for Nurses with Interpretive Statements.* [Pathway: http://goo.gl/mSPrD]

Delegation is always a gray area for new orientees. Mark knows it takes experience to know what to delegate and how, but he gives the orientees some good guidelines. He tells them to always use the five rights of delegation:

1. Right task
2. Right circumstance
3. Right person
4. Right direction
5. Right supervision

EXERCISE 8.12 Fill in the blanks (WORD BANK: *accountable* and *responsibility*):

The nurse is _________________________ but gives the immediate _________________________ to someone else while delegating.

The answer can be found on page 552

Poor communication is the number one cause of hospital errors. Transcribing orders correctly is very important to avoid communication mistakes.

EXERCISE 8.13 Select all that apply:

To correctly transcribe orders from a primary care practitioner, the nurse should:

A. Have another nurse listen on the phone
B. Use his or her cell phone
C. Repeat the order back
D. Just document the order once
E. Do not question an order

The answer can be found on page 552

One of the last issues that Mark addresses with the group is reporting misconduct. Most places have an incident reporting system that is separate from patient documentation.

EXERCISE 8.14 True/False:

An incident report should be completed for any incident that is not within the protocols or that is a potential incident, so that corrections can be put into place.

_____True
_____False

The answer can be found on page 552

UNFOLDING CASE STUDY 2: Janice Clark

Janice Clark is the nurse manager (NM) for Mark's unit. As budget preparation time is coming up, Janice asks her charge nurses to assist her in identifying staffing pattern requirements for the new personnel budget based on projections for patient volume and acuity. As night shift charge nurse, Mark reviews the budgeting process.

EXERCISE 8.15 Multiple-choice:

A plan that identifies how many and what kind of staff are needed shift by shift on a specific unit is called:

A. Patient classification system
B. Staffing pattern
C. Personnel budget
D. Strategic plan

The answer can be found on page 552

EXERCISE 8.16 Multiple-choice:

When considering patient acuity in relation to nursing resources needed, Mark uses data from a workload management tool called:

A. Patient classification system
B. Staffing pattern
C. Personnel budget
D. Strategic plan

The answer can be found on page 553

Because of reimbursement changes associated with pay for performance and other fiscal challenges, Janice has been directed by her nurse executive to reduce her unit's expense budget by 5% in the next fiscal year. Janice asks her charge nurses to help her decide where reductions can be made. Including staff in decisions is consistent with a *decentralized* decision-making process in management.

eRESOURCE

To reinforce your understanding of organizational structure, view the United Nations tutorial, *Structure of an Organization.* [Pathway: http://goo.gl/YZkQf]

Mark recognizes that he has a responsibility to ensure that adequate supplies and equipment are available for patients' needs and that cost-effectiveness and quality of care are both goals of the unit and the hospital. He decides to talk with his staff before making his recommendations.

EXERCISE 8.17 Select all that apply:

A key area where staff can make a difference in the costs associated with a patient's care is:

A. Taking only as much of a supply as is needed for the shift into a patient's room
B. Promptly returning equipment to central distribution when no longer in use
C. Periodically reevaluating stock levels of supplies on the unit based on usage
D. Participating in an evaluation of lower cost patient care supplies for possible adoption

The answer can be found on page 553

UNFOLDING CASE STUDY 3: Rachel

Rachel is one of Mark's staff on the night shift. She is a recent graduate who completed orientation last month. Having just taken her NCLEX-RN exam, Rachel is up to date in knowing the risks of cross-contamination to patients and staff alike. She also knows that hospital-acquired infection will be costly for her unit.

EXERCISE 8.18 Fill in the blanks:

Name at least two factors that increase the cost of care for hospital-acquired (nosocomial) infection.

1. ______________________________
2. ______________________________

The answer can be found on page 553

eRESOURCE

To reinforce your understanding of hospital-acquired infections, refer to Medscape on your mobile device. [Pathway: Medscape → enter "Hospital Acquired Infections" into the search field → select "Hospital Acquired Infections" and review content.]

EXERCISE 8.19 Select all that apply:

When delivering care to her patients, Rachel is careful to reduce the potential for patient and staff injury by:

A. Using standard precautions
B. Taking needle-stick precautions
C. Following good hand-washing technique
D. Wearing gloves when she delivers meal trays to her patients

The answer can be found on page 553

While on duty last night, Rachel noted that the electrical cord on the intravenous (IV) pump being used for one of her patients had a damaged plug. The wires inside the insulated covering were exposed.

EXERCISE 8.20 Ordering:

Rachel took the following actions to protect her patient from a hazardous situation. Place them in order of priority from 1 to 4:

_______ Disconnect the pump from the electrical outlet and place it on battery function
_______ Obtain a new pump from the unit storage area
_______ Place a sign on the defective pump that it requires repair
_______ Place a work order in the computer to the biomedical engineering department for repair of the unit

The answer can be found on page 553

UNFOLDING CASE STUDY 1 (CONTINUED): Mark

Mark's shift has gotten off to a busy start. The day charge nurse reported at shift change that the emergency department (ED) is holding a new admission for the unit and needs to transport the patient to the unit as soon as possible. She had asked them to wait until shift report had concluded, but was expecting the patient imminently. The expected patient is an 87-year-old man who had suffered a transient ischemic attack 6 hours ago. Still in the ED, he is now awake and alert and moving all extremities. His most recent pulse oximetry reading is 91%, he has mild pulmonary rales bilaterally, his temperature is 99°F, and he has been started on 2 L of oxygen by nasal cannula.

EXERCISE 8.21 Multiple-choice:

Mark needs to include this patient in the assignment of one of the nurses on duty that evening. Given the patient's expected needs, the most appropriate staff person to be assigned this patient is:

A. Latisha, a per diem RN with 5 years of experience
B. Rachel, an RN with 6 months of experience
C. Tom, a licensed practical nurse (LPN) with 15 years of experience
D. Rhonda, a certified nursing assistant (CNA) with 12 years of experience

The answer can be found on page 554

EXERCISE 8.22 Multiple-choice:

Mark needs to assign a room and bed number to the new patient, Mr. Sparks. The most appropriate placement for this patient is:

A. In a private room at the end of the unit, so that he can rest comfortably with little noise from unit activities
B. In a semi-private room at the end of the unit
C. In a private room across from the team center, so that he can have privacy but remain under close observation
D. In a semi-private room across from the team center

The answer can be found on page 554

EXERCISE 8.23 Multiple-choice:

In order to be able to give sufficient time to the admission assessment for Mr. Sparks, Rachel makes an initial rounding of all her six patients. Rachel's objective(s) for initial rounds is to:

A. Assess patient's overall condition relative to the ABCs (airway, breathing, circulation) of patient safety
B. Quickly assess her findings against the information she received in shift report
C. Identify tasks and priorities
D. Determine to whom specific care requirements will be delegated or assigned

The answer can be found on page 554

UNFOLDING CASE STUDY 4: Rachel and Palaka

Rachel's unit uses a team nursing model of care delivery. While still in her nursing education program, most of Rachel's exposure was to a total patient care model, so she is still struggling with effective delegation as a key skill of the professional nurse. *Huddles* is one of the activities done on her unit at the beginning and middle of the shift. In huddles, all personnel gather for 10 minutes to clearly identify those patients at risk for falls and other possible safety issues.

EXERCISE 8.24 Select all that apply:

While working through her issues with delegation, Rachel realizes that there are a number of reasons why nurses sometimes do not delegate. Identify some of the reasons.

A. Feelings of uncertainty
B. Concern about liability
C. Inability to organize work and manage others
D. A "do it myself" frame of mind

The answer can be found on page 555

EXERCISE 8.25 Select all that apply:

Delegation has many positive aspects in today's environment of care. These include:

A. The RN can spend more time at the desk if as much direct care as possible is carried out by team members.
B. Delegation increases the skill level and motivation of the team members.
C. Delegation increases efficiency of the team.
D. Delegation reinforces that the RN is "in charge."

The answer can be found on page 555

EXERCISE 8.26 Select all that apply:

Rachel delegates needed patient care and other tasks to Tom and Rhonda. In making her assignments, she considers what factors?

A. The five "rights" of delegation
B. Tom and Rhonda will also be delegated tasks by the other RN, Latisha
C. Tom just returned from family leave after the cancer death of his mother
D. Rhonda hates doing "icky" things

The answer can be found on page 555

eRESOURCE

Review the nurse's responsibilities in delegation, the five rights of delegation:

- The National Council of State Boards of Nursing's publication, *The Five Rights of Delegation.* [Pathway: www.ncsbn.org/fiverights.pdf]
- Nursing Currents, *Delegation as a Management Function.* [Pathway: http://goo.gl/RlSsy]

EXERCISE 8.27 Fill in the blanks:

Fill in Rachel's assignment of patients to the most appropriate caregiver that evening: Here are the choices: Tom, licensed practical nurse (LPN), or Rhonda, unauthorized personnel (UAP), or herself, RN:

Mrs. Elliot, who is stable 3 days post-transfer from the intensive care unit (ICU), who requires ambulation twice on the shift ____________________

Mr. Johnson, who requires an abdominal dressing change once during the shift ____________________

Mr. Carter, a diabetic whose most recent blood glucose was 470 mg/dL and is receiving an insulin infusion ____________________

Mr. Sharp, who, following his admission assessment, continues to show pulse oximetry readings in the low 90s ____________________

Mrs. Chou, an 80-year-old woman who speaks limited English, has a Foley catheter, is receiving nasogastric (NG) feedings, and is on bed rest ____________________

Dontell Murphy, a 16-year-old with sickle cell crisis, who is resting comfortably with as needed oral pain meds ____________________

The answer can be found on page 555

As Rachel has recently completed hospital orientation as a newly hired staff nurse, she is familiar with the hospital's policies regarding delegation and assignment of care. What patient care tasks can Rachel properly delegate or assign to the members of her team?

EXERCISE 8.28 Fill in the blanks:

Write "LPN" (licensed practical nurse)/"LVN" (licensed vocational nurse) or "CNA" (certified nursing assistant) after the task to designate the most appropriate care provider:

Tracheostomy care ____________________

Urinary catheter insertion ____________________

Ambulating ____________________

Vital signs ____________________

Intake and output ____________________

Tube feeding ____________________

Reinforce patient teaching ____________________

Specimen collection ____________________

The answer can be found on page 556

Although Rachel is the newest member of the team, she is aware that as the RN her responsibility for patient care extends to supervision of those to whom she delegates patient care tasks. This makes clear communication with her team members very important.

EXERCISE 8.29 Select all that apply:

Which of the following represents clear communication of a delegated task?

A. "Let me know what Mrs. Chou's 8 p.m. blood pressure is."
B. "Let me know whether Mrs. Chou's diastolic reading is greater than 90 when you take it."
C. "I'd like to look at Mr. Johnson's incision site before you redress it."
D. "Call me if it looks like Mr. Johnson's incision is still draining."
E. "Call me if there's anything I need to know."

The answer can be found on page 556

Reviewing the ED assessment of Mr. Sparks, Rachel notes the following: He was awake and alert and moving all extremities. His last ED pulse oximetry reading was 91%, mild pulmonary rales were noted bilaterally, his temperature was 99°F, and he had been started on 2 L of oxygen by nasal cannula. At the time of her initial assessment on the unit, her findings include the following:

- 87-year-old male status post-transient ischemic attack
- Blood pressure (BP) is 148/78 mmHg, pulse (P) is 90 beats per minute (bpm), respiratory rate (RR) is 16 breaths per minute and shallow, temperature is 99.5°F oral
- Pulse oximetry is 89%
- Soft diet order; the patient states he is hungry
- D_5NS at 100 mL/hr

EXERCISE 8.30 Exhibit-format:

On reviewing the emergency department (ED) assessment of Mr. Sparks, Rachel notes the following:

Assessment:

- 87-year-old male status post-transient ischemic attack
- He was awake and alert and moving all extremities.
- Pulse oximetry reading—91% on 2 L of oxygen by cannula
- Mild pulmonary rales bilaterally
- Temperature—99°F

Vital signs: Blood pressure (BP): 148/78 mmHg, pulse (P): 90 beats per minute (bpm), respiratory rate (RR): 16 breaths per minute and shallow, temperature: 99.5°F oral

Based on this information, to what findings should Rachel assign first priority?

A. Elevated temperature
B. Oxygen saturation level
C. Nutritional status
D. Lab results

The answer can be found on page 556

At 1 a.m., 6 hours into her shift, Rachel is working at the team center desk, performing the 24-hour chart check of all physician orders of the prior day. Her attention is drawn to a noise in Mr. Sparks's room across the hall. Entering the room, she finds Mr. Sparks on the floor next to his bed.

EXERCISE 8.31 Ordering:

In what order should Rachel carry out the following tasks?

___ Write up an incident report describing the occurrence
___ With assistance, carefully place Mr. Sparks in his bed
___ Check Mr. Sparks's pulse and respirations
___ Call the house physician to evaluate the patient
___ Perform a focused assessment to determine signs of injury
___ Ask the patient what caused him to get out of bed without using his call light to ask for help and reinforce the use of the call light for assistance
___ Notify Mark, the charge nurse, of the occurrence
___ Document the occurrence in the patient's medical record

The answer can be found on page 557

EXERCISE 8.32 Select all that apply:

When documenting the occurrence in the medical record, Rachel will include the following:

A. A description of what happened
B. The findings from her focused assessment
C. What actions were taken?
D. That an incident report was completed

The answer can be found on page 557

---

eRESOURCE

To review documentation standards, refer to:

- South Carolina Department of Health and Human Services' Documentation Guidelines. [Pathway: http://goo.gl/O4F6j]
- *Documentation,* presentation on nursing considerations related to documentation. [Pathway: http://goo.gl/WIzkI]

EXERCISE 8.33 Ordering:

Mark, as charge nurse, also has responsibilities in this situation. What are Mark's priorities in this case? Arrange them in the order in which they should be carried out.

____ Review with Rachel what elements in her initial assessment of Mr. Sparks may have contributed to his fall
____ Inform the nursing supervisor of the event and review the incident report with him

_____ Call the family to let them know of the occurrence and Mr. Sparks's current condition
_____ Call Mr. Sparks's attending physician
_____ Advise the nurse manager (NM) of the occurrence
_____ Place the patient on fall prevention protocol

The answer can be found on page 558

The house physician ordered x-rays for Mr. Sparks to determine whether he sustained any fractures as a result of his fall. In addition, he ordered a chest film and blood gases because of Mr. Sparks's low pulse oximetry reading. It is now close to 3 a.m., and Rachel feels stressed because of the amount of time that Mr. Sparks's care has required. She is behind in carrying out the tasks of patient care for her other patients. How can Rachel get back into control of her patient assignments?

EXERCISE 8.34 Select all that apply:

Rachel decides to review her previously set priorities. She will be determining which of the following:

A. Tasks that need to be completed immediately
B. Tasks that have a specific time for completion
C. Tasks that have to be completed by the end of the shift
D. Tasks that could be delegated to another team member
E. Tasks that could be delegated to the next shift

The answer can be found on page 558

Having identified the time frame in which tasks must be performed, Rachel can plan for completion of the activities based on priorities of patient care.

EXERCISE 8.35 Multiple-choice:

The most common time-management error is to:

A. Not asking other staff members for assistance
B. Not taking a break to relax and recover from patient care activities
C. Saving the hardest or longest tasks until the last part of the shift
D. Failing to develop a plan

The answer can be found on page 559

At the end of her shift, Rachel prepares to give the change-of-shift report on her patients to the oncoming RN, Palaka. Palaka, although an experienced nurse on the unit, has not worked for several days and knows none of the patients. Bedside shift report is the standard of practice on this unit. The evidence basis for bedside shift report is strong in the literature. Rachel remembers learning that patient care that promotes a culture of safety requires clear and accurate hand-off communication.

EXERCISE 8.36 Select all that apply:

In order to provide for effective continuity of care, Rachel's reports will need to include what information?

A. Patient's chief complaint
B. Any change in condition during the last shift
C. Patient's current status, including relevant diagnostic results
D. Expected diagnostic or treatment plans for the upcoming shift
E. Nursing diagnoses and plan of care, including safety needs

The answer can be found on page 559

EXERCISE 8.37 True/False:

A change-of-shift report most properly is conducted on walking rounds and takes place in the patient's room.

___True
___False

The answer can be found on page 559

EXERCISE 8.38 Multiple-choice:

Successful transfer of information between nurses has been demonstrated to prevent adverse events and medical errors. Patients and families can play a role to make sure these transitions in care are safe and effective. The involvement of the patient and family in the plan of care is called:

A. Primary nursing
B. Team nursing
C. Patient engagement
D. Discharge planning

The answer can be found on page 559

EXERCISE 8.39 True/False

Several of their patients are located in semiprivate rooms. To ensure that no Health Insurance Portability and Accountability Act (HIPAA) violation occurs in connection with bedside report, Rachel and Palaka do the following:

Ask the patient whether he or she wishes to participate in bedside shift report.

___True
___False

Request any visitors, other than those designated by the patient to remain, to leave the room temporarily.

___True

___False

The answer can be found on page 559

Exercise 8.40 Select all that apply:

While in the patient room, Rachel and Palaka promote patient engagement and ensure the accuracy of the report and patient safety by:

A. Introducing Palaka as the patient's oncoming nurse
B. Checking the patient's wrist band
C. Checking the status of intravenous (IV) drips and drains
D. Checking the position of bedside rails and access to the call light
E. Asking the patient about his or her pain level

The answer can be found on page 560

Based on the clinical pathway for sickle cell crisis, Palaka knows that Dontell will likely be going home shortly. Based on the information obtained on admission, Palaka requests that Dontell let her know when his mother comes to visit today, so that they can talk about his discharge planning.

EXERCISE 8.41 Fill in the blank:

Because Dontell will require ongoing care for his chronic illness, continuing care in the community will support him and his mother in managing his condition. Palaka calls ________________ to meet with her, Dontell, and his mother to discuss community supports.

The answer can be found on page 560

UNFOLDING CASE STUDY 5: Tameka Williams

Tameka Williams has been an RN on the mother–baby (M–B) unit for 3 years. She loves the supportive and teaching aspects of her role with new mothers. With her experience at the bedside, Tameka's confidence in herself as a professional and as a role model has grown. When her NM asked Tameka to lead the unit's Quality of Care Council and represent the unit in the nursing department's Patient Safety and Quality Council, she was happy to say yes.

EXERCISE 8.42 Multiple-choice:

A unit-based quality-of-care council led by a staff nurse with representation at a department-wide council is typical of what type of management structure?

A. Laissez-faire management style
B. Transformational leadership
C. Shared Governance Model
D. Magnet® status

The answer can be found on page 560

eRESOURCE

To reinforce your understanding of leadership styles, review these brief videos regarding leadership by CommLab India:

- *Leadership Styles.* [Pathway: http://goo.gl/001ns]
- *Inspirational Leader Vs Good Leader—What's the Difference?* [Pathway: http://goo.gl/dQ1AD]

eRESOURCE

To review leadership concepts, view the following video from CommLab India:

- Distinguishing Leadership and Management Activities. [Pathway: http://goo.gl/lJ6FU]

EXERCISE 8.43 Multiple-choice:

At the most recent Nursing Department Council meeting, the chief nursing officer reviewed the Hospital Consumer Assessment of Healthcare Providers and Systems (HCAHPS) scores for all units and discussed where targets were and were not being met.

In thinking about these results, Tameka remembers that HCAHPS is:

A. A Joint Commission program of required reporting of adverse events for hospitals
B. A standardized method of collecting information about patient perceptions of their hospital experience
C. A federally mandated program for acute care hospitals
D. Not applicable to maternity services

The answer can be found on page 560

EXERCISE 8.44 Multiple-choice:

The data showed that the mother–baby (M–B) unit was not meeting targets for two indicators: respect for patient privacy and pain relief. Tameka's next step is to:

A. Review the data with her nurse manager (NM)
B. Review the data with the M–B staff
C. Write a new policy for pain management for postpartum patients
D. Develop an educational plan for M–B staff about patient satisfaction

The answer can be found on page 561

In meeting with the Mother–Baby Quality Council, Tameka shows the team members a chart.

EXERCISE 8.45 Multiple-choice:

This form of chart is called:

A. A bar graph
B. A run chart
C. A pie chart
D. A spreadsheet

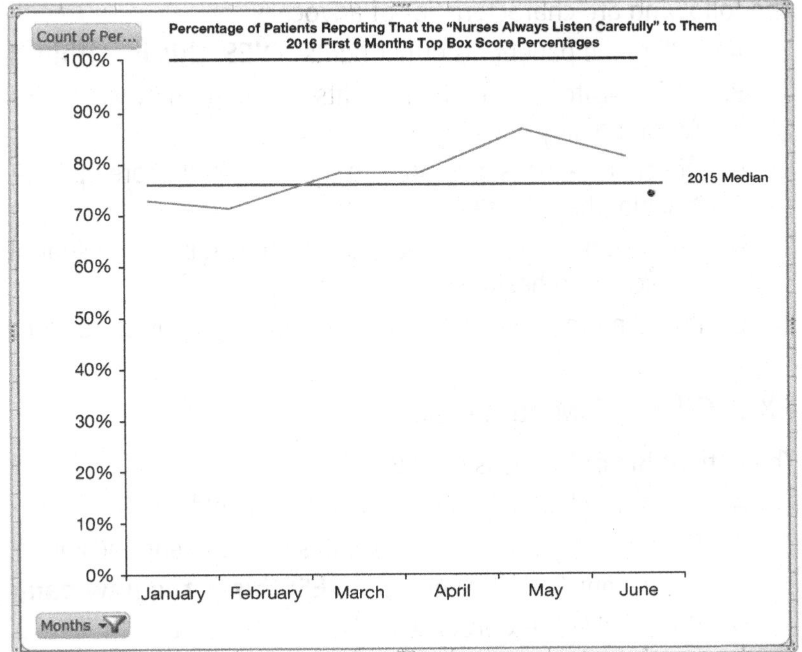

The answer can be found on page 561

EXERCISE 8.46 Multiple-choice:

Rosa, one of the RN members of the council, volunteers to search journals, nursing textbooks, and the worldwide web for current and best pain management practices for maternity patients and to prepare a presentation for the council on her findings. Using the literature to make decisions regarding nursing practice is called:

A. Primary nursing
B. Plan, Do, Check, Act
C. Transformational leadership
D. Evidence-based practice (EBP)

The answer can be found on page 562

Answers

EXERCISE 8.1 Select all that apply:

The following are characteristics of advocacy:

A. Telling the patient his or her rights—**YES; this is within the role of an advocate.**
B. Telling visitors the patient's rights—NO; this may violate Health Insurance Portability and Accountability Act (HIPPA).
C. Directing patients' decisions to the best health care option—NO; advocates assist patients in decision making; they do not direct them.
D. Explaining to patients that access to health is their responsibility—NO; advocates assist patients to get access to health care.
E. Providing the patient with information about his or her condition—**YES; advocates do teach!**

EXERCISE 8.2 Multiple-choice:

The Patient Bill of Rights is now titled:

A. The Family Bill of Rights—NO; this is the old name.
B. The Advocacy Document—NO; this is a different document.
C. The Patient Care Partnership—**YES; this is the new name.**
D. The Family Care Consensus—NO; this is not it.

EXERCISE 8.3 Fill in the blank:

Mark understands that under the Patient Self-Determination Act that was passed in 1991 he should ask Mr. B if he has what important document completed?

Advance directive

EXERCISE 8.4 Multiple-choice:

The following things might be found on a living will *except*:

A. Refusal of cardiopulmonary resuscitation—**YES; cardiopulmonary resuscitation can be refused.**
B. Refusal of artificial nutrition—**YES; nutrition to prolong life is often refused.**
C. Refusal of a ventilator—**YES; it is within a person's right to refuse artificial respiratory help.**
D. Refusal of pain medication—NO; pain medication is a humane treatment.

EXERCISE 8.5 True/False

In most cases, professional nurses can obtain a patient's informed consent.

__X__ **False;** the person doing the invasive procedure must obtain the consent; the nurse can be a witness to the signature.

EXERCISE 8.6 Multiple-choice:

The proper response to Mr. B's son-in-law is:

A. "The peripherally inserted central catheter (PICC) line was discussed with your mother-in-law and she agreed."—NO; too much information.
B. "The PICC line was decided on by the doctor, please call her."—NO; also too much information.
C. "This cannot be discussed because it would violate patient confidentiality."—**YES; this is the only option that does not violate giving patient information to those who are not entitled to it unless authorized by the patient in writing.**
D. "This happens many times once things are discussed and the PICC line is explained."—NO, it is not your place to inform them of any circumstances.

EXERCISE 8.7 Matching:

Match the standards of practice in Column A with the organizational levels that they originate from in Column B:

Column A	Column B
A. The Nurse Practice Act	C Facility
B. Standards of Practice	B Professional organization
C. Policies and Procedures	A State

EXERCISE 8.8 Select all that apply:

Which of the following words are often used in conjunction with negligence?

A. Acceptable—NO; what is acceptable to one may be different for another.
B. Best—NO; "best" is difficult to quantify.
C. Reasonable—**YES; negligence is usually discussed in terms of what is reasonable.**
D. Action—NO; they are looking at what the professional did or did not do.
E. Demonstrate—NO; they are looking at what the professional did or did not do.
F. Prudent—**YES; "prudence" is usually discussed in terms of what should have been done.**
G. Conscientious—NO; this is a personal attribute.

EXERCISE 8.9 Select all that apply:

Select the things that nurses can do to avoid negligence:

A. Follow the standard of care—**YES; always follow state and hospital guidelines.**
B. Give competent care—**YES; always be accountable and responsible at work.**
C. Follow the family's wishes—NO; they may differ from the patient.
D. Do not get too close to your patients—NO; establishing a rapport is needed but maintain professional boundaries.
E. Develop a caring rapport—**YES; this assists wellness.**
F. Document only what someone tells you—Possibly, but also try to witness things for yourself to increase the reliability.
G. Document fully—**YES.**

EXERCISE 8.10 Fill in the blanks:

Write an example of each of the following terms:

Assault **Threatening a patient with applying restraints that are not necessary or ordered for the patient's safety.**

Battery **Giving an intramuscular injection after the patient refuses.**

False imprisonment **Using restraints wrongly.**

EXERCISE 8.11 Multiple-choice:

Which scenario is within the nurse's scope of practice?

A. Nurse A is caring for a patient who is out of surgery and no longer needs his epidural catheter. She removes it and makes sure the tip is intact.—NO; this not within a nurse's standard of practice.

B. Nurse B is caring for a client who is out of surgery and no longer needs his epidural catheter. She calls the certified nursing assistant (CNA) to remove it.—NO; it is not appropriate to delegate this to a CNA.

C. Nurse C is caring for a patient who is out of surgery and no longer needs his epidural catheter. She calls the nurse anesthetist to remove it.—**YES.**

D. Nurse D is caring for a patient who is out of surgery and no longer needs his epidural catheter. She transfers him to the medical–surgical unit with the catheter in place.—NO; it is not needed and this would run the risk of dislodging it.

EXERCISE 8.12 Fill in the blanks (WORD BANK: *accountable and responsibility*):

The nurse is **accountable** but gives the immediate **responsibility** to someone else while delegating.

EXERCISE 8.13 Select all that apply:

To correctly transcribe orders from a primary care practitioner, the nurse should:

A. Have another nurse listen on the phone—**YES; this may be hospital policy.**

B. Use his or her cell phone—NO; use a clear land line if possible.

C. Repeat the order back—**YES; this is an established standard.**

D. Just document the order once—NO; document that you read it back.

E. Do not question an order—NO; always question it if it does not seem correct.

EXERCISE 8.14 True/False:

An incident report should be completed on any incident that is not within the protocols or that is a potential incident, so that corrections can be put into place.

X True

EXERCISE 8.15 Multiple-choice:

A plan that identifies how many and what kind of staff are needed shift by shift on a specific unit is called:

A. Patient classification system—NO; this is patient acuity.

B. Staffing pattern—**YES; this directly involves the staffing.**

C. Personnel budget—NO; this is full-time equivalency (FTE) related.

D. Strategic plan—NO; this involves short- and long-term planning strategies.

EXERCISE 8.16 Multiple-choice:

When considering patient acuity in relation to nursing resources needed, Mark uses data from a workload management tool called:

A. Patient classification system—**YES; this is patient acuity needed for decisions.**
B. Staffing pattern—NO; this is directly related to staffing.
C. Personnel budget—NO; this is full-time equivalency (FTE) related.
D. Strategic plan—NO; this involves short- and long-term planning strategies.

EXERCISE 8.17 Select all that apply:

A key area where staff can make a difference in the costs associated with a patient's care is:

A. Taking only as much of a supply as is needed for the shift into a patient's room—**YES; this helps budgeting.**
B. Promptly returning equipment to central distribution when no longer in use—**YES; this helps budgeting.**
C. Periodically reevaluating stock levels of supplies on the unit based on usage—**YES; this helps budgeting.**
D. Participating in an evaluation of lower cost patient care supplies for possible adoption—**YES; this too helps budgeting.**

EXERCISE 8.18 Fill in the blanks:

Name at least two factors that increase the cost of care for hospital-acquired (nosocomial) infection.

1. **Medicare and other third-party payers will not reimburse hospitals for the costs incurred for these patients' treatment.**
2. **Hospital-acquired infection increases the patient's length of hospital stay.**
3. **Treatment required often includes intravenous (IV) administration of antibiotics.**

EXERCISE 8.19 Select all that apply:

When delivering care to her patients, Rachel is careful to reduce the potential for patient and staff injury by:

A. Using standard precautions—**YES; this is a must to prevent the spread of infection.**
B. Taking needle-stick precautions—**YES; this is a must to prevent the spread of infection.**
C. Following good handwashing technique—**YES; this is a must to prevent the spread of infection.**
D. Wearing gloves when she delivers meal trays to her patients—NO; unless a patient is ordered special precautions; gloves are needed when there is a likelihood of blood or body fluid contact.

EXERCISE 8.20 Ordering:

Rachel took the following actions to protect her patient from a hazardous situation. Place them in order of priority from 1 to 4:

4 Disconnect the pump from the electrical outlet and place it on battery function—**YES; this action removes the potential harm from the patient and should be first.**

2 Obtaine a new pump from the unit storage area—**YES; this action ensures that the intravenous (IV) pump is continually functioning.**

__3__ Place a sign on the defective pump that it requires repair—**YES; this should be done to prevent anyone else from using the faulty pump.**

__1__ Place a work order in the computer to the biomedical engineering department for repair of the unit—**YES; this action initiates repair of the pump.**

EXERCISE 8.21 Multiple-choice:

Mark needs to include this patient in the assignment of one of the nurses on duty that evening. Given the patient's expected needs, the most appropriate staff person to be assigned this patient is:

A. Latisha, a per diem RN with 5 years of experience—NO; as the most experienced nurse on the shift, Latisha's assignment will comprise other patients with more complex needs.
B. Rachel, an RN with 6 months of experience—**YES; Rachel's experience at 6 months enables her to assess and prepare an initial plan of care for this patient.**
C. Tom, a licensed practical nurse (LPN) with 15 years of experience—NO; this patient's nursing assessment and care must be planned by an RN.
D. Rhonda, a certified nursing assistant (CNA) with 12 years of experience—NO; this patient's care is not within the scope of a CNA.

EXERCISE 8.22 Multiple-choice:

Mark needs to assign a room and bed number to the new patient, Mr. Sparks. The most appropriate placement for this patient is:

A. In a private room at the end of the unit, so that he can rest comfortably with little noise from unit activities—NO; this patient's condition does not warrant private room placement. The private rooms should be reserved for patients whose conditions require it.
B. In a semi-private room at the end of the unit—NO; Mr. Sparks is at moderate to high risk for falls because of his age and his condition. Assuming that the nursing unit layout includes a central nurses' station, this room assignment may place the patient at an increased risk of falling.
C. In a private room across from the team center, so that he can have privacy but remain under close observation—NO; again the patient's condition does not warrant private room placement.
D. In a semi-private room across from the team center—**YES; this room placement permits close observation of the patient during his early hospitalization, but does not unnecessarily make a private room unavailable for a patient who may need one.**

EXERCISE 8.23 Multiple-choice:

In order to be able to give sufficient time to the admission assessment for Mr. Sparks, Rachel makes an initial rounding of all her six patients. Rachel's objective(s) for initial rounds is to:

A. **Assess patient's overall condition relative to the ABCs (airway, breathing, circulation) of patient safety**
B. **Quickly assess her findings against the information she received in shift report**
C. **Identify tasks and priorities**
D. **Determine to whom specific care requirements will be delegated or assigned**

All these activities are appropriate for the initial rounding by the RN. This is an example of multitasking and critical thinking skills that are used in the clinical area for patient care.

EXERCISE 8.24 Select all that apply:

While working through her issues with delegation, Rachel realizes that there are a number of reasons why nurses sometimes do not delegate. Identify some of the reasons.

A. **Feelings of uncertainty**
B. **Concern about liability**
C. **Inability to organize work and manage others**
D. **A "do it myself" frame of mind**

All of these personal factors may play a role in a nurse's reluctance to delegate. In addition, other situational barriers come into play in the clinical area. For example, poor team relationships can inhibit a novice nurse's confidence or self-efficacy. This is usually overcome with experience, mentoring, and managerial support.

EXERCISE 8.25 Select all that apply:

Delegation has many positive aspects in today's environment of care. These include:

A. The RN can spend more time at the desk if as much direct care as possible is carried out by team members.—NO; a positive outcome of effective delegation is the ability to give time to those duties or responsibilities that only the RN can perform. However, these are not necessarily desk responsibilities.
B. Delegation increases the skill level and motivation of the team members.—**YES; through growth in ability and proficiency in the clinical area, team members increase in skill and motivation.**
C. Delegation increases efficiency of the team.—**YES; equal distribution assists in work completion.**
D. Delegation reinforces that the RN is "in charge."—NO; although the RN has authority with regard to team functions, overall effectiveness is the goal of appropriate delegation.

EXERCISE 8.26 Select all that apply:

Rachel delegates needed patient care and other tasks to Tom and Rhonda. In making her assignments, she considers what factors?

A. The five "rights" of delegation—**YES; the five "rights" are the standard for delegation of patient care and are the responsibility of the RN.**
B. Tom and Rhonda will also be delegated tasks by the other RN, Latisha—**YES; when a team member is overwhelmed, patient care suffers and the RN must consider this.**
C. Tom just returned from family leave after the cancer death of his mother—**YES; the RN may appropriately give consideration to a team member's situation and should ask Tom whether he feels able to care for this cancer patient tonight.**
D. Rhonda hates doing "icky" things—NO; team members must assume responsibility in performing all aspects of patient care. Failure to do this decreases the effectiveness of the team.

EXERCISE 8.27 Fill in the blanks:

Fill in Rachel's assignment of patients to the most appropriate caregiver that evening: Here are the choices:Tom, licensed practical nurse (LPN), or Rhonda, unauthorized personnel (UAP), or herself, RN:

Mrs. Elliot, who is stable 3 days post-transfer from the intensive care unit (ICU), who requires ambulation twice on the shift—**Rhonda, UAP. The patient is stable and improving and the UAP's job includes ambulating patients.**

Mr. Johnson, who requires an abdominal dressing change once during the shift—**Tom, LPN. Rachel can delegate the dressing change with instruction.**

Mr. Carter, a diabetic whose most recent blood glucose was 470 mg/dL and is receiving an insulin infusion—**Rachel, RN. This patient requires ongoing assessment of glucose levels throughout the shift and the infusing must be titrated.**

Mr. Sharp, who, following his admission assessment, continues to show pulse oximetry readings in the low 90s—**Rachel, RN. The patient's oxygenation is a concern and ongoing assessment is required.**

Mrs. Chou, an 80-year-old woman who speaks limited English, has a Foley catheter, is receiving nasogastric (NG) feedings, and is on bed rest—**Tom, LPN. The patient's care requirements include skilled procedures within the scope of LPN practice.**

Dontell Murphy, a 16-year-old with sickle cell crisis, who is resting comfortably with as needed oral pain meds—**Tom, LPN. Administering oral medications is within the LPN scope of practice.**

EXERCISE 8.28 Fill in the blanks:

Write "LPN" (licensed practical nurse)/"LVN" (licensed vocational nurse) or"CNA" (certified nursing assistant) after the task to designate the most appropriate care provider:

Tracheostomy care—**LPN**
Urinary catheter insertion—**LPN**
Ambulating—**CNA**
Vital signs—**CNA**
Intake and output—**CNA**
Tube feeding—**LPN**
Reinforce patient teaching—**LPN**
Specimen collection—**CNA**

EXERCISE 8.29 Select all that apply:

Which of the following represents clear communication of a delegated task?

A. **"Let me know what Mrs. Chou's 8 p.m. blood pressure is"**
B. **"Let me know whether Mrs. Chou's diastolic reading is greater than 90 when you take it."**
C. **"I'd like to look at Mr. Johnson's incision site before you redress it."**
D. **"Call me if it looks like Mr. Johnson's incision is still draining."**
E. "Call me if there's anything I need to know."

Depending on the RN's assessment of what is important in an individual patient's care, A, B, C, or D could be appropriate communication. However, E puts too much latitude in reporting back in the hands of the delegate, and represents an abandonment of the RN's duty of clear direction.

EXERCISE 8.30 Exhibit-format:

On reviewing the emergency department (ED) assessment of Mr. Sparks, Rachel notes the following:

Assessment:

- 87-year-old male status post-transient ischemic attack
- He was awake and alert and moving all extremities.

- Pulse oximetry reading—91% on 2 L of oxygen by cannula
- Mild pulmonary rales bilaterally
- Temperature—99°F

Vital signs: Blood pressure (BP): 148/78 mmHg, pulse (P): 90 beats per minute (bpm), respiratory rate (RR): 16 breaths per minute and shallow, temperature 99.5°F oral

Based on this information, to what findings should Rachel assign first priority?

A. Elevated temperature—NO; although this is important, it is not the priority.
B. Oxygen saturation level—**YES; according to Maslow's hierarchy and using the ABCs of assessment (airway, breathing, circulation), the patient's low oxygenation saturation level, which has decreased since the last read in the emergency department (ED) and despite the 2 L of oxygen, has to be Rachel's first concern.**
C. Nutritional status—NO; although this is important, it is not the priority.
D. Lab results—NO; although this is important, it is not the priority.

EXERCISE 8.31 Ordering:

In what order should Rachel carry out the following tasks?

__8__ Write up an incident report describing the occurrence—**Any patient event that is not within the normal and expected course of the hospital stay must be reported for risk-management purposes.**

__4__ With assistance, carefully place Mr. Sparks in his bed—**Assistance is required to stabilize the act of lifting and moving the patient, so as to prevent any further injury.**

__1__ Check Mr. Sparks's pulse and respirations—**Assess patient's ABCs—airway, breathing, and circulation.**

__5__ Call the house physician to evaluate the patient—**This change in the patient's status requires evaluation by a physician because the medical plan of care may need to be altered.**

__2__ Perform a focused assessment to determine signs of injury—**A focused assessment will reveal possible injury to the patient as a result of the fall—is there evidence of a head injury, limb injury?**

__6__ Ask the patient what caused him to get out of bed without using his call light to ask for help and reinforce the use of the call light for assistance—**If the patient is able to respond to this question, it may assist the nurse in enlisting the patient's cooperation in his own safety and may assist in revision of the patient's plan of care.**

__3__ Notify Mark, the charge nurse, of the occurrence—**The role of the charge nurse is to assist and/or intervene in circumstances that are not routine.**

__7__ Document the event in the patient's medical record—**All changes in patient's condition must be documented.**

EXERCISE 8.32 Select all that apply:

When documenting the occurrence in the medical record, Rachel will include the following:

A. A description of what happened—**YES; Rachel will document what she objectively knows about the incident. If the patient informs her why he left the bed or what he was doing when he fell, this may properly be included in the note. However, Rachel should not speculate in her charting.**

B. The findings from her focused assessment—**YES; Rachel will document physical findings and neurological assessment.**
C. What actions were taken—**YES; Rachel will document the actions taken to make the patient safe, to inform the physician of the occurrence, and will include the physician's visit to the patient.**
D. That an incident report was completed—NO; incident reports are confidential administrative records. A copy is not placed in the patient's chart, nor is it documented in the record.

EXERCISE 8.33 Ordering:

Mark, as charge nurse, also has responsibilities in this situation. What are Mark's priorities in this case? Arrange them in the order in which they should be carried out.

__4__ Review with Rachel what elements in her initial assessment of Mr. Sparks may have contributed to his fall—**Identifying risk for fall is an important aspect of the initial nursing assessment. By initiating the fall protocol immediately, this fall may have been prevented.**

__1__ Inform the nursing supervisor of the event and review the incident report with him—**Mark's duty as charge nurse includes the responsibility to follow administrative procedures of risk management. Informing his direct supervisor is required.**

__3__ Call the family to let them know of the occurrence and Mr. Sparks's current condition—**This responsibility can be carried out by any of a number of accountable persons depending on hospital policy. It may be the nurse who is caring for the patient, the house physician who evaluated the patient, the patient's attending physician, or the charge nurse. However, accreditation standards require that the family be informed.**

__2__ Call Mr. Sparks's attending physician—**In hospitals that use house physicians, it may be policy that the house physician places the call to the attending physician. Mark will need to be sure whether he or the physician will make this call.**

__6__ Advise the nurse manager (NM) of the occurrence—**Although Mark has informed the shift nursing supervisor of the occurrence, his direct superior is the NM, Janice Clark. Janice is accountable for the quality of care on her unit and is responsible for reviewing the circumstances of the occurrence with a goal of improving the climate of safety on the unit.**

__5__ Place the patient on fall prevention protocol—**Patients who fall once are likely to fall again. A single fall places the patient at increased risk; additional precautions are necessary to safeguard the patient and reduce liability for the hospital.**

EXERCISE 8.34 Select all that apply:

Rachel decides to review her previously set priorities. She will be determining which of the following:

A. Tasks that need to be completed immediately—**YES.**
B. Tasks that have a specific time for completion—**YES.**
C. Tasks that have to be completed by the end of the shift—**YES.**
D. Tasks that could be delegated to another team member—**YES.**
E. Tasks that could be delegated to the next shift—NO; all the above are correct priorities, except E. Priorities can change during the course of a nurse's typical 8- or 12-hour shift based on patient needs. However, "E" is not a good solution, as failure to complete priority tasks could compromise the patient's condition.

EXERCISE 8.35 Multiple-choice:

The most common time-management error is:

A. Not asking other staff members for assistance—NO; not the most common.
B. Not taking a break to relax and recover from patient care activities—NO; not the most common.
C. Saving the hardest or longest tasks until the last part of the shift—NO; not the most common.
D. Failing to develop a plan—**YES; all the preceding answers are elements of time-management errors. However, "D," failing to plan, is the most common. By failing to plan, it is not possible to make the best use of the people and resources that the nurse has on hand to accomplish patient care.**

EXERCISE 8.36 Select all that apply:

In order to provide for effective continuity of care, Rachel's reports will need to include what information?

A. Patient's chief complaint—**YES.**
B. Any change in condition during the last shift—**YES.**
C. Patient's current status, including relevant diagnostic results—**YES.**
D. Expected diagnostic or treatment plans for the upcoming shift—**YES.**
E. Nursing diagnoses and plan of care, including safety needs—**YES.**

All the answer options are characteristics of an effective shift report. Additional information needed includes the patient's demographics. Effective shift reports offer the oncoming nurse the opportunity to ask questions and seek clarification.

EXERCISE 8.37 True/False:

A change-of-shift report most properly is conducted on walking rounds and takes place in the patient's room.

_X_ **True; walking rounds that include the patient is a standard of practice.**

EXERCISE 8.38 Multiple-choice:

Successful transfer of information between nurses has been demonstrated to prevent adverse events and medical errors. Patients and families can play a role to make sure these transitions in care are safe and effective. The involvement of the patient and family in the plan of care is called:

A. Primary nursing—NO; this is a model of patient care that primarily includes RNs.
B. Team nursing—NO; this is a model of patient care that includes multiple nurses.
C. Patient engagement—**YES; this includes the patient and family.**
D. Discharge planning—NO; this is not the best answer, as discharge planning is only one aspect of the plan of care.

EXERCISE 8.39 True/False:

Several of their patients are located in semiprivate rooms. To ensure that no Health Insurance Portability and Accountability Act (HIPAA) violation occurs in connection with bedside report, Rachel and Palaka do the following:

Ask the patient whether he or she wishes to participate in bedside shift report.

_X_ **True—YES; the patient's decision whether to participate in bedside report is not a requirement. The patient's wishes must be respected in this regard.**

Request any visitors, other than those designated by the patient to remain, to leave the room temporarily.

_X_ **True—YES; the patient's wishes for who may be involved in his plan of care must be respected.**

Exercise 8.40 Select all that apply:

While in the patient room, Rachel and Palaka promote patient engagement and ensure the accuracy of report and patient safety by:

A. Introducing Palaka as the patient's oncoming nurse—**YES.**
B. Checking the patient's wrist band—**YES.**
C. Checking the status of intravenous (IV) drips and drains—**YES.**
D. Checking the position of bedside rails and access to the call light—**YES.**
E. Asking the patient about his or her pain level—**YES.**

All answers are correct. Positively identifying the patient and performing a focused assessment for accuracy and safety are essential to bedside report. Introducing the oncoming nurse and ensuring that the patient is comfortable involves the patient in his or her care immediately and for the next shift.

EXERCISE 8.41 Fill in the blank:

Because Dontell will require ongoing care for his chronic illness, continuing care in the community will support him and his mother in managing his condition. Palaka calls **the case manager** to meet with her, Dontell, and his mother to discuss community supports.

EXERCISE 8.42 Multiple-choice:

A unit-based quality-of-care council led by a staff nurse with representation at a department-wide council is typical of what type of management structure?

A. Laissez-faire management style—NO; these are leadership styles, rather than management models. Although leadership and management are related, they are not the same constructs.
B. Transformational leadership—NO; these are leadership styles, rather than management models. Although leadership and management are related, they are not the same constructs.
C. Shared Governance Model—**YES; Shared Governance is a management model in which staff nurses participate in making decisions that affect patient care on an individual unit.**
D. Magnet® status—NO; Magnet status is a program under the auspices of the American Nurses Association that measures quality and strength of nursing departments.

EXERCISE 8.43 Multiple-choice:

At the most recent Nursing Department Council meeting, the chief nursing officer reviewed the Hospital Consumer Assessment of Healthcare Providers and Systems (HCAHPS) scores for all units and discussed where targets were and were not being met.

In thinking about these results, Tameka remembers that HCAHPS is:

A. A Joint Commission program of required reporting of adverse events for hospitals—NO; The Joint Commission (TJC) has no connection with HCAHPS.

B. A standardized method of collecting information about patient perceptions of their hospital experience—**YES; this is correct. Before HCAHPS, health care organizations used many different types of surveys to assess "patient satisfaction" with services. HCAHPS provides a common basis that allows aggregation of data nationally regarding patient perceptions of their care.**

C. A federally mandated program for acute care hospitals—NO; this is not correct.

D. Not applicable to maternity services—NO; this is not correct. All acute care hospital patients are eligible to be surveyed for HCAHPS. See http://www.hcahpsonline.org/Files/HCAHPS_Fact_Sheet_June_2015.pdf

EXERCISE 8.44 Multiple-choice:

The data showed that the mother–baby (M–B) Unit was not meeting targets for two indicators: respect for patient privacy and pain relief. Tameka's next step is to:

A. Review the data with her nurse manager (NM)—**YES; this is correct because the NM is the accountable individual for unit performance, so should have first review of the new data. He or she will be an important ally for Tameka in working with staff to implement an improvement process.**

B. Review the data with the M–B staff—NO; this is not correct. The NM is afforded the courtesy of this information before sharing with staff.

C. Write a new policy for pain management for postpartum patients—NO; this is not correct. Whether the current policy is appropriate is a matter to be determined through evidence-based review.

D. Develop an educational plan for M–B staff about patient satisfaction—NO; this is not correct. Whether an educational plan is needed would be determined by assessing the current state of nurses' knowledge.

EXERCISE 8.45 Multiple-choice:

The form of this chart is called:

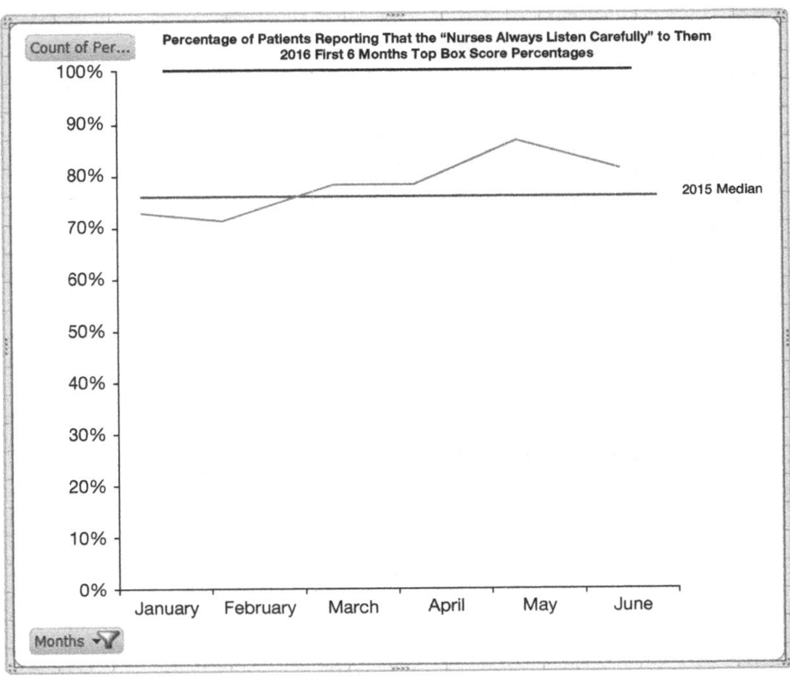

A. A bar graph—NO; a bar chart shows data as a horizontal or vertical bar that demonstrates the size of the value.

B. A run chart—**YES; a run chart is a line graph that runs horizontally over time for the same indicator.**

C. A pie chart—NO; a pie chart shows data as wedges within a circle or "pie."

D. A spreadsheet—NO; a spreadsheet is a digital document that shows data in rows and columns that can be manipulated for calculations.

EXERCISE 8.46 Multiple-choice:

Rosa, one of the RN members of the council, volunteers to search journals, nursing textbooks, and the worldwide web for current and best pain management practices for maternity patients and to prepare a presentation for the council on her findings. Using the literature to make decisions regarding nursing practice is called:

A. Primary nursing—NO; this is a care delivery model.
B. Plan, Do, Check, Act—NO; this is a model for performance improvement.
C. Transformational leadership—NO; transformational leadership is a leadership style.
D. Evidence-based practice (EBP)—**YES, EBP refers to the practice of using best practices based on research.**

Resources

Grossman, S. C., & Valigra, T. M. (2013). *The new leadership challenge: Creating the future of nursing* (4th ed.). Philadelphia, PA: F. A. Davis.

Rigolosi, E. L. (2012). *Management and leadership in nursing and health care an experiential approach* (3rd ed.). New York, NY: Springer Publishing.

CHAPTER 9

Men's Health

Tracy P. George

UNFOLDING CASE STUDY 1: John

John is a 65-year-old retired mechanic. He is obese and has been diagnosed with hypertension and diabetes. He comes to the family practice clinic because of urinary hesitancy and a decreased urine flow. This has been going on for 4 months. His friend told him that his prostate might be enlarged. The nurse explains that there are several symptoms associated with benign prostatic hyperplasia (BPH).

EXERCISE 9.1 Fill in the blanks:

List at least two symptoms other than urinary hesitancy and decreased urine flow that can be associated with benign prostatic hyperplasia (BPH):

1. ______________________
2. ______________________

The answer can be found on page 578

John asks the nurse why he developed BPH, and the nurse describes several risk factors for BPH.

EXERCISE 9.2 Fill in the blanks:

List at least two risk factors for benign prostatic hyperplasia (BPH):

1. ______________________
2. ______________________

The answer can be found on page 578

John asks the nurse about any tests than can be performed to diagnose BPH. He is concerned because his brother's prostate cancer symptoms were similar to his BPH symptoms.

EXERCISE 9.3 Select all that apply:

The patient understands the nurse's teaching on diagnostic tests for benign prostatic hyperplasia (BPH) when he says:

A. "I need to have a colonoscopy."
B. "I need to have a digital rectal examination."
C. "I need to have a liver biopsy."
D. "I need to have an alpha-fetoprotein test."
E. "I need to have a urinalysis."
F. "I need to have a prostate-specific antigen test."

The answer can be found on page 578

---

eRESOURCE

To reinforce your understanding of the clinical presentation of BPH and its diagnostic tests, refer to Medscape on your mobile device. [Pathway: Medscape → enter "BPH" into the search field → select "BPH" and review content, focusing on "Overview" and "Workup."]

John asks the nurse about any changes to his diet that are needed with BPH. The nurse discusses helpful dietary modifications.

EXERCISE 9.4 Multiple-choice:

A patient with benign prostatic hyperplasia (BPH) understands the nurse's teaching when he states that:

A. "I need to avoid drinking large amounts of fluids at bedtime."
B. "I need to increase my caffeine intake."
C. "I need to eat more fish."
D. "I need to increase my calcium intake."

The answer can be found on page 578

EXERCISE 9.5 Multiple-choice:

The nurse also discusses with John the need to avoid antihistamines and decongestants. What is the rationale for avoiding these medications with benign prostatic hyperplasia (BPH)?

A. They increase bladder tone.
B. They cause urinary tract infections.
C. They decrease bladder tone.
D. They can increase creatinine levels.

The answer can be found on page 579

After trying dietary changes and avoidance of antihistamines and decongestants, John has returned to the clinic with continuing symptoms of BPH. John's health care provider has discussed the risks and benefits of various treatments for BPH, including pharmacological therapy and surgical treatments. John has decided to take an oral medication to manage BPH. The nurse explains to John that alpha-adrenergic blockers and 5-alpha-reductase inhibitors are commonly used medications for BPH, and the nurse tells John about side effects associated with each class of medications.

eRESOURCE

To reinforce your understanding of the action of each class of medication, refer to Medscape on your mobile device. [Pathway: Medscape → enter "BPH" into the search field → select "BPH" → select "Medication" and review content.]

EXERCISE 9.6 Matching:

Match each medication in Column A with the possible side effect in Column B (medications could be used more than once):

Column A	Column B
A. Terazosin	____Dizziness
B. Finasteride	____Decreased libido
C. Doxazosin	____Postural hypotension
D. Dutasteride	____Headache
E. Tamsulosin	____Gynecomastia
F. Alfuzosin	____Flushing
	____Sexual dysfunction

The answer can be found on page 579

eRESOURCE

To reinforce your understanding of specific medications used in the treatment of BPH, refer to Epocrates Online. [Pathway: http://online.epocrates.com → under the "Drugs" tab, select "Genitourinary" in the "Classes" column under the subclass column, select "BPH" and review the drugs listed, focusing on "Adverse Reactions" and "Safety/Monitoring."]

John returns after a trial of several different medications over a 1-year period. His symptoms are not significantly improved, and he is now open to considering a procedure for BPH.

EXERCISE 9.7 Select all that apply:

The nurse educates John on procedures used to treat benign prostatic hyperplasia (BPH). Which of the following are procedures used for the treatment of BPH?

A. Transurethral microwave heat treatment (TUMT)
B. Teletherapy
C. Transurethral needle ablation (TUNA)
D. Transurethral resection of the prostate (TURP)
E. Brachytherapy
F. Transurethral incision of the prostate

The answer can be found on page 579

eRESOURCE

To reinforce your understanding of the procedures used to treat BPH, refer to Medscape on your mobile device. [Pathway: Medscape ➔ enter "BPH" into the search field ➔ select "BPH" ➔ "Treatment & Management" and review content under "Approach Considerations."]

UNFOLDING CASE STUDY 2: Melvin

Melvin is a 60-year-old African American male who has been referred to the urology practice because of blood in his urine, a weak urine stream, urinary hesitancy, and an elevated prostate-specific antigen (PSA) result. He works as a police detective, and his symptoms are interfering with his work activities. The nurse notes that he has had frequent bladder infections over the past 6 months, and his brother had prostate cancer at the age of 57 years.

EXERCISE 9.8 Fill in the blanks:

What are two risk factors for prostate cancer?

1. ______________________________
2. ______________________________

The answer can be found on page 579

EXERCISE 9.9 Select all that apply:

The nurse realizes that prostate cancer can metastasize to other areas of the body. Which of the following questions would be most important to ask as part of the patient history in order to elicit symptoms of metastasis?

A. "Do you have a backache?"
B. "Have you gained weight over the past 3 months?"
C. "Do you have hip pain?"

D. "Have you had a rash?"
E. "Have you felt weak?"
F. "Have you had rectal or perineal discomfort?"

The answer can be found on page 580

---

eRESOURCE

To reinforce your understanding of the clinical presentation of a person with suspected prostate cancer, refer to Medscape on your mobile device. [Pathway: Medscape ➔ enter "Prostate Cancer" into the search field ➔ select "Prostate Cancer" and review content, focusing on "Overview" and "Clinical Presentation."]

EXERCISE 9.10 Multiple-choice:

The nurse discusses with Melvin the need for the health care provider to perform a digital rectal exam (DRE) today to evaluate the prostate. The nurse realizes that the findings on the DRE in a patient with prostate cancer include which of the following?

A. Hard prostate with irregularities
B. Enlarged, smooth prostate
C. Small, smooth prostate
D. Prostate smooth with rectal drainage

The answer can be found on page 580

The urologist also obtains a biopsy of Melvin's prostate, which confirms that he has prostate cancer. Further studies confirm that there is no metastatic bone disease. Melvin is in good health and leads an active lifestyle. The health care provider discusses the treatment options for prostate cancer, and Melvin chooses to have radical retropubic prostatectomy.

EXERCISE 9.11 Select all that apply:

Which of the following are most important for the nurse to assess during the postoperative period after a radical prostatectomy?

A. Urine output
B. Electrolyte imbalances
C. Mini-nutrition assessment
D. Braden scale
E. Anxiety level
F. Fluid volume used for irrigation

The answer can be found on page 580

Melvin occasionally takes ibuprofen for headaches, but he discontinued this practice 2 weeks before his prostatectomy as instructed by the nurse. It is important that patients undergoing a radical prostatectomy stop taking all aspirin, nonsteroidal anti-inflammatory medications, and platelet inhibitors for 10 to 14 days before surgery in order to decrease the risk of excessive bleeding after surgery.

eRESOURCE

To reinforce your understanding of the radical retropubic prostatectomy procedure, refer to Medscape on your mobile device. [Pathway: Medscape enter "Prostatectomy" into the search field → select "Radical Retropubic Prostatectomy" and review content, focusing on "Overview" and "Technique."]

EXERCISE 9.12 Multiple-choice:

Melvin calls the nurse 12 hours after surgery because he notices reddish pink drainage. He remembers about the risk of bleeding after surgery. What is the most appropriate response for the nurse to make?

A. "You are hemorrhaging. Let me call the urologist now!"
B. "Often drainage begins as reddish pink then it becomes lighter pink 24 hours after surgery."
C. "You may have a urinary tract infection."
D. "We will need to check your hemoglobin because of this bleeding."

The answer can be found on page 581

EXERCISE 9.13 Select all that apply:

It is the first day after Melvin's radical prostatectomy. Which of the following are nursing interventions that may decrease the risk of deep vein thrombosis (DVT)?

A. Use of anti-embolism stockings
B. Low-fat diet
C. Ambulation
D. Use of subcutaneous enoxaparin
E. Adequate pain control
F. Increased fluid intake

The answer can be found on page 581

EXERCISE 9.14 Exhibit-format:

The nurse's assessment of Melvin on postoperative day 1 is as follows:

Awake and alert

Vital signs: Temperature: 99°F; heart rate (HR): 86 beats per minute (bpm); respiratory rate (RR): 22 respirations per minute; blood pressure (BP): 124/88 mmHg

Lung fields clear

HR regular

Bowel sounds positive, all four quadrants

Pedal pulses positive

Complains of the urgency to void and pressure and fullness in the bladder. What is the most likely cause of his symptoms?

A. Hemorrhage
B. Hyponatremia
C. Bladder spasms
D. Deep vein thrombosis (DVT)

The answer can be found on page 581

EXERCISE 9.15 Fill in the blanks:

The nurse provides discharge teaching on the risk of urinary tract infection and epididymitis after a radical prostatectomy. What are two symptoms that would require Melvin to notify the urologist?

1. ______________________
2. ______________________

The answer can be found on page 582

---

eRESOURCE

To reinforce your understanding of the radical retropubic prostatectomy procedure and associated periprocedural care, refer to Medscape on your mobile device. [Pathway: Medscape → enter "Prostatectomy" into the search field → select "Radical Retropubic Prostatectomy" and review content, focusing on "Periprocedural Care."]

After the removal of the catheter at his postoperative appointment, Melvin calls the urology office to report that he is having urinary incontinence after his radical prostatectomy. He is very disappointed about having incontinence. The nurse tells him that the majority of patients experience urinary incontinence, and that this symptom often decreases over a period of time.

EXERCISE 9.16 Fill in the blanks:

What are two ways that Melvin can prevent urinary incontinence after his radical prostatectomy?

1. ______________________
2. ______________________

The answer can be found on page 582

Melvin does not know how to perform pelvic floor exercises, and the nurse educates him on how to do them.

EXERCISE 9.17 Fill in the blank:

What is the proper technique for patients to use when performing pelvic floor exercises after a radical prostatectomy?

The answer can be found on page 582

eRESOURCE

To supplement your understanding of the management of urinary incontinence in adults, refer to the *Merck Manual.* [Pathway: www.merckmanuals.com/professional → enter "Incontinence" into the search field → select "Urinary Incontinence in Adults" → review content.]

UNFOLDING CASE STUDY 3: Joe

Joe is a 59-year-old African American male who is in the urology clinic to discuss his upcoming transurethral resection of the prostate (TURP). He is a high school teacher and football coach and has an active lifestyle. He has failed medical management of BPH with alpha-adrenergic blockers and 5-alpha-reductase inhibitors. He is ready to obtain relief from his urinary frequency, nocturia, and hesitancy with urination. The nurse explains how the TURP procedure is performed.

EXERCISE 9.18 Multiple-choice:

Joe needs additional education on transurethral resection of the prostate (TURP) when he states which of the following?

A. "The TURP procedure is a closed procedure."
B. "I'll need to stay in the hospital for 3 to 5 days."
C. "I cannot lift weights right after surgery."
D. "I'll have a catheter after surgery."

The answer can be found on page 582

Joe's urologist performs the TURP procedure by inserting a resectoscope through the urethra and removing excess prostate tissue.

eRESOURCE

To reinforce your understanding of the TURP procedure, refer to Medscape on your mobile device. [Pathway: Medscape → enter "Transurethral" into the search field → select "Transurethral Resection of the Prostate" and review content.]

Postoperatively, an indwelling three-way catheter is placed. The catheter drains urine and allows for continuous bladder irrigation (CBI) of normal saline or another irrigating solution. The nurse tells Joe that CBI is performed to prevent obstruction of the catheter.

EXERCISE 9.19 Multiple-choice:

The nurse who is caring for Joe notes that there is bright red bleeding with clots. How should the nurse modify the continuous bladder irrigation (CBI) rate, if indicated?

A. Decrease the CBI rate
B. Increase the CBI rate
C. Continue the CBI at the same rate
D. Stop the CBI and notify the urologist immediately

The answer can be found on page 582

EXERCISE 9.20 Fill in the blank:

How does the nurse calculate urine output with continuous bladder irrigation (CBI)?

____

The answer can be found on page 582

EXERCISE 9.21 Multiple-choice:

Joe asks the nurse why the catheter has a balloon that is taped to his leg. The nurse explains that the purpose of this intervention is which of the following?

A. To prevent deep vein thrombosis (DVT)
B. To prevent infection
C. To prevent bleeding
D. To prevent bladder spasms

The answer can be found on page 583

EXERCISE 9.22 Select all that apply:

While the three-way indwelling catheter is in place, Joe complains of pain, which is rated 6 of 10 on the pain scale. Which of the following interventions is most important for the nurse to perform?

A. Examine the tubing of the three-way catheter system
B. Irrigate the drainage system with irrigating fluid
C. Administer analgesics, if indicated
D. Obtain vital signs
E. Inspect the lower abdomen and bladder
F. Begin intravenous (IV) levofloxacin immediately

The answer can be found on page 583

EXERCISE 9.23 Matching:

The nurse administers several medications to Joe postoperatively. The nurse explains to Joe why each medication is being used. Match the medication classes in Column A with the rationales in Column B:

Column A	Column B
A. Analgesics	___ Prophylaxis of infection
B. Antibiotics	___ Prevention of bladder spasms
C. Antispasmodics	___ Prevention of straining with bowel movements
D. Stool softeners	___ Incisional pain

The answer can be found on page 583

EXERCISE 9.24 Select all that apply:

Joe is ready to go home after his transurethral resection of the prostate (TURP) procedure, and the nurse provides discharge teaching. Joe understands his patient education when he states which of the following?

A. "I need to drink 12 glasses of water per day."
B. "I need to avoid caffeine and alcohol."
C. "I can start jogging after 5 days."
D. "I need to call the urology practice if I have persistent bleeding."
E. "I need to contact my provider with any fever."
F. "I may resume sexual intercourse once I get home."

The answer can be found on page 583

eRESOURCE

To reinforce your understanding of the patient teaching following a TURP procedure, refer to MedlinePlus. [Pathway: www.nlm.nih.gov/medlineplus ➔ enter "TURP" into the search field ➔ select "Transurethral Resection of the Prostate—Discharge" and review content.]

UNFOLDING CASE STUDY 4: Preston

Preston is an 18-year-old White male who has been referred to the urology practice because of a painless "lump" in his right testicle. He noticed it 3 days ago while performing a monthly testicular self-examination (TSE). The transscrotal testicular ultrasound is suspicious for testicular cancer. He is embarrassed about being in the clinic, but his mother who is a nurse convinced him that he needed to have it evaluated. He is a senior in high school and plays tennis. He is going to college in the fall to pursue a computer science degree.

EXERCISE 9.25 Multiple-choice:

The nurse asks Preston several questions regarding the testicular mass. Which finding would be most concerning for metastasis?

A. Weight loss and backache for 6 months
B. Painless enlargement of the testis
C. History of chlamydia 8 months ago
D. Recent trip to Mexico on spring break

The answer can be found on page 584

Preston tells the nurse he has always been healthy and wonders why this is happening to him. He asks about the risk factors for testicular cancer. The nurse listens supportively to Preston, and she educates him on common risk factors for testicular cancer. She also tells him that testicular cancer is a highly treatable and curable form of cancer.

EXERCISE 9.26 Fill in the blanks:

What are two risk factors for testicular cancer?

1. ______________________________
2. ______________________________

The answer can be found on page 584

The nurse tells Preston that she needs to obtain tumor marker levels. She also tells him that a chest x-ray will be performed to rule out metastasis of the testicular cancer.

EXERCISE 9.27 Fill in the blanks:

What are two tumor markers that are often elevated in testicular cancer?

1. ______________________________
2. ______________________________

The answer can be found on page 584

---

eRESOURCE

To reinforce your understanding of testicular cancer, refer to Medscape on your mobile device. [Pathway: Medscape ➔ enter "Testicular" into the search field ➔ select "Testicular Cancer" and review content.]

The physician discusses the need to remove the testis by an orchiectomy, with the insertion of a testicular prosthesis.

eRESOURCE

To reinforce your understanding of the orchiectomy, refer to Medscape on your mobile device. [Pathway: Medscape ➔ enter "Orchiectomy" into the search field ➔ select "Radical Orchiectomy" and review content.]

The physician offers Preston the option of banking his sperm before the procedure. Preston is not in a relationship currently but desires to be a father after he gets married. He is unsure whether he wants to bank his sperm.

EXERCISE 9.28 Multiple-choice:

The nurse educates Preston on the need to consider sperm banking because of his diagnosis of testicular cancer. The nurse realizes that Preston understands the patient teaching when he states which of the following?

A. "Sperm banking is important for men who are ready to have children in 5 years or less."
B. "Many males with testicular cancer have decreased sperm quality, so I need to bank my sperm if I desire children at any point."
C. "I should bank my sperm if my testicular cancer has metastasized."
D. "I do not believe in being a sperm donor, so I do not need to bank my sperm."

The answer can be found on page 584

Preston begins chemotherapy for testicular cancer. The cancer responds to the chemotherapy treatments. The nurse educates Preston about the need for ongoing surveillance.

EXERCISE 9.29 Select all that apply:

Which of the following are common tests performed during surveillance for testicular cancer?

A. Chest x-rays
B. Beta-human chorionic gonadotropin (beta-hCG) and alpha-fetoprotein (AFP) levels
C. Examination of lymph nodes
D. Examination of testis
E. Testing for sexually transmitted infections
F. Sperm counts

The answer can be found on page 585

The nurse educates Preston on the need for monthly TSE following testicular cancer because of the risk of developing further tumors.

EXERCISE 9.30 Ordering:

Place the steps of the testicular self-examination (TSE) in the correct order.

____ Locate and palpate the epididymis
____ Locate and palpate the testis
____ Roll the testis horizontally between the thumb and fingers

____ Palpate the spermatic cord
____ Palpate upward along the testis
____ Report any lumps or swelling of the testis to your health care provider
____ Repeat for the other testis, epididymis, and spermatic cord

The answer can be found on page 585

---

eRESOURCE

To reinforce your understanding of the patient teaching related to performing a TSE, refer to MedlinePlus. [Pathway: www.nlm.nih.gov/medlineplus ➔ enter "Testicular Self-Exam" into the search field ➔ select "Testicular Self-Exam" and "How to Do a Testicular Self-Examination" and review content.]

Preston is concerned about body image and sexuality after testicular cancer. He tells the nurse, "I'll never date anyone again! I'm so embarrassed about having testicular cancer." The nurse talks to him about these issues, and reassures him that orgasm and libido are not usually affected by testicular cancer. The nurse tells him about a local support group for testicular cancer, and he agrees to go.

One year later, Preston returns to the office for a routine follow-up appointment. He has had a successful year at college, and he is now in a serious dating relationship. He has had no recurrence of testicular cancer, and he is now playing tennis on the college team.

UNFOLDING CASE STUDY 5: Pedro

Pedro is a 72-year-old Hispanic male who presents to the primary care clinic for a routine follow-up appointment. His wife died last year, and he lives alone. He is a retired welder. He has a history of diabetes and hypertension. At the end of the visit, Pedro tells the nurse practitioner that he is in a new relationship now, and he is having difficulty with achieving and maintaining erections.

EXERCISE 9.31 Select all that apply:

The nurse educates Pedro on common risk factors for erectile dysfunction (ED). Which of the following are risk factors for ED?

A. Chronic renal failure
B. Cardiovascular disease
C. Diabetes
D. Smoking
E. Hypothyroidism
F. Age younger than 40 years

The answer can be found on page 585

EXERCISE 9.32 Select all that apply:

In reviewing Pedro's medications, the nurse discovers that he is taking medications that are associated with erectile dysfunction (ED). Which of the following medications increase the risk of ED?

A. Nifedipine
B. Diphenhydramine
C. Hydrochlorothiazide
D. Ranitidine
E. Insulin
F. Fluoxetine

The answer can be found on page 585

After the nurse practitioner completes a comprehensive history and physical assessment, lab tests are obtained. The nurse practitioner also obtains a sexual history and asks Pedro to complete the International Index for Erectile Function (IIEF-5) questionnaire. Based on the results, Pedro is diagnosed with ED.

EXERCISE 9.33 Multiple-choice:

The nurse educates the patient on common treatment options for erectile dysfunction (ED). Which of the following are oral pharmacologic treatments for ED?

A. Busulfan
B. Leuprolide
C. Sildenafil
D. Papaverine

The answer can be found on page 586

EXERCISE 9.34 Fill in the blanks:

The nurse educates Pedro on the phosphodiesterase-5 (PDE-5) inhibitors used for erectile dysfunction (ED). What are three PDE-5 inhibitors used to treat ED?

1. ____________________
2. ____________________
3. ____________________

The answer can be found on page 586

EXERCISE 9.35 Select all that apply:

Pedro has heard on television that some patients should not take oral medications for erectile dysfunction (ED) because of the associated health risks. The nurse informs him that the patients taking the following medications or with the following conditions should not take the phosphodiesterase-5 (PDE-5) inhibitors:

A. Use of nitroglycerine
B. Use of isosorbide mononitrate (Imdur)

C. Myocardial infarction (MI) within the past 6 months
D. Kidney dysfunction
E. Hypothyroidism
F. Hypertension that is not well controlled

The answer can be found on page 586

EXERCISE 9.36 Multiple-choice:

The nurse informs Pedro that penile injections of vasoactive agents are another option for treatment of erectile dysfunction (ED). Which of the following is a complication that is related to penile injections?

A. Frequent urinary tract infections
B. Gynecomastia
C. Priapism
D. Benign prostatic hyperplasia (BPH)

The answer can be found on page 586

---

eRESOURCE

To reinforce your understanding of ED, refer to Medscape on your mobile device. [Pathway: Medscape ➔ enter "Erectile" into the search field ➔ select "Erectile Dysfunction" and review content.]

Pedro had excellent results with the oral medications for ED. He had a MI 4 months ago and was taken off sildenafil. Since being discharged from the hospital, he has been taking nitroglycerin as needed for chest pain. He is in cardiac rehabilitation regularly and feels well. His cardiologist has told him that he is healthy enough to consider sexual activity.

EXERCISE 9.37 Fill in the blanks:

Pedro returns to the office today to explore nonpharmacological options for erectile dysfunction (ED). List two therapies that can be used for ED in a patient who takes nitroglycerin.

1. ____________________
2. ____________________

The answer can be found on page 587

---

eRESOURCE

To learn more about nonpharmacological options for the treatment of ED, refer to Medscape on your mobile device. [Pathway: Medscape ➔ enter "Erectile" into the search field ➔ select "Erectile Dysfunction" ➔ select "Treatment & Management" ➔ select "External Erection-Facilitating Devices" and review content.]

Answers

EXERCISE 9.1 Fill in the blanks:

List at least two symptoms other than urinary hesitancy and decreased urine flow that can be associated with benign prostatic hyperplasia (BPH):

1. **Painless hematuria**
2. **Frequency of urination**

Other answers: nocturia, decrease in volume and force of urine, urinary retention, urgency with sensation that bladder has not emptied completely, abdominal straining, frequent bladder infections, and dribbling.

EXERCISE 9.2 Fill in the blanks:

List at least two risk factors for benign prostatic hyperplasia (BPH):

1. **Age older than 45 years**
2. **Smoking**

Other answers: heavy alcohol consumption, obesity, sedentary lifestyle, hypertension, heart disease, and diabetes.

EXERCISE 9.3 Select all that apply:

The patient understands the nurse's teaching on diagnostic tests for benign prostatic hyperplasia (BPH) when he says:

A. "I need to have a colonoscopy."—NO; this is not necessary for the diagnosis of BPH.
B. "I need to have a digital rectal examination."—**YES; a digital rectal exam will show an enlarged, smooth prostate in BPH.**
C. "I need to have a liver biopsy."—NO; this is not necessary for BPH.
D. "I need to have an alpha-fetoprotein test."—NO; this is not necessary for BPH.
E. "I need to have a urinalysis."—**YES; a urinalysis is needed to screen for hematuria and urinary tract infection.**
F. "I need to have a prostate-specific antigen test."—**YES; a prostate-specific antigen (PSA) should also be obtained for patients with at least a 10-year life expectancy and for patients for whom the diagnosis of prostate cancer would change their treatment. A frequency and volume chart should be obtained for patients with the main symptom of nocturia.**

EXERCISE 9.4 Multiple-choice:

A patient with benign prostatic hyperplasia (BPH) understands the nurse's teaching when he states that:

A. "I need to avoid drinking large amounts of fluids at bedtime."—**YES; drinking large amounts of fluids at bedtime can increase the symptoms of BPH.**
B. "I need to increase my caffeine intake."—NO; it is advisable to decrease caffeine and alcohol intake with BPH.
C. "I need to eat more fish."—NO; there are no recommendations on fish intake.
D. "I need to increase my calcium intake."—NO; there is no recommendation on calcium intake.

EXERCISE 9.5 Multiple-choice:

The nurse also discusses with John the need to avoid antihistamines and decongestants. What is the rationale for avoiding these medications with benign prostatic hyperplasia (BPH)?

A. They increase bladder tone.—NO; they decrease bladder tone.
B. They cause urinary tract infections.—NO; they have no impact on urinary tract infections.
C. They decrease bladder tone.—**YES; antihistamines and decongestants can decrease bladder tone, which increases BPH symptoms.**
D. They can increase creatinine levels.—NO; they do not increase creatinine levels.

EXERCISE 9.6 Matching:

Match each medication in Column A with the possible side effect in Column B (medications could be used more than once):

Column A	Column B	
A. Terazosin	**A, C, E, F**	Dizziness
B. Finasteride	**B, D**	Decreased libido
C. Doxazosin	**A, C, E, F**	Postural hypotension
D. Dutasteride	**A, C, E, F**	Headache
E. Tamsulosin	**B, D**	Gynecomastia
F. Alfuzosin	**B, D**	Flushing
	A, B,C, D, E, F	Sexual dysfunction

EXERCISE 9.7 Select all that apply:

The nurse educates John on procedures used to treat benign prostatic hyperplasia (BPH). Which of the following are procedures used for the treatment of BPH?

A. Transurethral microwave heat treatment (TUMT)—**YES; this is a procedure used to treat BPH.**
B. Teletherapy—NO; this is a type of radiation therapy used for prostate cancer.
C. Transurethral needle ablation (TUNA)—**YES; this is a procedure used to treat BPH.**
D. Transurethral resection of the prostate (TURP)—**YES; this is a procedure used to treat BPH.**
E. Brachytherapy—NO; this is a type of radiation therapy used for prostate cancer.
F. Transurethral incision of the prostate—**YES; this is a procedure used to treat BPH.**

EXERCISE 9.8 Fill in the blanks:

What are two risk factors for prostate cancer?

1. **African American race**
2. **Age older than 65 years**

Other answers: heredity, diet high in fat, and $BRCA_2$ mutation.

EXERCISE 9.9 Select all that apply:

The nurse realizes that prostate cancer can metastasize to other areas of the body. Which of the following questions would be most important to ask as part of the patient history in order to elicit symptoms of metastasis?

A. "Do you have a backache?"—**YES; this is a possible indication of the metastasis to the bone or lymph nodes.**
B. "Have you gained weight over the past 3 months?"—NO; weight loss is more indicative of metastasis than weight gain.
C. "Do you have hip pain?"—**YES; this is a possible indication of the metastasis to the bone or lymph nodes.**
D. "Have you had a rash?"—NO; a rash is not usually related to prostate cancer.
E. "Have you felt weak?"—**YES; this is a possible indication of the metastasis to the bone or lymph nodes.**
F. "Have you had rectal or perineal discomfort?"—**YES; this is a possible indication of the metastasis to the bone or lymph nodes. Other symptoms of metastasis may include anemia, decreased urine output, and spontaneous fractures.**

EXERCISE 9.10 Multiple-choice:

The nurse discusses with Melvin the need for the health care provider to perform a digital rectal exam (DRE) today to evaluate the prostate. The nurse realizes that the findings on the DRE in a patient with prostate cancer include which of the following?

A. Hard prostate with irregularities—**YES; typical findings with prostate cancer include a hard prostate with irregular areas noted.**
B. Enlarged, smooth prostate—NO; this is seen more commonly with benign prostatic hyperplasia (BPH).
C. Small, smooth prostate—NO; this is not a typical finding with prostate cancer.
D. Prostate smooth with rectal drainage—NO; this is not a typical finding with prostate cancer.

EXERCISE 9.11 Select all that apply:

Which of the following are most important for the nurse to assess during the postoperative period after a radical prostatectomy?

A. Urine output—**YES; the patient who is post-radical prostatectomy is at risk for imbalanced fluid volume because of the irrigation of the surgical site that occurred during and after surgery. It is important for the nurse to monitor urine output.**
B. Electrolyte imbalances—**YES; it is important to monitor for electrolyte imbalances postoperatively.**
C. Mini-nutrition assessment—NO; this is not the most important assessment during the postoperative period.
D. Braden scale—NO; this is not the most important assessment during the postoperative period.
E. Anxiety level—NO; this is not the most important assessment during the postoperative period.
F. Fluid volume used for irrigation—**YES; because of the risk of imbalanced fluid volume, it is important to monitor the fluid volume used for irrigation. Additional concerns postoperatively are increased blood pressure, confusion, and respiratory distress.**

EXERCISE 9.12 Multiple-choice:

Melvin calls the nurse 12 hours after surgery because he notices reddish pink drainage. He remembers about the risk of bleeding after surgery. What is the most appropriate response for the nurse to make?

A. "You are hemorrhaging. Let me call the urologist now!"—NO; this is a normal finding after surgery.
B. "Often drainage begins as reddish pink then it becomes lighter pink 24 hours after surgery."—**YES; this finding is normal after surgery and will decrease to reddish-pink drainage within 24 hours after surgery.**
C. "You may have a urinary tract infection."—NO; this is a normal finding after surgery, but it is important for the nurse to monitor for any signs or symptoms of a urinary tract infection in the patient.
D. "We will need to check your hemoglobin because of this bleeding."—NO; this is a normal finding after surgery.

EXERCISE 9.13 Select all that apply:

It is the first day after Melvin's radical prostatectomy. Which of the following are nursing interventions that may decrease the risk of deep vein thrombosis (DVT)?

A. Use of anti-embolism stockings—**YES; the use of anti-embolism stockings decreases the risk of a DVT.**
B. Low-fat diet—NO; this type of diet does not decrease the risk of a DVT.
C. Ambulation—**YES; early ambulation after surgery decreases the risk of a DVT.**
D. Use of subcutaneous enoxaparin—**YES; the use of subcutaneous enoxaparin decreases the risk of a DVT.**
E. Adequate pain control—NO; although this is important, it does not decrease the risk of a DVT.
F. Increased fluid intake—NO; this does not decrease the risk of a DVT.

EXERCISE 9.14 Exhibit-format:

The nurse's assessment of Melvin on postoperative day 1 is as follows:

Awake and alert
Vital signs: Temperature: 99°F; heart rate (HR): 86 beats per minute (bpm); respiratory rate (RR): 22 respirations per minute; blood pressure (BP): 124/88 mmHg
Lung fields clear
HR regular
Bowel sounds positive, all four quadrants
Pedal pulses positive

Complains of the urgency to void and pressure and fullness in the bladder. What is the most likely cause of his symptoms?

A. Hemorrhage—NO; a hemorrhage does not usually cause an urgency to void and pressure and fullness in the bladder.
B. Hyponatremia—NO; hyponatremia does not usually cause an urgency to void and pressure and fullness in the bladder.
C. Bladder spasms—**YES; these symptoms are consistent with bladder spasms, which are common after a radical prostatectomy. Antispasmodics can be administered to decrease the discomfort associated with bladder spasms.**
D. Deep vein thrombosis (DVT)—NO; a DVT does not usually cause an urgency to void and pressure and fullness in the bladder.

EXERCISE 9.15 Fill in the blanks:

The nurse provides discharge teaching on the risk of urinary tract infection and epididymitis after a radical prostatectomy. What are the two symptoms that would require Melvin to notify the urologist?

1. **Fever**
2. **Chills**

Other answers: sweating, body aches, dysuria, urinary frequency, or urgency.

EXERCISE 9.16 Fill in the blanks:

What are two ways that Melvin can prevent urinary incontinence after his radical prostatectomy?

1. **Increasing the frequency of urination**
2. **Decreasing fluid intake before activities**

Other answers: avoiding positions that increase the need to urinate and use of pelvic floor exercises.

EXERCISE 9.17 Fill in the blank:

What is the proper technique for patients to use when performing pelvic floor exercises after a radical prostatectomy?

Patients should tense the perineal muscles by pressing the buttocks together for 15 to 20 seconds, then relaxing them.

EXERCISE 9.18 Multiple-choice:

Joe needs additional education on transurethral resection of the prostate (TURP) when he states which of the following?

A. "The TURP procedure is a closed procedure."—NO; this is correct.
B. "I'll need to stay in the hospital for 3 to 5 days."—**YES; this is not correct as most TURP procedures do not require a 3- to 5-day hospitalization unless there are complications.**
C. "I cannot lift weights right after surgery."—NO; this is correct.
D. "I'll have a catheter after surgery."—NO; this is correct.

EXERCISE 9.19 Multiple-choice:

The nurse who is caring for Joe notes that there is bright red bleeding with clots. How should the nurse modify the continuous bladder irrigation (CBI) rate, if indicated?

A. Decrease the CBI rate—NO; the rate needs to increase.
B. Increase the CBI rate—**YES; the nurse needs to increase the CBI rate. The rate of CBI should be adjusted to keep the irrigation return pink or lighter.**
C. Continue the CBI at the same rate—NO; the rate needs to increase.
D. Stop the CBI and notify the urologist immediately—NO; the rate needs to increase.

EXERCISE 9.20 Fill in the blank:

How does the nurse calculate urine output with continuous bladder irrigation (CBI)?

The volume of irrigation solution instilled – the amount of irrigation return = urine output.

EXERCISE 9.21 Multiple-choice:

Joe asks the nurse why the catheter has a balloon that is taped to his leg. The nurse explains that the purpose of this intervention is which of the following?

A. To prevent deep vein thrombosis (DVT)—NO; the purpose is not to prevent DVT.
B. To prevent infection—NO; the purpose it not to prevent infection.
C. To prevent bleeding—**YES; hemorrhage is a possible complication after transurethral resection of the prostate (TURP). The balloon provides pressure to the prostatic fossa, which prevents bleeding.**
D. To prevent bladder spasms—NO; the purpose is not to prevent bladder spasms.

EXERCISE 9.22 Select all that apply:

While the three-way indwelling catheter is in place, Joe complains of pain, which is rated 6 of 10 on the pain scale. Which of the following interventions is most important for the nurse to perform?

A. Examine the tubing of the three-way catheter system—**YES; it is important to inspect the tubing.**
B. Irrigate the drainage system with irrigating fluid—**YES; it is important to irrigate the drainage system to clear any possible obstruction.**
C. Administer analgesics, if indicated—**YES; analgesics are an important intervention postoperatively.**
D. Obtain vital signs—**YES; it is important to assess vital signs when the patient reports pain postoperatively.**
E. Inspect the lower abdomen and bladder—**YES; it is important to inspect the lower abdomen and bladder. A rounded swelling above the pubis indicates that the bladder is overdistended.**
F. Begin intravenous (IV) levofloxacin immediately—NO; there is no indication yet of an infection.

EXERCISE 9.23 Matching:

The nurse administers several medications to Joe postoperatively. The nurse explains to Joe why each medication is being used. Match the medication classes in Column A with the rationales in Column B:

Column A	Column B
A. Analgesics	B Prophylaxis of infection
B. Antibiotics	C Prevention of bladder spasms
C. Antispasmodics	D Prevention of straining with bowel movements
D. Stool softener	A Incisional pain

EXERCISE 9.24 Select all that apply:

Joe is ready to go home after his transurethral resection of the prostate (TURP) procedure, and the nurse provides discharge teaching. Joe understands his patient education when he states which of the following?

A. "I need to drink 12 glasses of water per day."—**YES; water will keep the bladder functioning.**
B. "I need to avoid caffeine and alcohol."—**YES; caffeine and alcohol are bladder stimulants.**
C. "I can start jogging after 5 days."—NO; the patient should not jog for 2 to 6 weeks, depending on the specific instructions provided by his physician.

D. "I need to call the urology practice if I have persistent bleeding."—**YES; hemorrhage is a possible complication, and the patient should call with any bleeding that persists.**
E. "I need to contact my provider with any fever."—**YES; it is important for the patient to report any fever.**
F. "I may resume sexual intercourse once I get home."—NO; the patient should avoid sexual intercourse for 2 to 6 weeks, depending on the specific instructions provided by his physician.

EXERCISE 9.25 Multiple-choice:

The nurse asks Preston several questions regarding the testicular mass. Which finding would be most concerning for metastasis?

A. Weight loss and backache for 6 months—**YES; this is the most concerning finding. Weight loss, backache, abdominal pain, and weakness can indicate metastasis of testicular cancer.**
B. Painless enlargement of the testis—NO; this is a common finding with testicular cancer.
C. History of chlamydia 8 months ago—NO; this is important to note on the history but would not be the most concerning finding.
D. Recent trip to Mexico on spring break—NO; this would not indicate possible metastasis.

EXERCISE 9.26 Fill in the blanks:

What are two risk factors for testicular cancer?

1. **History of undescended testicles (cryptorchidism)**
2. **Family history of testicular cancer**

Other answers: personal history of testicular cancer, age (most common in 15–35 years of age), and Caucasian race.

EXERCISE 9.27 Fill in the blanks:

What are two tumor markers that are often elevated in testicular cancer?

1. **Alpha-fetoprotein (AFP)**
2. **Beta-human chorionic gonadotropin (beta-hCG)**

Other answers: lactic acid dehydrogenase (LDH). AFP and beta-hCG are often elevated in testicular cancer, and these two markers are used to diagnose, stage, and monitor the patient's response to treatment. Elevated LDH levels may indicate widespread metastasis.

EXERCISE 9.28 Multiple-choice:

The nurse educates Preston on the need to consider sperm banking because of his diagnosis of testicular cancer. The nurse realizes that Preston understands the patient teaching when he states which of the following?

A. "Sperm banking is important for men who are ready to have children in 5 years or less."—NO; all patients with testicular cancer should consider the option of sperm banking.
B. "Many males with testicular cancer have decreased sperm quality, so I need to bank my sperm if I desire children at any point."—**YES; all males should be given the option of sperm banking because of the risk of decreased sperm quality after testicular cancer.**

C. "I should bank my sperm if my testicular cancer has metastasized."—NO; all patients with testicular cancer should consider the option of sperm banking.
D. "I do not believe in being a sperm donor, so I do not need to bank my sperm."—NO; even if the patient does not plan to donate sperm, he may want to consider banking his sperm for his future use.

EXERCISE 9.29 Select all that apply:

Which of the following are common tests performed during surveillance for testicular cancer?

A. Chest x-rays—**YES; this is part of routine surveillance for testicular cancer.**
B. Beta-human chorionic gonadotropin (beta-hCG) and alpha-fetoprotein (AFP) levels—**YES; this is part of routine surveillance for testicular cancer.**
C. Examination of lymph nodes—**YES; this is part of routine surveillance for testicular cancer.**
D. Examination of testis—**YES; this is part of routine surveillance for testicular cancer.**
E. Testing for sexually transmitted infections—NO; this is not part of routine surveillance for testicular cancer.
F. Sperm counts—NO; this is not part of routine surveillance for testicular cancer.

EXERCISE 9.30 Ordering:

Place the steps of the testicular self-examination (TSE) in the correct order.

_4_ Locate and palpate the epididymis
_1_ Locate and palpate the testis
_2_ Roll the testis horizontally between the thumb and fingers
_5_ Palpate the spermatic cord
_3_ Palpate upward along the testis
_7_ Report any lumps or swelling of the testis to your health care provider
_6_ Repeat for the other testis, epididymis, and spermatic cord

EXERCISE 9.31 Select all that apply:

The nurse educates Pedro on common risk factors for erectile dysfunction (ED). Which of the following are risk factors for ED?

A. Chronic renal failure—**YES; this is a risk factor for ED.**
B. Cardiovascular disease—**YES; this is a risk factor for ED.**
C. Diabetes—**YES; this is a risk factor for ED.**
D. Smoking—**YES; this is a risk factor for ED.**
E. Hypothyroidism—**YES; this is a risk factor for ED.**
F. Age younger than 40 years—NO; ED is more common in men older than 40 years. In the United States, it is even more prevalent in men who are older than 70 years of age.

EXERCISE 9.32 Select all that apply:

In reviewing Pedro's medications, the nurse discovers that he is taking medications that are associated with erectile dysfunction (ED). Which of the following medications increase the risk of ED?

A. Nifedipine—**YES; calcium channel blockers like nifedipine can increase the risk of ED.**
B. Diphenhydramine—**YES; diphenhydramine increases the risk of ED.**
C. Hydrochlorothiazide—**YES; hydrochlorothiazide increases the risk of ED.**

D. Ranitidine—**YES; ranitidine increases the risk of ED.**
E. Insulin—NO; insulin does not increase the risk of ED.
F. Fluoxetine—**YES; fluoxetine increases the risk of ED.**

EXERCISE 9.33 Multiple-choice:

The nurse educates the patient on common treatment options for erectile dysfunction (ED). Which of the following are oral pharmacologic treatments for ED?

A. Busulfan—NO; this medication is not used for ED. It is a chemotherapeutic agent.
B. Leuprolide—NO; this medication is not used for ED. It is an antihormone used to treat prostate cancer.
C. Sildenafil—**YES; sildenafil (Viagra) is an oral medication used to treat ED.**
D. Papaverine—NO; this is not an oral medication. This medication is used as a penile injection for ED.

EXERCISE 9.34 Fill in the blanks:

The nurse educates Pedro on the phosphodiesterase-5 (PDE-5) inhibitors used for erectile dysfunction (ED). What are three PDE-5 inhibitors used to treat ED?

1. **Sildenafil (Viagra)**
2. **Vardenafil (Levitra)**
3. **Tadalafil (Cialis)**

EXERCISE 9.35 Select all that apply:

Pedro has heard on television that some patients should not take oral medications for erectile dysfunction (ED) because of the associated health risks. The nurse informs him that patients taking the following medications or with the following conditions should not take the phosphodiesterase-5 (PDE-5) inhibitors:

A. Use of nitroglycerine—**YES; patients who take nitroglycerine should not take PDE-5 inhibitors.**
B. Use of isosorbide mononitrate (Imdur)—**YES; patients who take isosorbide mononitrate (Imdur) should not take PDE-5 inhibitors.**
C. Myocardial infarction (MI) within the past 6 months—**YES; patients with a recent MI should not take PDE-5 inhibitors.**
D. Kidney dysfunction—**YES; patients with kidney dysfunction should not take PDE-5 inhibitors.**
E. Hypothyroidism—NO; patients with hypothyroidism can take PDE-5 inhibitors.
F. Hypertension that is not well controlled—**YES; patients with uncontrolled hypertension should not take PDE-5 inhibitors.**

EXERCISE 9.36 Multiple-choice:

The nurse educates Pedro that penile injections of vasoactive agents are another option for treatment of erectile dysfunction (ED). Which of the following is a complication that is related to penile injections?

A. Frequent urinary tract infections—NO; this is not a complication related to penile injections.
B. Gynecomastia—NO; this is not a complication related to penile injections.

C. Priapism—**YES; priapism is a persistent, abnormal erection that can occur with penile injections.**
D. Benign prostatic hyperplasia (BPH)—NO; this is not a complication related to penile injections.

EXERCISE 9.37 Fill in the blanks:

Pedro returns to the office today to explore nonpharmacological options for erectile dysfunction (ED). List two therapies that can be used for ED in a patient who takes nitroglycerin.

1. **Penile implant—YES; penile implants can be used. However, they require surgical placement.**
2. **Negative pressure vacuum devices—YES; these devices can be used.**

Other answers: counseling, lifestyle modifications (such as smoking cessation, exercise, and weight loss), and medication changes.

Resources

American Urological Association. (2010). American Urological Association guideline: Management of benign prostatic hyperplasia. Retrieved from http://www.auanet.org/common/pdf/education/clinical-guidance/Benign-Prostatic-Hyperplasia.pdf

Bankhead, C. (2012). TURP associated with lower risk of repeat procedures. *Urology Times, 40*(10), 17–21.

Bengall, P. (2014). Diagnosis and treatment of prostate cancer. *Nursing Times, 110*(9), 12–15.

Krader, C. G. (2012). Pelvic floor exercises post-RP, TURP may have value. *Urology Times, 40*(2), 24–25.

Lassen, B., Gattinger, H., & Saxer, S. (2013). A systematic review of physical impairments following radical prostatectomy: Effect of psychoeducational interventions. *Journal of Advanced Nursing, 69*(12), 2602–2612. doi:10.1111/jan.12186

Mobley, D., Feibus, A., & Baum, N. (2015). Benign prostatic hyperplasia and urinary symptoms: Evaluation and treatment. *Postgraduate Medicine, 127*(3), 301–307. doi:10.1080/00325481.2015.1018799

Mola, J. R. (2015). Erectile dysfunction in the older adult male. *Urologic Nursing, 35*(2), 87–93. doi:10.7257/1053–816X.2015.35.2.87

Russell, S. S. (2014). Testicular cancer: Overview and implications for health care providers. *Urologic Nursing, 34*(4), 172–176. doi:10.7257/1053–816X.2014.34.4.172

Smeltzer, S. C., Bare, B. G., Hinkle, J. L., & Cheever, K. H. (Eds.). (2014). *Brunner and Suddarth's textbook of medical–surgical nursing* (13th ed.). Philadelphia, PA: Lippincott Williams & Wilkins.

CHAPTER 10

Geriatric Health

Deborah L. Hopla

UNFOLDING CASE STUDY 1: Zadoc

Zadoc is a 66-year-old male who has herpes zoster virus (shingles). He is a widower who lives with his son and three grandchildren. The grandchildren have not been vaccinated for varicella (chicken pox) because of fear of side effects. The nurse is helping with Zadoc's care.

EXERCISE 10.1 Select all that apply:

The nurse understands that the following manifestations are associated with herpes zoster:

A. The onset of herpes zoster can be preceded by itching, tingling, or pain several days before eruption.
B. The onset of herpes zoster can be preceded by a pattern of papulovesicles along a dermatome.
C. Scarring may occur with herpes zoster.
D. Herpes zoster is infectious until it is crusty.
E. Removing the scabs decreases scarring.
F. There is a cure for herpes zoster.

The answer can be found on page 606

EXERCISE 10.2 Select all that apply:

The nurse understands in the case of Zadoc that:

A. The children are at risk of contracting varicella (chickenpox).
B. The children should be vaccinated as soon as possible to reduce the possibility of infection.
C. Vaccination at this stage would be pointless.
D. The possible side effects from vaccination should be avoided.
E. Vaccination should be done in 21 days when the family is sure the children are not infected.
F. Vaccines rarely cause autism.

The answer can be found on page 606

EXERCISE 10.3 Select all that apply:

The nurse understands that part of Zodac's teaching should include that he:

A. Should monitor the skin for secondary infections
B. Should avoid pregnant women
C. Is at risk for dementia
D. Is at risk for falls while taking pain medications
E. Should not drink grapefruit juice
F. Should stay confined for 21 days

The answer can be found on page 607

eRESOURCE

To reinforce your understanding of the clinical presentation of herpes zoster and the recommended patient teaching, refer to Medscape on your mobile device. [Pathway: Medscape ➔ enter "Herpes" into the search field ➔ select "Herpes Zoster" and review content, focusing on "Overview," "Clinical Presentation," and "Patient Education."]

UNFOLDING CASE STUDY 2: Jeannie

The nurse is caring for a 76-year-old patient, Jeannie, who has a recent history of coronary heart disease. Jeannie lives alone and has been widowed for 5 years. Jeannie sleeps on three pillows and has dyspnea with walking. On examining Jeannie, the nurse discovers she has not been taking her medications for hypertension, nor has she been taking her diuretic because, "I have to walk to the bathroom too much and sometimes I don't make it." Jeannie is currently taking:

- Lisinopril/hydrochlorothiazide (HCTZ) (Prinivil) 20/12.5 every day
- Metoprolol (Lopressor) 25 mg twice a day
- Tolterodine tartrate (Detrol) 2 mg
- Alprazolam (Xanax) 0.25 mg every day

EXERCISE 10.4 Select all that apply:

The nurse understands that consequences of coronary artery disease include:

A. Death in the elderly
B. Hypertension
C. Three-pillow orthopnea
D. Urinary incontinence
E. Dyspnea on exertion
F. Lack of libido

The answer can be found on page 607

EXERCISE 10.5 Select all that apply:

The nurse also understands that Jeannie is at risk for:

A. Postural hypotension
B. Falls
C. Undue sedative effects
D. Depression
E. Agitation
F. Pneumonia

The answer can be found on page 607

---

eRESOURCE

To reinforce your understanding of the risk factors for patients with coronary artery disease, refer to Medscape on your mobile device. [Pathway: Medscape → enter "Coronary Artery" into the search field → select "Risk Factors for Coronary Artery Disease" and review content.]

EXERCISE 10.6 Select all that apply:

Another concern the nurse has is Jeannie's urinary incontinence; the nurse understands the following about urinary incontinence:

A. It puts this patient at risk for urinary tract infections (UTIs)
B. Anticholinergics can cause constipation
C. Even mild symptoms of a UTI can lead to a septic infection
D. Urinary incontinence in this patient is caused by the diuretic in her Prinivil
E. Caffeine can increase its severity

The answer can be found on page 607

---

eRESOURCE

To supplement your understanding of assessment and management of urinary incontinence in adults, refer to:

- *Merck Manual.* [Pathway: www.merckmanuals.com/professional → enter "Incontinence" into the search field → select "Urinary Incontinence in Adults" → review "Pathophysiology" and "Signs & Symptoms."]
- Medscape on your mobile device. [Pathway: Medscape → enter "Incontinence" into the search field → select "Urinary Incontinence" and review content.]

EXERCISE 10.7 Select all that apply:

Priority nursing assessments for Jeannie include:

A. Potassium intake
B. Daily weight checks
C. Mental status checks

D. Sodium intake
E. Calcium level checks
F. Hemoglobin and hematocrit assessment

The answer can be found on page 608

UNFOLDING CASE STUDY 3: Marvin

Marvin is an 83-year-old male with a 65-year history of smoking. He has recently developed a cough, blood-tinged phlegm, shortness of breath (SOB), had a 20-lb weight loss in the past month, and worsening fatigue.

EXERCISE 10.8 Exhibit-format:

Assessment:

- Marvin's weight is 118 lb
- Resting heart rate (HR): 120 beats per minute (bpm)
- Respiratory rate (RR): labored and at 28 bpm
- Blood pressure (BP): 110/50 mmHg
- Oxygen saturation: 74% on room air

The nurse's priority concern is:

A. BP
B. HR
C. Weight
D. Oxygen saturation

The answer can be found on page 608

Marvin has a chest x-ray and a large mass is detected on his right lower lung. He is scheduled for a lung biopsy.

EXERCISE 10.9 Select all that apply:

The nurse's responsibility in preparing Marvin for a lung biopsy is to:

A. Ensure the patient understands his preoperative information
B. Teach the patient to cough and deep breathe
C. Inquire whether the patient has coping methods that were useful in the past
D. Inquire about the patient's support system
E. Ask the patient about financial resources
F. Ask the patient about an advance directive

The answer can be found on page 608

Marvin's biopsy reveals adenocarcinoma of the lung, stage V. The provider discusses surgery, radiation, and chemotherapy with Marvin.

EXERCISE 10.10 Multiple-choice:

The nurse finds Marvin anxious; he is asking questions about the treatment options and whether or not his smoking may have contributed to his diagnosis. The best therapeutic communication the nurse can use in this situation is:

A. "Many lung cancers have a good cure rate."
B. "Do you think smoking caused your cancer?"
C. "A stage V lung cancer is curable if you go through all the treatment."
D. "Your provider will be contacted and will answer all your questions."

The answer can be found on page 609

Marvin opts for lung resection, radiation, and chemotherapy.

eRESOURCE

To reinforce your understanding of the lung resection procedure and periprocedural care, refer to Medscape on your mobile device. [Pathway: Medscape ➔ enter "Lung Resection" into the search field ➔ select "Lung Segmentectomy and Limited Pulmonary Resection" and review content.]

EXERCISE 10.11 Select all that apply:

Marvin's collaborative care should include the following:

A. Increased caloric intake
B. Ambulation of the patient as soon as the patient is weaned from the ventilator
C. Tell the patient he will lose all his hair
D. Watch the patient's thorax for radiation burns
E. Advise that patient to avoid eating fruits

The answer can be found on page 609

---

eRESOURCE

To supplement your understanding of chemotherapy, consult the *Merck Manual.* [Pathway: www.merckmanuals.com/professional ➔ enter "Cancer Therapy" into the search field ➔ select "Modalities of Cancer Therapy" and review content, focusing on "Chemotherapy."]

Despite surgery, radiation, and chemotherapy, Marvin develops difficulty swallowing and a second scan reveals metastasis to the throat, liver, and bone.

EXERCISE 10.12 Multiple-choice:

Marvin opts to stop all treatment. The nurse knows the most important care issues for Marvin will be:

A. Nutrition
B. End-of-life issues
C. Comfort
D. Pain management

The answer can be found on page 609

---

eRESOURCE

To reinforce your understanding of palliative care, refer to Medscape on your mobile device. [Pathway: Medscape ➔ enter "Palliative" into the search field ➔ select "Palliative Cancer Care Guidelines" and review content.]

UNFOLDING CASE STUDY 4: Janora

Janora is an 83-year-old female with complaints of constipation. She has been self-treating by adding fiber and laxatives to her diet but reports she only has a bowel movement twice a week. Janora describes her bowel movements as dry and hard. She reports straining that has caused "my hemorrhoids to flare-up."

EXERCISE 10.13 Select all that apply:

The nurse knows important aspects of Janora's treatment will include:

A. Increasing physical activity to aid in evacuation
B. Increasing fluid in the diet
C. Taking time to go to the bathroom the same time each day
D. Ensuring fiber intake equals 25 to 30 g/day
E. Decreasing caffeine intake
F. Increasing dairy products

The answer can be found on page 609

---

eRESOURCE

To reinforce your understanding of constipation, refer to Medscape on your mobile device. [Pathway: Medscape ➔ enter "Constipation" into the search field ➔ select "Constipation" and review content.]

Janora adds the recommended treatments to her day and her constipation improves but her hemorrhoids continue to bother her.

EXERCISE 10.14 Select all that apply:

The nurse instructs Janora correctly when he recommends or teaches:

A. "Hemorrhoids are to be expected at your age."
B. "Warm water soaks may help ease discomfort."
C. "Having hemorrhoids increases your risk for cancer."
D. "Hemorrhoids improve with bulky stool so fiber and fluid intake is important."
E. "Reducing fruit juice intake will decrease swelling."
F. "Use ice when needed."

The answer can be found on page 610

eRESOURCE

To reinforce your understanding of hemorrhoids, refer to Medscape on your mobile device. [Pathway: Medscape ➔ enter "Hemorrhoids" into the search field ➔ select "Hemorrhoids" and review content.]

UNFOLDING CASE STUDY 5: Harley

Harley is a 78-year-old presenting with complaints of nocturnal dysuria. He reports a slow stream, hesitancy, and dribbling when trying to void. He reports he continues to have an active sex life with his wife but is concerned he might have cancer. The provider exams Harley's prostate by performing a rectal exam. The provider reports there were no nodules or masses, but an enlarged prostate is noted. A blood test for a complete blood count (CBC) and a prostate-specific antigen (PSA) is ordered. The provider requests a patient urinalysis.

EXERCISE 10.15 Multiple-choice:

The nurse suspects that Harley most likely is describing manifestations of:

A. A urinary tract infection
B. Benign prostatic hypertrophy (BPH)
C. Prostate cancer
D. Erectile dysfunction

The answer can be found on page 610

The provider orders an alpha-adrenergic blocker to treat Harley's symptoms.

EXERCISE 10.16 Select all that apply:

The nurse understands that the following should be taught to Harley about an alpha-adrenergic blocker. Harley should:

A. Increase his water intake
B. Be told his urine color will turn orange
C. Be told he will likely have erectile dysfunction from this medication
D. Be cautioned to rise slowly when first taking this medication
E. Protect his mattress with plastic
F. Consult a marriage therapist for relationship adjustments

The answer can be found on page 610

Harley's PSA comes back and is slightly elevated and he questions the nurse about the meaning of an elevated PSA.

EXERCISE 10.17 Multiple-choice:

Education about prostate cancer data may include:

A. The National Cancer Institute (NCI, 2013) reports cancer in half of all men older than the age of 70 years.
B. Only 3% of men older than the age of 70 years die from prostate cancer.
C. Surgical intervention is necessary to prevent prostate cancer from spreading in men older than the age of 70 years.
D. Erectile dysfunction is a result of prostate cancer.

The answer can be found on page 610

---

eRESOURCE

To supplement your understanding of BPH, consult the *Merck Manual*. [Pathway: www.merckmanuals.com/professional → enter "BPH" into the search field → select "Benign Prostatic Hypertroplasia (BPH)" and review content.]

UNFOLDING CASE STUDY 6: Daisy

Daisy is a 66-year-old widow brought in today by her daughter with complaints of "forgetfulness." Her daughter reports that her mom has been "getting lost" and she recently discovered her mom has bills stacked up. Decayed food in her refrigerator was also found by her daughter. Daisy recently has lost 10 lb and appears anxious.

EXERCISE 10.18 Select all that apply:

The nurse knows there can be many causes of this condition, including:

A. Depression
B. Hypothyroidism
C. Infection
D. Anemia
E. Stroke
F. Trauma

The answer can be found on page 611

Daisy is diagnosed with mild Alzheimer's disease.

EXERCISE 10.19 Select all that apply:

Patients with Alzheimer's disease:

A. Need total care
B. Have difficulty recognizing people
C. Get lost on familiar routes
D. Becomes anxious and/or depressed
E. Typically die within 2 years of diagnosis
F. Become extroverted

The answer can be found on page 611

EXERCISE 10.20 Select all that apply:

The nursing care priorities for a patient with Alzheimer's disease include:

A. Safety needs
B. Nutritional needs
C. Financial needs
D. Maintaining a medication regimen
E. Self-esteem
F. Autonomy

The answer can be found on page 611

---

eRESOURCE

To supplement your understanding of Alzheimer's disease, consult the *Merck Manual.* [Pathway: www.merckmanuals.com/professional ➔ enter "Alzheimer" into the search field ➔ select "Alzheimer Disease" and review content.]

The nurse understands that Alzheimer's is a progressive disease and will raise numerous issues in Daisy's future.

EXERCISE 10.21 Select all that apply:

Daisy's daughter asks, "What can I expect in the future?" The best response from the nurse includes:

A. "Death is usually caused by old age, not the disease."
B. "In early stages, most patients can be cared for at home by a family member or a caregiver."
C. "Late in the disease, patients may need assisted-living or nursing home placement."
D. "Patients with this diagnosis qualify for hospice."
E. "Patients are safest at home, where they are familiar."
F. "Family therapy that includes Daisy is appropriate."

The answer can be found on page 611

---

eRESOURCE

To supplement your knowledge of the resources and information available for Alzheimer patients and their families, refer to MedlinePlus. [Pathway: www.nlm.nih.gov/medlineplus → enter "Alzheimer" into the search field → select "Alzheimer's Disease" and review available content.]

Daisy is place on donepezil (Aricept) once a day and memantine (Namenda) twice a day.

EXERCISE 10.22 Select all that apply:

It will be important for the nurse to advise Daisy's daughter:

A. To give the medication about the same time every day
B. To report any side effects
C. To give the medications with food to reduce side effects
D. To know that over time the medications will cease to work
E. To have the patient stand for 30 minutes after ingesting the medication
F. To take the medication with a small amount of water

The answer can be found on page 612

---

eRESOURCE

To reinforce your understanding of the medications that Daisy is prescribed, refer to Epocrates Online. [Pathway: http://online.epocrates.com → under the "Drugs" tab, enter "Donepezil" in the search field → select "Donepezil" → review "Adult Dosing," "Adverse Reactions," and "Safety/Monitoring." Repeat with "Memantine."]

UNFOLDING CASE STUDY 7: Robert

EXERCISE 10.23 Exhibit-format:

Assessment

Robert, age 62 years, has come in with two complaints:

- Tremor of his hands that is worse at night
- His joints are growing steadily more stiff and difficult to move, and he states, "It takes me forever to get anywhere or even get my clothes on in the morning."

As Robert is speaking his face does not move and his hands are tremoring and his fingers are pill-rolling.

The clinical manifestations Robert is displaying are related to:

A. Stroke
B. Aging
C. Brain tumor
D. Parkinson's disease
E. Multiple sclerosis
F. Turret's syndrome

The answer can be found on page 612

Robert is started on levodopa-carbidopa (Sinemet) three times a day.

EXERCISE 10.24 Select all that apply:

Side effects of levodopa–carbidopa (Sinemet) include:

A. Tardive dyskinesia
B. Nausea and headache
C. Amnesia
D. Somnolence
E. Anorexia
F. Tremors or seizures

The answer can be found on page 612

---

eRESOURCE

To reinforce your understanding of Sinemet, refer to Epocrates Online. [Pathway: http://online.epocrates.com → under the "Drugs" tab, enter "Sinemet" in the search field → select "Sinemet" → review "Adult Dosing," "Adverse Reactions," and "Safety/Monitoring."]

EXERCISE 10.25 Select all that apply:

Common complications of Parkinson's disease include:

A. Constipation
B. Difficulty swallowing
C. Frequent falls
D. Frequent urination
E. Dry mouth
F. Headaches

The answer can be found on page 612

---

eRESOURCE

To reinforce your understanding of Parkinson's disease, refer to Medscape on your mobile device. [Pathway: Medscape → enter "Parkinson" into the search field → select "Parkinson Disease" and review content.]

UNFOLDING CASE STUDY 8: Dorothy

Dorothy is a 74-year-old who was brought into the emergency department by her son, who explains, "She was talking to me about a half hour ago and all of a sudden her speech was slurred and she seemed confused." In taking Dorothy's vital signs, the nurse notices the following:

- Blood pressure (BP): 162/102 mmHg
- Heart rate (HR): 90 bpm and irregular
- Respiratory rate (RR): 16 breaths per minute
- Temperature: 98.6°F

Dorothy tries to answer questions, but her answers are slurred and not comprehensible. The patient is not moving her right arm or hand to commandment. Dorothy has a history of hypertension and diabetes. Her medications include:

- Lisinopril (an angiotensin-converting-enzyme inhibitor) 10 mg once a day
- Metformin 500 mg twice a day

EXERCISE 10.26 Multiple-choice:

The nurse suspects that Dorothy's manifestations are a result of:

A. Hypertension
B. Trauma
C. Aneurysms
D. Bleeding abnormality

The answer can be found on page 613

Dorothy is sent for a head CT scan and an MRI of the brain.

eRESOURCE

To supplement your understanding of the MRI procedure, refer to the *Merck Manual.* [Pathway: www.merckmanuals.com/professional ➔ enter "MRI" into the search field select "Magnetic Resonance Imaging" ➔ review content.]

A diagnosis of a stroke and new-onset atrial fibrillation is made. The nurse knows it is important for Dorothy to be carefully, but rapidly, evaluated for the benefits and risk of thrombolytic therapy.

EXERCISE 10.27 True/False:

Dorothy is a candidate for thrombolytic therapy.

____ True

____ False

The answer can be found on page 613

Dorothy is stabilized and moved to the intensive care unit (ICU). Dorothy's symptoms gradually improve and she is observed for any further symptoms of stroke or cerebral vascular accident (CVA).

eRESOURCE

To supplement your understanding of the clinical presentation of a patient suffering from a stroke, refer to the *Merck Manual.* [Pathway: www.merckmanuals.com/professional ➔ enter "Stroke" into the search field ➔ select "Overview of Stroke" ➔ review content.]

The cardiologist adds metoprolol (Lopressor), which is a beta blocker, twice a day. Dorothy's current vital signs are:

- BP: 120/88 mmHg
- HR: 72 bpm
- RR: 16 breaths per minute

eRESOURCE

To reinforce your understanding of Lopressor, refer to Epocrates Online. [Pathway: http://online.epocrates.com ➔ under the "Drugs" tab, enter "Lopressor" in the search field ➔ select "Lopressor" ➔ review "Adult Dosing," "Adverse Reactions," and "Safety/Monitoring."]

Dorothy is evaluated for swallowing and speech. Physical therapy (PT) begins working with Dorothy to assist her in regaining her strength and range of motion (ROM) in her affected extremity and she states, "I am ready to go home!"

EXERCISE 10.28 Multiple-choice:

The nurse should use which ethical principle to guide her response to Dorothy?

A. Justice
B. Autonomy
C. Beneficence
D. Nonmalfeasance

The answer can be found on page 613

Dorothy is discharged and a nurse is assigned to visit her once a week for 4 weeks. In evaluating Dorothy's home, the nurse notices several scatter rugs, a second floor on which the patient's bedroom is located, and a bathroom with normal fixtures, including a tub and shower. Meals on Wheels is set up to deliver food once a day during the week and a family member comes on the weekend to assist the patient. Dorothy is experiencing a sense of loss of independence.

EXERCISE 10.29 Ordering:

Order the following priorities for Dorothy from 1 to 4:

____ Nutritional needs
____ Activities of daily living
____ Safety needs
____ Adaptive changes to loss of independence

The answer can be found on page 613

UNFOLDING CASE STUDY 9: Larry

Larry is a 67-year-old male patient who was admitted to the hospital for diverticulitis. He was stable on admission. Larry has lived with this disease for more than 10 years. He is currently experiencing abdominal pain, copious bloody diarrhea, and rectal irritation. Larry has had nothing by mouth (NPO). He is receiving morphine intravenously for pain control via a pump. His vital signs this morning are:

- Temperature: 100.2°F
- HR: 92 bpm
- RR: 12 breaths per minute
- BP supine: 100/58 mmHg

Larry's laboratory values are:

- Sodium: 132 mEq/L
- Potassium: 4.5 mEq/L

- Glucose: 120
- Calcium: 8.2
- Creatinine: 5.5
- Blood urea nitrogen: 40
- Carbon dioxide: 44
- White blood cells (WBC): 18,000
- Hemoglobin 10.2 and hematocrit 28
- Platelets: 25,000

After reviewing the patient's information the nurse calls the provider.

EXERCISE 10.30 Select all that apply:

For Larry's situation ("S" in SBAR [situation, background, assessment, recommendation]), the nurse should choose to report:

A. Rectal bleeding
B. Sodium and potassium results
C. Pulse and blood pressure
D. Information related to renal function
E. Information related to respiratory function
F. Hemoglobin and hematocrit results

The answer can be found on page 613

EXERCISE 10.31 Select all that apply:

For Larry's background ("B" in SBAR), the nurse should choose to report that the patient:

A. Has a new diagnosis of diverticulitis
B. Has had diverticulitis for more than 10 years
C. Was stable last evening
D. Is elderly
E. Understands his diagnosis
F. Is cooperative

The answer can be found on page 614

The provider decides to give the patient intravenous (IV) fluids and orders a type and cross-match for three units of packed red blood cells (PRBCs). A consult is ordered for a nephrologist. Larry's pain medication is increased and he is being considered for surgery for a ruptured diverticula.

EXERCISE 10.32 Ordering:

Place the following nursing interventions in their order of importance from 1 to 3:

___ Request an order for antibiotic therapy

___ Hang 0.9% normal saline

___ Place a urinary catheter

The answer can be found on page 614

eRESOURCE

To supplement your understanding of the clinical presentation associated with diverticulitis, refer to the *Merck Manual.* [Pathway: www.merckmanuals.com/professional ➔ enter "Diverticulitis" into the search field ➔ select "Diverticulitis" ➔ review "Symptom and Signs," "Diagnosis," and "Treatment."]

Larry continues to bleed and emergency surgery is done to remove the affected colon, which results in a temporary colostomy.

EXERCISE 10.33 Select all that apply:

Discharge planning for Larry should include:

A. Stoma care of a colostomy
B. Nutritional counseling
C. Pain management
D. Information about infection awareness

The answer can be found on page 614

Larry has had an uneventful healing time and is to undergo re-anastomosis of the colon. Larry has had some episodes of depression and adaptive changes related to body image and the colostomy.

eRESOURCE

To reinforce your understanding of a temporary colostomy, refer to Medscape on your mobile device. [Pathway: Medscape ➔ enter "Colostomy" into the search field ➔ select "Loop Colostomy" and review content.]

EXERCISE 10.34 Multiple-choice:

Larry remarks to the nurse, "I am sure I will be fine now. What do you think?" The best response the nurse can provide is:

A. "Sure, you will be just fine!"
B. "I hope you are right!"

C. "If your disease can be managed, you probably will not die from this disease!"
D. "Your surgeon feels you have done well, do you have concerns?"

The answer can be found on page 614

UNFOLDING CASE STUDY 10: Rebecca

Rebecca is an 83-year-old patient recently diagnosed with bacterial pneumonia. Her vital signs on admission are:

- Temperature: 103.3°F
- HR: 90 bpm
- RR: 30 breaths per minute
- BP: 142/90 mmHg

Rebecca is on oxygen at 2 L/min per nasal cannula. She is alert and oriented and sitting up in bed. She has an IV line with fluids at 75 mL/hr. The provider has ordered levofloxacin (Levaquin) IV every 12 hours. Rebecca has a Foley catheter in place.

EXERCISE 10.35 Select all that apply:

The nurse understands the following are consistent with the diagnosis of bacterial pneumonia:

A. It has a low mortality rate among the elderly
B. It has a high rate of mortality among the elderly
C. It can cause confusion and hypoxia
D. It has a greater risk of aspiration of foreign matter because it causes decreased sensitivity of pharyngeal reflexes
E. It may be preceded by a urinary tract infection
F. Antibiotics are effective in most cases

The answer can be found on page 614

eRESOURCE

To reinforce your understanding of the clinical presentation and treatment of bacterial pneumonia, refer to Medscape on your mobile device. [Pathway: Medscape → enter "Bacterial" into the search field → select "Bacterial Pneumonia" and review content.]

Rebecca becomes increasingly lethargic. It is determined she will require intubation. There is a do not resuscitate (DNR) living will from the patient. The nurse alerts the provider. No family members have been present and the provider is not willing to abide by the DNR.

EXERCISE 10.36 Select all that apply:

The nurse has the obligation(s) to:

A. Abide by the patient's do not resuscitate
B. Follow hospital policy
C. Notify the ethics committee
D. Follow the provider's orders
E. Keep searching for family members
F. Refer to the hospital's chaplin

The answer can be found on page 615

Answers

EXERCISE 10.1 Select all that apply:

The nurse understands that the following manifestations are associated with herpes zoster:

A. The onset of herpes zoster can be preceded by itching, tingling, or pain several days before eruption.—**YES; herpes can be preceded by itching, tingling, or pain for several days before eruption**.
B. The onset of herpes zoster can be preceded by a pattern of papulovesicles along a dermatome.—NO; the dermatome pattern of papulovesicles occurs after being infected for several days.
C. Scarring may occur with herpes zoster.—**YES; scarring may occur; especially if the patient does not have good hygiene or gets a bacterial infection.**
D. Herpes zoster is infectious until it is crusty.—**YES; the herpes zoster is infectious until it is scabbed over.**
E. Removing the scabs decreases scarring.—NO; this increases scarring.
F. There is a cure for herpes zoster.—NO; this is not true.

EXERCISE 10.2 Select all that apply:

The nurse understands in the case of Zadoc that:

A. The children are at risk of contracting varicella (chickenpox).—**YES; this is true.**
B. The children should be vaccinated as soon as possible to reduce the possibility of infection.—**YES; this is true**.
C. Vaccination at this stage would be pointless.—NO; the children need vaccination. If they contract varicella, the effects of the disease could be reduced by vaccination.
D. The possible side effects from vaccination should be avoided.—NO; the potential for side effects are minimal and usually limited to redness or pain at the injection site.
E. Vaccinations should be done in 21 days when the family is sure the children are not infected.—NO; the children should be vaccinated at their scheduled time.
F. Vaccines rarely cause autism.—NO; there is no link between autism and vaccines.

EXERCISE 10.3 Select all that apply:

The nurse understands that part of Zadoc's teaching should include that he:

A. Should monitor the skin for secondary infections—**YES; this is true.**
B. Should avoid pregnant women—**YES; this is true.**
C. Is at risk for dementia—NO; this is not true.
D. Is at risk for falls while taking pain medications—**YES; this is true.**
E. Should not drink grapefruit juice—NO; this is not true.
F. Should stay confined for 21 days—NO; this is not true. Once the scabbed areas are healing, the patient is not contagious.

EXERCISE 10.4 Select all that apply:

The nurse understands that consequences of coronary artery disease include:

A. Death in the elderly—**YES; it is the most common cause of death in the elderly.**
B. Hypertension—**YES; hypertension increases a patient's risk for myocardial infarction, cerebrovascular accident, and renal failure.**
C. Three-pillow orthopnea—**YES; this is related to shortness of breath during sleep, usually from left-side heart failure.**
D. Urinary incontinence—NO; incontinence is not related to coronary artery disease.
E. Dyspnea on exertion—**YES; this is true.**
F. Lack of libido—NO; this is not true.

EXERCISE 10.5 Select all that apply:

The nurse also understands that Jeannie is at risk for:

A. Postural hypotension—**YES; being older than 75 years and taking two hypertensive agents put this patient at risk for postural hypotension.**
B. Falls—**YES; taking more than four medications with one of the medications being an antianxiety agent puts this patient at risk for falls.**
C. Undue sedative effects—**YES; this patient is at risk for sedation because of the use of Xanax and the beta blocker metoprolol.**
D. Depression—**YES; this patient is widowed and is on a beta blocker which predisposes the patient to depression. A decline in health also puts this patient at risk for depression.**
E. Agitation—NO; this is not a risk factor.
F. Pneumonia—NO; this is not a risk factor.

EXERCISE 10.6 Select all that apply:

Another concern the nurse has is Jeannie's urinary incontinence; the nurse understands the following about urinary incontinence:

A. It puts this patient at risk for urinary tract infections (UTIs)—**YES; this is true.**
B. Anticholinergics can cause constipation—**YES; this is true.**
C. Even mild symptoms of a UTI can lead to a septic infection—**YES; this is true.**
D. Urinary incontinence in this patient is caused by the diuretic in her Prinivil—NO; the diuretic may cause urinary urgency but not incontinence.
E. Caffeine can increase its severity—**YES; this is true.**

EXERCISE 10.7 Select all that apply:

Priority nursing assessments for Jeannie include:

A. Potassium intake—**YES; because this patient is on a diuretic she could lose potassium, which could cause cardiac arrhythmia.**

B. Daily weight checks—**YES; monitoring weight gains can indicate worsening heart disease or the development of congestive heart failure.**

C. Mental status checks—**YES; the patient is taking Xanax, which can alter her mentation.**

D. Sodium intake—**YES; sodium intake should be reduced because of the patient's heart disease.**

E. Calcium level checks—**YES; this would be important because of the patient's age.**

F. Hemoglobin and hematocrit assessment—**YES; this would be important to assess as anemia can put the patient at risk for heart problems.**

EXERCISE 10.8 Exhibit-format:

Assessment:

- Marvin's weight is 118 lb
- Resting heart rate (HR): 120 beats per minute (bpm)
- Respiratory rate (RR): labored and at 28 bpm
- Blood pressure (BP): 110/50 mmHg
- Oxygen saturation: 74% on room air

The nurse's priority concern is:

A. BP—NO; the BP is fine.

B. HR—NO; even though the heart rate is elevated it is not the most important problem.

C. Weight—NO; even though the patient has had a significant weight loss this is not the most important problem.

D. Oxygen saturation—**YES; the oxygen saturation is dangerously low and needs to be addressed first.**

EXERCISE 10.9 Select all that apply:

The nurse's responsibility to prepare Marvin for a lung biopsy is to:

A. Ensure the patient understands his preoperative information—**YES; but if the patient has questions, the provider should be contacted.**

B. Teach the patient to cough and deep breathe—**YES; this is a nursing function before a surgery.**

C. Inquire whether the patient has coping methods that were useful in the past—**YES; establishing the patient's level of coping is important.**

D. Inquire about the patient's support system—**YES; ensuring the patient has a support system in place is important.**

E. Ask the patient about financial resources—NO; this is the social worker's responsibility.

F. Ask the patient about an advance directive—**YES; this is important.**

EXERCISE 10.10 Multiple choice:

The nurse finds Marvin anxious; he is asking questions about the treatment options and whether or not his smoking may have contributed to his diagnosis. The best therapeutic communication the nurse can use in this situation is:

A. "Many lung cancers have a good cure rate."—NO; lung cancer has only a 16% survival rate after 5 years of diagnosis.
B. "Do you think smoking caused your cancer?"—NO; smoking causes 90% of all lung cancers.
C. "A stage V lung cancer is curable if you go through all the treatment."—NO; lung cancer's 5-year survival rate is only 16%.
D. "Your provider will be contacted and will answer all your questions."—**YES; the patient should have all questions answered.**

EXERCISE 10.11 Select all that apply:

Marvin's collaborative care should include the following:

A. Increased caloric intake—**YES; the extra calorie intake will be needed for healing.**
B. Ambulation of the patient as soon as the patient is weaned from the ventilator—**YES; ambulation decreases secretions and aids in healing.**
C. Tell the patient he will lose all his hair—NO; not all patients lose their hair while undergoing chemotherapy.
D. Watch the patient's thorax for radiation burns—**YES; radiation burns to the skin are common.**
E. Advise the patient to avoid eating fruits—NO; fruits can be eaten if they are thoroughly washed or cooked.

EXERCISE 10.12 Select all that apply:

Marvin opts to stop all treatment. The nurse knows the most important care issues for Marvin will be:

A. Nutrition—NO; this is not the most important issue.
B. End-of-life issues—**YES; this is the patient's most important issue. End-of-life issues could include pain management, nutritional needs, comfort measures, possible hospice management, and mental health needs for end of life.**
C. Comfort—NO; this is important but not the most important.
D. Pain management—NO; this is important but not the most important issue facing this patient.

EXERCISE 10.13 Select all that apply:

The nurse knows important aspects of Janora's treatment will include:

A. Increasing physical activity to aid in evacuation—**YES; this is true.**
B. Increasing fluid in the diet—**YES; this is true.**
C. Taking time to go to the bathroom the same time each day—**YES; this is true.**
D. Ensuring fiber intake equals 25 to 30 g/day—**YES; this is true.**
E. Decreasing caffeine intake—**YES; this is true.**
F. Increasing dairy products—NO; this is not true.

EXERCISE 10.14 Select all that apply:

The nurse instructs Janora correctly when he recommends or teaches:

A. "Hemorrhoids are to be expected at your age."—NO; this is not true.
B. "Warm water soaks may help ease discomfort."—**YES; warm water soaks may relieve discomfort.**
C. "Having hemorrhoids increases your risk for cancer."—**YES; this is true.**
D. "Hemorrhoids improve with bulky stool so fiber and fluid intake is important."—**YES; this is true.**
E. "Reducing fruit juice intake will decrease swelling."—NO; this is not true.
F. "Use ice when needed."—NO; ice should only be used for 20 minutes.

EXERCISE 10.15 Multiple-choice:

The nurse suspects that Harley most likely is describing manifestations of:

A. A urinary tract infection—NO; this is possible but not likely.
B. Benign prostatic hypertrophy (BPH)—**YES; 80% of men at this age will suffer from an enlarged prostate.**
C. Prostate cancer—NO; this is being ruled out but not the likely cause of symptoms.
D. Erectile dysfunction—NO; this patient reports an active sex life with his wife.

EXERCISE 10.16 Select all that apply:

The nurse understands that the following should be taught to Harley about an alpha-adrenergic blocker. Harley should:

A. Increase his water intake—NO; although this is a healthy practice it is not necessary while taking this medication.
B. Be told his urine color will turn orange—NO; this is not a side effect.
C. Be told he will likely have erectile dysfunction from this medication—NO; this is not a side effect of this medication.
D. Be cautioned to rise slowly when first taking this medication—**YES; this is true.**
E. Protect his mattress with plastic—NO; this is not necessary.
F. Consult a marriage therapist for relationship adjustments—NO; this is not needed.

EXERCISE 10.17 Multiple-choice:

Education about prostate cancer data may include:

A. The National Cancer Institute (NCI, 2013) reports cancer in half of all men older than the age of 70 years.—**YES; this is true.**
B. Only 3% of men older than the age of 70 years die from prostate cancer.—**YES; this is true according to the NCI (2013).**
C. Surgical intervention is necessary to prevent prostate cancer from spreading in men older than the age of 70 years.—NO; this is not true according to the NCI (2013).
D. Erectile dysfunction is a result of prostate cancer.—NO; although this can happen, it is not usually true.

EXERCISE 10.18 Select all that apply:

The nurse knows there can be many causes of this condition, including:

A. Depression—**YES; this could be a possible cause**.
B. Hypothyroidism—**YES; this could be a possible cause.**
C. Infection—**YES; this could be a possible cause**.
D. Anemia—**YES; this could be a possible cause.**
E. Stroke—**YES; this could be a possible cause.**
F. Trauma—**YES; this could be a possible cause.**

EXERCISE 10.19 Select all that apply:

Patients with Alzheimer's disease:

A. Need total care—NO; this is severe/stage 3 Alzheimer's disease.
B. Has difficulty recognizing people—NO; this is moderate/stage 2 Alzheimer's disease.
C. Get lost on familiar routes—**YES; this is mild/stage 1 Alzheimer's disease.**
D. Becomes anxious and/or depressed—**YES; this is mild/stage 1 Alzheimer's disease.**
E. Typically die within 2 years of diagnosis—NO; this is not true.
F. Become extroverted—NO; this is not true.

EXERCISE 10.20 Select all that apply:

The nursing care priorities for a patient with Alzheimer's disease include:

A. Safety needs—**YES; this is the most important need for a patient with Alzheimer's disease.**
B. Nutritional needs—NO; this is important but not the most important need.
C. Financial needs—NO; this is important for the patient later in the disease because of the need for 24/7 care.
D. Maintaining a medication regimen—NO; this is important but medication only slows the progression and does not stop Alzheimer's disease.
E. Self-esteem—**YES; this is important.**
F. Autonomy—**YES; this is important.**

EXERCISE 10.21 Select all that apply:

Daisy's daughter asks, "What can I expect in the future?" The best response from the nurse includes:

A. "Death is usually caused by old age, not the disease."—NO; death is usually caused by septicemia, pneumonia, and/or complications from hip fractures.
B. "In early stages, most patients can be cared for at home by a family member or a caregiver."—**YES; this is true**.
C. "Late in the disease, patients may need assisted-living or nursing home placement."—**YES; this is true.**
D. "Patients with this diagnosis qualify for hospice."—**YES; this is true. Patients may go on and come off of hospice but an Alzheimer's diagnosis will qualify them for care.**
E. "Patients are safest at home, where they are familiar."—NO; as patients decline, they will need care 24/7.
F. "Family therapy that includes Daisy is appropriate."—**YES; this is true.**

EXERCISE 10.22 Select all that apply:

It will be important for the nurse to advise Daisy's daughter:

A. To give the medication about the same time every day—**YES; this is true.**
B. To report any side effects—**YES; this is true of all medications.**
C. To give the medications with food to reduce side effects—**YES; food will reduce side effects.**
D. To know that over time the medications will cease to work—**YES; over time these medications will cease to work.**
E. To have the patient stand for 30 minutes after ingesting the medication—NO; this is not necessary.
F. To take the medication with a small amount of water—NO; Aricept should be taken with a large glass of water.

EXERCISE 10.23 Exhibit-format:

Assessment

Robert, age 62 years, has come in with two complaints:

- Tremor of his hands that is worse at night
- His joints are growing steadily more stiff and difficult to move, and he states, "It takes me forever to get anywhere or even get my clothes on in the morning."

As Robert is speaking his face does not move and his hands are tremoring and his fingers are pill-rolling.

The clinical manifestations Robert is displaying are related to:

A. Stroke—NO; this is not true.
B. Aging—NO; this is not true. The patient is only 62 years old.
C. Brain tumor—NO; these are not the symptoms of a brain tumor.
D. Parkinson's disease—**YES; these are classic symptoms of Parkinson's disease.**
E. Multiple sclerosis—NO; this is not true.
F. Turret's syndrome—NO; patients with Turret's have movement disorders but do not exhibit pill-rolling.

EXERCISE 10.24 Select all that apply:

Side effects of levodopa–carbidopa (Sinemet) include:

A. Tardive dyskinesia—**YES; this can happen.**
B. Nausea and headache—**YES; this can be a common side effect.**
C. Amnesia—NO; this is not a side effect of the medication or the disease.
D. Somnolence—**YES; this is a potential side effect of the medication.**
E. Anorexia—**YES; though less common, this can be a side effect.**
F. Tremors or seizures—NO; this is not a side effect.

EXERCISE 10.25 Select all that apply:

Common complications of Parkinson's disease include:

A. Constipation—**YES; this results from the slowing of muscles and neurons and is a common problem.**
B. Difficulty swallowing—**YES; this is a common problem.**

C. Frequent falls—**YES; this is a common problem resulting from the cog-wheeling rigidity.**
D. Frequent urination—NO; this is not a common problem.
E. Dry mouth—NO; this is not true.
F. Headaches—NO; this is not a common problem.

EXERCISE 10.26 Select all that apply:

The nurse suspects that Dorothy's manifestations are a result of:

A. Hypertension—**YES; this can be a cause.**
B. Trauma—**YES; this can be a cause.**
C. Aneurysms—**YES; this can be a cause.**
D. Bleeding abnormality—**YES; this can be a cause.**

EXERCISE 10.27 True/False:

Dorothy is a candidate for thrombolytic therapy.

_X_ True; Dorothy's blood pressure is less than 185/110 mmHg; she is younger than 80 years and has had no recent trauma or gastrointestinal bleeds.

EXERCISE 10.28 Multiple-choice:

The nurse should use which ethical principle to guide her response to Dorothy?

A. Justice—NO; this is giving what is due.
B. Autonomy—**YES; this is personal freedom for decision making.**
C. Beneficence—NO; this is an attempt to do good.
D. Nonmalfeasance—NO; this means avoiding harm.

EXERCISE 10.29 Ordering:

Order the following priorities for Dorothy from 1 to 4:

_3_ Nutritional needs—**YES; this is related to cardiovascular accident (CVA) and patient's reduction of meals.**
_2_ Activities of daily living—**YES; this is related to number 1.**
_1_ Safety needs—**YES; safety needs are the most important. This would include removal of scatter rugs and adding elevated toilet seats and handrails for safety.**
_4_ Adaptive changes to loss of independence—**YES; although important, this is not the most important need for this patient.**

EXERCISE 10.30 Select all that apply:

For Larry's situation ("S" in SBAR [situation, background, assessment, recommendation]), the nurse should choose to report:

A. Rectal bleeding—**YES; this is a concern.**
B. Sodium and potassium results—**YES; this is a concern.**
C. Pulse and blood pressure—**YES; this is a concern.**
D. Information related to renal function—**YES; this is a concern.**
E. Information related to respiratory function—NO; this is not a concern.
F. Hemoglobin and hematocrit results—**YES; this is a concern.**

EXERCISE 10.31 Select all that apply:

For Larry's background ("B" in SBAR), the nurse should choose to report that the patient:

A. Has a new diagnosis of diverticulitis—NO; this is not true.
B. Has had diverticulitis for more than 10 years—**YES; this is true.**
C. Was stable last evening—**YES; this is true.**
D. Is elderly—**YES; this is true.**
E. Understands his diagnosis—**YES; Larry has had this diagnosis for 10 years.**
F. Is cooperative—**YES; Larry is cooperative.**

EXERCISE 10.32 Ordering:

Place the following nursing interventions in their order of importance from 1 to 3:

__2__ Request an order for antibiotic therapy; **this is next because the patient is at risk for infection from ruptured diverticula.**
__1__ Hang 0.9% normal saline; **this is first because the patient is bleeding and has symptoms of shock.**
__3__ Place a urinary catheter; **this can be done last; it will provide an accurate intake and output.**

EXERCISE 10.33 Select all that apply:

Discharge planning for Larry should include:

A. Stoma care of a colostomy—**YES; this is important.**
B. Nutritional counselling—**YES; a shortened colon can lead to vitamin deficiency.**
C. Pain management—**YES; this is an important part of postop care.**
D. Information about infection awareness—**YES; this is important in case the patient has postoperative complications.**

EXERCISE 10.34 Multiple-choice:

Larry remarks to the nurse, "I am sure I will be fine now. What do you think?" The best response the nurse can provide is:

A. "Sure, you will be just fine!"—NO; this may not be true.
B. "I hope you are right!"—NO; this is not the best response.
C. "If your disease can be managed, you probably will not die from this disease!"—NO; this is not the best response.
D. "Your surgeon feels you have done well, do you have concerns?"—**YES; this is an open-ended question that allows the patient to express his feelings.**

EXERCISE 10.35 Select all that apply:

The nurse understands the following are consistent with the diagnosis of bacterial pneumonia:

A. It has a low mortality rate among the elderly—NO; this is not true.
B. It has a high rate of mortality among the elderly—**YES; this is true.**

C. It can cause confusion and hypoxia—**YES; this is true**.
D. It has a greater risk of aspiration of foreign matter because it causes decreased sensitivity of pharyngeal reflexes—**YES; this is true.**
E. It may be preceded by a urinary tract infection—NO; bacterial pneumonia is usually caused by *Staphylococcus aureus.*
F. Antibiotics are effective in most cases—**YES; once the organism has been identified antibiotics are effective except in the very elderly and immunocompromised, for whom the mortality rate is 30%.**

EXERCISE 10.36 Select all that apply:

The nurse has the obligation(s) to:

A. Abide by the patient's do not resuscitate—NO; this is the goal but may have to be delayed according to the hospital policy.
B. Follow hospital policy—**YES; the nurse is bound to abide by the hospital policy. The nurse may state his or her objections to being assigned to participate in something he or she feels is unethical.**
C. Notify the ethics committee—**YES; this would be the best option.**
D. Follow the provider's orders—**YES; this is necessary until the ethics committee can resolve this issue. The nurse could state his or her objections and request to be reassigned.**
E. Keep searching for family members—**YES; this would be important.**
F. Refer to the hospital's chaplin—**YES; usually the hospital's chaplin is a part of the ethics committee.**

Resources

Eliopoulos, C. (2014). *Fast facts for the gerontology nurse: A nursing care guide in a nutshell.* New York, NY: Springer Publishing.

Hirth, V., Wieland, D., & Denver-Bumba. (2011). *Case-based geriatrics: A global approach.* New York, NY: McGraw-Hill.

National Cancer Institute. (2013). Screening for prostate cancer: A guidance statement. Retrieved from http://www.guideline.gov

Touhy, T. A., & Jett, K. F. (2014). *Ebersol and Hess' gerontological nursing and health aging* (4th ed.). St. Louis, MO: Elsevier.

Toy, E. C., Dentino, A. N., Johnson, L. S., & Williams, M. M. (2014). *Case files: Geriatrics.* New York, NY: McGraw-Hill.

Winland-Brown, J. E., & Dunphy, L. M. (2013). *Adult-gerontology and family nurse practitioner certification examination: Review questions and strategies.* Philadelphia, PA: F. A. Davis.

CHAPTER 11

Veterans' Health

Karyn E. Holt

UNFOLDING CASE STUDY 1: Steve

Steve, a 31-year-old single man, served as an improvised explosive device (IED) technician in the U.S. Army and was deployed to Iraq once and to Afghanistan twice. His last deployment was in 2011. During that last deployment 7 days before Steve was due to return home after active duty in Afghanistan for 18 months, he was out on patrol and discovered and was unsuccessful at defusing an IED. Steve saved his platoon, but he himself received extensive blast injuries that resulted in bilateral leg amputations. He was sent to a Mobile Army Surgical Hospital (MASH) unit and then evacuated via air to a hospital in Washington, DC, where he resided for 1½ years.

Patient's Health Care History Before Injury

- Allergy: penicillin
- Lifestyle: cigarette smoking; 1.5 packs per day since 2008 (his first deployment)
- Alcoholic beverages: beer "when stressed"
- Past medical history: noncontributory before blast injuries

Patient's Blast Injury History

"I was due to return home in 7 days—a long 7 days. I had been in Afghanistan for 18 months, or two Christmases, and I was looking forward to joining some friends back home. I was really looking forward to eating a big juicy burger. The day of the blast, I was the lead in our IED patrol, the first one out front. About 30 minutes into our patrol, I saw an IED in the road about 20 feet away. I stopped our patrol's forward progress and pointed out the IED, which had a remote activation and yelled 'Remote! Remote!' After that, I remember nothing until I woke up in the hospital in Landstuhl, Germany, awaiting my return to the United States. That is when I discovered that I had no legs anymore and multiple tubes in me so that I did not know what was working and what was not. You know, like my plumbing? And the pain, my goodness I cannot tell you how much my legs, my head, my stomach, my arms, and my back hurt. I felt so alone. I hurt, a lot. My buddies, what happened to them? There was no one around to tell me. It was awful."

Steve's record indicates that the blast resulted in the need for bilateral above-the-knee amputation. Steve experienced a temporary hearing loss that has completely resolved at this time.

Steve was fitted with bilateral prostheses 2 years after his injury. Over the past 4 years, the fit has been a problem, causing discomfort such that Steve now prefers to use a wheelchair.

Patient's Current History

The patient presents to the Veterans Affairs (VA) clinic for a checkup and bilateral prosthetic fittings of the lower extremities. When asked about the reason for his visit by the intake RN, Steve replied, "I am at the VA clinic in this wheelchair with no legs and getting fitted with two new prostheses so that perhaps I can learn to walk again. It was 6 years, 5 months, and 23 days ago that my life was stolen." Steve's health care record indicates that he has suffered depression since his injuries, for which he takes an antidepressant daily, and has done so for 3 years. His scripts have been refilled regularly and on time.

A social history today reveals that Steve's mom and dad now live next door to Steve so that they can help provide some of his physical care. In fact, his mother has quit her job as an administrative assistant to help with and organize Steve's health care. Steve's mother is waiting in the patient waiting area, as Steve does not want her to come into the exam room for his physical examination. In fact, Steve became quite agitated and loud when his mother tried to wheel him into the examination room and he told her to "stay out!"

EXERCISE 11.1 Fill in the blanks:

What questions would the nurse ask to determine whether Steve has problems with the fit of the prosthetic devices?

____

____

____

____

What questions would the nurse ask to determine whether Steve has problems with the function of the prosthetic devices?

____

____

____

The answer can be found on page 627

Steve tells the nurse, "At first the legs functioned fine—it felt good to be able to move around at least a little more normally. I was even able to go up and down stairs without feeling like a 2-year-old. But lately, the prostheses hurt my legs and I'm almost at the point where I'd rather not put them on. I saw that some guys even learned to run on them, and I got excited about doing that, but there's no way I can run on these."

EXERCISE 11.2 Select all that apply:

Steve is asking for better fitting prostheses. His current prostheses were fitted 3 years ago, 2 years after his injuries were sustained. Steve needs new prostheses for the following reasons:

A. His stumps have shrunk bilaterally and the prostheses form no longer fits well.
B. Steve wants to try to learn to jog again and his current prostheses will not articulate in that way.
C. Steve is becoming more and more agitated and angry toward his family and caregivers.
D. He is eligible for new prostheses every 3 years with the Veterans Affairs (VA).

The answer can be found on page 627

The nurse noted that Steve referred to the pain he remembered when he became aware of his injuries and again now with the poorly fitting prostheses. The nurse needs to know how Steve manages pain.

EXERCISE 11.3 Multiple-choice:

What question by the nurse is appropriate to explore how Steve manages the pain?

A. "Do you think you're addicted to pain medication now?"
B. "Do you use narcotics for the pain?"
C. "You said earlier that you drink beer when stressed; do you drink to cope with your prostheses?"
D. "It sounds like there's a lot of pain and frustration involved with using the current prostheses. How do you manage that pain and frustration?"

The answer can be found on page 627

Research indicates that 11% of Iraq and Afghanistan veterans using VA health care for the first time were diagnosed with substance abuse disorders. Risk factors for substance abuse that Steve shares include never being married, severe combat exposure, and a depression diagnosis (Seal et al., 2011).

Steve replies, "Drugs and alcohol abuse are a huge issue for us vets. I've met some guys, and even when we were deployed, who it seemed must have been high most of the time. Not in my unit, my superior ran a tight unit. But now I can understand how easy it would be to just take stuff to reduce the physical—and emotional—pain. Yeah, I probably am drinking a little more beer than I used to—probably about four beers a week now—but I just take over-the-counter pain pills for the pain the legs cause. Sometimes I'll put ice or a heat pack on the stumps and that seems to help, too. I've seen what happens when guys let that kind of thing get out of control, and I don't want to go there."

eRESOURCE

To review how to conduct a pain assessment, refer to Medscape on your mobile device. [Pathway: Medscape ➔ enter "Pain" into the search field ➔ select "Pain Assessment" and review content.]

Physical Assessment

EXERCISE 11.4 Select all that apply:

What area(s) deserve special inspection for skin breakdown?

A. Thighs
B. Stumps
C. Elbows
D. Buttocks

The answer can be found on page 628

The nurse notes no abnormalities on inspection of the skin. The nurse understands that prosthetic care, if not done, is costly and time-consuming. The nurse tells Steve that before he goes to the prosthetics office he should review how to care for the new prosthesis. Would he like his mother to join them for this part of the visit? Steve is silent for quite a while. The nurse repeats the question, saying, "Sometimes it's good to have an extra set of ears listening to this kind of thing, so everyone understands, but it's up to you whether you want her here or not." Steve still hesitates, and then angrily says, "I do and I don't! I know she's going to need to know this, but she's so … She's just so… AGGRAVATING!!"

EXERCISE 11.5 Fill in the blank:

The nurse decides that direct questioning is the best way to uncover any problem and asks, "Steve, you seem anxious and uncomfortable with your mother. How are things at home?" Steve replies, "They're fine." The nurse pursues this direction and asks whether something has happened that makes him feel uncomfortable with his mother, to which he replies, "Well, how would you feel if at 31 years of age you were still depending on your mother to take you to the bathroom? Plus, she calls me 'Stevie' and, like I'm 2 years old, talks about the 'potty.' I know I need her help but sometimes I think I'm going to explode! Sometimes I feel like I might actually hurt her." What is the best communication strategy to use to continue this discussion with Steve?

____

The answer can be found on page 628

Steve agrees that his mother should join the session and she is invited in for the teaching portion. She seems completely accepting of the situation, and does not ask Steve why he looks so angry.

EXERCISE 11.6 Select all that apply:

What are the priorities for care of the prosthetics?

A. Schedule maintenance visits three to four times per year
B. Wash the prosthesis daily with water
C. Make daily adjustments to the socket until it is completely comfortable
D. Never use water on a prosthesis
E. Clean the prosthesis with alcohol
F. Keep the prosthetic away from weather extremes
G. Keep the prosthetic away from all liquid

The answer can be found on page 628

---

eRESOURCE

To supplement your understanding of limb prosthetics, refer to the *Merck Manual.* [Pathway: www.merckmanuals.com/professional → enter "Limb Prosthetics" into the search field → select "Overview of Limb Prosthetics" → review content.]

Psychosocial

Steve is angry and extremely verbal today. His chart states a diagnosis of depression, but the nurse suspects he also has posttraumatic stress disorder (PTSD), based on history and symptoms.

EXERCISE 11.7 Select all that apply:

What are the clinical manifestations for posttraumatic stress disorder (PTSD)?

A. Trauma-related thoughts or feelings
B. Nightmares
C. Flashbacks of the event
D. Feeling anxious
E. Experiencing a sense of panic
F. Difficulty sleeping
G. Difficulty concentrating
H. Establishing long-term relationships

The answer can be found on page 628

EXERCISE 11.8 Select all that apply:

What techniques should be used by the nurse while communicating with a patient diagnosed with post-traumatic stress disorder (PTSD)?

A. Repeat back the information to the patient
B. Tell the patient to think about pleasant times before the incident
C. Discuss alternative methods for the patient to keep busy
D. Paraphrase what the patient already stated

The answer can be found on page 629

eRESOURCE

To review the clinical presentation of an individual suffering from PTSD, refer to Medscape on your mobile device. [Pathway: Medscape ➔ enter "PTSD" into the search field ➔ select "Posttraumatic Stress Disorder" and review content.]

KEY TAKEAWAY POINTS

Posttraumatic Stress Disorder (PTSD)

- One of the most important points in PTSD is realizing that you need help. This is not something that can always be done independently.

Depression

- The rate of depression in veterans is one in three, whereas in the general American population it is one in 10.
- Depression is significantly more prevalent in persons with a traumatic brain injury (TBI) than in those without.
- Depression pre-TBI correlates with a higher risk of developing depression post-TBI.
- Those with post-TBI depression exhibit:
  - Poorer rehabilitation outcomes
  - Greater functional disability
  - Reduced activities of daily living
  - Less social and recreational activity
  - Less employment potential
  - Elevated divorce rates
  - Greater caregiver burden

(continued)

- Greater sexual dysfunction
- Lower ratings of health
- Poorer subjective well-being
- Poorer quality of life
- Increased rates of suicidal ideation

EXERCISE 11.9 Select all that apply:

What helpful strategies have been implemented to assist Steve to deal with the diagnosis of depression?

A. He has set up a routine for his day and sticks with it even if he does not feel like it.
B. He has continued to be involved in activities that used to give him pleasure, even if they no longer do.
C. He began using technology to reconnect with his friends.
D. He has been treated successfully with antidepressants for 3 years.

The answer can be found on page 629

eRESOURCE

To review the clinical presentation of an individual suffering from depression, refer to Medscape on your mobile device. [Pathway: Medscape ➔ enter "Depression" into the search field ➔ select "Depression" and review content.]

Steve attempts to complete a 10-minute body image survey at this clinic visit, but he stops midway through and tears up. He leaves the clinic.

EXERCISE 11.10 Select all that apply:

What actions, if any, would be most helpful now?

A. Nothing, Steve needs to cool down
B. Call out to Steve verbally and ask whether you can help
C. Catch up to Steve, make eye contact, and ask whether you can accompany him to the prosthetics office to begin the fitting for his new prostheses
D. Chart these events and request that Steve be evaluated for additional diagnoses such as posttraumatic stress disorder (PTSD) or traumatic brain injury (TBI)

The answer can be found on page 629

eRESOURCE

To reinforce your understanding of therapeutic communication, refer to Nursing Planet. [Pathway: http://nursingplanet.com ➔ select "Mental Health Nursing" ➔ scroll down to the "Assessment & Evaluation" section and select "Therapeutic Communication" and review content.]

Steve did allow the nurse to catch up with him and walk him to the prosthesis clinic where he will be fitted for two new prostheses so that he can begin a running program. The nurse asked Steve to please stop by the office when he finished with the fitting. The nurse plans to reopen the conversation about his anger and encourage him to participate in group therapy and possibly family therapy with his parents.

EXERCISE 11.11 Select all that apply:

What should the nurse do next?

A. Complete a referral to the prosthetic clinic for adjustment to physical activity and improved body image
B. Complete a request for evaluation of posttraumatic stress disorder (PTSD)/traumatic brain injury (TBI)
C. Recommend family therapy, either through the Veterans Affairs (VA) or privately
D. Complete a request for evaluation of depression therapy
E. Have another veteran with prosthetics speak with him

The answer can be found on page 629

Steve's original trip to the health center today was to obtain services for bilateral prostheses of his lower extremities. Although the goal of limb loss care is to improve functioning of the affected part, high-level quality of life (QOL) is equally important. For veterans of Steve's service era, researchers have identified that QOL is worse when it is associated with combat-associated head injury, combat-associated injury to nonamputated limbs, and assistance needed in daily living. Improved satisfaction with prostheses, improving mental health, and treating other combat-associated injuries are recommended to improve overall QOL for these veterans (Epstein, Heinemann, & McFarland, 2010).

eRESOURCE

Veterans Affairs has many options to treat patients with PTSD, such as cognitive processing therapy (CPT) and prolonged exposure therapy. Pathway: http://goo.gl/bcCf9H ➔ review list of "Treatment Basics," "Getting Started with Treatment," and "Treatment Information for Veterans."

UNFOLDING CASE STUDY 2: Joe

Joe is a 30-year-old veteran who returned from active duty in Afghanistan 2 weeks ago.

EXERCISE 11.12 Exhibit-format:

Subjective data: Joe seeks medical attention for symptoms, which he describes as headaches, occasional dizziness, and difficulty concentrating. He states that he decided to "tough it out" because he thought it would resolve after he returned home.

He was exposed to multiple nearby blasts and explosions during his tour. He denies sustaining any known physical injuries.

Objective data: Blood pressure (BP): 128/78 mmHg, heart rate (HR): 68 beats per minute (bpm), respiratory rate (RR): 22 breaths per minute, pupils equal and reactive to light accommodation (PERLA); there is no limitation of movement in the upper or lower extremities.

What findings have been identified as indicators of traumatic brain injury (TBI) in veterans and which ones are being exhibited by Joe?

A. Loss of energy
B. Change in sense of taste or smell
C. Difficulty speaking
D. Forgetfulness
E. Repeating things
F. Difficulty making decisions
G. Becoming frustrated easily
H. Acting without thinking
I. Overeating

The answer can be found on page 630

Joe was provided with an appointment to be examined by a neurologist. The neurologist determined that Joe had TBI resulting from a concussion sustained from explosions while in Afghanistan. A plan of care was discussed. The social worker and psychologist will be involved in assisting Joe to determine short-term and long-term goals. Joe's wife works part time but attends as many appointments as possible. She would like to have an active role in his treatment.

EXERCISE 11.13 Select all that apply:

What recommendations would the nurse provide to aid in the recovery of postconcussion syndrome?

A. Exercise during the day to promote sleep at night
B. Use relaxation exercises twice a day
C. Avoid alcohol
D. Use the self-assessment tool to measure symptoms

The answer can be found on page 630

eRESOURCE

To supplement your understanding of TBI, refer to the *Merck Manual.* [Pathway: www.merckmanuals.com/professional ➔ enter "Traumatic Brain Injury" into the search field ➔ select "Traumatic Brain Injury" ➔ review content.]

Ritalin is sometimes used for the treatment ofTBI. It increases the release of norepinephrine and dopamine, which has demonstrated positive results for some patients. Research with Ritalin has shown decreased recovery time, increased concentration, and improvement in memory.

EXERCISE 11.14 Multiple-choice:

Joe is taking methylphenidate (Ritalin) 10 mg twice daily. What symptom reported by Joe's wife needs immediate action?

A. Decreased appetite
B. Nervousness
C. Aggressive behavior
D. Trouble sleeping

The answer can be found on page 630

---

eRESOURCE

To reinforce your understanding of methylphenidate, refer to Epocrates Online. [Pathway: http://online.epocrates.com ➔ under the "Drugs" tab, enter "Methylphenidate" in the search field ➔ select "Methylphenidate" ➔ review "Black Box Warnings."]

EXERCISE 11.15 Select all that apply:

Joe becomes stressed when he cannot find something, remember information, or complete a task. What guidelines can the nurse provide?

A. Keep a notepad and pen in his pocket
B. Place items, such as glasses, in the same location
C. Avoid the challenge and do something else more enjoyable
D. Continue to try, even if fatigued
E. Perform tasks in a quiet environment

The answer can be found on page 631

Answers

EXERCISE 11.1 Fill in the blanks:

What questions would the nurse ask to determine whether Steve has problems with the fit of the prosthetic devices?

Have you had any blisters or skin breakdown on your stumps?
Have your stumps changed size?
Do you wear your prosthesis?
Are you able to perform the same activities with your prosthesis now that you could when they were new?

What questions would the nurse ask to determine whether Steve has problems with the function of the prosthetic devices?

Do your knees bend as they are supposed to?
Has the prosthesis been damaged in any way?
Where do you store your prosthesis?

EXERCISE 11.2 Select all that apply:

Steve is asking for a better fitting prostheses. His current prostheses were fitted 3 years ago, 2 years after his injuries were sustained. Steve needs new prostheses for the following reasons:

A. His stumps have shrunk bilaterally and the prostheses form no longer fits well.—**YES; this is a reason for a refitting.**
B. Steve wants to try to learn to jog again and his current prostheses will not articulate in that way.—**YES; this means the patient is moving on in his activity level.**
C. Steve is becoming more and more agitated and angry toward his family and caregivers.—NO; this is not a result of the prosthesis.
D. He is eligible for new prostheses every 3 years with the Veterans Affairs (VA).—NO; this is not universally true, he may need a replacement sooner.

EXERCISE 11.3 Multiple-choice:

What question by the nurse is appropriate to explore how Steve manages the pain?

A. "Do you think you're addicted to pain medication now?"—NO; the nurse would not suggest the patient is addicted, the patient may become defensive.
B. "Do you use narcotics for the pain?"—NO; the nurse would not suggest the patient uses narcotics, the patient may become defensive.
C. "You said earlier that you drink beer when stressed; do you drink to cope with your prosthesis?"—NO; the nurse would not suggest the patient is self-medicating with alcohol.
D. "It sounds like there's a lot of pain and frustration involved with using the current prostheses. How do you manage that pain and frustration?"—**YES; this is open-ended and does not suggest or imply the patient is using medication or alcohol.**

EXERCISE 11.4 Select all that apply:

What area(s) deserve special inspection for skin breakdown?

A. Thighs—NO; his thighs should not be rubbing against the sides of the wheelchair.
B. Stumps—**YES; his stumps are at risk because the prostheses do not fit properly.**
C. Elbows—NO; his elbows should be moving freely.
D. Buttocks—**YES; his buttocks are at risk because of sitting in a wheelchair.**

EXERCISE 11.5 Fill in the blank:

The nurse decides that direct questioning is the best way to uncover any problem and asks, "Steve, you seem anxious and uncomfortable with your mother. How are things at home?" Steve replies, "They're fine." The nurse pursues this direction and asks whether something has happened that makes him feel uncomfortable with his mother, to which he replies, "Well, how would you feel if at 31 years of age you were still depending on your mother to take you to the bathroom? Plus, she calls me 'Stevie' and, like I'm 2 years old, talks about the 'potty.' I know I need her help but sometimes I think I'm going to explode! Sometimes I feel like I might actually hurt her." What is the best communication strategy to use to continue this communication with Steve?

Open-ended questions

EXERCISE 11.6 Select all that apply:

What are the priorities for care of the prosthetics?

A. Schedule maintenance visits three to four times per year—NO; visits are scheduled depending on the patient's needs.
B. Wash the prosthesis daily with water—NO; never use water on prostheses.
C. Make daily adjustments to the socket until it is completely comfortable—**YES; this is needed in order for the prosthetic to be comfortable.**
D. Never use water on a prosthesis—**YES; never use water on prostheses.**
E. Clean the prosthesis with alcohol—**YES; do not wash with water.**
F. Keep prosthetic away from weather extremes—**YES; this may warp the prostheses.**
G. Keep prosthetic away from all liquid—**YES; it should remain dry.**

EXERCISE 11.7 Select all that apply:

What are the clinical manifestations for posttraumatic stress disorder (PTSD)?

A. Trauma-related thoughts or feelings—**YES.**
B. Nightmares—**YES.**
C. Flashbacks of the event—**YES.**
D. Feeling anxious—**YES.**
E. Experiencing a sense of panic—**YES.**
F. Difficulty sleeping—**YES.**
G. Difficulty concentrating—**YES.**
H. Establishing long-term relationships—NO; many times establishing relationships is difficult because of the psychological impact of the PTSD.

EXERCISE 11.8 Select all that apply:

What techniques should be used by the nurse while communicating with a patient diagnosed with posttraumatic stress disorder (PTSD)?

A. Repeat back the information to the patient—**YES; reflective listening confirms that the patient was understood.**
B. Tell the patient to think about pleasant times before the incident—NO; avoidance is not a useful technique.
C. Discuss alternative methods for the patient to keep busy—NO; avoidance is not a useful technique.
D. Paraphrase what the patient already stated—**YES; reflective listening confirms that the patient was understood.**

EXERCISE 11.9 Select all that apply:

What helpful strategies have been implemented to assist Steve to deal with the diagnosis of depression?

A. He has set up a routine for his day and sticks with it even if he does not feel like it.—**YES; this provides consistency and predictability.**
B. He has continued to be involved in activities that used to give him pleasure, even if they no longer do.—**YES; this adds to the familiarity of life as it was and is.**
C. He began using technology to reconnect with his friends.—**YES; this provides him with a method of communication and provides a sense of belonging.**
D. He has been treated successfully with antidepressants for 3 years.—**YES; medication is helpful for many patients.**

EXERCISE 11.10 Select all that apply:

What actions, if any, would be most helpful now?

A. Nothing, Steve needs to cool down—NO; this is not an effective strategy because he may get increasingly agitated.
B. Call out to Steve verbally and ask whether you can help—NO; this may inflame the situation if it is brought out in the open for the public to hear.
C. Catch up to Steve, make eye contact, and ask whether you can accompany him to the prosthetics office to begin the fitting for his new prostheses—**YES; being present is therapeutic.**
D. Chart these events and request that Steve be evaluated for additional diagnoses such as PTSD or TBI—**YES; referrals are needed to access the proper help for patients.**

EXERCISE 11.11 Select all that apply:

What should the nurse do next?

A. Complete a referral to the prosthetic clinic for adjustment to physical activity and improved body image—**YES; this will assist Steve to meet his goals.**
B. Complete a request for evaluation of posttraumatic stress disorder (PTSD)/traumatic brain injury (TBI)—**YES; he may need to deal with these issues to improve his qualities of life.**
C. Recommend family therapy, either through the Veterans Affairs (VA) or privately—**YES; he and his mother need to be able to communicate effectively.**
D. Complete a request for evaluation of depression therapy—NO; he is already being treated.
E. Have another veteran with prosthetics speak with him—**YES; peer support is effective.**

EXERCISE 11.12 Exhibit-format:

Subjective data: Joe seeks medical attention for symptoms, which he describes as headaches, occasional dizziness, and difficulty concentrating. He states that he decided to "tough it out" because he thought it would resolve after he returned home.

He was exposed to multiple nearby blasts and explosions during his tour. He denies sustaining any known physical injuries.

Objective data: Blood pressure (BP): 128/78 mmHg, heart rate (HR): 68 beats per minute (bpm), respiratory rate (RR): 22 breaths per minute, pupils equal and reactive to light accommodation (PERLA); there is no limitation of movement in the upper or lower extremities.

What findings have been identified as indicators of traumatic brain injury (TBI) in veterans and which ones are being exhibited by Joe?

A. Loss of energy—**YES; this is a physical symptom.**
B. Change in sense of taste or smell—**YES; this is a physical symptom.**
C. Difficulty speaking—**YES; this is a physical symptom.**
D. Forgetfulness—**YES; this is a cognitive symptom.**
E. Repeating things—**YES; this is a cognitive symptom.**
F. Difficulty making decisions—**YES; this is a cognitive symptom.**
G. Becoming frustrated easily—**YES; this is a behavioral symptom.**
H. Acting without thinking—**YES; this is a behavioral symptom.**
I. Overeating—NO; this has not been identified as a symptom of TBI.

EXERCISE 11.13 Select all that apply:

What recommendations would the nurse provide to aid in the recovery of postconcussion syndrome?

A. Exercise during the day to promote sleep at night—NO; rest during the day is important to promote healing.
B. Use relaxation exercises twice a day—**YES; frustration is decreased by relaxation exercises.**
C. Avoid alcohol—**YES; should not be consumed during the healing process.**
D. Use the self-assessment tool to measure symptoms—**YES; a mobile app self-assessment tool is effective in tracking symptoms over time.**

EXERCISE 11.14 Multiple-choice:

Joe is taking methylphenidate (Ritalin) 10 mg twice daily. What symptom reported by Joe's wife needs immediate action?

A. Decreased appetite—NO; this is common and usually resolves.
B. Nervousness—NO; this is common and usually resolves.
C. Aggressive behavior—**YES; this may be a symptom of overdose of Ritalin and needs immediate medical attention.**
D. Trouble sleeping—NO; this is common and usually resolves if the medication is taken earlier in the day before sleep.

EXERCISE 11.15 Select all that apply:

Joe becomes stressed when he cannot find something, remember information, or complete a task. What guidelines can the nurse provide?

A. Keep a notepad and pen in his pocket—**YES; this will help him to be successful.**
B. Place items, such as glasses, in the same location—**YES; this will help him to be successful.**
C. Avoid the challenge and do something else more enjoyable—NO; he should attempt to complete the task so there is a sense of accomplishment.
D. Continue to try, even if fatigued—NO; fatigue will increase his stress and frustration.
E. Perform tasks in a quiet environment—**YES; this will help him to be successful.**

Resources

Epstein, R. A., Heinemann, A. W., & McFarland, L. V. (2010). Quality of life for veterans and service members with major traumatic limb loss from Vietnam and OIF/OEF conflicts. *Journal of Rehabilitation Research & Development, 47*(4), 373–385.

Seal, K. H., Cohen, G., Waldrop, A., Cohen, B. E., Maguen, S., & Ren, L. (2011). Substance use disorders in Iraq and Afghanistan veterans in VA healthcare, 2001–2010: Implications for screening, diagnosis, and treatment. *Drug and Alcohol Dependence, 116*(1–3), 93–101. Retrieved from http://digitalcommons.unl.edu/publichealthresources/198

Index

Printed in the United States
By Bookmasters